P9-DUM-959

A REFERENCE COMPANION TO THE HISTORY OF ABNORMAL PSYCHOLOGY

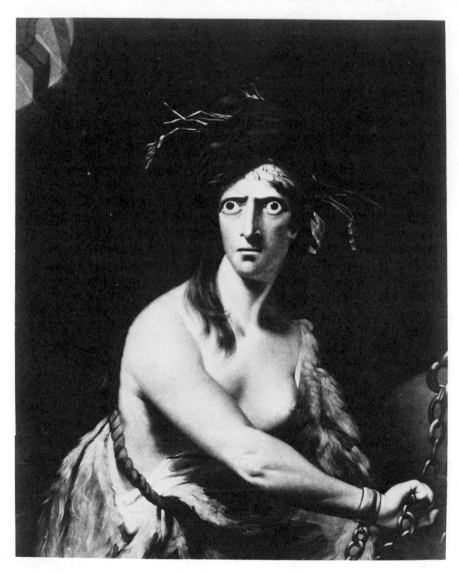

MADNESS. A dramatic representation of the breakdown of the mind: Agitation demands restraint by chains and ropes; the inappropriate clothing and the straw in the hair reflect disordered thought and the staring eyes suggest hallucination. Mezzotint by W. Dickson after R. E. Pine, 1775. By courtesy of the Wellcome Trustees, Wellcome Institute for the History of Medicine, London.

A REFERENCE COMPANION TO THE HISTORY OF ABNORMAL PSYCHOLOGY

John G. Howells
and
M. Livia Osborn

A — L

GREENWOOD PRESS
Westport, Connecticut • London, England

Library of Congress Cataloging in Publication Data

Howells, John G.
  A reference companion to the history of abnormal
psychology.

  Includes index.
  1. Psychology, Pathological—Miscellanea.
2. Psychology, Pathological—Early works to 1900-
Miscellanea. I. Osborn, M. Livia, joint author.
II. Title.
RC454.4.H68   616.89   80-27163
ISBN 0-313-22183-9 (lib. bdg.)
ISBN 0-313-24261-5 (lib. bdg. : v. 1)
ISBN 0-313-24262-3 (lib. bdg. : v. 2)

Library of Congress Catalog Card Number: 80-27163
ISBN: 0-313-22183-9

First published in 1984

Greenwood Press
A division of Congressional Information Service, Inc.
88 Post Road West
Westport, Connecticut 06881

Printed in the United States of America

10 9 8 7 6 5 4 3 2 1

Contents

Illustrations

Acknowledgments

It gives us pleasure to record our grateful appreciation of help received from Miss Jessica Smith, Mrs. Patricia Smith, and the Department of Medical Illustration of the Ipswich Hospital.

Introduction

A Reference Companion to the History of Abnormal Psychology is a source book and a channel to the history of abnormal psychology. As it gleans from the pastures of the literature of abnormal psychology, it is also an analecta. As many of its entries were selected for their fascination, it is a delectus. As It hopes to be a ready servant to the reader, it is an ancilla. The book provides within its covers material of historical interest in the field of abnormal psychology that is not found in a single volume. By the term "abnormal" we mean the unusual as well as the frankly pathological. These two terms are taken in their historical context. For example, although conditions such as mental retardation and epilepsy are not now considered part of the field of abnormal psychology, they were in the past. Because they were not understood, the behavior they engendered was linked to psychiatric disorders.

The *Companion* paints on a broad canvas packed with holy springs, sacred plants, old superstitions, ancient fears, amulets, potions, strange beliefs, madhouses, scientific ideas, instruments of therapy, legal edicts, famous books, poets, painters, politicians, kings, queens, humble folk, popes, and debauchers, saints and sinners, healers and the healed, exploiters and the exploited, the wise and the foolish. A male soprano, FARINELLI, who, with his golden voice, cured Philip V of Spain of his melancholy, precedes an entry on FARMING, a method of therapy imposed on mental patients in eighteenth-century Scotland. MAHLER's emotional difficulties and the diagnosis of his condition by Freud give a new dimension to the understanding of his music. SPIRIT OF SKULL, as administered to Charles II of England, the SPINNING CHAIR, TOBACCO and its history, the strange symptoms of TARANTISM and the psychopathic activities of the THUGS are some of the entries that throw an unusual, intriguing, and often unexpected light on the history of abnormal behavior, its explanation and its treatment. Should the reader require brief biographical details and data on the major achievements of famous physicians of antiquity, psychiatrists, or psychologists and relatively modern workers in allied disciplines, especially in neurology, these will be found within the *Companion*, as well as entries on major hospitals of historical interest and material, which, although not abnormal or unusual, is relevant to the field. Again, the relevance of some entries is to be found in their historical context; a belief or a practice that today is considered commonplace, was once unusual, originated from a unexpected source, or was in advance of its time.

Whenever the opportunity presented, we have added a touch of human interest. We have deliberately paused on any unusual, intriguing, or humorous note; flesh has been added to bare bones, without deviating from the truth. Most entries have been completed with a bibliographical reference that the reader can consult for further information or use to begin the study of a particular subject.

The reasons for the selection of some entries are obvious, particularly in those entries concerning famous contributors to the field of abnormal behavior. There is, however, always some room for a difference of opinion, as each individual has a personal store of cherished particles of knowledge. Some of the material that is not directly a part of abnormal psychology leaves latitude for a personal element in selection. We hope our choice meets the requirements of most readers. The weight given to each entry called for considerable judgment. The key factor was its usefulness to the reader. Some material is readily available elsewhere, thus we have given it short space. Less accessible material that is likely to intrigue the reader is given more space. With a few exceptions, living people have been omitted.

The book is intended for those readers who have an interest in abnormal psychology in its broadest sense. The general reader will find not only pleasure but also information in the *Companion*. We believe the *Companion* will be equally at home on the shelves of professional and general libraries as on the private desk. As a reference work, it will, of course, have a particular appeal to the writer, researcher, teacher, and student in the field of abnormal psychology.

The foundation of the book rests on material gathered over the last twenty-five years. A still growing collection of books, articles, and notes accumulated for a quarter of a century seemed too precious to be left unused and its excitement unshared. Thus, over the last ten years, we set out to marshal the material in an easily retrievable form before offering to share it with others, who, like us, worship at the shrine of Clio.

Over 4200 entries are arranged in alphabetical order with frequent cross references. Structured reading is made possible by the category appendix. For example, a reader interested in the history of hypnosis will find categorized in the appendix those items referring to it. Another reader may wish to abstract items that would give him a collection of names of artists noted for their abnormal behavior. Yet another may wish to collect the names of saints invoked by the insane. All this and more is possible. Each reader can easily compile a bibliography for further reading in his field of interest by collecting the relevant references provided in each entry.

We have been particularly careful to assure the accuracy of our facts, but, like others before us, we have learned that sources sometimes disagree. Whenever posible, we have consulted original sources or those most likely to be exact. Nevertheless, we are bound to have made errors both of ommission and commission.

We found our material in the most unexpected places. We went from old texts to daily newspapers, from sacred books to profane manuals, from biographies to works of art, and all of them yielded a particle for inclusion. In the quest for relevant, useful, and intriguing material hundreds of books have been searched. Not unlike Burton's *Anatomy of Melancholy*, the *Companion* casts its net wide in time and place and harvests a multitude of facts, ranging from unusual objects and strange beliefs to brief biographies and little known anecdotal curiosities. We were fascinated, awed, amused, and, at times, depressed by what we found. It was impossible to record it all. Every reader will know of material he would like to see included; some— we hope most—he will find among our selection. Inevitably some material will not appear due to the limitations of our experience, or it may have been unavailable to us, or it may have been omitted to meet the constraints of space. Every reader, therefore, can find pleasure in adding to the items we make available.

Journal Abbreviations

Acta Paedopsychiat.	Acta Paedopsychiatrica
Acta Psychiatrica Scandinavica	Acta Psychiatrica Scandinavica
Allg. Zeitschr. f. Psych.	Allgemeine Zeitschrift für Psychiatrie
Amer. Anthropologist	American Anthropologist
Am. Imago	American Imago
Am. J. Clin. Hypn.	American Journal of Clinical Hypnosis
Am. J. Dis. Chil.	American Journal of Diseases of Childhood
Am. J. of Medical Sciences	American Journal of Medical Sciences
Am. J. Obstetr.	American Journal of Obstetrics
Am. J. Psychiat.	American Journal of Psychiatry
Am. J. Psychol.	American Journal of Psychology
Anatomischer Anzeiger	Anatomischer Anzeiger
Ann. med. psychol.	Annales medico-psychologiques
Annals of Medical History	Annals of Medical History
Archive de Psychologie	Archive de Psychologie
Archive für pathologische Anatomie und Physiologie	Archive für pathologische Anatomie und Physiologie
Archiv. für Psychiatrie	Archives für Psychiatrie
Arch. Gen. Psychiat.	Archives of General Psychiatry
Arch. Neur. Paris	Archives of Neurology, Paris
Berliner Klinische Wchnschr.	Berliner Klinische Wochenschrift
Brain	Brain
Bristol Med.-Chir. J.	Bristol Medico-Chirurgical Journal
Brit. J. Dermatol.	British Journal of Dermatology
Brit. J. Psychiat.	British Journal of Psychiatry

Bull. Hist. Med.	Bulletin of the History of Medicine
Bull. Menninger Clinic	Bulletin of the Menninger Clinic
Bull. Soc. d'anthrop. de Paris	Bulletin de la Societé d'anthropologie de Paris
Bull. Univer. de Lyon	Bulletin de l'Université de Lyon
Bulletins de la Societé de psychologie physiologiques	Bulletins de la Societé de psychologie physiologiques
Can. Med. Assn. J.	Canadian Medical Association Journal
Can. Psychiat. Ass. J.	Canadian Psychiatric Association Journal
Clin. Lect. Rep. London Hosp.	Clinical Lecture Report, London Hospital
Confinia Psychiat.	Confinia Psychiatrica
Developmental Medicine and Child Neurology	Developmental Medicine and Child Neurology
Encéphale	Encéphale
Epilepsia	Epilepsia
Episteme	Episteme
Essays in Applied Psychoanalysis	Essays in Applied Psychoanalysis
Hamdard	Hamdard
Hist. Med.	Histoire de la Médicine
Hist. Sci. Med.	History of Scientific Medicine
Indian Antiquary	Indian Antiquary
Indian J. Psychiat.	Indian Journal of Psychiatry
Int. J. Psychoanal.	International Journal of Psychoanalysis
Int. J. Psychoanal. Psychoth.	International Journal of Psychoanalytic Psychotherapy
Int. J. Soc. Psychiat.	International Journal of Social Psychiatry
Irrenfreund	Irrenfreund
Journal de Psichologie	Journal de Psichologie
J. Ethno-pharmacology	Journal of Ethno-pharmacology
J. Experimental Medicine	Journal of Experimental Medicine
J. Homosex.	Journal of Homosexuality
J. Ment. Sci.	Journal of Mental Sciences
J. Psychol. Med. Ment. Pathol.	Journal of Psychological Medicine and Mental Pathology

J. Psychol.	Journal of Psychology
J. Sex. Res.	Journal of Sexual Research
J. Hist. Behav. Sci.	Journal of the History of Behavioral Sciences
J. Hist. Med. & All. Sci.	Journal of the History of Medicine and Allied Sciences
J. Hist. Philosophy	Journal of the History of Philosophy
J. of the Polynesian Society	Journal of the Polynesian Society
Lancet	Lancet
Life Threatening Behavior	Life Threatening Behavior
Med. Hist.	Medical History
Med. J. Australia	Medical Journal of Australia
Med. Klin., Berlin	Medizine Klinik, Berlin
Medical Women's Federation J.	Medical Women's Federation Journal
Medico-Chirurgical Transactions	Medico-Chirurgical Transactions
Mem. Nat. Acad. Sci.	Memorandum of National Academy of Sciences
Milbank Memorial Fund Quarterly	Milbank Memorial Fund Quarterly
Minerva Medica	Minerva Medica
Mod. Lang. Rev.	Modern Language Review
Neurology	Neurology
New Zealand Med. J.	New Zealand Medical Journal
Practitioner	Practitioner
Proceedings of the Society of Psychical Research	Proceedings of the Society of Psychical Research
Proc. Roy. Soc. Med.	Proceedings of the Royal Society of Medicine
Psychiatric Annals	Psychiatric Annals
Psychiat. Neurol.	Psychiatria, Neurologia, Neurochirurgia
Psychiatric News	Psychiatric News
Psychiatry	Psychiatry
Psychoanal. Quart.	Psychoanalytic Quarterly
Psychol. Bull.	Psychological Bulletin
Psychol. Med.	Psychological Medicine
Psychological Rev.	Psychological Review
Review of English Studies	Review of English Studies
Revue Philosophique	Revue Philosophique
Rivista Sperimentale di Freniatria	Rivista Sperimentale di Freniatria

Soc. Psychiatry — Social Psychiatry

Spike Wave — Spike Wave

Trans. Stud. Coll. Physicians Phila. — Transactional Studies of the College of Physicians of Philadelphia

Transactions of the Amer. Ophthalmol. Soc. — Transactions of the American Ophthalmological Society

Trans. Ophthal. Soc. U.K. — Transactions of the Ophthalmological Society of the United Kingdom

Transcultural Psychiatric Research Review — Transcultural Psychiatric Research Review

World Medicine — World Medicine

World Psychiatric Assn. Bulletin — World Psychiatric Association Bulletin

Yale J. Biol. Med. — Yale Journal of Biology and Medicine

Zeitschrift für die gesamte Neurologie und Psychiatrie — Zeitschrift für die gesamte Neurologie und Psychiatrie

A REFERENCE COMPANION TO THE HISTORY OF ABNORMAL PSYCHOLOGY

A

AARON. A Shakespearian character, a Moor responsible for murder, execution and mutilation. He depicts a classic psychopath who lives to do harm:

> Even now I curse the day . . .
> Wherein I did not some notorious ill.
>
> [*Titus Andronicus*, 5.1]

Aaron inspired the first known illustration of a Shakespearian character, a drawing by the Reverend Henry Peacham (c. 1576-1643). For other psychopaths *see* IAGO, EDMUND, RICHARD III(q.v.), CALIBAN, LADY MACBETH (*see* MACBETH, LADY) and GONERIL.
Bibliography: Halliday, F.E. 1964. *A Shakespeare companion.*

ABANO, PIETRO D' (1250-1315). Also known as Petrus Aponensis, an Italian physician, philosopher, and teacher at the University of Padua. Using dogma and syllogisms, he attempted to solve the contradictions between dialectic Arabian medicine and speculative philosophy. He was a follower of Averröes (q.v.) and Avicenna (q.v.) and believed that the soul and the intellect were united during life. This theory became corrupted into a belief in a common soul for all mankind. Opposed to magic practices, Pietro d' Abano advised simple therapeutic measures, which frequently employed cold water. Despite this harmless approach, the literature of his time claimed that his cures were made with the help of the devil. He was persecuted by the Inquisition (q.v.) and died while being tried for the second time on charges of sorcery and necromancy (q.v.). His dead body was condemned to be burned at the stake, but his followers concealed it, and the sentence

was carried out on an effigy. His worldwide fame and influence persisted long after his death.
Bibliography: Castiglioni, A. 1946. *A history of medicine*, trans. and ed. E.B. Knumbhaar.

ABBOTT, JOHN STEVENS CABOT (1805-1877). An American clergyman, author of a book on child rearing, *The Mother at Home: Or the Principles of Maternal Duty Familiarly Illustrated*. This early "Spock", published in 1833 in Boston, was a best seller which sold over 125,000 copies in several editions. Abbott was concerned with child neglect and advised mothers to show more warmth and indulgence toward their infants, especially during the early years. However, as soon as the child was old enough to understand, his rebelliousness was to be firmly controlled. He thought that the children of his time were spoilt.
Bibliography: 1973. *History of childhood quarterly.* 1:24.

ABDERA. A Greek city on the coast of Thrace. Its inhabitants were said to have been stricken with insanity after remaining too long in the sun watching Euripides' (q.v.) play *Andromeda*. They became proverbial for their stupidity; yet Democritus (q.v.), Protagoras (q.v.) and Anaxarchus (fl. 350 B.C.), three celebrated philosophers, were born there. The term *abderite* was used derogatorily to mean simpleton.
Bibliography: Tuke, D. H. 1892. *A dictionary of psychological medicine.*

ABÉLARD, PIERRE (1079-1142). A brilliant theologian and philosopher, born near Nantes, France. He advocated rational theological inquiry and denied that the devil had the power to produce mental disorders. He fell in love with Héloïse, a highly intelligent and learned woman. Fulbert, her uncle and canon of Notre Dame, discovered their association and had his hirelings cruelly castrate him. Abélard withdrew to a monastery but was persecuted and declared an heretic. He died on the way to Rome, where he was going to present his defense. His body was given to Héloïse, who was eventually buried in the same grave in 1163.
Bibliography: Pernoud, R. 1973. *Heloïse and Abélard.*

ABENDBERG INSTITUTION. A colony for cretins (*see* CRETINISM) located near Interlaken, Switzerland, more than 4,000 feet above sea level. The famous colony was established in 1842 by Dr. Jakob Guggenbühl (q.v.) at the instigation of Karl Kasthofer (q.v.), a Swiss forester. Kasthofer had observed that while cretinism was common in the valleys, it was not prevalent in the mountains and thought that it could be ameliorated by living at the top of a mountain. The patients were housed in cottages dotted around a central building that contained an assembly hall and other communal facilities. Their nursing was entrusted to the Diakonissen, Evangelican Sisters

of Mercy. The institution became world famous; physicians and philan-
thropists flocked to it and reported back in glowing terms. Similar institutions modelled on it were established in many countries. The initial
enthusiasm, however, quickly waned, and conditions in the mountainside
cottages deteriorated. After an adverse report by the British minister to
Berne, the Swiss Association of Natural Sciences withdrew its sponsorship,
and the institution closed. It was sold in 1867 and became an hotel and later
a dairy.

Bibliography: Kanner, L. 1964. *A history of the care and study of the mentally retarded.*

ABERDEEN ROYAL MENTAL HOSPITAL. One of the Scottish royal
asylums (q.v.) opened in 1800. The building was originally a leper hospital
(*see* LEPROSY). Until its opening, the mentally ill had been housed in cells
attached to the general hospital. Funds for a new hospital building, which
opened in 1820, were provided by a rich merchant John Forbes, to whom
a memorial was erected on the hospital grounds. The first superintendent
physician was Dr. Macrobin who was followed by Dr. Robert Jamieson in
1852. Jamieson instituted lectures in psychiatry and advocated nonrestraint
of the patients, but retained the whirling chair (q.v.) as a form of therapy.

Bibliography: Henderson, D. K. 1964. *The evolution of psychiatry in Scotland.*

ABERDEEN WITCHCRAFT. An outbreak of obsession (q.v.) with witchcraft (q.v.) in Aberdeen, Scotland in 1596. The publication of *Daemonologie
In Forme of a Dialogue* (q.v.) by King James I of England and VI of Scotland
had such power of suggestion on the inhabitants of Aberdeen that they
became obsessed with what they believed to be supernatural phenomena
caused by witchcraft. Twenty-four people were accused of being allied with
the devil and were burned at the stake.

Bibliography: Robbins, R. H. 1959. *The encyclopedia of witchcraft and demonology.*

ABLUTOMANIA. A morbid impulse to continuously wash or bathe. One
famous example of ablutomania is Lady Macbeth (q.v.) who, guilt ridden
after the murder of Duncan, was afflicted by it; with her it took the form
of hand-washing mania:

> It is an accustomed action with her,
> to seem thus washing her hands;
> I have known her continue in this a
> quarter of an hour.

[Shakespeare, *Macbeth*, 5.1]

Bibliography: Salzman, L. 1968. *The obsessive personality: origins, dynamics and therapy.*

ÅBO (TURKU). A town in Finland. An institution caring for the mentally
ill existed there as early as 1396. The patients included lepers (*see* LEPROSY)

as well as the poor. It was called, as were other later institutions of this type, House of the Holy Ghost. In 1623 the patients were transferred to Seili Hospital (q.v.).

Bibliography: Retterstøl, N. 1975. Scandinavia and Finland. In *World history of psychiatry*, ed. J. G. Howells.

ABOIMENT. An obsolete term derived from the French and meaning "barking." It was used to denote involuntary animal-like sounds often produced by schizophrenic (*see* SCHIZOPHRENIA) patients in advanced stages of the disease. It is also present in nervous conditions. Billy Swansea "with the dog's voice" is an illustration of the latter in Dylan Thomas's *Under Milk Wood*. In 1885 Georges Gilles de la Tourette (q.v.) described this syndrome, and his name is associated with it.

ABORTIVE INSANITY. *See* INSANITY, ABORTIVE.

ABRAHAM, KARL (1877-1925). A psychoanalyst, born in Bremen, Germany from an old Jewish family. He was originally interested in philosophy and linguistics and later used both in his psychoanalytic (*see* PSCHOANALYSIS) work. A scrupulously honest man in both his work, and his personal relationships, he impressed all who knew him with his friendliness and tolerance. He was a close friend of Sigmund Freud (q.v.) whom he met in 1907. Freud called him the first German psychoanalyst. He used dream (q.v.) symbolism in the exploration of many mythological subjects and pioneered the study of libido development, the influence of progenital fixation on character formation, alcoholism (q.v.), and drug addiction, as well as of schizophrenia (q.v.) and manic-depressive psychoses (q.v.). He worked at Eugen Bleuler's psychiatric clinic, the Burghölzli Hospital (q.v.), in Zürich, Switzerland with Carl Jung (q.v.), and became editor of the *Psychoanalytic Year Book*. In 1908 he founded the Psychoanalytic Society in Berlin. During World War I he ran a clearing house for psychiatric casualties from the eastern front. Much of his clinical work has been incorporated into modern psychiatry (q.v.).

Bibliography: Abraham, K. 1954. *Selected papers on psychoanalysis*. Edited by D. Bryan and A. Strachey.

Alexander, F.; Eisenstein, S; and Grotjahn, M., eds. 1966. *psychoanalytic pioneers*.

ABRAHAM-MEN. Beggars. The name may be derived from Abraham ward in Bethlem Hospital (*see* BETHLEM ROYAL HOSPITAL). Some may have been genuine lunatics (q.v.), but others were thieves or beggars who decorated their hats and coats with tattered colored ribbons in order to appear insane. Robert Burton (q.v.) mentioned them in his *The Anatomy of Melancholy*

(q.v.) and expressed the opinion that their lunacy was counterfeited. Tom O'Bedlam (q.v.) was another name for them.
Bibliography: O'Donoghue, E. G. 1914. *The story of Bethlehem Hospital.*

ABREACTION. Term first used by Sigmund Freud (q.v.) in a letter to Wilhelm Fliess (q.v.) dated June 28, 1892, to indicate a verbal reaction to past trauma. It first appeared in literature in the paper entitled "On the Psychical Mechanism of Hysterical Phenomenon: Preliminary Communication," written by Freud in collaboration with Joseph Breuer (q.v.) in 1893.
See also TALKING CURE.
Bibliography: Freud, S. 1964. *The complete psychological works of Sigmund Freud.* Vol. 2. Edited by J. Strachey.

ABSINTHE. A plant native to Europe, also known as wormwood. A French liqueur, yellow-brown in appearance and very strong, is made from it. In addition to anise and other aromatic oils, the liqueur Absinthe contains oil of thuja, a powerful cerebral convulsant. Chronic intoxication, delirium (q.v.), complete paralysis, and dementia can result from addiction to it. In 1915, following a number of deaths caused by its excessive consumption, the French government prohibited its manufacture. Vincent Van Gogh (q.v.) was addicted to it and under its influence cut off the lobe of his ear. Edgar Degas (1834-1917) and Pablo Picasso (1881-1973) are among the artists who observed and depicted the plight of the absinthe drinker.
Bibliography: Lehner, E., and Lehner, J. 1973. *Folklore and odysseys of food and medicinal plants.*

ABU BAKR [EL SIDDIG] (573-634). Islamic leader and first caliph of Mecca. His daughter Aisha married Mohammed (q.v.). As one of Mohammed's first followers, he was so distressed by the Prophet's death that he died of sorrow, thus providing an example of psychosomatic death. His death also illustrates an important teaching in Arabian psychiatry that is based on the Prophet's saying: "He who is overcome by worries will have a sick body."
Bibliography: Baasher, T. 1975. The Arab countries. In *World history of psychiatry*, ed. J. G. Howells.

ACADÉMIE DES SCIENCES. A society of learned men founded in Paris in 1666. It played an important part in the historical beginnings of dynamic psychiatry (q.v.). On February 13, 1882, Jean Martin Charcot (q.v.) persuaded the Académie to hear his paper on the diverse nervous states occurring in hypnotized hysterics (*see* HYSTERIA). This event had great historical significance as the Académie had previously refused to hear any paper dealing with animal magnetism (q.v.), mesmerism (q.v.) or any form of hypnotism

(q.v.), Charcot's paper forced the Académie to yield to the pressure of events and change its passive policy into one more attuned to scientific integrity.
Bibliography: Zilboorg, G. 1941. *A history of medical psychology.*

ACADEMY, THE. A college named from "Academia," a grove near Athens, where Plato (q.v.) founded his school of philosophy around 387 B.C. On completion of their studies, the pupils, Aristotle (q.v.) among them, often remained at the Academy as teachers. On Plato's death in 347 B.C., his nephew Speusippus took over the leadership of the Academy. The second Academy was founded by Arcesilaus c. 250 B.C. He taught a modified Platonic doctrine. Carneades founded a third in 213 B.C. The Academy came to an end when the Emperor Justinian closed all pagan schools in A.D. 529. Its influence left an indelible mark on the development of psychology (q.v.) in the Western world.
Bibliography: Watson, R. I. 1963. *The great psychologists.*

ACEDIA *or* **ACCIDIA.** A syndrome of "not caring." The term was employed to describe spiritual sloth or melancholy (*see* MELANCHOLIA). Originally described in the Middle Ages (q.v.), it is still referred to in the twentieth century. Clerics regarded it as the fourth cardinal sin, the seven sins being: Superbia (pride), Invidia (jealousy), Ira (temper), Accidia (sloth), Avaritia (greed), Gula (gluttony), and Luxuria (extravagance). It seems to describe a clinical state of apathy due to anxiety states, neurosis (q.v.), depression, or schizophrenia (q.v.). Philosophers and physicians of the Middle Ages recognized that it could lead to despair and suicide (q.v.), and attributed its causes to emotional disorders, such as excessive grief or frustration, or to melancholic humors or viewed it as a sin prompted by the devil. Robert Burton (q.v.) in his *Anatomy of Melancholy* (q.v.) stated that accidia "proceeds from flegm, it stirs up dull symptoms, and a kind of stupidity or impassionate hurt, they are sleepy saith Savonarola, dull, slow, cold, blockish and asslike."
Bibliography: Wenzel, S. 1967. *The sin of sloth—acedia in medieval thought and literature.*

ACH, NARZISS J. (1871-1946). A psychologist born in Ermershausen Germany. He worked with Georg E. Muller (q.v.) at Göttingen in 1900 and in 1904 with Oswald Külpe (q.v.) at Würzburg before becoming a professor at Konigsberg in 1907. He continued the work of Henry J. Watt (q.v.) on unconscious "determining tendencies," as he called them, and contributed to the study of the will process with his thorough description of volition. Ach also worked on problems of action and thought. "Systematic experimental introspection" and "awareness" (*Bewusstheit*) are among some of his terms. He was a strong defender of the method of self-observation and created the Ach-Ducker law of special determination. He also devised

a new tool for experimental psychology (q.v.), the chronotyper. He was a prolific writer of papers and books and wrote, among other things, *Uber die Willenstatigkeit und das Denken* (1905) and *Analyse des Willens* (1935).
Bibliography: Flugel, J. C. 1945. *A hundred years of psychology.*

ACHILLES. A patient of Pierre Janet's (q.v.). He was perhaps one of the most outstanding examples of Janet's clinical success. Considered the victim of demonic possession (q.v.), Achilles was brought to Salpêtrière (q.v.) in 1893. Instead of the time-honored practice of exorcism (q.v.), Janet used his new technique of dynamic psychotherapy (q.v.), which produced a cure.
Bibliography: Janet, P. 1894. Un cas de possession et l'exorcisme modern. *Bull. Univer. de Lyon.* 8:41-57.

ACID FASCISM. A type of violence in which extreme political viewpoints are inculcated by the use of mind-altering drugs. It is illustrated by the murders directed by Charles Manson in California in 1969.
Bibliography: Bugliosi, V., and Gentry, C. 1975. *The Manson murders: helter skelter.*

ACRASIA. A figure in Edmund Spenser's (q.v.) *Faerie Queene.* She represented intemperance, and her name meant "lack of self-control". In the sixteenth century, the term was used to indicate a type of abnormal behavior.
Bibliography: Hamilton, A. C. 1961. *The structure of allegory in the Faerie Queen.*

ACTE GRATUIT. A term used by the French writer André Gide (q.v.) to denote an impulsive, inconsequent action. An example occurs in Gide's tale *Les Caves du Vatican*, where the protagonist takes a dislike to the man sitting in front of him on the train and decides to throw him out if he sees a light before he has finished counting to twelve. He sees a light in the time allotted, and the unfortunate man is thrown out.

ACTION THEORY OF CONSCIOUSNESS. A theory developed by Hugo Münsterberg (q.v.). It stresses the significance of motor discharge.
Bibliography: Flugel, J. C. 1945. *A hundred years of psychology.*

ACT PSYCHOLOGY. An approach developed in 1874 by Franz Brentano (q.v.). It concentrated on mental processes and investigated the relationship between activities and objects. Brentano's approach was directed toward establishing psychology as a scientific discipline. *See also* PSYCHOLOGY.
Bibliography: Flugel, J. C. 1945. *A hundred years of psychology.*

ACTUARIUS, JOHANNES (?-1283). A physician at the court of Constantinople (q.v.). He wrote an important volume on urinoscopy and another on mental diseases. He followed the doctrine of humors (*See* HUMORAL THEORY) derived from Hippocrates and Galen (qq.v.) and opposed de-

monological explanations of mental disorders in vogue at his time. He believed that all cases of melancholia (q.v.) could be treated by correct dieting, which included food that was "of good flavour, lightly cooked and toothsome, in order to make sure that the head is neither overfed nor starved."
Bibliography: Whitwell, J. R. 1936. *Historical notes on psychiatry.*

ADAMITES. Members of a Christian heretical sect with strange erotic tendencies. They believed that nudity and sexual promiscuity would lead humanity back to primitive innocence. The sect originated in Africa and was sporadically active between the second and the sixteenth centuries. In the fifteenth century a similar sect appeared in Bohemia and Moravia. Hieronymus Bosch (q.v.) is said to have belonged to the Adamites, whose views influenced his choice of subjects for his paintings.
Bibliography: Douglas, J. D., ed. 1978. *The new international dictionary of the Christian church.*

ADENOMA SEBACEUM. In 1890 John J. Pringle (q.v.) presented a case of "congenital adenoma sebaceum." In 1908, H. Vogt first established that it constitutes a triad always present in tuberous sclerosis (q.v.) when it is accompanied by convulsions and mental defect.
Bibliography: Kanner, L. 1964. *A history of the care and study of the mentally retarded.*

ADIE, WILLIAM JOHN (1886-1935). British neurologist whose name is associated with a condition known as Adie pupil, or tonic pupil, in which the pupil shows poor response to light. The tonic pupil is sometimes termed the Holmes-Adie syndrome as both Gordon Holmes and Adie described the anomaly independently in 1931. However, John Hughlings Jackson (q.v.) had already described the syndrome in 1881.
Bibliography: Haymaker, W., and Schiller, F. 1970. *The founders of Neurology.* 2d. ed.

ADLER, ALFRED (1870-1937). A psychologist, born in Penzing, a suburb of Vienna, Austria, the second son of a grain merchant. Because he suffered from rickets, which caused him to experience terrifying attacks of spasm of the glottis, he could not walk until he was four years old. He felt inferior to his elder brother, who was his mother's favorite child, and always was aware of his brother's athletic achievements, which he could not hope to emulate. As a small child he was involved in several street accidents. His interest in botany and biology found an outlet in cultivating flowers and collecting pigeons. When he was five years old he decided to become a physician, and he eventually graduated in medicine from the University of Vienna in 1895. Two years later he married Raisse Tinofejewna, a Russian with very progressive ideas on the rights of women. The life of the cafe society of Vienna suited him well; he enjoyed informality and made friends from all walks of life. Adler was particularly troubled by the frequency of eye disorders among tailors; he wrote and lectured on the subject and was able to bring about some social reforms for them. Eventually his interest turned to neurology (q.v.). His defense of Sigmund Freud's (q.v.) *Interpretation of Dreams* led to an invitation to join Freud's Wednesday evening discussion group in 1902. In the *Study of Organ Inferiority and Its Physical Compensation*, published in 1907, Adler expressed his belief in the importance of the individual's inner image in regard to his defective functioning. By 1911 his criticism of Freud's sexual theories caused a break between the two men. Freud attempted a reconciliation by making Adler president of the Viennese Psychoanalytic Society and coeditor with Wilhelm Stekel (q.v.) of its journal, but the attempt failed. Adler and nine other members resigned and founded the Society for Free Psychoanalysis (q.v.), which changed its name to the Society for Individual Psychology in 1912. In 1919, he founded, in Vienna, the first child guidance clinic (q.v.). His fame spread and his views became widely known. In 1934, after many lecture tours in the United States and after an appointment as professor of medical psychology at Long Island College of Medicine, he decided to move to New York. During a European lecture tour in 1937 he died of a heart attack while walking in the streets of Aberdeen, Scotland.

Supportive psychotherapy (q.v.) owes much to his theories and to his belief that the role of the therapist should be that of interpreting for the patient. "Individual psychology" (q.v.), "inferiority complex" (q.v.), "compensation" and "overcompensation" are only a few of the terms he coined.
Bibliography: Ansbacher, H. H., and Ansbacher, R. R. 1956. *The individual psychology of Alfred Adler*.
Bottome, P. 1939. *Alfred Adler*.
Roazen, P. 1975. *Freud and his followers*.

ADOLPHE. A novel by the French writer Benjamin Constant de Rebecque (1767-1830). It is considered a landmark in the history of psychological analysis in fiction. The novel describes in detail the changing feelings of the hero who seduces a woman out of vanity. She falls in love with him and dies of grief when she realizes that his protestations of love are false.
Bibliography: Constant, B. 1816. *Adolphe*.

ADOPTIO. A legal act in ancient Roman law, under it a citizen could enter another family and become subject to the authority of its chief. It also took into account the right of succession and property. The emotional tie between parents and adopted children was particularly strong in Roman families.
Bibliography: Buckland, W. W. 1964. *A textbook of Roman law from Augustus to Justinian*.

ADVERTISING. In the eighteenth century it was common for owners of private asylums (q.v.) to place advertisements in local newspapers to attract clients. Their inflated claims were seldom factual. Daniel H. Tuke (q.v.) quoted the following advertisement, which appeared in the London *Post Boy* in 1700, for a madhouse run by James Newton (q.v.):

In Clerkenwell-Close, where the figure of mad people are over the gate; liveth one, who by the blessing of God, cures all lunatick distracted or mad people, he seldom exceeds 3 months in the cure of the maddest person that comes in his house, several have been cur'd in a fortnight, and some in less time; he has cur'd several from Bedlam and other mad-houses in and about this city, and has conveniency for people of what quality soever. No cure — no money.
Bibliography: Parry-Jones, W. Ll. 1972. *The trade in lunacy.*

ADYNAMIAS. One of four orders listed under class two (neuroses) in William Cullen's (q.v.) classification of mental disorders. It included pathological prostration.
Bibliography: Cullen, W. 1800. *Nosology of a systematic arrangement of diseases by classes, orders, genera, and species.*

AESCULAPIUS (*or* ASCLĒPIOS). The Greek god of medicine, considered to be son of Apollo (q.v.). Aesculapius was probably a human being who was deified after his death. The cult of Aesculapius was influential in Greece for centuries. Hundreds of Aesculapian temples were built in the ancient world, mainly in Greece but also in Rome, where the first temple was erected in 293 B.C. on an island in the Tiber. The cult had great appeal because it provided for a personal relationship with the divine. Survival of the cult depended on its reputation, and therefore the severely ill were denied treatment. Diet (q.v.), bath, and exercise were employed, but the most important treatment was temple or incubation sleep (q.v.). Exhausted after a long fast and drugged, the patient, while sleeping in the temple, would receive dream (q.v.) inspirations or instructions from the Aesculapian priests accompanied by the sacred snakes. The dream was supposed to reveal to the patient what he needed to do to be cured. In the powerfully suggestive atmosphere of the temple, cures were often claimed. Slabs have been found near the temple of Aesculapius at Epidaurus (q.v.) listing the names of men and women who had been healed. The Aesculapian cult particularly emphasized the emotional aspect of illness. Using anxiety and hope of recovery to influence the patient's mind, the Aesculapian priests employed a technique very similar to present-day psychotherapy (q.v.). A humorous account of a visit to a temple can be found in Aristophanes' (q.v.) *Plutus.*
Bibliography: Rogers, B. B., trans. 1972. *Aristophanes.* Vol. 3.
Sigerist, H. E. 1961. *A history of medicine.* Vol. 2.

AESTHESIOMETER. An instrument used by Ernst H. Weber (q.v.) in his compass test (q.v.) experiment to determine at what distance two simultaneous touches on the skin are perceived as two rather than one.
Bibliography: Flugel, J. C. 1933. *A hundred years of psychology.*

AETIUS OF AMIDA (A.D. 502-575). The first Christian physician of note, born in Mesopotamia. He was appointed physician to Justinian I at the court of Byzantium (q.v.). He collected the writings of previous authors and compiled original treatises on medicine. He distinguished three types of phrenitis (q.v.), each of which corresponded to defects of memory (q.v.), reason or imagination, depending on the location of the dysfunction in the brain. He thought that mania (q.v.) was due to an excess of blood going to the head; melancholy (*see* MELANCHOLIA) was attributed to faulty diet (q.v.), which led to black or yellow bile (q.v.). He advised against purging (q.v.) epileptics (*see* EPILEPSY) as he believed them to be too weak, and suggested clysters (q.v.) or gargles instead. Magnets (q.v.) were used by him in the treatment of mental disorders.
Bibliography: Whitwell, J. R. 1936. *Historical notes on psychiatry.*

AFTER-CARE MOVEMENT. A movement that tried to provide financial, medical, and emotional assistance to patients recently discharged from mental hospitals, thus helping to prevent relapses. It was strongly supported by all workers in the mental health field. First introduced in 1829 in Nassau, Germany, by Dr. Lindpainter and in France in 1841 by Jean Falret (q.v.), it was established in England in 1871 by a society called the Guild of Friends of the Infirm in Mind (q.v.). Toward the end of the nineteenth century it reached the United States, where it was vigorously championed by the American Neurological Association (q.v.).
Bibliography: Deutsch, A. 1949. The mentally ill in America.

AGATE. A semiprecious stone, which was said to have certain medical properties. Saint Hildegard of Bengen (q.v.) advised epileptics (*see* EPILEPSY) to put an agate in the water in which their food was cooked.
See also PRECIOUS STONES.
Bibliography: Evans, J. 1922. *Magical jewels.*

AGAVE. Mother of Pentheus (q.v.) in Euripides' (q.v.) drama *Bacchae.* Struck with madness by Dionysus (q.v.), she joined the women of Thebes, in an orgy and took part in the killing of her son, returning to the palace carrying his head. Once her ecstasy (q.v.) was over, she returned to her senses and realized the enormity of her actions.
Bibliography: Way, A. S., trans. 1912. *Euripides.* Vol. 3.

AGER (*or* AGERIUS), NICHOLAS (1568-1634). A physician and bota-

nist, born in Alsace. He studied medicine in Switzerland and France and became professor of medicine and botany at Strasbourg in 1618. He investigated psychological disorders, including insomnia. His many writings include descriptions of new plants and their use in medicine.
Bibliography: Debus, A. G., ed. 1968. *World who's who in science.*

AGORAPHOBIA. A term derived from the Greek, meaning "dread of open spaces" (literally "fear of markets") and credited to Carl Westphal (q.v.). The condition was first noticed by a hydrotherapist, Anton Bruck (1798-1885), but Westphal gave the first clinical description of it in 1871 in the German journal *Archives Psychiatrie Nervenkrankh.* His article appeared in English in 1873.
See also PHOBIAS.
Bibliography: Westphal, C. 1873. *J. Ment. Sci.* 29: 456.

AGRIMONY. Herb used in the treatment of mental disorders by John Wesley (q.v.), who suggested that lunatics (q.v.) should be given a decoction of this herb four times a day.
Bibliography: Wesley, J. 1747. Reprint. 1960. *Primitive physic.*

AGRIOTHYMIA. A term derived from the Greek and introduced into medical psychology (q.v.) by De Valenzi (1728-1813). In agriothymia the mania (q.v.) has become so severe that the patient is dangerous and menancing.
Bibliography: MacNalty, A. S. ed. 1965. *Butterworths medical dictionary.*

AGRIPPA, HENRICUS, CORNELIUS VON NETTESHEIM (1486?-1535). German physician, student of the occult and theology. A restless, aggressive, but brilliant individual, he was also a scientist and soldier who went into battle with a rucksack full of books and manuscripts. He was a lonely man whose only companion was a black poodle called Monsieur, which many of his contemporaries considered to be an incarnation of the devil. He was much disliked and slandered. He married three times, and his third wife proved to be a harlot, but nevertheless he wrote *On the Nobility and Preeminence of the Femine Sex* in which he defended women against the misogyny of the monks (q.v.) and the witch-hunting fanaticism of the Inquisition (q.v.). He clashed with the medical profession of his day and openly denounced the Dominican Inquisitor Nicholas Savin. Johann Weyer (q.v.) studied under him at Bonn, and Weyer's enlightened views on mental disorders reflect Agrippa's influence. Agrippa recognised four forms of madness: 1) madness produced by the Muse; 2) madness produced by Dionysus (q.v.); 3) madness produced by Apollo (q.v.); and 4) madness produced by Venus (q.v.).

Although he was an office holder in the city of Metz, he was forced to flee to London, where he died poor and alone, still persecuted by the monks, who devised a cruel and slanderous epitaph for his tomb.

Bibliography: Morley, H. 1856. *The life of Henry Cornelius Agrippa von Nettesheim.* Zilboorg, G. 1941. *A history of medical psychology.*

AGRIPPINA THE ELDER (c. 12 B.C.-A.D. 33). The daughter of M. Vipsanius Agrippa and Julia, who was the daughter of Augustus. She married Germanicus Caesar, and was the mother of Caligula (q.v.). Because she was too well liked by the people, Tiberius (q.v.) sent her into exile on the island of Pandataria near Naples. The stress of her hopeless situation led to depression and she committed suicide (q.v.) by starving herself to death.
Bibliography: Charlesworth, M. P. 1951. *The Roman empire.*

AGRIPPINA THE YOUNGER (c. A.D. 16-A.D. 59). The daughter of Agrippina the Elder (q.v.), and the mother of Nero (q.v.) She was a paranoid (*see* PARANOIA), homicidal, and psychopathic (*see* PSYCHOPATHY) woman, who was completely ruthless in her drive for power. She poisoned her rivals, including her uncle, the Emperor Claudius, and murdered enemies to gain the throne for her son Nero, but he too found her intolerable and had her put to death.
Bibliography: Hyslop, T. B. 1925. *The great abnormals.*

AGUESSAU, HENRI FRANÇOIS D' (1668-1751). A celebrated French jurist who became chancellor of France. He realized that abnormal behavior required treatment, not punishment, and advised the parliament that witchcraft (q.v.) would cease when it stopped talking about it and instead committed the so-called sorcerers and witches to the care of the physicians.
Bibliography: Esquirol, J. E. D. 1845. Reprint. 1965. *Mental maladies: a treatise on insanity.*

AHITHOPHEL. A Biblical character who committed suicide (q.v.). He was counselor to King David, but became a traitor and deserted to Absalom. Unable to withstand the frustration of having his advice rejected he went home and "set his house in order and hanged himself."
Bibliography: 2 Sam. 17: 23.

AICHHORN, AUGUST (1878-1949). A psychoanalyst born in Vienna, Austria. He had his first contact with delinquent behavior by mixing with the adolescents and children who lingered around his father's bakery. As a schoolteacher he was noted for his ability to deal with aggressive youngsters. In 1918 he established and directed a reformatory for adolescents at Ober-Hollabrunn; two years later he founded another house at St. Andra. Anna Freud (q.v.), who was impressed with his work, suggested that he should undertake psychoanalytic training, which he did at the Viennese Psychoanalytic Institute. He believed that a child's asocial behavior was the consequence of his unsatisfactory relationship with a parent. In place of punishment,

he advocated warm and supportive relationships with trusting adults. Aichhorn's enlightened views on the treatment of delinquents inspired the founding of residential treatment centers not only for behaviorally disordered children but also for children with other forms of emotional disturbances.
Bibliography: Aichhorn, A. 1935. *Wayward youth.*
Mohr, G. 1966. August Aichhorn. In *Psychoanalytic pioneers*, eds. Alexander, F.; Grotjahn, M.; and Eisenstein, S.

AIX-EN-PROVENCE NUNS. In 1611 the convent of the Ursuline nuns in Aix-en-Provence became the scene of mass hysteria (q.v.). Many nuns were believed to be possessed (*see* POSSESSION) by the devil, following the manifestations of Sister Madeleine de Demandolx (q.v.).
Bibliography: Robbins, R. H. 1959. *The encyclopedia of witchcraft and demonology.*

AJAX. A Greek hero depicted by Homer (q.v.) in the *Odyssey* (q.v.) and by Sophocles (q.v.) in his play *Ajax.* He displays an anomaly of perception when, maddened with resentment because the arms of Achilles were awarded to Odysseus, he becomes so confused that he slaughters a flock of sheep, mistaking them for the enemy. On recovering his senses, shame and remorse overcome him, and he commits suicide (q.v.) by impaling himself on his sword.
Bibliography: Simon, B. 1978. *Mind and madness in ancient Greece.*

AKERFELDT, S. A Swiss biochemist who, in 1957, found that the blood of schizophrenic patients contained ceruloplasmin, a copper-carrying enzyme. This was thought at first to be an important factor in the diagnosis of schizophrenia (q.v.), but it was discovered that the same substance is present in the blood of all individuals suffering from vitamin C deficiency.
Bibliography: Alexander, F. G., and Selesnick, S. T. 1966. *The history of psychiatry.*

ALBERT B. An eleven-month-old child who was the subject of a series of experiments conducted by John B. Watson (q.v.). He was made to fear rats, rabbits, and then all furry objects by sudden loud sounds occurring every time he handled the animals. Watson called this reaction a transfer or spread of conditioned response.
Bibliography: Watson, J. B., and Watson, R. R. 1921. Studies in infant psychology. *Science Monitor.* 13: 493-515.

ALBERTUS MAGNUS, SAINT (ALBERT VON BOLLSTÄDT)(1193-1280). A German natural scientist, the son of Count Von Bollstädt. He studied in Padua and became a Dominican monk in 1222. He was a pioneer in the scholastic (*see* SCHOLASTICISM) method of study which was developed still further by Thomas Aquinas (q.v.), one of his pupils. Relying on observation and reason, rather than deduction, he wrote extensively on a large

number of subjects, including the interpretation of dreams (q.v.) and brain localization. According to him, the anterior ventricle of the brain was responsible for feeling, and the posterior ventricle was responsible for memory (q.v.). His *Opera Omnia* were collected and published in 1651.
Bibliography: Castiglioni, A. 1946. Translated by V. Gianturco. *Adventures of the mind*.

ALBINOS. Persons with a congenital deficiency of pigment in skin and hair. For many years they were thought to be of inferior intelligence. As late as 1824, J.E. Belhomme (q.v.) found it necessary to point out this error by citing examples of intelligent albinos.
Bibliography: Kanner, L. 1964. *A history of the care and study of the mentally retarded*.

ALCHEMY. The chemistry of the Middle Ages (q.v.) and sixteenth century. It was based on the belief that all matter is made up of four elements and a fifth entity, which can change the whole. Physical and mental health depended on the balance of the elements in the body. Alchemists became associated with magic (q.v.) and witchcraft (q.v.) and were often subjected to excommunication, torture, and death at the stake. In 1317, Pope John XXII had forbidden the study of alchemy, but its mixture of scientific inquiry and superstition continued to excite the imagination of men until the end of the sixteenth century.
Bibliography: Thompson C. J. Reprint. 1974. *Alchemy: source of chemistry and medicine*.

ALCMAEON. In Greek mythology he was the son of Amphiaraus and Eriphyle. By command of his father and encouraged by the oracle of Apollo (q.v.), he killed his own mother. As a punishment for matricide the Erinyes (q.v.) pursued him from place to place until he became mad. The King of Psophis in Arcadia partially purified him and gave him his daughter in marriage. But, the land became infertile because a matricide was being harbored there. Alcmaeon was forced to leave, and his madness returned. He found peace and sanity on an island newly formed at the mouth of the river Acheleus, where the land had been submerged at the time of his crime. Here he married again and by trickery obtained from the king of Psophis the necklace he had given to his first wife. The king discovered the deception and had him killed but was slain in turn by Alcmaeon's sons. The fatal necklace eventually was dedicated to Apollo and was said to bring bad luck to whoever possessed it.
See also ORESTES.
Bibliography: Harvey, P. 1966. *The Oxford companion to classical literature*.

ALCMAEON OF CROTONA(c.500 B.C.). A pupil of Pythagoras (q.v.) and the founder of the Sicilian school. His experiments with animal brains led him to believe that the brain was the site of intellect, understanding, and sensation. He enucleated the eye of a corpse and discovered the course of the optic nerve to the brain. Remarkably, Alcmaeon postulated that each sensation has its own territory of localization in the brain — a concept not revived until the twentieth century. He also investigated functional disorders caused by brain injuries. Although most of his book *On Nature* has been lost, small parts of it can be found as quotations in other authors, especially Plato (q.v.).

Bibliography: Zilboorg, G. 1941. *A history of medical psychology.*

ALCOHOLICS ANONYMOUS (AA). An organization founded in 1935 by a physician and a broker, both former alcoholics. Carl G. Jung (q.v.) was indirectly responsible for the venture because he told one of his patients, who was an alcoholic, that psychiatry (q.v.) could not help him but a religious experience might. The patient eventually experienced spiritual conversion and was cured. He proceeded to help other alcoholics, and the idea for a society of alcoholics who could help each other came into existence. It has since become an international movement. Members of the organization dedicate themselves to the rescue and support of those who desire to conquer their addiction to alcohol.

Bibliography: Ellenberger, H. F. 1970. *The discovery of the unconscious.*

ALCOHOLISM. Preoccupation with alcohol and uncontrollable desire to consume it. Although Asclepiades (q.v.) and his followers prescribed large doses of vintage wine as medication, this practice was condemned by Soranus (q.v.), who thought that mania (q.v.) often resulted from excessive drinking of wine and wrote, "inflammation of an organ as delicate and sensitive as the brain and its membranes is increased by the slight excitation. . . . How can it occur to the mind of any man to dispel intoxication by intoxication." William Shakespeare (q.v.) referred to alcohol intoxication in several passages and described how it impaired memory (q.v.) and reason, produced euphoria, indiscretion, and heightened perception, and produced a temporary improvement in performance that ended in loss of consciousness. (*Macbeth,* I, iii and VII; *Henry IV,* pt. 2, IV, iii; *Twelfth Night,* I, v; *Othello,* II, iii.) In the eighteenth and nineteenth centuries alcohol was regarded as one of the main causes of mental disorders.

See also ABSINTHE and GIN.

Bibliography: Zilboorg, G. 1941. *A history of medical psychology.*

ALCORTA, DIEGO(1807-1842). An Argentinian physician. He was the first person in Latin America to write a thesis on psychiatry (q.v.). He chose as his subject "acute mania (q.v.)". As an admirer of Philippe Pinel (q.v.), he supported humanitarian reforms in mental hospitals, including the introduction of moral medicine (q.v.).

Bibliography: Leon, C. A. and Rosselli, H. 1975. Latin America. *World history of psychiatry*, ed. J. G. Howells.

ALCOTT, AMOS BRONSON(1799-1888). An American educationalist and father of Louisa May Alcott (1832-1888), who wrote *Little Women*. He used his first daughter, and later her two sisters, in an experiment aimed at producing perfect individuals by good nurturing, loving warmth, and great permissiveness. The experiment was not a success, and the children became demanding and aggressive. He recorded the progress of the children and his own observations and feelings under the title of "Observations of Phenomena of Life, as Developed in the Progressive History on an Infant, during the First Year of its Existence." The manuscript was nearly twenty-five hundred pages long, and he could find no publisher for it. After failing to make a living as a pedlar, he started a progressive school, but his ideas were too advanced for his time, and this venture also met with failure. He then tried to establish a vegetarian community. It too did not succeed. After these somewhat eccentric ventures, he found a more stable occupation as superintendent of a school in Concord, Massachusetts, where he founded a school of philosophy and literature that reflected his transcendental beliefs. He wrote a number of books on child-rearing practices, but a truer picture of the Alcott family is to be found in his daughter's *Little Women*.
Bibliography: Shepard, O. 1937. *Pedlar's progress: the life of Bronson Alcott*.

ALEMAN, ANDREW(c. 1480). A Danish physician who entered the service of James III (q.v.) of Scotland. He had a great reputation as an astrologer (*see* ASTROLOGY) and a soothsayer. He predicted the manner of the king's death by interpreting a lion being strangled by its cub as a sign that James would be murdered by a member of his own family. His prediction had great influence on the behavior of the emotionally unstable James III.
Bibliography: Talbot, C. H., and Hammond, E. A. 1965. *The medical practitioners in medieval England*.

ALEXANDER III, *known as* **ALEXANDER THE GREAT**(356-323 B.C.). A Macedonian king who achieved great renown as general and ruler. His father had an ungovernable temper and his mother was a woman of debauched character. From his parents he acquired unpleasant personality traits and a taste for vulgar and debased experiences. His head appeared to be lopsided because of a contraction of the muscles of the neck, probably of psychosomatic origin.
Bibliography: Fox, R. L. 1973. *Alexander the great*.

ALEXANDER, FRANZ(1891-1964). A psychologist born in Budapest, Hungary. He graduated from the University of Budapest in 1912 and the Berlin Psychoanalytic Institute in 1919. In 1929 he was appointed the first

professor of psychoanalysis at the University of Chicago. Alexander differentiated the psychology (q.v.) of guilt from the psychology of shame. Because of his studies on unconscious motivation, a German criminal court asked his opinion in the case of a kleptomaniac girl, who stole cheap reproductions of the Madonna. He was able to convince the judges that she was motivated by her intense wish to have a child. As she could not gratify this desire because of the position of her lover, she identified with the Virgin Mary and virgin birth. This episode led to Alexander's thesis *The Criminal, the Judge and the Public*, written in 1929 with the Berlin lawyer Hugo Staub. Alexander's other contributions were in the field of brief analytic therapy and of psychosomatic medicine (q.v.). A prolific writer, he wrote sixteen books and over 250 articles. For a time he was president of the American Psychoanalytic Association and the American Society for Research in Psychosomatic Medicine. At the time of his death he was president of the Academy of Psychoanalysis.
Bibliography: Alexander, F. 1957. *Psychoanalysis and psychotherapy.*

ALEXANDERISM. A condition defined by Daniel H. Tuke (q.v.) as "the insanity of conquest, the irrepressible desire to destroy or exterminate nations." It is derived from the name of Alexander the Great (q.v.).
Bibliography: Tuke, D. 1892. *A dictionary of psychological medicine.*

ALEXANDER OF APHRODISIAS(fl. A.D. 200). An early commentator on the works of Aristotle (q.v.). He regarded the passive intellect as a faculty of the human soul and the active intellect as separated from it and limited to extrinsic mystical illuminations.
Bibliography: 1959. *The history and philosophy of the brain and its functions.*

ALEXANDER OF HALES(d.1245). An English scholastic (*see* SCHOLASTICISM) theologian and philosopher who tried to correlate the ideas of Saint Augustine (q.v.) with those of Aristotle (q.v.) and the Arabs (q.v.). He was interested in the problems posed by the human conscience and in how scruples and feelings of remorse were produced. He wrote *Summa Theologiae*, a vast work, left unfinished.
Bibliography: Zilboorg, G. 1941. *A history of medical psychology.*

ALEXANDER OF TRALLES(A.D. 525-605). A physician born in Tralles, Lydia. He studied in Alexandria and after much traveling settled in Rome, where he practiced and taught medicine. After Hippocrates (q.v.), he was one of the best Greek physicians. His works were translated in Hebrew, Latin, and Arabic. He classified mental disorders into phrenitis (q.v.), lethargus, epilepsy (q.v.), and six types of melancholy (*see* MELANCHOLIA). He claimed that melancholy due to excess of blood was most common in slim people with dark hair. He considered melancholy due to blocking of the blood extremely serious because it could turn into mania (q.v.). Alexander advocated humane treatment of the mentally ill and recommended baths, diets (q.v.), wines, and sedatives. He recognized that depression and mania may be present in the same individual. His treatment of deluded (*see* DE-LUSION) patients included a prescription for a hat made of lead for a man who thought he had lost his head and a deftly produced snake for a patient who believed she had swallowed one.

Bibliography: Brunet, F. 1933. *Oeuvres médicales d'Alexandre de Tralles.*

ALEXANDRA OF BAVARIA. A paternal aunt of Maximilian Joseph I, king of Bavaria (1727-1777). In 1850 she was treated for insanity in the asylum (q.v.) of Illenau. She believed that she had swallowed a glass sofa.

Bibliography: Ireland, W. W. 1889. *Through the ivory gate.*

ALEXIS OF PIEDMONT(c.1471-1565). A physician born in Piedmont, Italy. He mentioned "lunatic disease" in children — probably an early description of either delirium (q.v.) in children or childhood psychosis (q.v.). He attributed the cause of it to a double-headed worm in the body.

Bibliography: Whitwell, J. R. 1936. *Historical notes on psychiatry.*

ALFIERI, VITTORIO(1749-1803). A wealthy Italian dramatist, born in Piedmont, Italy. He traveled a great deal. His numerous love-affairs included a deep involvement with the wife of the Young Pretender, Charles Edward Stuart. His most famous works are his tragedies (*Maria Stuarda, Saul,* and *Abele,* among others) and his masterly autobiography, which relates his frequent episodes of deep melancholy (*see* MELANCHOLIA) and, on one occasion, the experience of seeing his own image coming toward him. At the age of eight in a fit of depression, he tried to commit suicide (q.v.) by eating what he believed to be hemlock. It made him very sick, he was shut up in his room and then taken to church, still in his nightcap. Because he found that driving a coach made his depression more bearable, he did so frequently, an eccentric activity in an age of coachmen and servants.

Bibliography: Alfieri, V. 1953. *Life of Vittorio Alfieri, written by himself,* trans. Molinaro and Corrigan.

ALICE-IN-WONDERLAND SYNDROME. A term applied to phenomena of derealisation. It is a reference to the experiences of the character Alice in Charles L. Dodgson's (q.v.) classic, *Alice's Adventures in Wonderland* (1865).

Bibliography: Todd, J. 1955. The syndrome of Alice in Wonderland. *Canada med. Ass. J.* 73, 701-704.

ALIENIST. A nineteenth-century term for doctors dealing with the mentally ill. It is derived from the expression "mental alienation," which was first used in France by Jean Pierre Falret (q.v.) to imply the estrangement of the mentally ill from the community.

ALLEGED LUNATICS' FRIEND SOCIETY. A society founded in England in 1845 through the instigation of John Thomas Perceval (q.v.), who was its honorary secretary. Although it did not gain much public support, it did influence reform in the legislation relating to the certification and treatment of mental patients. It published reports in 1851 and in 1858.

ALLEN, FREDERICK(1890-1964). An American psychiatrist, born in San Jose, California. For many years he was the director of the Philadelphia Child Guidance Clinic. His therapeutic approach was influenced by the theories of August Aichhorn (q.v.), and he believed that disturbed children needed a warm and supportive relationship if they were to relate satisfactorily to adults. Unlike Aichhorn, he thought that children have a natural potential for healthy development.
Bibliography: Allen, F. 1942. *Psychotherapy with children.*

ALLEN, MATTHEW (?-1845). A physician who obtained his degree in Aberdeen, Scotland. Early in his career he became interested in the problems of mental disorders and visited many asylums (q.v.) from 1807 onwards. Between 1816 and 1819 he undertook lecture tours, speaking on the subject "Mind and its Diseases." During one of these tours, he met and formed a friendship with Thomas Carlyle (q.v.), who was impressed by his lecture on phrenology (q.v.). In 1819 he became resident medical officer of the York Lunatic Asylum (q.v.). During his five years there, he was instrumental in establishing what he called "a mild system of treatment." In 1825, he founded a licensed house for private patients near Epping in Essex. He was the first to consider the home background of his patients, attributing mental breakdowns to "the demon of domestic strife." In accordance to the belief of nineteenth-century psychiatry (q.v.), he considered his neurotic (*see* NEUROSIS) patients insane and "delicately but candidly" told them so. He was the first to suggest a system of voluntary patients and indeed admitted uncertified patients to his madhouse, thus incurring the displeasure of the Commissioners in Lunacy (q.v.). The poet John Clare (q.v.) was one of his patients but escaped from his establishment. Allen seems to have had many connections with the literary world, as Alfred Lord Tennyson (q.v.) lent him money for an ill-fated venture involving wood-carving by machine, which ended in bankruptcy.
Bibliography: Hunter, R., and Macalpine, I. 1963. *Three hundred years of psychiatry.*

ALLEN, THOMAS (?-1684). English physician to Charles II and Bethlem Royal Hospital (q.v.). He objected to submitting patients in the hospital to experiments in blood transfusions (q.v.) that used sheep's blood. He also

owned a private asylum, Finnesbury Madhouse. One of his patients was James Carkesse (q.v.), who later described his experiences there.
Bibliography: Hunter R., and Macalpine, I. 1963. *Three hundred years of psychiatry.*

ALL HALLOWS HOSPITAL. A proposed institution near Barking, London for the care of priests and others "who suddenly fell into a frenzy and lost their memories." In 1369 Robert Denton, an English chaplain, obtained a license from Edward III for its foundation, but through lack of funds the venture came to nothing. However, John Stow (q.v.) in his *The Survey of London* referred to it as Denton's Hospital, founded in the forty-fourth year of Edward III, only to be suppressed later in his reign or that of Henry V.
Bibliography: Talbot, C. H. 1967. *Medicine in medieval England.*

ALLPORT, GORDON W. (1897-1967). An American psychologist, born in Montezuma, Indiana. After graduating from Harvard University, he studied in Germany and in England. His work covered the psychology (q.v.) of race relations, expressive movement, and prejudice. He is considered an authority on the psychology of personality.
Bibliography: Allport, G.W. 1951. *Personality.*————. 1961. *Pattern and growth of personality.*

AL-MANSUR HOSPITAL. The most important of the Cairo lunatic asylums (q.v.), also known as "the great hospital of Al-Mansur." From its beginnings in 1284 it had a proper system of treatment for the mentally ill. Each patient was cared for by two attendants under the supervision of well-paid physicians. Musicians and storytellers were employed to sooth restless patients and to provoke sleep in them. Convalescents were housed in separate quarters, and dancing and plays were part of their therapy. On discharge, each patient received five gold pieces.
Bibliography: Browne, E. G. 1921. *Arabian medicine.*

ALPHA TESTS. A series of intelligence tests devised in the United States during World War I. A committee for psychology (q.v.) under the auspices of the surgeon general was organized to find ways of using psychology in the training and selecting of army recruits. Hundreds of intelligence tests were reviewed, and finally a series of tests (alpha tests) based on those submitted by A. S. Otis of Stanford University were developed. 1,727,000 men were tested, and it then was discovered that 30 percent of the recruits were illiterate. Special tests (beta tests [q.v.]) were developed for them, and it was found that 46,000 men had a mental age of less than ten years. These men were discharged as untrainable.
Bibliography: Yerkes, R.H., ed. 1921. Psychological examining in the United States Army. *Mem. Nat. Acad. Sci.* Vol. 15.

ALPINI, PROSPERO (1553-?1616). An Italian physician and botanist. He was professor of botany at the University of Padua, where he personally cared for the herb garden. After an expedition to Egypt (q.v.), he wrote a treatise on Egyptian medicine and, later, a book on prognosis (q.v.). He is also said to have introduced coffee to Europe. From his visits to Japan in 1616 he brought back moxa (q.v.) which were to become the most common means of cauterizing (see CAUTERIZATION) the insane.
Bibliography: Garrison, F.H. 1929. *An introduction to the history of medicine.*

ALT-SCHERBITZ ASYLUM. A public institution in Saxony, Prussia. It was well known in the nineteenth century for its pioneer work in the treatment of the insane with enlightened methods.
Bibliography: Letchworth, W. P. 1889. *The insane in foreign countries.*

ALUSIA. A term meaning illusion. It was used by John Mason Good (q.v.) in his classification of mental disorders. It was a subdivision of the class Neurotica.

ALVAREZ, BERNARDINO (1517-1584). A Spanish philanthropist, born in Andalusia. He became a lieutenant of Hernando Cortes (1485-1547) and went with him to Mexico, where his behavior eventually deteriorated into delinquency. Drinking, gambling, and thievery finally led to his imprisonment, but he escaped and reached Cuzco in Peru, where he made a fortune. At that point in his life he remembered his family in Spain. He sent for them but learned that his father had died, and his mother and sisters had become nuns and had no wish to leave their convent. His mother admonished him to change his way of life and to use his wealth for a Christian purpose. In 1556, perhaps driven by remorse, he returned to Mexico City still rich but subdued and given to prayer and fasting. He dedicated himself to the founding of a hospital for the mentally ill, and thus the San Hipólito Hospital (q.v.), the first mental hospital in Latin America, came into existence in 1567. He then founded two chains of hospitals, one reaching the Atlantic Ocean and one reaching the shores of the Pacific. Each hospital was run by the Hipólitos (q.v.), members of a religious order he had founded. Alvarez lived the remainder of his life in a little cell in the San Hipólito Hospital and died there, loved and respected. In 1967 the Republic of Mexico named a new and modern mental hospital after him.
Bibliography: Rumbaut, Ruben D. 1971. Bernardino Alvarez: New World Psychiatric Pioneer. *Am. J. Psychiat.* 127: 1217-221.

ALZHEIMER, ALOIS (1864-1915). A psychiatrist born in Markbreit, Germany. In 1912 he was appointed professor of psychiatry (q.v.) and neurology (q.v.) at Breslau University in Poland. His investigations in the pathology of senile dementia led to the discovery of the disorder now known as Alzheimer's disease, a presenile condition characterized by progressive mental deterioration and associated with cortical cerebral sclerosis. His studies also included research in the symptomatology of schizophrenia (q.v.) and of manic depressive psychoses (q.v.).

Bibliography: Lewey, F.H. 1953. Alois Alzheimer (1864-1915). In *The founders of neurology*, eds. W. Haymaker and F. Schiller.

AMASIS II (568-525 B.C.). A king of Egypt. Herodotus (q.v.) reported that he deliberatedly used relaxation as a means of reducing nervous tension. Amasis answered those who criticized his revels by stating that, like a bow which if kept permanently strung will break and be of no use when need arises, so he would go mad or suffer a stroke, if he did not relax.

Bibliography: Brothwell, D., and Sandison, A. T. 1967. *Diseases in antiquity.*

AMAUROTIC FAMILIAL IDIOCY. A term used by Bernard Sachs (q.v.) in his study of infantile cerebromacular degeneration, which was published in 1887. He regarded it as a congenital defect of development. Because Warren Tay (q.v.), a British ophthalmologist, had described the retinal changes that occur in this condition in 1881, the disease is often referred to as Tay-Sachs disease.

Bibliography: Jablonski, S. 1969. *Illustrated dictionary of eponymic syndromes and diseases and their synonyms.*

AMAZONS. A mythical race of female warriors, possibly from southwest Asia. They were said to kill or maim their male children. The females had their right breast amputated to facilitate the use of bows in battle. The race was perpetuated by periodic mating with men of other races. The term is now used for masculine-looking women.

Bibliography: Forsdyke, J. 1956. *Greece before Homer.*

AMBER. The fossilized resin of conifers. It was used to diagnose disorders of the nervous system. Wearing it against the body was said to preserve nervous energy.

See also PRECIOUS STONES.

Bibliography: Bonser, W. 1963. *The medical background of Anglo-Saxon England.*

AMBIVALENCE. A term coined by Eugen Bleuler (q.v.) to indicate the simultaneous presence of two opposing tendencies in certain psychotics (*see* PSYCHOSIS).

AMENOMANIA. A term coined by Benjamin Rush (q.v.) to describe a state of "partial intellectual derangement accompanied with pleasure, or not accompanied with distress."

Bibliography: Rush, B. 1812. Reprint. 1962. *Medical enquiries and observations upon diseases of the mind.*

AMERICAN ASSOCIATION ON MENTAL DEFICIENCY. Originally entitled the Association of Medical Officers of American Institutions for Idiots and Feebleminded Persons. It was founded by a group of superintendents in June 1876, in Media, Pennsylvania. It changed its name in 1906 to the American Association for the Study of the Feebleminded and again in 1933 to the American Association on Mental Deficiency. Among its chartered members were such outstanding pioneers in the care and treatment of the mentally defective as G.A. Doren (q.v.), George Brown, Isaac N. Kerlin (q.v.), Henry M. Knight (q.v.), Joseph Parrish, Edouard O. Seguin (q.v.), H.B. Wilbur (q.v.), and C.T. Wilbur. Its official journal is the *American Journal of Mental Deficiency* (q.v.).
Bibliography: Deutsch, A. 1949. *The mentally ill in America.*

AMERICAN BREEDERS' ASSOCIATION. An association concerned with animals and dedicated to maintaining breeding standards. In 1911, worried by the increasing number of mentally defectives, a committee of this association, produced a ten point document. Its objective was the "purging from the blood of the race the innately defective strains." Their main recommendations were segregation and sterilization (q.v.).
Bibliography: Kanner, L. 1964. *A history of the care and study of the mentally retarded.*

AMERICAN JOURNAL OF INSANITY. See AMERICAN JOURNAL OF PSYCHIATRY.

AMERICAN JOURNAL OF MENTAL DEFICIENCY. The official organ of the American Association on Mental Deficiency (q.v.) since 1940. Originally the association published a quarterly journal *The Journal of Psycho-Asthenics*, which was founded in 1896 and edited by Dr. A. C. Rogers of the Minnesota School for the Feebleminded at Faribeult, but its publication ceased in 1918.
Bibliography: Kanner, L. 1964. *A history of the care and study of the mentally retarded.*

AMERICAN JOURNAL OF PSYCHIATRY. Originally the *American Journal of Insanity.* It was founded in 1844 by Amariah Brigham (q.v.). He published it as a quarterly at his own expense and edited it in collaboration with his colleagues at Utica State Hospital (q.v.). The hospital print shop, which was operated by the patients, printed it. It was the first journal devoted to psychiatry (q.v.) that was written in English. Annual subscription was one dollar. In the first issue Brigham invited support not only from physicians but also from lawyers and clergymen. He hoped to make the general public aware of the need for more facilities for the care of the insane. At the end of the nineteenth century, the American Psychiatric Association

(q.v.) adopted it as its official journal and moved its publishing headquarters to Baltimore, Maryland. In 1921 it changed its title to the *American Journal of Psychiatry*.
Bibliography: Arieti, S., ed. 1974. *American handbook of psychiatry*. vol. 1.

AMERICAN JOURNAL OF PSYCHOLOGY. The first American journal dedicated to psychology (q.v.). It was founded in 1887 by G. Stanley Hall (q.v.) after a visit to Wilhelm M. Wundt's (q.v.) new laboratory in Leipzig, Germany. Unlike other journals of its time, it was not biased in favor of any one school of psychology.
Bibliography: Boring, E. G. 1950. *A history of experimental psychology*.

AMERICAN NEUROLOGICAL ASSOCIATION. An association founded in 1875. Dr. J. S. Jewell of Chicago, Illinois, was its first president. Its predecessor was the New York Neurological Society, which had been established by a group of distinguished neurologists in 1872. The official organ of the association is the *Journal of Nervous and Mental Diseases*, which was also founded by Dr. Jewell.
Bibliography: Deutsch, A. 1949. *The mentally ill in America*.

AMERICAN ORTHOPSYCHIATRIC ASSOCIATION. An association founded in 1924 "to meet the needs for a central organization of those dealing with the psychiatric aspects of delinquency." Its scope and membership later were expanded to include all fields of study and treatment of human behavior.
Bibliography: Deutsch, A. 1949. *The mentally ill in America*.

AMERICAN PSYCHIATRIC ASSOCIATION. The first national society of medical men in the United States. The idea for its formation developed in a conversation between Dr. Francis T. Stribling (q.v.) and Dr. Samuel B. Woodward (q.v.) in 1844. Later in that year, on October 16, a founding meeting was held at Jones' Hotel in Philadelphia, Pennsylvania, attended by thirteen distinguished medical superintendents: Samuel B. Woodward, Samuel White, Thomas Kirkbride, Amariah Brigham, Isaac Ray, Pliny Earle, Luther V. Bell, William M. Awl, Nehemiah Cutter, Francis T. Stribling, John S. Butler, John M. Galt, and Charles H. Stedman (qq.v.). From then on they were referred to as "the original thirteen." The society was known as the Association of Medical Superintendents of American Institutions for the Insane. For over half a century it remained a small organization with a membership of approximately 200. In 1893 it changed its name to the American Medico-Psychological Association. During this period, its presidents included such distinguished men as Adolf Meyer, William Alanson White, Ernest Southard, and Thomas W. Salmon (qq.v.). By 1921 its membership had increased to 1,000, and the name changed to the present American Psychiatric Association, which in 1977 had an estimated membership of

24,000. From its beginning, the association has regarded mental disorders as a part of general medicine, and its primary aims have been the improvement of hospital facilities for the mentally ill and the unification and dissemination of all knowledge relating to psychiatry (q.v.). The association's central office is now in Washington, D.C.; its official organs are the *American Journal of Psychiatry* (q.v.) and *Psychiatric News*. It is also responsible for other publications, for a modern library, and for a major collection of historical works in psychiatry.

Bibliography: American Psychiatric Associations 1977. *Biographical directory of the American psychiatric association.*

AMERICAN PSYCHOLOGICAL ASSOCIATION. An association of psychologists originally planned in 1892 in G. Stanley Hall's (q.v.) study; it came into being during the same year with Hall (q.v.) as its first president. From an initial membership of 26, it has grown to over 20,000 members, grouped into divisions according to scientific or professional interests. It publishes some twelve journals, of which the oldest and best known are the *American Journal of Psychology* (q.v.) and the *Psychological Review* (q.v.).

Bibliography: Boring, E. G. 1950. *A history of experimental psychology.*

AMERLING, KARL. The founder of *diasophy*, an abstruse doctrine, and head of the Bohemian Physiocratic Society. He was the director of an institution for 300 mentally retarded children, established in Prague in 1871 by the Saint Anna Women's Organization.

Bibliography: Kanner, L. 1964. *A history of the care and study of the mentally retarded.*

AMETHYST. A gem, which in the Middle Ages (q.v.) was believed to preserve its wearer from bad dreams (q.v.) and was said to possess medical qualities. As late as the nineteenth century it was believed that an amethyst inserted under the skin would cure epilepsy (q.v.).

See also PRECIOUS STONES.

Bibliography: Esquirol, J. E. D. 1845. Reprint. 1965. *Mental maladies: a treatise on insanity.*

AMIDAS. A Japanese divinity whose followers were bent on self-destruction. During religious festivities dedicated to the god, men and women, encouraged by applauding onlookers, jumped into the sea in a state of frenzy; others were buried alive, their shouts of "Amidas, Amidas" continuing until hunger and exhaustion silenced them in death.

Bibliography: Fedden, H. R. 1938. *Suicide.*

AMIEL, HENRI-FRÉDÉRIC (1821-1881). A Swiss philosopher, born in Geneva. He kept a diary for many years, and it was its posthumous publication as *Journal Intime* (1821-1881) that made the author known. In a

remarkable, introspective analysis lasting some thirty years, Amiel wrote about his weak will and lack of strength, which destroyed his creativity and imprisoned him. Action was a torment to him. An English translation of his diary was published in 1885.
Bibliography: Harvey, P., and Heseltine, J. E. 1959. *Oxford companion to French literature.*

AMNESIA. A term for loss of memory (q.v.). It was introduced into medical psychology (q.v.) by De Valenzi (1728-1813).
Bibliography: Zilboorg, G. 1941. *A history of medical psychology.*

AMNON. A Biblical (*see* BIBLE) character, son of David (q.v.). He became enamored of his sister Tamar and seduced her. His guilty love so affected him that he became ill, thus providing an example of incest (q.v.) followed by guilt, leading to psychosomatic illness.
Bibliography: 2 Sam. 13: 1-2.

AMOK. An indiscriminate and motiveless act of aggression. It is common in Malaysia and the surrounding area where tradition, religion, and social structure favor this behavior as a means of tension reduction. A similar version of this syndrome is found in Papua and New Guinea, usually among healthy young adults who, after an initial period of unusual quietness, arm themselves and kill or wound anyone around. The inhabitants claim that the amok individual suffers from amnesia (q.v.) during these acts of destruction, which they regard as an attempt to reduce unbearable tension. Eugen Bleuler (q.v.) in his *Textbook of Psychiatry* mentioned "the running amok of the Malays, in which the patients run through the streets with drawn daggers, cut people down at random until they collapse, or, which is more frequent, are shot down or made harmless in some other way."
Bibliography: Burton-Bradley, B. G. 1968. The amok syndrome in Papua and New Guinea. *Med. J. Australia.* 1: 252.

AMOUR MÉDECIN, L'. A French comedy by Molière, first produced at Versailles in 1665. The heroine, Lucinde, suffers from melancholia (q.v.) when she is forbidden by her father to see her lover, Clitandre. He pretends to be a doctor, gains admission to her and persuades the father that he can cure Lucinde through the mind by performing an imaginary marriage; the marriage turns out to be real and binds the two lovers. The play ridiculed the court doctors yet underlined the importance of the emotions in the aetiology of illness.

AMOURS DU CHEVALIER DE FAUBLAS, LES. A French novel by Louvet de Couvray (1760-1797). It recounts the adventures of a young man who is irresistible to women and leads a licentious life. His many loves leave

a trail of tragedies, including suicide (q.v.). He is so haunted by hallucinations (q.v.) in which he sees the people he has wronged seeking revenge
that he finally loses his reason.
Bibliography: Harvey, P. & Heseltine, J. E. 1959. *The Oxford companion to French
literature.*

AMPUTATION DOLL. A doll that can be taken to pieces. It was introduced by the American psychiatrist David Levy as a tool in play therapy
for young children. It represents a mother figure, and the child is encouraged
to project his feelings on to it.
Bibliography: Bender, L. 1952. *Child psychiatric techniques.*

AMULETS. Charms or objects worn for their magical (*see* MAGIC) protection against witchcraft (q.v.) sickness, or accidents. A belief in amulets has
been present from antiquity in all populations and still persists today in the
form of mascots. The type of amulet, the place where it is found and the
circumstances surrounding its acquisition are considered of special significance. The amulet may take the form of a ring, nail, stone, plant or human
bones from someone who has died violently. It may have been found at
crossroads (q.v.), burialplaces, or may have been collected under appropriate
stellar influences. The comfort and support amulets offer to those who
believe in them, including the emotionally ill, are used as a proof of their
worth. Robert Burton (q.v.) in his *Anatomy of Melancholy* (q.v.) discusses
at length the evidence of this cure of "head-melancholy": "Amulets and
things to be borne about I find prescribed, taxed by some, approved by . . .
others."
See also TALISMAN.
Bibliography: Evans, J. 1922. *Magical jewels.*

ANACLITIC DEPRESSION. A term introduced by René Spitz (q.v.) in
1946 to describe the syndrome found in infants deprived of love objects.
Anaclitic depression is commonly observed in institutionalized infants.
Bibliography: Spitz, R. 1946. Anaclitic depression. In *Psychoanalytic study of the
child.* Vol. 2.

ANAGOGIC INTERPRETATION. In psychoanalysis (q.v.) the interpretation of psychic material as expressive of ideas. H. Silberer first described
the anagogic interpretation of dreams in 1914 in a work entitled *Probleme
der Hystik und ihrer Sympolik.* He felt that dreams (q.v.) should be interpreted in a spiritual, nonsexual manner in order to discover their more serious
nature and the idealistic strivings of the unconscious.
Bibliography: Eidelberg, L. 1968. *Encyclopedia of psychoanalysis.*

ANALYTIC GROUP THERAPY. E.W. Lazell first experimented with
psychoanalytic techniques in group therapy at St. Elizabeth's Hospital (q.v.)

in Washington, D.C., in 1921. He was followed by Louis Wender and Paul Schilder (q.v.) in the 1930s and by S.R. Slavson in the 1950s.
Bibliography: Goldenson, R. M. 1970. *Encyclopedia of human behaviour.*

ANALYZING INSTRUMENT. The analyst's frame of mind during psychoanalysis (q.v.) as described by Sigmund Freud (q.v.) in *The Interpretation of Dreams* (1900).
Bibliography: Freud, S. 1974. *The complete psychological works of Sigmund Freud.* Vol. 4. Ed. J. Strachey.

ANANIZAPTA. A word used in medieval England as a charm against epilepsy (q.v.). Sometimes it was engraved on rings or bracelets to be worn by those afflicted with the disease.
Bibliography: Evans, J. 1922. *Magical jewels.*

ANANKE. A Greek term introduced by Sigmund Freud (q.v.) in a lecture in 1917 to mean an external necessity or fate. He defined it as "the pressure of vital needs — Necessity."
Bibliography: Freud, S. 1963. *Introductory lectures in psycho-analysis.*

ANATOMY OF MELANCHOLY, THE. A medical work written by Robert Burton (q.v.) in 1621. It is more a collection of anecdotes, historical quotations of about a thousand authors, and items of general interest than a medical textbook. The volume was meant to entertain whilst offering the reader a source of references not only on the subject of melancholy (*see* MELANCHOLIA) but also on a miscellaneous field of knowledge. It has been widely read and referred to despite its many inaccuracies. The work is divided into three parts: aetiology and symptomatology; treatment; melancholy of love (q.v.) and melancholy of religion. Physical and mental health are discussed within a framework of social and political reform, and the entire book is suffused with a sense of religious toleration as well as a sense of humor. It has run to many editions, five of them in Burton's own lifetime, each containing changes by author, editors, and printers.
(See Plate 1.)
Bibliography: Burton, R. 1621. Reprint. 1964. *The anatomy of melancholy.*

ANAXAGORAS OF CLEOMENES (c.500-428 B.C.). A Greek philosopher and scientist and a contemporary of Hippocrates (q.v.). He was the first to describe the lateral ventricles of the brain and believed that the soul resided there. According to him an independent spirit of intelligence (*Nous*) was the supreme moving force in the universe. This concept revolutionized Greek philosophy and became the origin of the doctrine that mind and matter are two distinct entities. He was also the first to explain solar eclipses, but he was accused of blasphemy when he stated that the sun was made of

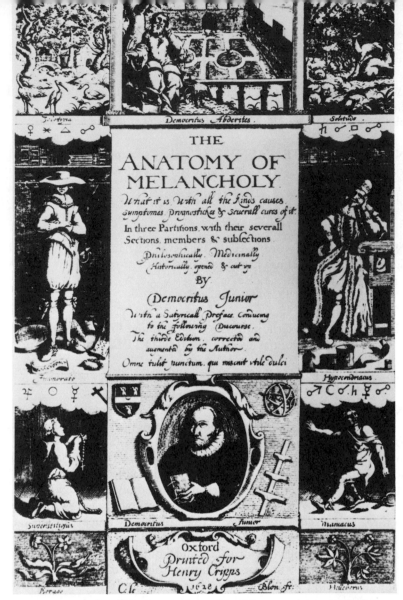

1. *THE ANATOMY OF MELANCHOLY*, frontispiece for the 3rd edition. At the top, in the center, Democritus of Abdera, a Greek philosopher of the fifth century B.C., is represented surrounded by the animals he anatomized while searching for blackbile; allegorical representations of jealousy and solitude, two aspects of melancholy, are depicted in the top corners. In the middle, the four figures on the left and on the right of the page, are types of melancholics—the gloomy lover, the hypochrondriac, the superstitious, and the manic, each with appropriate symbols. Borage and hellebore, "to purge the veins of melancholy and cheer the heart," fill the bottom corners. The portrait is captioned "Democritus Junior," the pseudonym of the author. The sign of Saturn, the planet of melancholy, recurs here and there on the page. By courtesy of the Department of Medical Illustration, Ipswich Hospital.

a flaming matter and the gods were merely inventions of the human mind. For these beliefs he was heavily fined and expelled from Athens.
Bibliography: Guthrie, W. K. C. 1960. *The Greek philosophers.*

ANDERSEN, HANS CHRISTIAN (1805-1875). A Danish author. He was the only child of a cobbler who wanted him to be a tailor, but he hoped to be an opera singer or a dancer. As a child he was a daydreamer, and the despair of his teachers, who thought him dull. He wandered about, lost in his own thoughts, with his eyes shut. He went to University and wrote his first book when he was twenty-four years old, but his most famous writings are his fairy tales, which reveal his sensitivity and psychological insight.
Bibliography: Bredsdorff, E. 1975. *Hans Christian Andersen: the story of his life and work.*

ANDERSEN, TRYGGVE (1866-1920). A Norwegian novelist and short-story writer, best known for his historical novel *I Cancelliraadens dage* (1897) set in Norway, in the early nineteenth century. He was deeply depressed and suffered from hallucinations (q.v.) and obsessions (q.v.). His state of mind is reflected in his writings, especially in his novel *Mod Kvaeld* (1900) and the posthumously published *Dagbog* (1923).

ANDREAS-SALOMÉ, LOU (1861-1937). A psychoanalyst of German origin. She was brought up in Russia, where her father was in business. She was a prolific novelist, and also wrote many theoretical papers on psycho-analysis (q.v.), after she had become a disciple and personal friend of Sigmund Freud (q.v.) whom she first met in 1911. She claimed that her early writing had anticipated Freud's work. Friedrich Nietzsche (q.v.) was fascinated by her and even proposed marriage, but she rejected him. She married an Oriental scholar, Andreas, in 1887. She then became the mistress of the poet Rainer Maria Rilke (1875-1926), who remained dependent on her to the end of his life. Lou Andreas-Salomé has been regarded by many as a genius (q.v.) in spite of her hysterical and unconventional behavior.
Bibliography: Binion, R. 1968. *Frau Lou: Nietzsche's wayward disciple.*
Pfeiffer, E., ed. *Freud/Andreas-Salomé: letters.*

ANDRÉ CORNÉLIS. A French novel by Paul Bourget (1852-1935). Written in 1887, it provides a psychological analysis of the hero's feelings of anguish and indecision when he discovers that his stepfather, unknown to his mother, killed his father. He demands that his stepfather commit suicide (q.v.) and when he refuses, stabs him. The dying man leaves a note for his wife asserting that he has killed himself because he is incurably ill. André remains in his anguish, unable to decide whether to tell his mother the truth.
Bibliography: Bourget, P. 1887. *André Cornélis.*

ANEMOMANIA. A term coined by Benjamin Rush (q.v.) to describe paranoia (q.v.). He derived it from the Greek meaning of "fear of the wind," an unfounded fear.
Bibliography: Rush, B. 1812. Reprint. 1962. *Medical enquiries and observations upon diseases of the mind.*

ANESTHESIA. A term derived from the Greek, meaning "insensibility to pain." Hippocrates (q.v.) commented that anesthesia was a sign of brain injury. The demonologists gave particular significance to anesthesia of the skin and of mucous membranes; it was regarded as a stigma (*stigmata* [q.v.] *diaboli*) imposed by the devil on his associates. As late as the nineteenth century, Jean Charcot (q.v.) listed skin anesthesia as a permanent characteristic of major hysteria (q.v.).
Bibliography: Zilboorg, G. 1941. *A history of medical psychology.*

ANGELL, JAMES ROWLAND (1869-1949). An American psychologist and educator. After graduating from Harvard, he studied abroad, mainly in Germany. His intellectual life was influenced by an early interest in philosophy and logic and later by the work of William James (q.v.). His name is closely connected with that of A. W. Moore in the study of the reaction time, which combined with his studies in functional psychology and comparative psychology gives him an important place in the history of experimental psychology (q.v.). The development of the Chicago school of psychology was especially influenced by his strong personality. He became chairman of the National Research Council, president of the Carnegie Corporation, president of Yale University, and educational counsellor of the National Broadcasting Company.
Bibliography: Murchison, C., ed. 1936. *A history of psychology in autobiography.* Vol. 3.

ANGLO-SAXON HERBAL. A medieval collection of remedies handed down through the ages and reflecting the folklore of the time. Among other prescriptions, it suggests the use of peony and clovewort in the treatment of insanity, and indicates the right seasons and lunar phases for gathering the ingredients.
Bibliography: Bonser, W. 1963. *The medical background of Anglo-Saxon England.*

ANHEDONIA. A term referring to a chronic state of lack of pleasure, with an absence of pain, but often with acute anxiety. Théodule Ribot (q.v.) was the first to employ this concept in describing insensibility to pleasure.
Bibliography: Eidelberg, L. 1968. *Encyclopedia of psychoanalysis.*

ANIMA. A Jungian term. Its original meaning was soul or life-force. It was used by Carl Jung (q.v.) to describe an archetype (q.v.) in a man's collective unconscious that described his inherited collective image of all women. Later, Jung introduced an analogous term, *animus* to describe the archetype in a woman's collective unconscious that described her inherited, collective image of all men.

Bibliography: Jacobi, J. 1962. *Psychology of C.G. Jung*, trans. by R. Mannheim.

ANIMAL MAGNETISM. A fluid that was believed to pass from the operator to the subject during the production of hypnotic (*see* HYPNOTISM) phenomena. This theory originated with Franz A. Mesmer (q.v.) in the eighteenth century.

Bibliography: Buranelli, V. 1975. *The wizard from Vienna—Franz Anton Mesmer and the origin of hypnotism.*

ANIMALS. The ancients perceived that animals, like humans, are subject to mental disorders and emotional upsets. Robert Burton (q.v.) wrote, "of all other [animals], dogs are most subject to this malady, insomuch some hold their dream as men do, and through violence of melancholy run mad; I could relate many stories of dogs that have died for grief, and pined away for loss of their masters. . . . "

In more recent times, Jane Goodall's studies of chimpanzees have contributed greatly to the knowledge of animal behavior. Among the many examples of emotional disorders that she cites, there is one of psychosomatic death, which occurred when an 8-year-old chimpanzee lost his will to live after the death of his mother.

Bibliography: Burton, R. 1621. Reprint. 1964. *Anatomy of melancholy.*
Goodall, J. 1979. Life and death at Gombe. *National Geographic*, 155: 592-622.

ANIMAL SOUL. Regarded by Galen (q.v.) as the rational soul. He located it in the brain. He concluded after experimenting on animals that the rational soul was divided in two parts, the external and the internal. The external was responsible for the five senses, while the internal regulated imagination, judgment, memory (q.v.), apperception, and movement.

Bibliography: Temkin, O. 1973. *Galenism.*

ANIMAL SPIRITS. Distillations from the blood in the brain, according to Thomas Willis (q.v.) who believed that animal spirits would escape from the brain by rising and expanding and invade the nervous paths. They were said to excite the intellect to a torment that led to mania (q.v.).

Bibliography: Willis, T. 1672. *De anima brutorum.*

ANIMA SENSITIVA. A term used by Georg E. Stahl (q.v.) to indicate a kind of unconscious perception that causes dreams (q.v.) to reflect abnormal bodily states.

Bibliography: Zilboorg, G. 1941. *A history of medical psychology.*

ANIMISM. A belief, still existent in primitive cultures, that objects in nature have souls or spirits or are inhabited by them. Georg E. Stahl (q.v.) used

the term animism to indicate that the soul is the vital principle and responsible for organic development.
Bibliography: Smart, N. 1971. *The religious experience of mankind.*

ANNA BOLENA. An opera by the Italian composer Gaetano Donizetti (q.v.). It is loosely based on the historical figure of Anne Boleyn, the second wife of Henry VIII of England. In the opera, Anna's mind gives way on the day of her execution. She hallucinates (*see* HALLUCINATION), imagining that it is her wedding day, and chides her companions for not being cheerful.
Bibliography: Harewood, ed. 1969. *Kobbé's complete opera book.*

ANNA KARENINA. The name of the heroine in a novel by Leo Tolstoy (q.v.). She leaves her husband and child to be with her lover. As he tires of her, she becomes increasingly depressed. Eventually she commits suicide (q.v.) by throwing herself under a train. Passions, doubts, and torments are described by Tolstoy and reflect his own emotional problems.
Bibliography: Tolstoy, L. 1873-1877. Reprint 1954. *Anna Karenina,* trans. by R. Edmonds.

ANNALES MÉDICO-PSYCHOLOGIQUES. The first French journal dedicated to psychological medicine. It was founded in 1843 by Jules Baillarger (q.v.).

ANNA O. (1859-1936). The pseudonym used by Joseph Breuer (q.v.) for his patient, Bertha Pappenheim. She is regarded as the first patient in the history of psychoanalysis (q.v.). Breuer treated her in 1880 for classic hysterical (*see* HYSTERIA) symptoms. Each symptom was made to disappear under hypnosis (*see* HYPNOTISM) by recalling the original traumatic event that had caused it. The girl's recollections were accompanied by violent expressions of emotion that had been repressed at the time of the event. Breuer called his therapeutic technique *catharsis* (q.v.). The patient also had a double personality, one living in the present and one living exactly one year earlier and both coexisting. Sigmund Freud (q.v.) heard about the case from Breuer in November 1882 and was much impressed by it.
Bibliography: Breuer, J., and Freud, S. 1895. Reprint. 1960. *Studies on hysteria,* trans. by A. A. Brill.
Freud, S. 1964. *The complete psychological works of Sigmund Freud,* ed. J. Strachey. Vol. 2.

ANNÉE PSYCHOLOGIQUE, L'. A leading French journal of psychology (q.v.) originally founded in 1895 by Alfred Binet (q.v.) in cooperation with

Henri E. Beaunis (q.v.) and Victor Henri (1872-1940), as an outlet for the publication of his research.
Bibliography: Zusne, L. 1975. *Names in the history of psychology.*

ANNÉE SOCIOLOGIQUE, L'. The first sociological journal. It was founded in France in 1898 by Émile Durkheim (q.v.).

ANNIVERSARY REACTION. A breakdown in health on the anniversary of a significant event in the past life of an individual. These anniversary dates, months, or even seasons may have significance for whole populations as well as for particular individuals. For example, a higher incidence of suicide (q.v.) is reported among the Mormons of Salt Lake City, Utah at Christmas than at other times, hence the term, "Christmas Disease."
Bibliography: Hilgard, J.R., and Newman, M.F. 1968. Anniversary in Mental Illness. In *Theory and practice of family psychiatry*, ed. J.G. Howells.

ANOMIA. A term originally meaning "lack of the usual social standards." Benjamin Rush (q.v.) used it to indicate little appreciation of or complete lack of morality — a condition typical of the psychopath. The sociologist Emile Durkheim (q.v.) used *anomie* to cover society's loss of its commonly accepted normative code. It has been used more loosely to describe an individual who is prone to disorientation or psychic disorder.
Bibliography: Durkheim, E. 1952. *Suicide*, trans. by J. A. Spaulding and G. Simpson.

ANOREXIA NERVOSA. A term first used by William Gull (q.v.) in 1873 to denote a disorder characterized by a refusal to eat, which leads to extreme emaciation. Gull thought that it was due to "a morbid mental state."
Bibliography: Gull, W. W. 1874. *Transactions of the clinical society of London*, 7:22.

ANTENEASMON (*sometimes called* **ENTHUSIASMOS**). A form of choromania (q.v.) seen in the Middle Ages (q.v.) and described by Gariopontus (q.v.). According to him, the victim hears voices or music and is impelled by these to rush about or dance; he may become violent and hurt himself and others. Gariopontus attributed this abnormal behavior to the influence of "a legion of devils."
Bibliography: Whitwell, J. R. 1936. *Historical notes on psychiatry.*

ANTHONY, *or* ANTONY, SAINT (c. A.D. 250-350). An Egyptian Christian hermit and ascetic. He withdrew from society to live in complete isolation, emerging occasionally to organize religious communities. Legends about him tell of his struggle against evil forces and his temptations in the form of dreadful hallucinations (q.v.), which may have been caused by privation and isolation.
Bibliography: Butler, A. 1956. *Butler's lives of the saints.*

ANTHROPOLOGIE. The title of a book by Immanuel Kant (q.v.) published in 1798. In this work, Kant described a system of classifying mental illness and discussed the aetiology of insanity. According to him, inability to adapt to the environment was the cause of mental illness. Although he particularly emphasized the intellectual aspects of stress, he neglected the emotional aspects. He considered the study of primitive people to be an approach to the understanding of mental disorders. Kant wrote that he knew of no child who was insane and therefore it seemed likely that the germ of insanity developed at the same time as the germ of procreation, that is, at or after puberty.
Bibliography: Kant, I. 1798. *Anthropologie.*

ANTHROPOLOGIUM. A term first used in 1501 by Magnus Hundt (q.v.) to indicate the study or knowledge of man. Hundt published a book in 1502 entitled *Anthropologia.*

ANTHROPOMETRIC LABORATORY. A laboratory opened in 1884 by Sir Francis Galton (q.v.) for the study of the comparative measurements of the human body and its parts. It was located at the South Kensington Museum in London. In the six years that it functioned nearly ten thousand people were examined there.
Bibliography: Forrest, D. W. 1974. *Francis Galton: the life and work of a Victorian genius.*

ANTICYRA. Modern Aspraspitia, a Greek peninsula on the Gulf of Corinth. Because the best black hellebore (q.v.) was said to grow there, patients were sent there for treatment. Those needing treatment for madness were advised "Naviget Anticyram" [Sail to Anticyra].
Bibliography: Whitwell, J. R. 1946. *Anlecta psychiatrica.*

ANTIMONY. A mineral found in France, Italy, and China (q.v.). It was used in medicine for the treatment of insanity, as it caused the desired violent vomiting and purging (q.v.). In the sixteenth century, Conrad Gesner (q.v.) used it for treating patients suffering from melancholia (q.v.) and patients contemplating suicide (q.v.) "with happiest results."

ANTINOUS (?-A. D. 130). A beautiful youth loved by the emperor Hadrian. The homosexual relationship probably was imposed on Antinous. He was always represented as sad and died by drowning himself in the Nile. Hadrian deified him and founded a city in his memory.
Bibliography: Yourcenar, M. 1955. *Memoirs of Hadrian.*

ANTIOCHUS I (324-261 B.C.). Son of the first king of the Seleucid dynasty. He was said to suffer from melancholy (*see* MELANCHOLIA) caused by love

for his stepmother, Stratonice. Erasistratus (q.v.) cured him by persuading his father to renounce Stratonice, who then married Antiochus.
Bibliography: Tarn, W. W. 1952. *Hellenistic civilisation.*

ANTIPALUS MALEFICIORUM. A book about witches (*see* WITCH-CRAFT) written toward the end of the fifteenth century by Johannes Trithemius (q.v.). It antedates the *Malleus Maleficarum* (q.v.). Trithemius regretted that there were too few judges and inquisitors (*see* INQUISITION) to deal with witches. The work stressed that all illness was caused by demonic possession (q.v.): "Many suffer constantly from the most severe diseases and are not even aware that they are bewitched."

ANTIPHON (480-411 B.C.). A Greek orator, of the fifth century B.C., he is considered the first professional psychotherapist. According to Plutarch (q.v.), he displayed his qualifications on the doorplate of his house in Corinth and stated that he could treat those afflicted with grief and melancholy (*see* MELANCHOLIA). His method of therapy was to enquire into the causes of the patients' sufferings and comfort them with words.
Bibliography: Entralgo, P. L. 1970. *The therapy of the word*, trans. by L. J. Rather and J. M. Sharp, 1970.

ANTI-PSYCHOSIS. A term used by Daniel H. Tuke (q.v.) to indicate a substance that he hoped would be discovered one day, which would as "safely and speedily cut short an attack of mania (q.v.) or melancholia (q.v.) as bark an attack of ague."
Bibliography: Zilboorg, G. 1941. *A history of medical psychology.*

ANTON REISER. The title of the first psychological novel in German literature. It was written by Karl Philipp Moritz (q.v.) and published in four volumes between 1785 and 1790. It was an autobiographical work in which Moritz related his struggle to understand his relationship with his father whose character was a mixture of mysticism and rigidity. The author's interest in psychopathology was a result of his search for solutions to his own problems.
Bibliography: Moritz, C. P. 1785. Reprint. 1926. *Anton Reiser. A psychological novel*, trans. by P. E. Matheson.

ANTON SYNDROME. A syndrome first described by the Czech neurologist and psychiatrist Gabriel Anton (1858-1933). It is the failure of a patient who is blind to recognize the fact.
Bibliography: Jablonski, S. 1969. *Eponymic syndromes and diseases and their synonyms.*

ANUMANTHAPURAM. A corruption of the Indian term Aran Amaranathapuran meaning "Lord Shiva's abode," a temple in Tamil Nadu, India.

In the belief that they will be cured, sufferers from mental disorders journey there to be dipped in the sacred waters, which are contained in the temple tank.
Bibliography: 1973. *Indian Journal of Psychiatry*, 15:38.

APANTHROPIA. A term derived from the Greek and indicating a pathological desire to be alone. It was introduced into medical psychology (q.v.) by De Valenzi (1728-1813).
Bibliography: Zilboorg, G. 1941. *A history of medical psychology.*

APASARA. A term for epilepsy (q.v.) used in the seventh century B.C. in Hindu medicine.
Bibliography: Whitwell, J. P. 1936. *Historical notes on psychiatry.*

APHANISIS. The total extinction of the ability to enjoy sexual activities. It was introduced by Ernest Jones (q.v.) in a paper on psychoanalysis (q.v.) in 1938. He considered aphanisis to be at the root of all neuroses (*see* NEUROSIS).
Bibliography: Jones, E. 1948. *Collected papers on psychoanalysis.*

APHELXIA. A term for reverie used by John Mason Good (q.v.) in his classification of mental disorder. He placed it under the class Neurotica.
Bibliography: Good, J. M. 1817. *A physiological system of nosology.*

APHEMIA. A term introduced by Paul Broca (q.v.) in 1861 to describe motor aphasia.
Bibliography: Broca, P. 1861. *Bull. Soc. d'anthrop. de Paris*, ii 235-36.

APOLLO. A Greek god associated with medicine and prophecy. The Greeks believed him to be the father of the healer god Aesculapius (q.v.). Apollo's temple at Delphi was also known to the Romans, who adopted him as a god of healing, oracles, and prophecy. Divination by his priests and priestesses was through possession (q.v.); the medium was said to receive inspiration through the god.
Bibliography: Guthrie, W. K. C. 1950. *The Greeks and their gods.*

APOLLONIUS OF TYANA. A Greek Neo-Pythagorean philosopher of the first century A.D. He traveled throughout India and acquired a reputation for magical (*see* MAGIC) cures, which he achieved through his extraordinary power of suggestion.
Bibliography: Hammond, N. G. L. and Scullard, H. H., eds. 1973. *The Oxford classical dictionary.*

APOPHRADES. A term used for days dedicated to gloomy rites. In ancient Greece, these days were considered unlucky because the dead were believed

to visit their former houses. People smeared the doors with pitch for protection against spirits. The belief in unlucky days still persists in most cultures, and may be an indication of widespread insecurity.
See also ANNIVERSARY REACTION.
Bibliography: Hammond, N. G. L., and Scullard, H. H., eds. 1973. *The Oxford classical dictionary.*

APPLES. John Wesley (q.v.) advised that patients suffering from "raving madness" should "eat nothing but apples for a month."
Bibliography: Wesley, J. 1747. Reprint. 1960. *Primitive physics.*

APPLIED PSYCHOLOGY. The first example of applied psychology is provided by the doctrine of Johann F. Herbart (q.v.) who advocated its use in the educational field.
See also PSYCHOLOGY.
Bibliography: Misiak, H. and Sexton, V. S. 1966. *History of psychology.*

AQUINAS, SAINT THOMAS (1225?-1274). An Italian scholastic (*see* SCHOLASTICISM) philosopher, born near Aquino, Italy, in the family castle at Roccasecca. He was educated by the Benedictine monks at Monte Cassino and later attended the University of Naples. In 1243 he became a Dominican friar and subsequently traveled to France and Germany. He was a pupil of Albertus Magnus (q.v.) and established a school of theology at Cologne. Saint Thomas developed a philosophical school called Thomism that systematized Catholic theology and reconciled the natural philosophy of Aristotle (q.v.) with Christian dogma. In his theological and philosophical works he tried to harmonize faith and reason, which he did not consider dependent on the brain or any other organ in the body. His acceptance of dogma precluded any free inquiry, and was an obstacle to scientific development for a long time. Thus, his influence on psychiatry (q.v.) was negative in spite of his clear deductive intellectual approach, which puts his works far above those of his medieval contemporaries. Often called the "Angelic Doctor," he was known to his school companions as "the Dumb Ox," which suggests his taciturn nature.
Bibliography: Chesterton, G. K. 1956. *St. Thomas Aquinas.*

ARABS. After the rise of their empire in the sixth century A.D., the Arabs contributed greatly to medical knowledge. They had a particularly enlightened attitude toward the mentally ill whom they considered to be inspired by God. They recognized mania (q.v.), compulsions and obsessions (q.v.), depression, and persecutory psychosis (q.v.). Najab ud din Unhammad, a physician who based his deductions on the direct observation of patients, devised a classification of mental disorders that was divided into approximately thirty different syndromes.

Arab asylums (q.v.) were pleasant buildings surrounded by gardens and fountains, which contributed to their relaxing atmosphere. As early as the ninth century, the Baghdad hospital had a division for the mentally ill. Treatment included drugs (q.v.) such as poppy seed, attention to diet (q.v.), baths, and change of climate. Altercation with patients was also used as a form of psychotherapy (q.v.).

See also AVERRÖES, AVICENNA, DAR-UL-MARAFTAN, and RHAZES.
Bibliography: Browne, E. G. 1921. *Arabian medicine.*
Ullman, M. 1978. *Islamic medicine.*

ARBEIT [WORK]. The name of an institution for the mentally retarded founded in 1875 in Budapest, Hungary. Its director was a Dr. Frim. By 1879 the original nine patients had increased to thirteen. At that time, it was the only institution for retarded children in Hungary, which was said to have over 18,000 mentally retarded individuals, nearly half of whom were of school age.
Bibliography: Kanner, L. 1967. *A history of the care and the study of the mentally retarded.*

ARBUTHNOT, JOHN (1667-1735). A successful Scottish physician. He practiced and taught in London, where he was the idol of the Tories. He became physician to Queen Anne and attended her in her last illness. Jonathan Swift (q.v.) was a close friend of his, as were many other literary figures of his time. He wrote poetry, literary works, and essays in medicine. He believed the seasons influenced physical and emotional development and blamed the climate for diseases, including mental illness.
Bibliography: Arbuthnot, John. 1733. *An essay concerning the effect of air on human bodies.*

ARCHER, JOHN (fl. 1660-1684). An English physician at the court of Charles II. Although he had no qualifications, he styled himself "One of His Majesties Physitians in Ordinary." He wrote a book entitled *Everyman his own doctor* (1673), which contained a section on "melancholy [see MELANCHOLIA] and distraction" and offered advice on its management and treatment. He opened one of the earliest private madhouses in London.
Bibliography: Parry-Jones, W.L1. 1972. *The trade in lunacy: a study of private madhouses in England in the eighteenth and nineteenth century.*

ARCHETYPE. A term used by Carl G. Jung (q.v.) to indicate the representation of thoughts and patterns of reaction derived from the experience of the race in the collective unconscious.
See also ANIMA.
Bibliography: Hannah, B. 1977. *Jung: his life and work.*

ARCHEUS. The vital force that Paracelsus (q.v.) claimed regulated human life. He believed that understanding it was essential to the proper diagnosis

and treatment of all disorders. Franciscus Van Helmont (q.v.) placed it at the pyloric opening of the stomach.
Bibliography: Pachter, H. M. 1951. *Paracelsus.*

ARCHIGENES. A Greek eclectic physician of the first century A.D.. He practiced in Rome at the time of Trajan. Alexander of Tralles (q.v.) called him divine. He was considered an excellent prognostician and believed amulets (q.v.) to be infallible remedies for mental disorders.
Bibliography: Phillips, E. D. 1973. *Greek medicine.*

ARCHIVES OF NEUROLOGY. A journal founded by Jean-Martin Charcot (q.v.) in 1880. He edited it until his death in 1893.

ARCTIC HYSTERIA. A disorder characterized by extreme suggestibility. An individual so affected is only able to act by imitating the movements of those around him. It was first observed in Siberia in the early 1900s and was reported also by explorers of Canada, Alaska, and Greenland. The Museum of Natural History in Washington, D.C., has a collection of pictures taken during a 1907 expedition that show an Eskimo woman in a state of hysteria (q.v.), mimicking local animals, having convulsions, and suffering from spasms, tremor, and exhaustion.
Bibliography: Foulks, E. F. 1972. *The Arctic hysterias of the North Alaskan Eskimo.*

ARCULANUS, JOHANNES (or ARCOLANI, GIOVANNI)(?-1484). An Italian professor of medicine and surgery at Padua. He recognized the following mental disorders: phrenesis, true and false; lethargy; epilepsy (q.v.); melancholia (q.v.); and mania (q.v.). Barley water, which was to be taken once or twice a day, and anointment of the head with oil of violets mixed with woman's milk were among the remedies he recommended.
Bibliography: Whitwell, J. R. 1936. *Historical notes on psychiatry.*

ARETAEUS OF CAPPADOCIA. A Greek physician of the first and second century A.D. Born in eastern Asia Minor, he studied in Alexandria and Egypt before going to Rome to practice medicine. He was a contemporary of Galen (q.v.). His vivid clinical descriptions of diseases are unusually free from dogma and superstition and clearly indicate his deep concern for his patients. He was the first to describe the premorbid personality of mental patients. He classified mental disorders under the following categories: 1) epilepsy (q.v.), ordinary and hysterical (*see* HYSTERIA) occurring in women; 2) melancholia (q.v.), including anxiety and sadness; 3) mania (q.v.) ordinary, recurrent, and divine; 4) phrenitis (q.v.), or delirium (q.v.) with fever; 5) drug (q.v.) delirium, temporary, 6) senile dementia; 7) secondary dementia. This classification recognized the relationship between mania and melancholia, which he located in the hypochondrium. He considered mel-

ancholia to be the basis from which all other psychotic disorders (*see* PSY-CHOSIS) developed. In a sense, he anticipated Emil Kraepelin (q.v.) by about two thousand years. He described mania as "a lowness of spirits from a single fantasy without fever; and it appears to me that melancholy is the commencement and a part of mania." He included in his treatment of epilepsy trepanation (q.v.). *De Causis et Signis Morborum* is the only one of his works that has survived.
Bibliography: Allbutt, T. C. 1921. *Greek medicine in Rome.*

ARGOS. The mythological Greek kingdom of Proetus (q.v.) whose female population was stricken with madness following the frenzy of Proetus' three daughters. They were cured by Melampus (q.v.).
Bibliography: Hammond, N. G. L., and Scullard, H. H. 1973. *The Oxford classical dictionary.*

ARGUS. A giant in Greek mythology with one hundred eyes whom Juno, in her jealousy, set to watch Io. He was slain by Mercury and his eyes were set in the peacock's tail. It provides a vivid image of the feelings of paranoid (*see* PARANOIA) individuals, who believe themselves perpetually under scrutiny.
Bibliography: 1978. *Brewer's dictionary of phrase and fable.*

ARGYLL AND BUTE HOSPITAL. A mental hospital in Scotland that opened in 1864. It was the first hospital to follow the recommendations of the 1857 Act for the Regulation of Care and Treatment of Lunatics in Scotland, and set a pattern for future hospital building. Its records show that as early as 1880 it implemented an open-door policy (unlocked wards) with success.
Bibliography: Burdett, H. C. 1891. *Hospitals and asylums of the world.*

ARGYLL ROBERTSON, DOUGLAS MORAY COOPER LAMB (1837-1909). A Scottish physician. In 1869 he described a pupil that reacts to accommodation but not to light, which sometimes is characteristic of syphylitic (*see* SYPHILIS) disorders. His findings were published in a paper entitled *Four Cases of Spinal Myosis; with remarks on the action of light on the pupil.*
Bibliography: Haymaker, W., and Schiller, F. 1970. *The founders of neurology.* 2d ed.

ARISTIDES, PUBLIUS AELIUS. A Greek rhetorician of the second century A.D. A chronic invalid for many years, he went to Aesculapius (q.v.) after all other physicians had failed to help him. He followed the instructions given to him in a dream (q.v.) and was healed. By command of Aesculapius he wrote his religious autobiography *Sacred Discourses* in which he described

how mentally and emotionally ill people could become adequately adjusted to society if cultural and religious practices made provision for them.
Bibliography: Wright, W.C., trans. 1952. Lives of the sophists. In *Philostratus and Eunapius.*

ARISTOPHANES (c.448-380 B.C.). A Greek poet, born in Athens. He courageously satirized the society of his time, including its form of democracy and the government then in power. In his play *Birds*, he suggested that mentally ill people were chased away from the temples with stones, a reference to the fact that those who are most in need of help, are often denied it. In *Plutus* he gave a farcical account of the proceedings at the temple of Aesculapius (q.v.) in Athens, where incubation (q.v.) was practised.
Bibliography: Bickley, B., trans. 1924. *Aristophanes.* Vols. 2 and 3.

ARISTOTLE (394-322 B.C.). A Greek philosopher, born at Stageria, the son of a physician. At the age of seventeen he became a pupil of Plato (q.v.). Philip of Macedonia invited him to become the tutor of his son Alexander III (q.v.). His Peripatetic school was so called because he taught while walking around the lyceum. Tradition describes Aristotle as an unattractive man who was bald with thin legs, small eyes, a lisp in his speech, and a mocking manner. This last attribute is reflected in his writings. He believed that all motion had its origin in the soul. *Pneuma* (q.v.) acted as an agent between soul and body. He regarded the heart rather than the brain as the seat of sensation and intelligence. He considered the brain to be a cold organ that acted as moderator, tempering the great heat generated in the region of the heart. Understanding, he thought, was built out of sensuous materials, each particular sensation giving rise to a sensuous state; and the permanence of these states was memory (q.v.). Memory gave rise to distinctions, experience, after repetition, and science, developing from experience. He recognized association (*see* ASSOCIATIONISM) as an essential part of mentation and divided it into three divisions, similarity, contrast, and contiguity. Aristotle recognized the frequent occurrence of melancholia (q.v.), especially in philosophers, artists, and poets and cited Plato, Socrates, and Empedocles (qq.v.) as examples. He believed mental character was not independent of and unaffected by bodily processes but rather conditioned by the state of the body. Conversely, he believed the body was sympathetically influenced by affections of the soul. The former of these propositions is well exemplified by drunkenness and sickness in which altered bodily conditions produce obvious mental modifications. The second proposition can be exemplified by the emotions of love (q.v.) and fear and the states of pleasure and pain.

Aristotle's works covered a wide field and were the results of findings based on experiments. His main contributions to psychology (q.v.) can be found in *De Anima* (q.v.), which contains unsurpassed descriptions of affective states, *De Sensu et Sensili* in which he describes the doctrine of sensation, and *De Memoria et Reminiscentia*, a discussion on the laws of memory and imagination, which he defined as the ability to produce a mental image in the absence of the original object. Finally, in *De miraculis auscultationibus*, he referred to the many beliefs then current about epilepsy (q.v.) and mental disease. His greatest error was his refusal to recognize the importance of the brain.

Bibliography: Hammond, W.A. 1902. *Aristotle's psychology.*

ARLIDGE, JOHN THOMAS (1822-1899). An English apothecary and physician. As a student he was a pupil of John Conolly (q.v.). He traveled widely at home and abroad, visiting asylums (q.v.) and writing about them in professional journals. In 1859 he wrote "On the state of Lunacy and the Legal Provision for the Insane" in which he pointed out that mental disorders frequently were fostered and made worse by a number of factors in the community and in the asylums. He was unequivocally opposed to the practice of bleeding (q.v.) the insane and was an advocate of moral medicine (q.v.).

Bibliography: Parry-Jones, W. Ll. 1972. *The trade in lunacy: a study of private madhouses in England in the eighteenth and nineteenth century.*

ARMENIAN STONE. A blue calcerous stone containing quartz, mica, and copper. It was used as a purgative in preference to hellebore (q.v.) in the treatment of mental disorders. Alexander of Tralles (q.v.) and Rhazes (q.v.) were both enthusiastic prescribers of it.

See also PRECIOUS STONES.

Bibliography: Zilboorg, G. 1941. *A history of medical psychology.*

ARMILLA. An iron bracelet with the mark of Bethlem Royal Hospital (q.v.). Although the hospital did not issue bracelets to its patients, beggars in seventeenth-century England often wore them on their left arms to make people believe that they were insane and had been licensed to beg by the hospital. This fraud was so widespread that in 1675 and again in 1676 the governors of Bethlem gave official notice that they had never sent patients out to collect alms, nor did they issue bracelets, plates, or any other marks.

See also ABRAHAM-MEN, BESS O'BEDLAM, and TOM O'BEDLAM.

Bibliography: O'Donoghue, E. G. 1914. *The story of Bethlehem Hospital.*

ARNDT, RUDOLF GOTTFRIED (1835-1900). A German physician, born in Bialken. He studied medicine in Greifswald and Halle. After serving as an army physician, he became head of the asylum (q.v.) at Greifswald in

1867 and professor of psychiatry in 1873. He studied the progress of psychoses (q.v.) and tried to give a scientific basis to psychiatry (q.v.).
Bibliography: Arndt, R. G. 1883. *Lehrbuch der Psychiatrie fur Arzte und Studierende.*
————. 1892-1895. *Biologische Studien.* 2 vols.

ARNOLD, THOMAS (1742-1816). An English physician, born in Leicester. He gained his degree in Edinburgh, where he studied under William Cullen (q.v.). Returning to Leicester, he became a successful practitioner and opened a private house for lunatics (q.v.). His first book was *Observations on the Nature, Kinds, Causes and Prevention of Insanity, Lunacy or Madness* (1782). He dedicated the first volume of his work completely to nosology, and his classification is based mainly upon symptoms. He divided insanity (*see* INSANIA) into ideal (disorders of perception) and notional (delusional disorders) and discussed the frequency and distribution of insanity in England in comparison with the frequency and distribution of insanity in other countries. In his defense of the idea that melancholia (q.v.) and suicide (q.v.) were more common in England than elsewhere, he pointed out that England was prosperous, and prosperity, or wealth and luxury, was a common cause of insanity. He further claimed that the national temperament was more sensitive to the misfortunes of love (q.v.), which was another common cause of mental disorders. Despite his misconceptions, Arnold represents a crucial point in the history of the development of professional psychiatry (q.v.). His second book *A Case of Hydrophobia Successfully Treated* appeared in 1793 and *Observations on the Management of the Insane* in 1809.
Bibliography: Leigh, D. 1961. *The historical development of British psychiatry.*

ARNOLD OF VILLANOVA (1240?-?1313). A doctor of several disciplines, probably born in Catalonia, Spain. He taught theology, law, philosophy, and medicine at Barcelona, Paris, and the University of Montpellier. He vividly described hallucinations (q.v.) and epilepsy (q.v.) and recommended perforation of the cranium as a treatment for mania (q.v.) so that devils and vapors could escape. Although he adhered to the beliefs of the time, he had a great understanding of emotional phenomena. A prolific and elegant writer, he disdained to revise his work. His most important medical contributions are the *Breviary of Practice* and the *Parabolae*, 345 aphorisms. An even greater contribution to the welfare of man was his invention of brandy, which he called *aqua vitae*. The Inquisition (q.v.) condemned him for attempting to amalgamate Hippocratic (*see* HIPPOCRATES) principles with demon worship, but he was saved from burning at the stake through his friendship with Pope Boniface VIII.
Bibliography: Graham, T. F. 1967. *Medieval minds.*

ARO. A village near Abeokuta, Nigeria where mentally ill patients are boarded out in the community with at least one relative and attend the hospital during the day. The scheme was initiated by Dr. Adeoye Lambo in 1954 in order to combine modern forms of treatment with traditional elements of Yoruba culture.

Bibliography: Lambo, T. A. 1975. Mid and West Africa. In *World history of psychiatry*, ed. J. G. Howells.

ART. The products of arts, like fantasies and dreams (q.v.), are regarded as expressions of the psyche and as such are of interest in normal and abnormal psychology. Sigmund Freud (q.v.) investigated this field and concluded that "the artist is originally a man who turns from reality because he cannot come to terms with the demand for the renunciation of instinctual satisfaction as it is first made, and who then in phantasy-life allows full play to his erotic and ambitious wishes." Carl Jung (q.v.) stated "Art, like every other human activity, proceeds from psychic motives. . . ." Many artists have expressed their feelings through art. The depression and agitation of Vincent Van Gogh (q.v.), the suicidal wish of Dylan Thomas (q.v.), the basic insecurity of the surrealist, and the contented stability of Pierre Renoir are all easily seen in their works. Insanity (*see* INSANIA) too can be discerned in artistic production: Louis Wain's (q.v.) series of paintings of cats, the art of Richard Dadd (q.v.), the hallucinatory illustrations to his autobiography by Daniel Paul Schreber (q.v.) and the perseveration in the architectural designs of Antonio Gaudí (q.v.) offer more than adequate examples.

See also GUTTMAN-MACLAY COLLECTION.

Bibliography: Jakab, I., ed. 1971. *Psychiatry and art.*
Reitman, F. 1950. *Psychotic art.*

ARTAUD, ANTONIN (1896-1948). A French poet, born at Marseille, He was a drug (q.v.) addict. In 1936 he visited Mexico, and it was after his experience there that his already unbalanced thoughts took shape. His aggression and defiance of an orderly society are reflected in his writings, *Le Retour d'Artaud le Mômo* and *Van Gogh ou le suicide de la société*. These books brought him some fame, but he did not live long enough to enjoy it. He died in 1948, the year of their publication.

Bibliography: Esslin, M. 1976. *Artaud.*

ARTEMIDORUS. A Greek soothsayer, born in Ephesus in the latter half of the second century A.D. He is often called Daldianus after his mother's birthplace, Daldis in Lydia. He was interested in the interpretation of dreams (q.v.). To collect as many descriptions of them as he could, he traveled extensively. His treatise *The Interpretation of Dreams* is still extant and filled with material that is important to the study of ancient folklore (q.v.).

Bibliography: Blum, C. 1936. *Studies in the dream-book of Artemidorus.*

ARTEMISIA (?-c.350 B.C.). The queen of Caria in Asia Minor. She married her brother Mausolus whom she loved deeply. When he died she had him

cremated, mixed his ashes in a liquid, and drank them. She remained in mourning for the rest of her life. The mausoleum she erected to her husband's memory was one of the seven wonders of the ancient world.
Bibliography: Boccaccio, G. 1964. *Concerning famous women*, trans. G. A. Guarino.

ARUNDELL, JOHN (?-1477). A master of Bethlem Royal Hospital (q.v.) and chaplain, confessor, and first physician to Henry VI (q.v.) whom he cared for during the latter's periods of insanity (*see* INSANIA). In 1458 he became bishop of Chichester.
Bibliography: O'Donoghue, E. G. 1914. *The story of Bethlehem Hospital*.

ASAFOETIDA. A gum resin with strong acrid smell. It is obtained from the stem of an umbelliferous plant *Ferula foetida* found in Persia and Afghanistan. It was used in the treatment of hysteria (q.v.).
Bibliography: Morton, J. F. 1977. *Major medicinal plants*.

ASCETICS. The followers of various doctrines that demand the mortification of the flesh. Some ascetics carried the practices to such extremes that they eventually became mad and died of their intense privations. The Hindu fakirs (q.v.) are examples of ascetics practicing acute self-mortification. They may spend whole days hanging upside down from a tree or lying on a bed of nails.
See also ANTHONY, SAINT, and GYMNOSOPHISTS.
Bibliography: Hastings, J., ed. 1908. *Encyclopedia of religion and ethics*.

ASCLEPIADES OF BITHYNIA (*or* OF PRUSA) (124 B.C.-?). A Greek adventurer trained in philosophy and medicine in Alexandria and Athens. He found his way to Rome but was not allowed to practice medicine because of the prejudice against Greek physicians. He was allowed to exercise his profession after he rescued from a funeral procession a man previously presumed dead. He promised that the treatment he would offer not only would be safe but also pleasant in order to elevate the patients' morale. He recognized the importance of emotional disorders and his mental patients were prescribed warm baths, massage, and vintage wines in sunlit rooms. He distinguished hallucinations (q.v.) from delusions (q.v.), acute from chronic diseases, and in general opposed Hippocratic (*see* HIPPOCRATES) reasoning. Asclepiades is said to have promised that he would renounce the title of physician if he ever fell ill. He kept his promise and did not die of illness but by falling down a flight of stairs.
Bibliography: Sigerist, H. E. 1933. *Great doctors*.

ASHBOURNE, JOHN (c.1611-1661). An English cleric and "practitioner in phisycke." In the seventeenth century he was a "clerical mad-doctor," that is, an unqualified practitioner, probably licensed by his bishop, who chose to treat the melancholy (*see* MELANCHOLIA) and the mad. He accepted patients in his own house at Norton, near Woolpit, in Suffolk. Ashbourne was killed by one of his patients who met him in a meadow and stabbed him in the neck with a pitchfork.

Bibliography: Hunter, R., and Macalpine, I. 1972. The Reverend John Ashbourne (c.1611-61) and the origins of the private madhouse system. *Lancet.* 2:513-15.

ASHLEY, LORD. *See* SHAFTESBURY, EARL OF.

ASMODEUS. In the Apocrypha, he was the evil spirit who killed the seven successive husbands of Sarah in an effort to gain her for himself. He was driven away by Tobias with the smoke produced by the burning heart and liver of a fish. Asmodeus represented the demon of matrimonial unhappiness.

Bibliography: *The Book of Tobit* 3:8.

ASP. A small snake, probably the Egyptian horned viper. Cleopatra (q.v.) was said to have used its poisonous bite to commit suicide (q.v.).

ASPATIA. A character in *The Maid's Tragedy* (1611) by Francis Beaumont (1584-1616) and John Fletcher (1579-1625). Deserted by her lover, ridiculed by all, and weighed down by sorrows, she remains patient in the face of many adversities. She is an example of the apathy of depression.

See also GRISELDA.

ASSASSINS. A secret Moslem sect founded in Persia by Hasan i Sabbah around 1090. For two centuries its sadistic (*see* SADISM) members terrorized Persia and Syria, until the sect was destroyed by the Mongols in Persia in 1256 and by the sultan of Egypt in Syria around 1270. Lower orders of devotees carried out the murders in strict obedience and without knowing why they were ordered. Devotees were given hashish (q.v.) to produce intoxication and ecstasy (q.v.), hence they were called hashashins, which was later corrupted to assassins.

Bibliography: Daraul, A. 1965. *Secret societies.*

ASSES' MILK. Dr. Friedrich Hoffmann (q.v.), physician to Frederick the Great (q.v.) advocated asses' milk for nervous disorders. An English translation of his *Treatise of the Extraordinary Virtues and Effects of Asses' Milk* was published in London in 1754, and it is likely that this work influenced the royal physicians' decision to prescribe the remedy for George III (q.v.).

Bibliography: Macalpine, I., and Hunter, R. 1969. *George III and the mad-business.*

ASSOCIATIONISM. A theory of memory (q.v.) introduced by Aristotle (q.v.). Plato (q.v.) had referred to similarity and continuity as two factors

in recollection previously, but Aristotle recognized and developed these principles into three links: similarity, contrast, and contiguity. The recalling of an object is followed by recalling one similar to it, one contrary to it, and one contiguous to it. He also mentioned three more relevant factors: frequency, emotional effect, and degree of meaningfulness. All of these factors find a place in modern learning theory. The phrase "association of ideas" is credited to Aristotle. In the seventeenth century, Thomas Hobbes (q.v.) and John Locke (q.v.) used the same terms to indicate the connection of ideas in the flow of consciousness.
Bibliography: Randal, J. H. 1960. *Aristotle.*
Warren, H. C. 1921. *A history of association psychology.*

ASSOCIATION OF MEDICAL OFFICERS OF AMERICAN INSTITUTIONS FOR IDIOTS AND FEEBLEMINDED PERSONS. *See* AMERICAN ASSOCIATION ON MENTAL DEFICIENCY.

ASSOCIATION OF MEDICAL OFFICERS OF ASYLUMS AND HOSPITALS FOR THE INSANE. The professional association of British psychiatrists founded in 1841. It is the oldest of its kind. In 1865 it called itself the Medico-Psychological Association of Great Britain and Ireland. In 1926, it again changed its name to the Royal Medico-Psychological Association, and finally in 1971 it became the Royal College of Psychiatrists.
Bibliography: Howells, J. G. 1971. *Royal college of psychiatrists.*

ASSOCIATION OF MEDICAL SUPERINTENDENTS OF AMERICAN INSTITUTIONS FOR THE INSANE. *See* AMERICAN PSYCHIATRIC ASSOCIATION.

ASS'S HOOF. In the Renaissance pieces of ass's hoof were set into rings, which were then worn as amulets (q.v.) against epilepsy (q.v.).
See also ELK.
Bibliography: Evans, J. 1922. *Magical jewels.*

ASSUEFACTION. A term used in the seventeenth century by Sir Kenelm Digby (q.v.) to describe what is now termed "conditioning." He gave examples of animal behavior that demonstrated how animals could be trained to act in ways contrary to their natures, thus reversing "any aversion of the fantasy."
Bibliography: Hunter, R., and Macalpine, I. 1963. *Three hundred years of psychiatry.*

ASTHENIC TYPE. One of the four physical types distinguished by Ernst Kretschmer (q.v.). Tall and thin in body structure, this type was said by him to have schizoid (*see* SCHIZOPHRENIA) tendencies.
See also ATHLETIC TYPE, and PYKNIC TYPE.
Bibliography: Kretschmer, E. 1944. *Körperbau und charakter.*

ASTROLOGY. In ancient thought heaven and earth were bound in a universal sympathy; thus it was believed that if the recurrence of heavenly phenomena could be predicted, earthly events could also be predicted. Astrology, which was a mixture of religion and science that spread from Mesopotamia to Egypt and then to Greece and Rome, dealt with these predictions. Planets (q.v.) were believed to influence human destiny as well as the personality, health, and actions of men. Astrology dominated medical theory in the Middle Ages (q.v.) and even later. The influence of the moon (q.v.) and certain planets was thought to be a cause of many mental disorders. Shakespeare gives many examples:

> "It is the stars,
> The stars above us, govern our conditions."
>
> (*King Lear*, IV, iii.)
>
> "As if some planet had unwitted men."
>
> (*Othello*, II, iii.)

See also ZODIAC.
Bibliography: Bram, J. R., trans. 1975. *Firmicus maternus: ancient astrology, theory and practice.*

ASYLUM JOURNAL, THE. 1) An intramural publication of the Vermont Asylum (q.v.) at Brattleboro, Vermont. It was founded in 1842 by a seventeen-year-old printer, who was a patient at the hospital. It began as a weekly publication and then was issued monthly. It ceased publication after a four-year run when the young founder and other patients involved in its preparation were discharged.
See also JOURNALS BY PATIENTS, THE OPAL, MOONBEAMS, NEW MOON, and RETREAT GAZETTE.
2) A journal of the same title was first published in Great Britain in 1853. It was the official organ of the Association of Medical Officers of Asylums and Hospitals for the Insane (q.v.) (now the Royal College of Psychiatrists). The first editor was John C. Bucknill (q.v.). It later changed its title to *Journal of Mental Science* and now is known as the *British Journal of Psychiatry.*

ASYLUMS. Originally, places of refuge offering inviolable sanctuary, such as churches. Later, institutions for the insane were so designated. Throughout the Middle Ages (q.v.) there were provisions for the care of the insane in general hospitals. A few special houses were built for them with the purpose of detention rather than treatment; these buildings seem to have been especially numerous in Germany where they were called *Narrturmer* (tower-of-fools). Most cities agreed to care for the local insane, but those wandering in from other places were usually driven away. Royal hospitals, voluntary hospitals, and hospitals developed under the laws of each country were sometimes available for the insane in the seventeenth and eighteenth centuries. Many of these hospitals were in the hands of private individuals who had no medical qualifications at all. The nineteenth century saw the erection of many institutions and the passage of legislation that attempted to insure proper treatment for the insane and the protection of their rights in the community. (For more information concerning a specific asylum, look under asylum name or location.)

See also ASYLUMS, ONE-MAN, CAIRO LUNATIC ASYLUMS, COUNTY ASYLUMS, DOLL-HAUS, FREE HOUSES, HOLY GHOST HOUSE, LICENSED HOUSES, PETITES MAISONS, PRIVATE MADHOUSES, PROBATIONARY ASYLUMS, REGISTERED HOSPITALS, ROYAL ASYLUMS, TOLLKISTE, and TOLLOKOBEN.

Bibliography: Rothman, D. 1971. *The discovery of the asylum.*

ASYLUMS, ONE-MAN. In the colonial United States, madmen were regarded as a danger to the community and as such were incarcerated. Court records testify to the provision of buildings specially erected for just one person afflicted with insanity (*see* INSANIA). The following entries are respectively from the Upland, Pennsylvania, court records of 1676 and the 1689 town records of Braintree, Massachusetts.

Jan Vorelissen of Amesland, Complayning to ye Court that his son Erik is bereft of his naturall Senses and is turned quyt madd and yt, he being a poore man is not able to maintaine him; Ordered: yt three or four persons bee hired to build a little block-house at Amesland for to put in the said m dman.

That Samuel Speere should build a little house 7 foote long & 5 foote wide & set it by his house to secure his Sister good wife Witty being distracted & provide for her.

Bibliography: Pennsylvania, Delaware County, Upland court records, 1676-1681. Quoted in A. Deutsch. 1949. *The mentally ill in America.*

ASYLUM VISITING. Until the beginning of the nineteenth century asylum (q.v.) visiting was considered a legitimate form of entertainment. Samuel Pepys (q.v.) remarked in his diary entry for February 19, 1669, that he had sent some young relatives to see the sights of Bedlam (q.v.), then located in Bishopsgate Without. Whole families would go to stare and to tease the unfortunate inmates. Admission tickets were issued, and attendants and porters regarded the tips they received from the visitors as a considerable part of their earnings. William Hogarth (q.v.) satirized the morbid curiosity and lack of feeling exhibited by visitors in a series of engravings that depicted the insane and the visitors in Bedlam. In 1799 Immanuel Kant (q.v.)

warned those of nervous disposition against such visits, lest they become similarly affected.
Bibliography: Kraepelin, E. 1962. *One hundred years of psychiatry.*

ATHAMAS. In Greek mythology, the son of Aelus, and king of Orchomenus in Boeotia. He incurred the displeasure of Juno, who punished him by causing him to become insane. Plagued by hallucinations (q.v.), Athamas mistook his son Learchus for a stag and slew him.
Bibliography: Graves, R. 1960. *The Greek myths.*

ATHENAEUS OF ATTALEIA (lst Century A.D.). A physician. He practiced in Rome at the time of Claudius (A.D. 41-54) and was the founder of a new school of thought, that of the Pneumatists, so called from the *pneuma* (q.v.), a fifth element that he added to the traditional four (air, earth, water, and fire). He explained health and disease in terms of the right or wrong proportion of the elements in the body. Athenaeus regarded a knowledge of medicine as a necessary part of general education. His rules for healthy living were differentiated according to age and included educational precepts as well as dietetic rules. Galen (q.v.) thought very highly of his ideas.
Bibliography: Scarborough, J. 1969. *Roman medicine.*

ATHLETIC TYPE. One of the four physical types distinguished by Ernst Kretschmer (q.v.). It referred to a person with a strong skeletal structure, broad chest, and powerful muscles.
See also ASTHENIC TYPE, and PYKNIC TYPE.
Bibliography: Kretschmer, E. 1944. *Körperbau und charakter.*

ATLANTA. A wooden figurehead representing the half-naked body of a golden-haired woman. It was found in 1866 floating in the Atlantic Ocean, but there was no sign of the ship whose prow she had adorned. The Italian sailors who recovered the figure were so fascinated by her beauty that they spent hours gazing at her and eventually began to fight over her, until the captain had to lock her away. She then was taken to the naval museum in Genoa. There the middle-aged caretaker became so obsessed (*see* OBSESSION) with her that people began to wonder about his sanity. Depressed by the hopelessness of his infatuation he drowned himself in the ocean. In 1944 a German officer, Eric Kurz, came under the spell of Atlanta and hid the figurehead in his room. He was found dead at her feet. He had shot himself through the head, leaving a farewell note pinned to her wooden body. The figure has since been returned to the naval museum at Genoa.

ATREUS. A legendary hero, king of Mycenae. He killed his brother Thestes' sons and fed their flesh to him in revenge for the seduction of his wife. The

deed was so horrible that the sun turned back on its course, and the whole family of Atreus was cursed for all time.
Bibliography: Whitwell, J. R. 1946. *Analecta psychiatrica.*

ATTIS. A character in Greek mythology. In one form of the myth, he castrated himself with a flint while in a religious frenzy. Others in states of ecstasy (q.v.) followed his example. He became the leader of an order of eunuch priests devoted to the cult of Cybele, the mother-goddess. Catullus, the Roman poet, wrote one of his best poems about Attis. It is pervaded by his horror of this self-mutilation.
Bibliography: Vermaseren, M. J. 1966. *The legend of Attis in Greek and Roman art.*

AUBERT, HERMANN (1826-1892). A German physician, professor of physiology at Breslau and at Rostock. He conducted extensive research on visual adaptation and perception. He was the first to measure correctly the zonal changes of color sensitivity. He was also one of the early editors of *Zeitschrift für Psychologie.*
Bibliography: Aubert, H. 1876. *Grundzüge der physiologischen.*

AUBREY, JOHN (1626-1697). An English antiquary. His best-known work, *Brief Lives of Contemporaries*, was first published in 1813. A humorous, gossipy, lively production, it contains references to William Harvey (q.v.), at whose funeral Aubrey was pallbearer, Robert Hooke (q.v.), architect of Bethlem Royal Hospital (q.v.), and Robert Burton (q.v.). It also contains a few references to psychopathological events: "Lady Jordan being at Cirencester, when it was besieged was so terrified with the shooting, that her understanding was so spoyled, that she became a tiny-child, that they made babies for her to play withall."

His book *An Idea of Education of Young Gentlemen* displayed an outlook on progressive education not only far ahead of his time but rarely equalled today. He wrote: "A Schoole should be indeed the house of play and pleasure; and not of feare and bondage and pupils should take so great a delight in their studies, that they would learn as fast as one could teach them." This letter is suggestive of such progressive educationalists as Alexander S. Neill (q.v.).
Bibliography: Dick, O. L. 1949. *Aubrey's brief lives.*

AUDE. A girl betrothed to Roland in the *Chanson de Roland* [*Song of Roland*], a medieval romance. She is an example of death brought about by emotion. She died of grief when she heard that Roland was dead.
Bibliography: *The song of Roland* (11th century). 1959, trans. by C. K. Scott-Moncrieff.

AUENBRUGGER VON AUENBRUGG, LEOPOLD (1722-1809). An Austrian physician, remembered as the discoverer of immediate percussion of the chest in diagnosis. He was a modest, unassuming, and honest scientist. He wrote a monograph on suicide (q.v.), which he regarded as a disease, and related it to emotional disorder.
Bibliography: Rosen, S. 1971. History in the study of suicide. *Psychol. Med.* 1:267.

AUGUSTINE OF HIPPO, SAINT (354-430). A leader of the early Christian church, born at Tagaste in the province of Numidia, North Africa. He belonged to a family divided by religious differences. His father, Patricius, was a pagan and his mother, Monica, a devout Christian. He studied rhetoric at Carthage and was greatly influenced by the writings of Cicero (q.v.). Augustine then went to Milan to teach rhetoric; there he was influenced by Bishop Ambrose (340?-397). Guided by Alypius, a friend of Ambrose, and moved by the Epistles of Saint Paul, he was able to end the conflict between his religious tendencies and his love of material pleasures. He left his concubine, entered the church, and founded a religious order. He became a priest and eventually the bishop of Hippo. Saint Augustine was the first writer to give vivid and detailed descriptions of personal emotional experiences. His *Confessions*, written in 406, shows an introspective self-analysis and insight that give the work a unique place in the history of personal analysis. He used introspection as a source of psychological knowledge but accepted the dogmas and superstitions of the church at that time. He categorically denied that man could find the truth by the use of his own faculties. He died at Hippo during the seige of the Vandals.
Bibliography: Battenhouse, R. W., ed. 1955. *The life of St. Augustine.*
Pusey, E. B., trans. 1949. *St. Augustine: Confessions.*

AURA IN EPILEPSY. A sensation occurring immediately before an epileptic seizure. The first recorded mention of the aura in epilepsy (q.v.) is found in the works of Aretaeus of Cappadocia (q.v.). Fyodor Dostoevsky (q.v.), also an epileptic, described the onset of an attack as "a feeling of happiness which I never experience in my normal state and of which I cannot give the idea. . . . complete harmony with myself and with the whole world."
Bibliography: Temkin, O. 1971. *The falling sickness.*

AURELIANUS, CAELIUS. *See* CAELIUS AURELIANUS.

AUSTRIAN SCHOOL. A school of psychology (q.v.) founded by Franz Brentano (q.v.) toward the end of the nineteenth century. It concerned itself with psychic acts rather than with psychic contents.
Bibliography: Eysenck, H. J. 1972. *Encyclopaedia of psychology.*

AUSTRIUS, SEBASTIANUS (?-1550). An Alsatian medical writer. In 1540 he wrote a treatise on pediatrics, *De Infantium Morborum Diagnotione,*

that contained a great deal of material from an earlier tract by Cornelius Roelans (q.v.). Austrius' work included remarks on psychological disorders in children and stressed that bad mental habits could be corrected by channeling thoughts in the right direction.
Bibliography: Walk, A. 1964. Prehistory of psychiatry. *Brit. J. Psychiat.* 110:754-67.

AUTENRIETH, FERDINAND (1772-1835). A German physician. Johann C. Reil (q.v.) was closely associated with him. He was interested in mental disorders and advocated a practical and vigorous approach in their treatment. Unlike others of his time, he believed that acute psychosis (q.v.) could be cured. Among the devices he invented to restrain mental patients is a metal mask, which prevented patients from being too noisy. He was also interested in the legal aspects of psychiatry (q.v.). The poet Johann Christian Friedrich Hölderlin (q.v.) was one of his patients.
Bibliography: Mora, G. 1972. Anniversaries. *Am. J. Psychiat.* 129:653.

AUTISM. A primitive form of thought process, which was regarded by Eugen Bleuler (q.v.) as one of the main characteristics of psychosis (q.v.). Bleuler claimed that for him the term *autism* was "the positive aspect of what (Pierre) Janet (q.v.) called, on the negative side, 'loss of feeling of reality.' "
Bibliography: Galdston, I., ed. 1967. *Historic derivations of modern psychiatry.*

AUTOCHIRIA. A term meaning self-destruction. It was used before the eighteenth century, when the term *suicide* (q.v.) was coined.
Bibliography: Esquirol, J. E. D. 1845. Reprint. 1965. *Mental maladies: a treatise on insanity.*

AUTO-DA-FÉ. A term meaning "act of faith." During the Inquisition (q.v.) in Spain and Portugal, the auto-da-fé was the ceremony at which heretics and witches were condemned. A public procession and a church service were part of the proceedings before punishment. Its severest form of punishment was death by burning at the stake, which was carried out in the presence of high dignitaries of the state and the church. Those responsible for the sentence felt no guilt because they believed that saving a soul from the devil justified the destruction of the body. The victims of the Inquisition often endured torture and death in a kind of ecstasy (q.v.) as an act of devotion. The opera *Don Carlo* by Giuseppe Verdi (1813-1901) has a scene representing an auto-da-fé attended by Philip II (q.v.).
Bibliography: Hauben, P. J. 1969. *The Spanish inquisition.*

AUTOEROTISM. A term first employed by Havelock Ellis (q.v.) to denote a libido (q.v.) related solely to the self.
Bibliography: Ellis, H. 1933. *Psychology of sex.*

AUTOMATIC TALKING. A technique for the exploration of the subconscious used by Pierre Janet (q.v.). Sigmund Freud (q.v.) later employed a similar approach with his method of free association.

AUTOSUGGESTION. Self suggestion, especially in hypnosis (q.v.). The term was first used by Émile Coué (q.v.), who based his method of psychotherapy (q.v.) on it.

AUXONNE NUNS. In 1658 the Ursuline nuns in Auxonne were believed to be possessed by devils. Hysterical (*see* HYSTERIA) symptoms lasted for over five years and led to accusations of lesbianism (q.v.), seduction, and witchcraft (q.v.). Exorcism (q.v.) was tried frequently, but the hysteria abated only when the Mother Superior was sent to another convent. Many physicians examined the nuns, but only one believed them to be sick rather than possessed.
See also DEMONAIC POSSESSION.
Bibliography: Robbins, R. H. 1970. *The encyclopedia of witchcraft and demonology.*

AUZOUY, M. The author of a paper describing in moving terms the life of the cagots (q.v.) of southern France, a tribe afflicted with cretinism (q.v.). He considered them to be different from most cretins because of their proficiency as a community. He was convinced that if they were brought into contact with the people around them and allowed to participate in the usual community activities, they would become useful citizens.
Bibliography: Auzouy, M. 1967. Les crétins et les cagot des Pyreneés. *Ann. méd. psychol.* 4th series. 9: 1-31.

AVELING, FRANCIS ARTHUR POWELL (1875-1941). An English psychologist. He investigated the part played by the will in the feelings and expression of emotions. The process involved in choice was also analyzed by him.
Bibliography: Aveling, F. A. P. 1931. *Personality and will.*

AVENARIUS, RICHARD (1843-1896). A German philosopher, born in Paris, France, nephew of Richard Wagner (q.v.). He was professor of philosophy at the University of Zürich from 1877 to 1896. Avenarius developed a complicated theory of the bodily system upon which consciousness depends. His concepts were published in 1888 and 1890 in two volumes entitled *Kritik der reinen Erfahrung.* The difficulty and effort involved in explaining his theories so affected his health that he died soon after the publication of the second volume.
Bibliography: Boring, E. G. 1950. *A history of experimental psychology.*

AVENZOAR (IBN ZUHR) (1091?-1162). An Arab physician, born in Seville, Spain. He was the teacher of Averröes (q.v.) and a great admirer and follower of Galen (q.v.). He rejected superstitious quackery and strongly objected to the use of cauterization (q.v.) as a form of treatment in mental disorders.
Bibliography: Ullman, M. 1978. *Islamic medicine.*

AVERRÖES (1126-1198). A Muslim philosopher and physician, born in Cordova, Spain. He was banished from Spain for a number of years because of his freethinking. He was the principal Arab commentator on Aristotle (q.v.). Averröes regarded the intellect as separate from the body. He maintained that there was a double truth, which was based half on science and half on faith. His philosophy (Averroism) had great impact on Christian thought and made it legitimate to study natural phenomena without contradicting scriptural dogma. He was the author of many works on jurisprudence, astronomy, medicine, and philosophy as well as commentaries on Aristotle.
Bibliography: Graham, T. F. 1967. *Medieval minds.*

AVERSA. A small town near Naples, Italy. It is famous for its mental hospital, which was founded in the thirteenth century as a leprosarium. In 1420 the hospital was turned into a convent for the nuns of Saint Mary Magdalene, and remained a convent until the early nineteenth century when it became an asylum (q.v.) for the mentally ill. Its superintendent was a priest, Giovanni Linguiti (q.v.) who advocated moral medicine (q.v.) and occupational therapy (q.v.). Printing, translating, music, husbandry, and the manufacture of woolen cloth were among the activities of the patients. Linguiti was followed by Biagio Miraglia (q.v.), who further improved conditions and abolished all forms of restraint (q.v.). The hospital was recognized throughout Europe as an enlightened center of treatment. Henry C. Burdett (q.v.) in his *Hospitals and Asylums of the World* (q.v.) showed it to be one of the largest mental hospitals in Italy. It is now called Ospedale Psichiatrico S. Maria Maddalena.
Bibliography: La Pegna, E. 1913. *Il R. Manicomio di Aversa.*

AVERSION THERAPY. An early experiment in this form of treatment was conducted by Benjamin Rush (q.v.). The subject was a Negro, and the aim was to cure his fondness of alcohol. He was given some rum to which tartar emetic had been added. Rush reported that the beverage "sickened and puked him to such a degree, that . . . he could not bear the sight, nor the smell of spirits, for two years afterwards."
Bibliography: Rush, B. 1812. *Medical inquiries.*

AVICENNA (980-1037). The Western name of abu 'Ali-al-Husayn ibn-Sinā. Born in Bukhara, Persia, the son of a tax collector, he was a child prodigy who had memorized the entire Koran (q.v.) by the time he was ten years old. He was at first attracted to theology, which he mastered before his eighteenth birthday. At the age of eighteen he also had written a compendium of the scientific knowledge of his time. He turned to medicine and, while still in his teens, became physician to the king. Avicenna's life was full of adventures: one moment he was rewarded and feted, the next he had to seek safety in flight. He was a restless individual in constant pursuit of knowledge, but this did not quench his thirst for life, or his love of gaiety, women, and wine. He found time to write over one hundred books on a great variety of subjects. His most famous work is *The Canon*, a complete system of medicine, which became the standard textbook for physicians in the East and in Europe throughout the seventeenth century. It ran into fifteen Latin editions and was translated into numerous languages. Avicenna, who said that "the different kinds of madness are countless", did not separate mental illness from physical illness. Instead, he observed the effect of emotion on bodily states, for example on the pulse. Like Hippocrates (q.v.), he considered the stomach, liver, and spleen as the seats of melancholia (q.v.). He also studied the influence of emotional factors, diet (q.v.), climate (q.v.), and housing, among other things, on the development of disease, analyzing all the factors that impinge on man's health. Like his contemporaries, he related brain activities to the ventricles. He described five psychological faculties and related them to distinct brain areas. These were the composite (or commonsense), imagination, instinct, memory (q.v.), and understanding. His classification of mental disorders was divided into 1) Phrenitis (q.v.); 2) Lethargus (stupor); 3) Delirium (q.v.); 4) Fatuitas (amentia); 5) Oblivio (loss of memory); 6) Disorders of imagination (hallucinations [q.v.]); 7) Mania (q.v.); 8) Melancholia (q.v.); 9) Lycanthropy (q.v.); 10) Amor insanus (love sickness); 11) Incubus (q.v.); 12) Mollities (effeminacy). He emphasized prevention. His theories were based on the work of Galen, Hippocrates, and Aristotle (qq.v.) and influenced medicine, and at times retarded its progress, for many centuries. Even in his own time he was known as "The Prince of Physicians." According to tradition he died at the age of fifty-seven as the result of his life of pleasure.

Bibliography: Shah, Mazhar H. 1966. *The general principles of Avicenna's canon of medicine*.
Ullman, M. 1978. *Islamic medicine*.

AWL, WILLIAM M. (1799-1876). An American physician, born in Harrisburg, Pennsylvania. After some years in general practice, he became interested in psychiatry (q.v.) and advocated the establishment of institutions controlled by the state for the care of the insane. After the passage of the 1835 law, which provided for such institutions, he helped to found the Ohio State Asylum for the Insane (q.v.) and in 1838 became its first superintendent. He believed that he could control any mental patient by merely gazing

into his eyes. His statistical report to the year 1843 ended, "per cent of recovery on all recent cases discharged the present year, 100"—an extreme example of the then fashionable institutional claims for impressive recovery rates. He remained in office for twelve years, until political factions removed him. He then became physician to the Ohio Institution for the Blind. Awl was one of the original thirteen founders of the American Psychiatric Association (q.v.).
Bibliography: Deutsch, A. 1949. *The mentally ill in America.*

AXEL. A nineteenth-century drama by the French writer Villiers de l'Isle Adam (1840-1889). In the work, suicide (q.v.) is presented as a positive act. After much searching, the hero finds his ideal woman, and they imagine the wonderful life they will live together. They decide life would be only an illusion, best left to poor fools, "who can only measure reality by sensation," and choose to die by poison before their "real" dream is destroyed by earthly "illusion."
Bibliography: Fedden, H. R. 1938. *Suicide.*

AYESHA. A character in a novel by Rider Haggard (q.v.). Haggard claimed he had written the novel in a kind of trance, after sudden inspiration. Ayesha was an ancient white African queen who had survived for two thousand years by a process of magic (q.v.). She destroyed men unless they overcame her spells. She dies while encouraging the young Englishman who discovered her to pass through a pillar of fire that would have made him immortal. The character of this enigmatic and diabolic woman inspired popular imagination and psychological study. Jung (q.v.) referred to her as the *Anima Gestalt,* or anima (q.v.) figure, who attracts and destroys men.
Bibliography: Haggard, H. R. 1887. *She. A history of adventure.*

AYHUASCA. A powerful hallucinogen. It is used to make a drink consumed in ritualistic healing ceremonies in Peru. The healers, called *ayahuasqueros,* use the resulting hallucinations (q.v.) to determine the cause of an illness and then apply counter magic to alleviate the anxiety of their patients, who have also consumed the hallucinogen.
Bibliography: Emboden, W. 1972. *Narcotic plants.*

AYUR-VEDA. The most ancient Hindu system of medicine dating from circa 1400 B.C.. It is ascribed to Brahma and therefore considered to be of divine origin. It contains a classification of mental disorders, which were believed to be caused by malevolent spirits.
Bibliography: Sharma, P.V. 1972. *Indian medicine in the classical age.*

AZAM, ETIENNE EUGÈNE (1822-1899). A French surgeon, professor of surgery at the University of Bordeaux. He was intensely interested in hypnotism (q.v.). One of his patients, Felida X. (q.v.) was a case of double personality; he followed her for thirty-five years and published her case history with an introduction by Jean Martin Charcot (q.v.).

Bibliography: Azam, E. E. 1887. *Hypnotisme, double conscience et altération de la personnalité.*

AZUCENA. A character in *Il Trovatore*, an opera by Giuseppe Verdi (1813-1901). She was a gypsy torn between love and a thirst for vengeance. Verdi made it clear in his notes that such feelings would cause her to become emotionally upset but not mad. He wrote to the librettist: "Do not make Azucena mad. Overwhelmed by care, grief, terror, sleeplessness, she is incapable of consecutive utterance. Her senses are oppressed, but she is not mad."

Bibliography: Osborne, 1971. *Letters of Giuseppe Verdi.*

B

BABINSKI, JOSEPH FRANÇOIS FELIX (1857-1932). A clinical neurologist, born in Paris; his parents were Polish exiles. After qualifying in medicine, he became assistant to Jean Martin Charcot (q.v.) at the Salpêtrière (q.v.) but failed to achieve the professorial chair there, obtaining instead the post of chief of the neurological clinic at the Pitié. A big, tall man, strikingly handsome, he had a quiet manner but could produce dramatic clinical demonstrations. He was a perfectionist who attacked neurological problems with refined clinical techniques and published his findings in succinct, systematic, and factual papers. He described the plantar response—Babinski's sign—in a contribution of twenty-eight lines. His methods of neurological examination, which were based on physical findings, are still routine practice. He distinguished hysterical (*see* HYSTERIA) from organic symptomatology, noted the disappearance of hysterical symptoms in patients at the Salpêtrière after Charcot's death, and acknowledged the difficulty in distinguishing between true hysteria and malingering. With Alfred Frohlich (q.v.), he investigated endocrine disorders; adiposogenital dystrophy is now known as Babinski-Fröhlich syndrome. He helped to found the Societé de Neurologie de Paris. His personal interests included opera, ballet, and gastronomy, this latter giving rise to the story that he abruptly broke off a ward round to rush home, where he had been summoned by a message that the soufflé was nearly ready. He lived with his brother, a distinguished engineer and famous cook.
Bibliography: Haymaker, W., and Schiller, F. 1970. *The founders of neurology.* 2d ed.

BABYLONIAN MEDICINE. Cuneiform records of ancient Babylonia (first mentioned in c.2700 B.C.) have been preserved in clay tablets and contain some information about medicine. The Babylonians believed that living persons were composed of soul and body. The intellect was located in the

heart, and the liver served as a central organ for the blood, which they considered the true life principle. They divided the blood into two kinds: blood of the daytime (bright arterial) and blood of the night (dark venous). They regarded disease as something of the nature of a demon that invaded the body, and each disease had its own special demon. Many symptoms of mental illness were described by the Babylonians, including delusions (q.v.), hallucinations (q.v.), anxiety, mania (q.v.), hysterical (*see* HYSTERIA) states, apathy, and phobias (q.v.). Schizophrenia (q.v.), suicide, and epilepsy (qq.v.) were also described. Mental illness was believed to be caused by evil demons, witchcraft (q.v.), spells, and magic (q.v.). *Asakku* was the demon that brought trouble to the head. The priests then employed elaborate rituals and incantations to counteract his spells. The great treatise of *Maqlû* (q.v.) was one of the main text books of Babylonian psychiatry. *Šurpu* (q.v.), another ancient Babylonian book, deals with what now is known as neurosis (q.v.).
Bibliography: Wilson, V. J. K. n.d. *An introduction to Babylonian psychiatry.* Assiriological Studies, no. 16.

BACCHANALIA. Orgies celebrated in ancient Rome in connection with the cult of Bacchus, a god of wine, vegetation, and fertility. Intoxication, possession (q.v.), and ecstasy (q.v.) were experienced by those taking part in the celebrations, which were banned in 186 B.C., possibly for political rather than moral reasons.
Bibliography: Nilsson, M. P. 1957. *The Dionysiac mysteries of the Hellenistic and Roman age.*

BACCHANALS. A play by the Greek dramatist Euripides (q.v.). In it the Maenads (q.v.) are seized by a frenzy sent by Dionysus (q.v.) as punishment for Pentheus' (q.v.) ban on his cult in Thebes.
Bibliography: *Euripides.* Vol. 3, trans. A. S. Way, 1912.

BACHOFEN, JOHANN JAKOB (1815-1887). A Swiss jurist and historian. His interest in archaeology led him to study symbols recording primitive history. He evolved a theory that early society had been ruled by women. According to him, matriarchy had been a complete social system that embraced all aspects of life. During this period, night was more important than day, the moon and the dead were worshipped, and daughters were preferred to sons. The symbol of the matriarchy was the sphinx. He expressed these views in his book *Das Mutterrecht* in 1861. Because his theories were obscure, he gained little following among his contemporaries, but he influenced Friedrich Nietzsche (q.v.) and the Neo-Romantic poets of Germany a half century later. Many similarities can be found between Bachofen's interpretation of symbols and that of Sigmund Freud's (q.v.). Alfred Adler (q.v.) and Carl G. Jung (q.v.) probably either had read his work or had been influenced by it through secondary sources. The sup-

porters of equal rights for women have often quoted his work to justify
their theories.
Bibliography: Bachofen, J. J. 1948. *Das Mutterrecht*, ed. Karl Meuli. Vols. 1 and
2.

BACKUS, FREDERICK. An American doctor. His interest in mental retardation culminated in the introduction of a bill in the 1846 session of
Congress for the provision of residential schools for mentally retarded children. The bill was not accepted, but Samuel Gridley Howe (q.v.) reintroduced it later and it was approved.
Bibliography: Kanner, L. 1964. *A history of the care and study of the mentally
retarded.*

BACON, FRANCIS (1561-1626). An English philosopher and statesman
with the titles of Verulam and Viscount St. Albans. He was born at York
House in the Strand, London. After his education at Trinity College, Cambridge, he entered the legal profession and then dedicated himself to politics,
eventually becoming lord chancellor. His cynicism masked a deep sense of
insecurity. He was often acutely depressed, and, when under pressure, he
suffered fits of nervous prostration. John Aubrey (q.v.) believed that he was
a pederast, but there is no proof that he was a homosexual (*see* HOMOSEX-
UALITY), although it would explain his coldness toward women. He was
accused of bribery and corruption, and sent to the Tower, but was soon
released. He wrote many philosophical, legal, and literary works. In his
essays on science, he refuted the belief that mental illness was caused by
physical disorder or divine punishment and urged investigations based on
the study of individual cases, the correlation of body and mind, postmortem
findings, and the interaction between the individual and society. His writings, in elegant Latin or English, are sometimes obscure.
Bibliography: Bowen, C. D. 1963. *Francis Bacon: the temper of a man.*

BACON, ROGER (1214?-1294). An English philosopher, a learned scholar,
and a man of science, referred to as "Doctor Mirabilis" (the Admirable
Doctor). He was educated in Oxford and Paris, where he may have obtained
a doctorate in medicine. As a Franciscan friar, his views incurred the displeasure and suspicion of his order and caused him to be kept under continuous surveillance. He believed that experience rather than deduction led
to truth and opposed the philosophy of Saint Thomas Aquinas (q.v.). Contrary to the views of his time and of his church, he held that mental illness
was due to natural causes. His experiments in chemistry and alchemy (q.v.)
were considered heretical practices. Nevertheless, Pope Clement IV commissioned him to write Latin treatises on the sciences. He invented spec-
tacles, came very near to the concept of a telescope, and prepared a rectified

calendar in 1263. To him is also attributed the construction of a "brazen head," which could talk.
Bibliography: Easton, S. C. 1952. *Roger Bacon and his search for a universal science.*

BADIANO'S CODEX. A treatise written in Mexico in the sixteenth century by the Indian physicians Martin de la Cruz and Juan Badiano, who also translated it. It contains a number of medical precepts of psychiatric interest. It advises the use of certain plants for melancholy, emetics and spells for epilepsy, and prescribes ointments made of animal parts for anxiety.
Bibliography: Leon, C. A., and Rosselli, H. 1975. Latin America. In *World history of psychiatry*, ed. J. G. Howells.

BAD NEWS. A sixteenth-century therapeutic technique used in Bethlem Royal Hospital (q.v.) whereby patients in a state of mania (q.v.) were given frequent unpleasant sad news to dampen their spirits.
Bibliography: O'Donoghue, E. G. 1914. *The story of Bethlehem Hospital.*

BAGHDAD ASYLUM. *See* DÁR-UL-MARAFTAN.

BAGLIVI, GIORGIO (1668-?1707). An Italian physician, pupil of Marcello Malpighi (1628-1694), the Italian anatomist. Pope Clement XI appointed him to the chair of medical theory in the Collegio della Sapienza in Rome. He propounded the theory of solidism, which regarded solid parts of the body as the seat of disease. He considered the body a machine made up of smaller machines. He distinguished between smooth and striped muscles and described heart stroke and the acute organic psychosis (q.v.) resulting from the bite of a tarantula (tarantism [q.v.]). He emphasized the role of emotion, especially hysteria (q.v.), in pathogenesis and believed that gastrointestinal symptoms were a manifestation of mental disorders. His theories were often unproven, but his clinical practice was insightful, sensitive, and considerate. He said that "to frequent societies, to visit libraries, to own valuable unread books or shine in all the journals does not in the least contribute to the comfort of the sick." He advised physicians to offer support to patients and to include travel, music, and dancing in their treatment. It is said that he died of hard work.
Bibliography: Sigerist, H. E. 1971. *The great doctors.*

BAILLARGER, JULES (1806-1891). A French psychiatrist, pupil of Jean Esquirol (q.v.). Baillarger, like Esquirol, became interested in hallucinatory phenomena and described the hallucinations (q.v.) occurring in the hypnagogic state and the hallucinations accompanying alcoholic delirium (see DELIRIUM TREMENS). He investigated manic-depressive psychoses (q.v.), which he called *folie à double forme* (q.v.), and cretinism (q.v.). The first French journal dedicated to psychological medicine, *Annales Médico-psychologiques* (q.v.) was founded by him in 1843.

Bibliography: Pelicier, Y. 1975. France. In *World history of psychiatry*, ed. J. G. Howells.

BAILLY, JEAN SYVAIN (1736-1793). A French scholar, politician, and astronomer born in Paris. In 1784 the Académie des Sciences (q.v.) appointed him to a committee of five, which then joined with the committee of the faculty of medicine to investigate the practice of magnetism (q.v.). After seeing the work of Charles D'Eslon (q.v.) the joint committee presented its report, which was written by Bailly. The report condemned magnetism and declared the animal magnetic fluid nonexistent. Bailly became mayor of Paris in 1791, but his passionate revolutionary ideas, which included drastic hospital reforms, eventually led to his downfall and execution by guillotine.
Bibliography: Zilboorg, G. 1941. *A history of medical psychology*.

BAIN, ALEXANDER (1818-1903). A psychologist, born in Aberdeen, Scotland. He was one of five children in a poor working-class family. As a boy he worked as a weaver, like his father, and educated himself, leaning toward mathematics and science and finally becoming attracted to metaphysics. He managed to enter and graduate from Marischall College in Aberdeen. When the college amalgamated with the university, he obtained the chair of logic and English, which he retained until he resigned twenty-five years later because of poor health. Despite opposition he was elected rector of the University three times. In 1855 he published *The Senses and the Intellect* followed by *The Emotions and the Will* in 1859. Then, because of the post he held, he dedicated himself to writing grammar and rhetoric for the next nine years before returning to his primary interest with *Mental and Moral Science* (1868) and *Mind and Body* (1872). He was the first psychologist to dedicate his life work to psychology (q.v.), which he reoriented toward physiological methods and away from the empiricism of the past. In 1876 he founded *Mind* (q.v.), the first psychological journal. Despite ill health, he lived to be eighty-five.
Bibliography: Boring, E. G. 1950. *A history of experimental psychology*.

BAKER, MARY. *See* EDDIE, MARY BAKER.

BAKER, RACHEL (1794-?). American religious fanatic, born in Massachusetts. As a child she became preoccupied with religion. She grew into a shy, melancholic girl, who was overwhelmed by a feeling of unworthiness. When she was seventeen years old she started to talk in her sleep, shrieking and relating terrible visions. These paroxysms later changed, and she started to preach in her sleep. The sermons were rational, vivacious, and compelling, although Rachel in her waking state was a quiet, rather dull, girl. People came from far and wide to hear her. Doctors were consulted and she was treated to no avail with laudanum (q.v.), bleeding (q.v.), and a change of environment. Books about her and collections of her sermons began to appear. She was thought by some to be divinely possessed (*see* POSSESSION), by others to be mad, but her doctors remained puzzled, tentatively suggesting hysteria (q.v.) or somniloquism, talking during sleep. Sometime after 1815 a group of people took charge of her; she was protected from the public and no more was heard of her.

Bibliography: Baker, Rachel. 1815. *The remarkable sermons of Rachel Baker . . . taken down in shorthand by C. Mais.*

BAKEWELL, THOMAS (1761-1835). The English owner of a private asylum (q.v.), Spring Vale, which opened in Staffordshire in 1808. He was a weaver by trade, but his grandfather and his uncle had been proprietors of madhouses. In 1809 he wrote *The Domestic Guide in Cases of Insanity*, addressing himself to the general public and clergy and giving a review of the course, symptoms, and therapy of insanity (*see* INSANIA). His son, Samuel Glover Bakewell (1811-1866) studied medicine and specialized in disorders of the mind. Samuel Glover Bakewell's *An Essay on Insanity* (1833), which he dedicated to his father, paid tribute to his father's practical experience and success with the mentally ill.

Bibliography: Parry-Jones, W. Ll. 1972. *The trade in lunacy.*

BALDI, CAMILLO (1547?-1634). An Italian physician, professor of medicine and philosophy and professor of theoretical medicine at the University of Bologne. He wrote on the Aristotelian (*see* ARISTOTLE) theory of physiognomy. Another of his books was on graphology (q.v.) and was entitled *Tratto come da una lettera missiva si cognoscano la natura e qualità del scrittore* [How to know the nature and quality of the writer from his letter]. It was published in 1622 and was the first book on handwriting analysis.

Bibliography: Rand, H. A. 1962. *Graphology.*

BALDWIN, JAMES MARK (1861-1934). A psychologist, born at the beginning of the American Civil War in Columbia, South Carolina, he came from a prominent family. Educated at Princeton University, he completed his studies in Germany and gained a doctorate in philosophy. After teaching metaphysics and logic at the University of Toronto, he returned to Princeton in 1893 as professor of psychology (q.v.). Although he had written a number of philosophical works before returning to psychology (*Senses and Intellect* published in 1889; *Feeling and Will* published in 1891), the ten years he spent at Princeton were the most productive of his life. The evolutionary principle in psychology, which he did much to advance, is represented in many of his works, for example, *Mental Development in the Child and the Race* (1895). His lighter book *The Story of the Mind* was very popular and

went into many editions. In 1894, with James Cattell (q.v.), he founded the *Psychological Review* (q.v.), and a number of other psychological journals, but the two men, due to their uncompromising natures, were incapable of cooperation. They finally agreed that each would assume responsibility for the journals in alternate years. When that arrangement also broke down, they bid against each other for the sole ownership, which was won by Baldwin for $3,505. His pioneer work in experimental psychology (q.v.) was reflected in his founding of psychological laboratories at both Princeton and Toronto and his restoration of G. Stanley Hall's (q.v.) laboratory at Johns Hopkins University. After leaving Princeton, he traveled widely and worked for some years in Mexico and in France.
Bibliography: Boring, E. G. 1950. *A history of experimental psychology.*

BALINT, MICHAEL (1896-1970). A Hungarian psychiatrist. He was analyzed by Sandor Ferenczi (q.v.). In 1939 he settled in England and worked at the Tavistock Clinic (q.v.) in London. He pioneered the organization of seminars for general practioners in psychiatry and published the findings resulting from these meetings in 1957.
Bibliography: Balint, M. 1957. *The doctor, his patient and his illness.*

BALM. The botanical name of this woodland plant, *Mellisa*, derives from its connection with bees. Paracelsus (q.v.) believed it to be an elixir of life that would prevent senility and impotency; the Arabs more realistically made perfume from it. It was used in the treatment of mental disorders and as a remedy against sleep disorders.
Bibliography: De Baïracli Levy, J. 1974. *The illustrated herbal handbook.*

BALMY. A term meaning "mad." It is said to be derived from Balmes House, later called Whitmore House (q.v.), a private madhouse in England.
Bibliography: Morris, A. D. 1958. *Hoxton madhouses.*

BALSAMO, GIUSEPPE (1743-1795). The real name of Alessandro di Cagliostro, a self-styled Italian count, born of a poor family in Palermo, Italy. He is an illustration of *pseudologia fantastica* (q.v.). His knowledge of chemistry and medicine consisted of what he had learned as assistant apothecary in a monastery. He traveled widely with Lorenza Feliciani, his wife and assistant, and profitably swindled the many credulous people who bought his love philters and elixirs of youth. He held seances attended by the nobility of France, England, and Italy, and exploited to the full the then fashionable belief in animal magnetism (q.v.). His many adventures include involvement in the famous diamond necklace affair in Paris. In Rome he was condemned to death for heresy, but his sentence was commuted to life imprisonment.
Bibliography: Gervaso, R. 1974. *Cagliostro*, trans. by C.O. Cuilleanain.

BALZAC, HONORÉ DE (1799-1850). One of the greatest novelists of France. As a child he was stubborn and difficult. Although one of his teachers stated that he went around in a state of intellectual coma, he was, in fact, a voracious reader. He was given to daydreaming and through overconfidence attempted grandiose business ventures, including publishing and printing, which left him in debt until almost the end of his life. He was extravagant and pathologically vain, but as a writer, he was observant, sensitive, and imaginative. He planned to amalgamate his various writings, describing many sides of life, in one gigantic work entitled *La Comédie Humaine*. The first series of it was published in 1842; a posthumous publication consisted of forty-seven volumes. Considered the founder of the realistic novel, his descriptions of the unhealthy aspects of life have given him a reputation for exposing what is sordid, while at the same time moralizing against it.
Bibliography: Zweig, S. 1970. *Balzac*. English translation, by W. & D. Rose.

BANSHEE. Phonetic spelling of the Irish *bean sidhe*, an invisible female spirit whose presence is revealed by a mournful scream called keening. In Celtic folklore she is believed to wail outside a house where a death is about to occur. Similar beliefs can be found in many cultures; they demonstrate how acute anxiety causes misinterpretation of phenomena and aural hallucinations (q.v.).
Bibliography: Borges, J. L. 1970. *The book of imaginary beings*.

BANTING, SIR FREDERICK GRANT (1891-1941). A Canadian physician. In 1922, with Charles H. Best (1899-), he discovered insulin, which became the first systematic biological form of treatment for schizophrenia (q.v.), as well as the standard remedy for diabetes. Small doses of insulin (modified insulin therapy) were also administered to neurotic (*see* NEUROSIS) patients to stimulate their appetite.
Bibliography: Alexander, F. G., and Selesnick, S. T. 1966. *The history of psychiatry*.

BAQUET. A trough-like contraption devised by Franz Mesmer (q.v.) to be used in magnetic treatment séances (*see* PLATE 2.) It was first filled with water, then mirrors and iron rods were attached to it. People sat in a circle around it holding hands, and Mesmer touched or stroked the patients with his magnetic wand or rubbed himself against them.
Bibliography: Buranelli, V. 1975. *The wizard from Vienna: Franz Anton Mesmer and the origins of hypnotism*.

BARBA-JACOB, PORFIRIO (1883-1942). Pseudonym of the Columbian lyric poet Miguel Angel Osorio. Following a sad childhood—abandoned by his father when he was three years old—he became an eccentric vagabond,

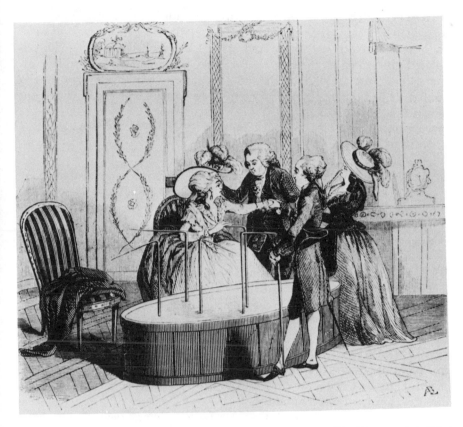

2. THE BAQUET DEVISED BY FRANZ ANTON MESMER. The trough is filled with water from which iron rods protrude. From a French print of 1784. By courtesy of the Department of Medical Illustration, Ipswich Hospital.

neurotic homosexual and an alcoholic. He rejoiced in his reputation of moral turpitude. He was described as an "Adam and Eve," who changed his opinions and his loyalties from day to day.
Bibliography: Jaramillo Meza, J. B. n.d. *Vida de Porfirio Barba-Jacob*.

BARBITURATE. A salt of barbituric acid with hypnotic qualities much used in psychiatry. It was synthetized in 1903. The name was given to malonylurea, which was discovered in 1864 by Adolf von Bayer, who celebrated his finding by visiting a tavern that was popular with artillery officers. It was the day of Saint Barbara, the patron saint of artillerymen, and von Bayer had the inspiration of combining Barbara and urea to name the new substance.
Bibliography: Goodman, L. S., and Gilman, A. 1965. *The pharmacological basis of therapeutics*.

BARLEY WATER. A decoction of pearl barley was recommended by many medical writers as a treatment for insanity. Johannes Arculanus (q.v.) thought that it would cool the brain in cases of phrenetic mania and prescribed one or two doses of it a day.
Bibliography: Whitwell, J. R. 1936. *Historical notes on psychiatry*.

BARMY. Barm is the froth that forms on top of fermenting malt liquors, and the term "barmy" in the sense of mad is derived from it. It is a reference to the spittle on the lips of defective or insane individuals.
Bibliography: 1978. *Brewer's dictionary of phrase and fable*. Ed. Evans, I. H.

BARONY PAROCHIAL ASYLUM. A pauper asylum (q.v.) built in 1875 in a pleasant country site near Glasgow, Scotland. Its enlightened management of patients, who were not restrained by locked doors or walled enclosures, attracted much attention.
Bibliography: Letchworth, W. P. 1889. *The insane in foreign countries*.

BARR, MURRAY LLEWELLYN (1908-   ). A professor of anatomy, born in Belmont, Ontario, Canada. He is an outstanding worker in the field of cytology. His extensive research in mental retardation and sex chromosome abnormalities has led to the discovery of sex chromatin (Barr body), which is a special mass of chromatin found in females only. He also has developed the technique of nuclear sexing from a buccal smear.
Bibliography: Barr, M. L. 1968. The significance of nuclear sexing. In *Modern perspectives in world psychiatry*, ed. J. G. Howells.

BARROUGH, PHILIP (fl.1560-1590). An English physician. His textbook *The Methode of Phisicke, Conteyning the Causes, Signes, and Cures of Inward Diseases in Mans Body From the Head to the Foote* was published in

London in 1583 and was reissued several times until 1652. Barrough classified diseases according to Galen's (q.v.) method and described frensie (madness with fever), lethargus, which he defined as a "dull oblivion," fatuitas (foolishness), catalepsy, coma, apoplexia (palsy), mania (q.v.), and melancholia (q.v.), which he described as "an alienation of the mind troubling reason, and waxing foolish." As treatments he advised the use of white wine, walking, riding or sailing, baths, moist diet, plenty of sleep, "moderate carnal copulation," music (see MUSIC THERAPY), and singing. He suggested bleeding (q.v.) and purging (q.v.) only when the melancholic blood was in the whole body, rather than in the brain only.

Bibliography: Hunter, R., and Macalpine, I. 1964. *Three hundred years of psychiatry.*

BARRY, JAMES (1741-1806). An Irish painter of historical subjects. In his childhood he was considered a juvenile delinquent. As an adult, he was irascible, stubborn to the point of perversity, erratic, and peculiar in his mode of dress. His striking talent brought him the protection of the British statesman and philosopher Edmund Burke (1729-1797) and the painter Joshua Reynolds (1723-1792). He became professor of painting at the Royal Academy, but his quarrels and antagonism, aimed at everybody, made him unpopular. His miserly habits caused him to be robbed, which so upset him that he accused his fellow academicians of the robbery, thus bringing about his own expulsion from the academy in 1799. He retired to his house and lived alone in a state of filth and squalor, sleeping on a bedstead with a blanket nailed to one side. He became firmly convinced that people were plotting against him and planning to kill him. Eventually, a friend rescued him and took care of him.

Bibliography: Winslow, L. S. 1898. *Mad humanity.*

BARTHEZ, PAUL JOSEPH (1734-1806). A French medical writer and philosopher who gave impetus to the idea of a life-force. The idea became known as vitalism (q.v.) and was an important factor in the development of medical psychology and hospital psychiatry. It also stimulated research in neurology and the theory of instincts. Barthez was one of the contributors to the *Encyclopédie*, the famous work containing exhaustive information on all branches of knowledge, compiled in France between 1751 and 1772.

Bibliography: Zilboorg, G. 1941. *A history of medical psychology.*

BARTHOLD, F. The first director of a school for defective children founded in 1859 in München-Gladbach, Germany. The institution was sponsored by the church, the government, and civic organizations. It collected children from the Rhineland and Westphalia. In 1868 Barthold wrote a book on mental retardation, entitled *Der Idiotismus und seine Bekämpfung* [Idiocy and its control].

Bibliography: Kanner, L. 1964. *A history of the care and study of the mentally retarded.*

BARTHOLOMAEUS ANGLICUS (d. 1260?). An English Franciscan friar who became professor of theology in Paris. Between 1230 and 1240 he compiled an encyclopedia, *De. Proprietatibus Rerum* (*The Properties of Things*), which was translated into English by John of Trevisa in 1398 and printed by Wynkyn de Worde in 1495. The work included a dissertation on the brain. According to the author the brain is white because it is a *tabula rasa* (q.v.) ready to receive images; round in shape to afford maximum protection and volume; located at the top of the body because that is the most distinguished place; and moist and cold to counteract the heat of the heart. Its three ventricles contain respectively imagination, rational thinking, and memory. Temperament and character depend on the brain. A hot brain makes a man quick and brave; a cold one produces forgetfulness and laziness; a dry brain encourages good memory; and too much fluid in the brain causes disease.

Bartholomaeus Anglicus also recognized that mental disorders can have a physical or psychological cause:

Madness cometh sometime of passions of the soul, as of business and of great thoughts, of sorrow and of too great study, and of dread; sometime of the biting of a wood-hound [mad dog], or some other venomous beast; sometime of melancholy meats, and sometime of drink of strong wine. And as the causes be diverse, the tokens and signs be diverse. For some cry and leap and hurt and wound themselves and other men, and darken and hide themselves in privy and secret places. The medicine of them is, that they be bound, that they hurt not themselves and other men. And namely such shall be refreshed, and comforted, and withdrawn from cause and matter of dread and busy thoughts. And they must be gladded with instruments of music and some deal be occupied.

De Proprietatibus Rerum was the first book to be printed on paper made in England. It was reprinted many times and had great influence on English thoughts and writings until the end of the sixteenth century.
Bibliography: Bartholomeus Anglicus. 1495, Reprint. 1975. *On the Properties of Things.*

BARTHOLOMÄI, F. A German educator who, in 1870, made a psychological survey of preschool children by gathering information based on parental observations of their children's behavior up to the time of school entrance.
Bibliography: Bartholomäi, F. 1870. Der Vorstellungskreis der Berliner Kinder beim Eintritt in die Schule. Berlin und seine Entwicklung. *Städtisches Jahrbuch für Volkswirtschaft und Statistik.* 4: 59-77. English translation in U.S. Committee on Education. 1902. *Reports for Year 1900-1901.*

BARTLEBY THE SCRIVENER. A short story by Herman Melville (q.v.) published in 1856 as a part of *The Piazza Tales*. The story describes the strange personality and behavior of a scrivener, who gradually becomes more and more withdrawn until finally he spends most of his time standing motionless and silent in the middle of the room. The attitudes, postures, and stuporous state of the scribe offer an accurate picture of catatonia (q.v.). It is a remarkable description because the first clinical account of the condition, which was given by Karl Kahlbaum (q.v.), was not published until 1874.

BARTLETT, SIR FREDERIC CHARLES (1886-1969). A psychologist, born at Stow-on-the-World, England. He is particularly well known for his work on memory. Although he was originally interested in anthropology, World War I prevented him from doing field work, and he turned to psychology (q.v.) and its practical application. He believed that psychology could develop properly only through experimentation and observation and that it should be applied to industry, medicine, the armed services, and legal procedures. He became professor of psychology at Cambridge University in 1931. He was the author of many books including *Psychology and Primitive Culture* (1923), *Remembering: a Study in Experimental and Social Psychology (1932)*, *The Problem of Noise* (1934), and *The Mind at Work and Play* (1951). A leader in experimental psychology, he devised many aptitude tests for servicemen during World War II.
Bibliography: Murchinson, C., ed. 1936. *A history of psychology in autobiography*, vol. 3.

BARUK, HENRI MARC (1897-?). A French neuropsychiatrist. He wrote on many subjects, including mental disorders and brain tumors, catatonia (q.v.), and moral medicine (q.v.). He conducted research on moral consciousness, social psychiatry, and on delusions of passion.
Bibliography: Hirsch, S. R. and Shepherd, M., eds. 1974. *Themes and variations in European psychiatry.*

BASEDOWOID TYPE. One of the personality types described by Erich Jaensch (q.v.). The basedowoid type is said to be given to eidetic imagery, distinguished by an enlarged thyroid gland, and liable to overreactions of the sympathetic nervous system; artists are assigned to this type. Sometimes the term *B Type* was employed by Jaensch. The other type of personality is the *T* (Tetanoid) *Type* (q.v.).
Bibliography: Flugel, J. C. 1945. *A hundred years of psychology.*

BASEDOW'S DISEASE. Exophthalmic goiter. It was first described by the German physician Karl A. von Basedow (1799-1854) in 1840.
Bibliography: Tuke, D. H. 1892. *A dictionary of psychological medicine.*

BASHKIRTSEFF, MARIE (1860-1884). A Russian diarist who lived mostly in France and Italy. She wrote a remarkable diary, in French, which she began when she was thirteen years old and continued until eleven days before her death. In it she recorded with extreme candor her experiences and those of her family. She felt frustrated by her meaningless existence and filled her days with romantic fantasies. She died of consumption when she was only twenty-four years old.
Bibliography: Harvey, P. 1959. *The Oxford companion to French literature*.

BASILISK. An imaginary animal, also known as a cockatrice (q.v.). It is linked with the superstition of the evil eye (q.v.).
Bibliography: Mode, H. 1976. *Fabulous beasts and demons*.

BASIL THE GREAT, SAINT (c. 329-379). A prominent bishop who greatly influenced Eastern monasticism. He had a sympathetic attitude to the insane and built a town hospital with a special unit for the insane.
Bibliography: Prestige, G. L. 1956. *St. Basil the great and Apollinaris*.

BASKET MEN. Male attendants at Bethlem Royal Hospital (q.v.). The name, which was used in the seventeenth century, was derived from the time when the hospital was a monastery and the monks went out begging for alms and food, which they placed in the baskets they carried.
Bibliography: O'Donoghue, E. G. 1914. *The story of Bethlehem Hospital*.

BASSANO, FRANCESCO (1549-1592). An Italian painter, son of Jacopo da Bassano (1517-1592), the famous Venetian painter. His mother was said to be mentally deranged. He, himself, was an anxious man who was often depressed, and deluded. Writing in 1775, Verci, his biographer, noted that Bassano "tormented by this weakness, his spirit worn out. . . . fell into a fierce hypochondria which often drove him out of his senses." He suffered from severe paranoia (q.v.) and suspected his friends, his servants, and even his wife of plotting his arrest. One day when he was left alone briefly a violent knock at the door so frightened him that he threw himself out of the window and died from his injuries.
Bibliography: Rosen, G. 1968. *Madness in society*.

BASTIAN, ADOLF (1826-1905). A German ethnologist, born in Bremen. Soon after completing his studies in medicine, he traveled in every continent and then published the results of his worldwide observations in a three volume book entitled *Man in History: Towards the Foundation of a Psychological Conception of the World*. This was followed by *Comparative Linguistic Studies* in 1870, and *Ethnological Research* (1871-73). His concepts were based on social psychology (q.v.) and the understanding of the religions, legal systems, and social lives of the people studied. He was professor

of ethnology at the University of Berlin and director of the folklore museum there.
Bibliography: Lowie, R. G. 1937. *History of ethnological theory.*

BASTIAN, HENRY CHARLTON (1837-1915). A British neurologist who is considered the founder of neurology (q.v.) in Britain. Bastian investigated aphasia and other speech defects, paralyses, and brain disorders. He objected to the confused use of the terms "hysterical" and "functional," and pointed out that they were not synonymous; he regarded hysteria (q.v.) as a neurosis. He was interested also in the evolution of life and believed in the doctrine of spontaneous generation.
Bibliography: Haymaker, W., and Schiller, F. 1970. *The founders of neurology.* 2d ed.

BATH MENTAL DEFICIENCY COLONY. The first institution for fee-bleminded to be established in Britain. It was a private institution founded and maintained by two women, the Misses White, in Bath, England. It was opened in 1846 and could accommodate only a small number of defective children.
Bibliography: Barr, M. W. 1904. *Mental defectives.*

BATH OF SURPRISE. A sudden and totally unexpected plunge into cold water. Many medical authorities advocated this form of treatment, which was regarded as "efficacious in overcoming sensibility." Jean Esquirol (q.v.) explained that the patient was precipitated into a reservoir, a river, or the sea, and added "we can conceive the vivid impression the patient experiences, who falls unexpectedly into the water, with the fear of being drowned."
See also IMMERSION.
Bibliography: Esquirol, J.E.D. 1845. Reprint. 1965. *Mental maladies: a treatise on insanity.*

BATHORY, ELIZABETH(?-1614). A member of a noble Hungarian family that was notorious for its pathological cruelty. It was rumored that she preserved her great beauty by bathing in the blood of girls murdered for this purpose. She was brought to trial in 1610 and condemned to spend the rest of her life walled up in a tiny cell in the palace of Csejte. The allegations against her have never been adequately proven. She may have been a victim of the genetic disorder *erythropoietic protoporphyria*, which produces reddening of eyes and teeth and bleeding of the skin when exposed to light. It was then undiagnosed, and doctors treated it by keeping their patients in darkness and making them drink blood to replace the blood they lost. Elizabeth Bathory's case has connections with tales of werewolves (q.v.).
Bibliography: Baring-Gould, W. S. 1865. *Book of were-wolves.*

BATHS. At various times baths have been employed in the treatment of mental disorders. Mustard and other substances were often added to the water, which varied from extremely cold to very hot, according to the therapeutic fashion of the time.
Bibliography: Tuke, D. H. 1892. *A dictionary of psychological medicine.*

BATTEN, FREDERICK EUSTACE (1865-1918). An English neurologist. In 1903 he described a juvenile form of amaurotic familial idiocy (q.v.) in two members of a family who showed "cerebral degeneration with symmetrical changes in the maculae."
Bibliography: Schmidt, J. E. 1959. *Medical discoveries: who and when.*

BATTIE, WILLIAM (1703-1776). An English physician and classical scholar, born at Modbury in Devon, England and educated at Eton and Cambridge. His first medical practice was in Cambridge, where he was also an anatomy demonstrator for the university. After moving to London, he became a Fellow of the Royal College of Physicians. In 1742 his interest in psychiatry (q.v.) caused him to pay £50 for election to the board of governors of the Bethlem Royal Hospital (q.v.). In 1751 he founded Saint Luke's Hospital for Lunatics (q.v.) and became its first physician. This venture was followed by the acquisition of a house in Islington Road, London, where he treated his private patients, and a madhouse in Wood's Close, that had previously belonged to James Newton (q.v.).

Battie's personal qualities did much to raise the status of psychiatry as a profession, and his reforms improved treatment and conditions in the hospitals. He advocated research into the causes and effects of madness, first-hand experience for students, and special training courses for the "servants" (mental nurses) in the institutions. His passionate belief in his own methods led to notorious public wrangling with John Monro (q.v.), the superintendent of the Bethlem Royal Asylum, who, with Battie, was the leading psychiatrist of his day. In 1764 Battie was elected president of the Royal College of Physicians, a reflection of the esteem in which he was held as he was the first and only psychiatrist to hold that office. His published work included editions of the works of Isocrates and Aristotle (q.v.), a treatise on physiology, aphorisms on medical practice, and his famous *Treatise on Madness* (q.v.) published in 1758. This treatise did much to further progress of psychiatry by denouncing old methods and advocating a more rational approach to the problems of insanity. Endowed with a keen sense of humor, Battie was also a shrewd business man who made good use of his success. He died a rich man.
Bibliography: Hunter, R., and Macalpine I., eds. 1962. *A psychiatric controversy of the eighteenth century.*

BATTUS (550-530 B.C.). A king of Cyrene. He was lame and afflicted with stammering. The term *battarismus*, meaning stammering or the babbling of an imbecile, is derived from his name.
Bibliography: Tuke, D. H. 1892. *A dictionary of psychological medicine.*

BAUBLE. The fool's (q.v.) emblem; a short stick decorated with ass's ears and ribbons and carried by court jesters. It was carried sometimes by beggars feigning insanity.
See also TOM O'BEDLAM.
Bibliography: 1978. *Brewer's dictionary of phrase and fable.* Ed. I. H. Evans.

BAUDELAIRE, CHARLES PIERRE (1821-1867). A French poet, born in Paris. As a student, he contracted venereal disease. His parents removed him from the university and sent him on a voyage to India but when he reached Mauritius he decided that he could not go through with the trip and returned home. The experience left a vivid impression on his mind and a nostalgic longing for the East. His life was dissolute and extravagant. He lived with Jeanne Duval, the mulatto woman he celebrated in the erotic poem *Black Venus*; *White Venus* and *Green-Eyed Venus* were similarly inspired by Madam Sabotier and Marie Daubrun. Baudelaire was addicted to hashish (q.v.) and opium (q.v.), which he took in enormous quantities. He regarded drug addiction as moral suicide (q.v.) but had no wish to break the habit. Of his many works, *Les Fleurs du Mal*, a collection of poems underlining the abnormal, the depraved, and the morbid is his most famous; the poems were banned in France for their obscenity. Richard von Krafft-Ebing (q.v.) described him as a masochist (*see* MASOCHISM) and sadist (*see* SADISM) in his *Psychopathia Sexualis*, but later studies have shown Baudelaire to be a hypersensitive, tortured, and self-destructive individual. He died in poverty and obscurity, a victim of syphilis (q.v.) and drugs.
Bibliography: Ruff, M. A. 1965. *Baudelaire*, trans. A. Kertesz.

BAYEZID (BAJAZET) II (1447-1513). An Arab sultan responsible for several fine buildings, including a mental hospital in Adrianopolis, erected in 1500. The hospital was surrounded by gardens and fountains, and the patients were treated by special diets, perfumed baths (q.v.), drugs, and music therapy (q.v.), which was played on specially tuned instruments. It was an example of the enlightened views of the Arabs (q.v.) towards the mentally ill.
Bibliography: Galdston, I., ed. 1967. *Historic derivations of modern psychiatry.*

BAYLE, ANTOINE LAURENTE JESSÉ (1799-1858). A French physician. In his doctoral thesis, written in 1822, he correlated the mental symptoms of progressive dementia with paralytic manifestations, thus demonstrating conclusively that some mental derangements have organic causes. His work was an important breakthrough in neuropsychiatry. As a result of his work, general paralysis of the insane (q.v.) in France is often referred to as "la maladie de Bayle." His *Traité de maladies du cerveau et des ses membranes* was published in Paris in 1826.
Bibliography: Zilboorg, G. 1941. *A history of medical psychology.*

BAYLE, FRANÇOIS (1662-1709). A French physician and a member of the Lanternistes (q.v.). He had an excellent reputation as a clinician and a teacher. In 1681 the parliament of Toulouse, with great enlightenment for that time, asked him to examine a woman accused of witchcraft (q.v.). On inquiry, Bayle found that the woman had been roaming aimlessly, dancing and talking to herself and attracting so much attention that a crowd had followed her to a church. There she had undressed and had danced in a frenzy until she had collapsed in a convulsion. Some of the women in the crowd then imitated her and claimed that the devil spoke through them. Bayle, after examining the woman, reported that she was not possessed, nor were the other women victims of demoniac possession (q.v.). He stated that all those involved in the affair would recover if they were sent somewhere peaceful, where demonic possessions and witchcraft were not topics of interest.
Bibliography: Semelaigne, R. 1930. *Les pionniers de la psichiatrie française.*

BAZZI, GIOVANNI ANTONIO DE' (1477-1549). An eccentric Italian painter, nicknamed Sodoma because of his vices. Giorgio Vasari, in his *Lives of the Artists,* wrote that Bazzi was

a merry and licentious man who kept others diverted and amused by leading a life of scant chastity, in consequence of which—and because he always surrounded himself with boys and beardless youths whom he loved beyond measure—he acquired the nickname of Sodoma. This not only failed to trouble or anger him, but he took pride in it, making stanzas and satirical poems on it which he sang very prettily to his lute. Apart from this he delighted in having in his house many kinds of extraordinary animals. . . .
Bibliography: Wittkower, R., and Wittkower, M. 1963. *Born under Saturn.*

BEARD, GEORGE M. (1839-1883). An American psychiatrist, born in Montville, Connecticut. He introduced the term *neurasthenia* (q.v.) and explained it in a paper entitled "Neurasthenia or Nervous Exhaustion," published by the *Boston Medical and Surgical Journal* in 1869. For some time, Neurasthenia was referred to as "Beard's disease" and was attributed to a toxic state of the nervous system. Beard was a pioneer in pointing out the importance of emotion on the aetiology, course, and outcome of disease, and in advocating the use of psychotherapy (q.v.). His paper "The Influence of Mind in the Causation and Cure of Disease and the Potency of Definite Expectation," presented in New York in 1876, was considered very controversial.
Bibliography: Schneck, J. M. 1975. United States of America. In *World history of psychiatry,* ed. J. G. Howells.

BEATTIE, JAMES (1735-1803). A Scottish poet and philosopher, best remembered for his poem *The Minstrel*, which anticipated Romanticism (q.v.).
His mind became permanently deranged following the death of his eldest
and favorite son. His physicians diagnosed dementia with paralysis.
Bibliography: Forbes, M. 1902. *Beattie and his friends.*

BEAUCHAMP, CHRISTINE (1875-?). A patient of Morton Prince (q.v.).
Following psychological traumas in childhood and adolescence, she developed a number of psychosomatic symptoms. When Prince was consulted
about these, he chose to use hypnosis (*see* HYPNOTISM) in her treatment.
She was an easy subject to hypnotize, and under hypnosis, revealed a number
of different personalities quite at variance from her waking self. Prince
eventually managed to fuse these multiple personalities. The patient married,
and the rest of her life seems to have been uneventful.
Bibliography: Prince, M. 1906. *Dissociation of a personality.*

BEAUNIS, HENRI E. (1830-1921). A physiologist and psychologist, born
in Amboise, France. He was professor of physiology at the University of
Nancy. With the help of Alfred Binet (q.v.), Beaunis founded the first French
laboratory of physiological psychology in 1889 at the Sorbonne. He also
wrote notes on military medicine covering the years 1871 to 1872 and textbooks on physiology. He studied both the psychology of dreams (q.v.) and
hypnotism (q.v.) and opposed the concepts of Jean Martin Charcot (q.v.).
He was an exponent of the School of Nancy (q.v.). In 1895 and again with
Binet he founded the first French journal of psychology *L'Année psychologique* (q.v.).
Bibliography: Watson, R. I. 1974. *Eminent contributors to psychology*, vol. 1.

BECCARIA, CESARE BONESANA DI (1738-1794). An Italian economist and jurist who held enlightened views on suicide (q.v.). He advocated
prevention of crime by education and condemned capital punishment, torture, and confiscation.
Bibliography: Rosen, G. 1971. History in the study of suicide. *Psychol. Med.* 1:
267-85.

BECK, SAMUEL JACOB (1896-   ). A psychologist born in Tecuciu,
Romania. He was educated in the United States at Harvard and Columbia
universities and became head of the psychology laboratory at the Michael
Reese Hospital in Chicago, Illinois. His well-known work on schizophrenia
(q.v.) was based on Rorschach (q.v.) studies, and his name is associated
with that test. He developed the test and published the first research work
on the Rorschach in the United States.
Bibliography: Beck, S. 1965. *Psychological processes in the schizophrenic adaptation.*

BEDDOES, THOMAS LOVELL(1803-1847). An English poet and physician, who lived mostly in Europe, where he participated in liberal political movements. His writings were inclined toward the macabre and the supernatural. He found it difficult to come to terms with reality as shown in his poem *Dream Pedlary* in which he wrote, "If there were dreams to sell, what would you buy?" His main work was *Death's Jest-Book*, which was altered many times and finally published posthumously. In it he referred to an attempted suicide (q.v.) with beautiful simplicity: "It was his choice; and why should he be breathing Against his will?" Beddoes committed suicide in Basel, Switzerland.
Bibliography: Snow, R. H. 1928. *Thomas Lovell Beddoes: eccentric and poet.*

BEDLAM. A corruption of Bethlem the derivation of Bethlem Royal Hospital (q.v.). The term is used to indicate any madhouse or any form of pandemonium and wild excitement.
Bibliography: 1978. *Brewer's dictionary of phrase and fable.* Ed. I. H. Evans.

BEDLAM POEMS. Poetry dealing with Bethlem Royal Hospital (q.v.) and its inmates. Many such writings appeared in the eighteenth century. They usually reflected the popular concepts of madness and described the building, the patients, and their symptoms. Almost all of them concluded with an exhortation to the reader who wished to avoid sharing the fate of the Bedlam patients. A perfect example is *Bedlam: A poem 1776* written by the Reverend Thomas Fitzgerald (1695-1752).
Bibliography: Hunter, R., and Macalpine, I. 1963. *Three hundred years of psychiatry.*

BEECHER, HENRY KNOWLES(1904-   ). A distinguished American physician and educator, born in Wichita, Kansas. His work has been in the field of anesthesia with particular regard to placebo (q.v.) reactions.
Bibliography: Beecher, H. K. 1959. *Measurement of the subjective response.*

BEERS, CLIFFORD W. (1876-1943). An American businessman, born in New Haven, Connecticut. As an undergraduate at Yale University, he was much affected by the sudden onset of epilepsy (q.v.) in an older brother. Eventually an obsessional fear of epilepsy dominated his life, and at the age of twenty-four he attempted suicide (q.v.) by jumping out of a fourth-floor window. Although his physical injuries were minor, his mental breakdown was complete and required his admission to a mental hospital. He spent three years in institutions. On recovery, the harsh treatment he had received caused him to devote his life to the improvement of conditions in mental hospitals. His autobiographical book *The Mind that Found Itself* (1908) did much to forward a program of reforms and led to the organization in 1909

of the National Committee for Mental Hygiene, later called National Association for Mental Health (q.v.).
Bibliography: Deutsch, A. 1949. *The mentally ill in America.*

BEETHOVEN, LUDWIG VAN (1770-1827). A German composer. His father was an alcoholic (*see* ALCOHOLISM) whose ruthless determination to present him as a child prodigy made him miserable and frustrated. Beethoven may have harbored the illusion that he was the illegitimate child of a royal personage out of rejection of his father. He eventually became established in Vienna, but his arrogance, bad manners, and unkempt appearance hindered social acceptance, although his music was received enthusiastically. He had a number of inconclusive love affairs with his pupils. His health was never good and deafness added to his hypochondriasis (q.v.) and his bouts of depression, which were aggravated by family troubles. His nephew and ward, Karl, caused him great anxiety by his way of life and his attempted suicide (q.v.). Beethoven's persistent gastric disorders may have had a psychic aetiology, and he, himself, attributed the beginnings of his deafness to having thrown himself on the floor in a rage when a tenor, who wanted his notes changed, kept interrupting his work. In his final years Beethoven was extremely isolated, and excessive drinking in the company of social inferiors became his refuge from anguish. The extreme contrasts in his personality are reflected in his work, which is full of emotion ranging from delight to despair. He named the final movement of his sixth string quartet *La Malinconia*, Italian for sadness, a term which was then employed in psychiatry to denote manic-depressive disorders.
Bibliography: Solomon, M. 1978. *Beethoven.*

BEHAN, BRENDAN (1923-1964). Irish writer and playwright. At the age of sixteen he was arrested in England as a terrorist for the Irish Republican Army and became an inmate of a Borstal institution (q.v.) in Hollesley Bay, Suffolk, England, before his deportation at the age of nineteen. He used this experience as the basis of his autobiographical work *Borstal Boy* (1958). The book is an entertaining, compassionate, and revealing account of the institutional management of delinquents. A lifelong alcoholic, he died of alcoholism (q.v.) and diabetes when he was forty-one years old.
Bibliography: Jeffs, Rae. 1968. *Brendan Behan: man and showman.*

BEHAVIORISM. A term first used by John B. Watson (q.v.) in 1913 to indicate a school of psychology (q.v.) that took human behavior and activities as its subject matter, basing its observations on reflex reactions without reference to the mind.
Bibliography: Watson, J. B. 1930. *Behaviorism.* 2d ed.

BEKHTEREV, VLADIMIR M. (1857-1927). A psychologist, born in the Viatka Province (U.S.S.R.). He received his medical education at the Mil-

itary Academy of St. Petersburg (now Leningrad) in 1881; this was followed by study abroad, first in Germany in Wilhelm Wundt's (q.v.) laboratory, and then in Paris with Jean Martin Charcot (q.v.). On his return to Russia, he became director of the psychophysiological laboratory at Kazan and in 1907 founded the psychoneurological institute in Leningrad. He studied physiological phenomena in relation to hypnosis (*see* HYPNOTISM) and experimented in psychosurgery (q.v.). He contributed greatly to the knowledge of the anatomy and physiology of the brain by correlating the motor areas of the cerebral cortex with acquired learned movements. His systematic exposition of behaviourism (q.v.) may antedate the work of his contemporary Ivan P. Pavlov (q.v.). It established the theory of both normal and pathological reflexes. He was the first to use the term *reflexology*. He wrote a number of papers and books, among which are *Objective Psychology* (1910) and *General Principles of Humor Reflexology: An Introduction to the Objective Study of Personality* (1917), which was translated into English by A. Gerver in 1932. Toward the end of his life he became interested in parapsychology and thought suggestion.
Bibliography: Boring, E. G. 1950. *A history of experimental psychology.*

BELGIAN CAGE. A wooden cage on short posts. It was exhibited at the national fair held in Brussels in 1880. Its purpose was the restraint (q.v.) of insane patients, who could be fed by passing food through small openings in its framework.
Bibliography: Letchworth, W. P. 1889. *The insane in foreign countries.*

BELHOMME, J. E. (1800-1880). A French physician who advocated education for the mentally retarded. In 1835, he wrote an angry letter to the Academie des Sciences (q.v.), claiming that his own writings were not given enough prominence and that others took credit for his suggestions. He established a private asylum (q.v.) for paying patients. Philippe Pinel (q.v.) was a frequent visitor to it.
Bibliography: Belhomme, J. E. 1843. Reprint. 1924. *Essai sur l'idiote, propositions sur l'education des idiots, mise en rapport avec leur degré d'intelligence.*

BELL, SIR CHARLES (1774-1842). A scientist born in Edinburgh, Scotland, the son of an Episcopal clergyman. He became a leading anatomist, physiologist, and neurologist. In 1804 he went to London and taught anatomy in his own house. He also gave lectures to artists and was himself a gifted illustrator, who produced exquisite sketches for many of his works. He retired when he was sixty-two because he wanted to dedicate more of his time to research. His many discoveries, which were deduced from anatomy because he disliked vivisection, included the description of the separate functions of the sensory and motor nerves (Bell-Magendie law [q.v.]), the localization in the brain of the respiratory reflex, and a paralysis of the face

due to neuropathology (q.v.), which is now known as Bell's palsy. He wrote, among other works, *Anatomy of the Brain* in 1811 and *Nervous System of the Human Body* in 1830. The study of the higher nervous system through reflexology was much advanced by his work. He was considered a dandy, a man of many friends and a person of great generosity. He was held in such high international esteem that the French physiologist Roux is said to have dismissed his class of medical students without a lecture after a visit from him, saying, "You have seen Bell, that is enough."
Bibliography: Boring, E. G. 1950. *A history of experimental psychology.*

BELL, LUTHER V. (1806-1862). An American physician who qualified at the age of twenty and practiced in New Hampshire, where he also served on the legislature. He was instrumental in establishing a state asylum (q.v.) at Concord. In 1826 he became superintendent of the McLean Asylum (q.v.) in Somerville, Massachusetts. He retained that position for twenty years and caused many valuable structural alterations to be made in the hospital. Although he wrote on several clinical subjects, he is best remembered for his descriptions of a form of acute mania (q.v.) now known as Bell's disease. By his actions he influenced the movement for better conditions in insane asylums, and was much quoted by his friend, the reformer Dorothea Dix (q.v.). Bell was one of the original thirteen founders of the American Psychiatric Association (q.v.). In 1856 he resigned his post at the McLean Asylum because of illness. He subsequently volunteered in the Union Forces during the Civil War and died while serving as brigade surgeon with General Joseph Hooker.
Bibliography: Deutsch, A. 1944. *The mentally ill in America.*

BELLADONNA. The common name for *Atropa belladonna*, an hallucinogenic herb particularly associated with abnormal behavior. It is also called deadly nightshade or enchanter's nightshade, devil's herb, and Sodom's apple. The Greeks linked the term *atropa* with the name of Atropos, the third Fate who was responsible for cutting the thread of life. Hippocrates (q.v.) used it as a narcotic. In the ancient Norse language its name *dwale* meant trance or sleep. Roman priests drank it to induce frenzy before making sacrifices to Bellona, the goddess of war. In medieval times it was associated with witches (*see* WITCHCRAFT), and it was believed that the devil himself tended it. John Gerard (q.v.) warned against having such a dangerous plant in domestic gardens. The atropine in it causes enlargement of the pupils, which was once considered a mark of beauty. Its use by Italian women to enhance the beauty of their eyes led to its name, Belladonna, or beautiful woman.
Bibliography: Emboden, W. 1972. *Narcotic plants.*

BELLE VUE ASYLUM. A small asylum (q.v.) for about forty patients. It is a good example of the privately run institutions for the insane that were

common in England during the nineteenth century. Belle Vue Asylum was located in Ipswich, Suffolk, England and was opened on the Woodbridge Road in 1835, by James Shaw, surgeon. On his death his widow took charge of it.
Bibliography: 1885. *History gazetteer and directory of Suffolk.*

BELL-MAGENDIE LAW. A law that differentiates between sensory and motor nerves. It takes its name from the two workers who did independent investigations on sensory and motor nerves: the English physician Charles Bell (q.v.), who was first to write on it, and François Magendie (q.v.) of France, who later clarified the issue.
Bibliography: Watson, R. I. 1963. *The great psychologists.*

BELMONT HOSPITAL. A neurosis (q.v.) hospital, still functioning in Surrey, England. It began in 1853 as a workhouse for vagrant children; fifty years later it became a workhouse for men and a colony for epileptics. The paupers were harshly treated. A diet of bread and water and confinement was common punishment for trivial misdemeanours and eventually led to riots. During World War I, the institution held prisoners of war and in 1928 it became a rehabilitation training center. In anticipation of an increase in neurotic disorders during World War II, it was converted into a neurosis unit.
Bibliography: Hospital brochure. 1973. *Belmont Hospital, 1853-1973.*

BENDER, LAURETTA (1897-   ). A leading American neuropsychiatrist well known for her work in child psychiatry (q.v.). She devised the Visual Motor Gestalt Test. The use of puppets to reenact traumatic events is a feature of her work with children. She has contributed to research in childhood schizophrenia (q.v.) and brain damage.
Bibliography: Bender, L. 1952. *Child psychiatry techniques.*

BENEDICT, RUTH (1887-1948). An American social anthropologist. In her work she demonstrated how every culture has an ideological pattern, which not only determines the social functioning of the group and the way in which children are brought up but also influences mental development.
Bibliography: Benedict, R. 1952. *Patterns of culture.*

BENEDICT OF NURSIA, SAINT (A.D. 480?-?543). The founder of the oldest monastic order in Western Europe. He laid the foundation of the monastery of Monte Cassino in southern Italy and formulated strict rules for the monks, stating, "the care of the sick is to be placed above and before every other duty. . . . the infirmarian must be thoroughly reliable, known for his piety and diligence, solicitous for his charges." His prescription

BENIGN STUPORS / 87

envisaged the physical and psychological care of the sick that became the basis of hospital medicine in the Middle Ages (q.v.).
Bibliography: MacKinnzy, L. C. 1937. *Early medieval medicine.*

BENEDICTSSON, VICTORIA MARIA (1850-1888). A Swedish novelist who used the pseudonym Ernst Ahlgren. Her unhappy marriage to a village postmaster is said to have been responsible for her mental breakdown and subsequent lifelong neurosis. She left Sweden and lived in Copenhagen, supporting herself by writing. She became the mistress of Georg Brandes (1842-1927), but the relationship did not change her outlook on life. She committed suicide in Copenhagen. Her best known works are *Fran Skåne* (1884) and *Fru Marianne* (1887).
Bibliography: Blankner, F. 1938. *The history of Scandinavian literature.*

BENEDIKT, MORITZ (1835-1920). A Viennese physician who made many contributions to neurology (q.v.)., criminology, electrotherapy, and dynamic psychiatry (q.v.). He emphasized the importance of the inner life of the individual and corrected the erroneous belief that hysteria (q.v.) was linked to disease of the uterus (q.v.) by describing cases of hysteria in males and correlating them to repressed or pathological sexual behavior. He termed the sexual instinct *libido* (q.v.) and believed that the pathogenesis of neuroses (*see* NEUROSIS) originated in "guilty secrets," which gave rise to physical symptoms.
Bibliography: Galdston, I., ed. 1967. *Historic derivations of modern psychiatry.*

BENEKE, FRIEDRICH EDUARD (1798-1854). A German psychologist and philosopher. His empirical approach to psychology (q.v.) shows the influence of the philosophical thought of his time. He was accused of epicureanism (*see* EPICURUS) because he proposed that ideas could be expressed by physical reactions. He differentiated men from animals by endowing them with "powers of the soul" or "faculties," a concept similar to the ego functions of present-day psychology. His works covered the fields of psychology, logic, ethics, and pedagogy. In *Lehrbuch der Psychologie als Naturwissenschaft* (1833), he linked psychology to natural science and insisted that it should have its own laws independent from other sciences.
Bibliography: Zilboorg, G. 1941. *A history of medical psychology.*

BENÊT. French term for an idiot or a possessed (*see* POSSESSION) person. It was derived from *eau benite* meaning "holy water," a reference to exorcism (q.v.) during which the possessed individual was sprinkled with holy water.
Bibliography: Tuke, D. H. 1892. *A dictionary of psychological medicine.*

BENIGN STUPORS. A term used by August Hoch (1868-1919) (q.v.) to indicate certain forms of manic-depressive psychoses (q.v.).
Bibliography: Zilboorg, G. and Henry, G. W. 1941. *A history of medical psychology.*

BENIVIENI, ANTONIO (c. 1440-1502). An Italian physician, surgeon, and anatomist. He stressed the importance of observation rather than theory in the practice of medicine. He gave a description of a girl suffering from the petit mal type of epilepsy.
Bibliography: Whitwell, J. R. 1936. *Historical notes on psychiatry.*

BENTHAM, JEREMY (1748-1832). An English philosopher and jurist, born in London. The eighteenth-century psychological theory of hedonism (q.v.) is associated with his name. His many books, usually on economic and legislative matters, brought about reforms in government and criminal law. Vote by secret ballot owes much to his theories. His essay on "Paederastry", which was written around 1785, is the first known argument for homosexual (*see* HOMOSEXUALITY) law reform in England. Unfortunately Bentham's anxiety about expressing his views in the light of eighteenth-century legal opinion prevented its publication. It finally was published in 1978.
Bibliography: Bentham, J. 1978. Offences against one's self: paederastry. *J. Homosex.* 3 and 4:389-405.

BENUSSI, VITTORIO (1878-1927). An Austrian experimental psychologist. He worked on the theory of perception and published his findings in about fifteen papers between 1902 and 1920. He was a pupil of Alexius Meinong (q.v.) and lived and worked in Graz for many years. He died in Padua, Italy.
Bibliography: Boring, E. G. 1950. *A history of experimental psychology.*

BEOBACHTUNGEN ÜBER DEN CRETINISMUS. The first journal entirely devoted to mental deficiency. It was founded by Heinrich K. Rösch (q.v.) as an organ of communication for workers in this field. The first issue, which appeared in 1850, was financed and edited at the Mariaberg Institution (q.v.). In 1851 and 1852 two more issues were published, containing reports of original investigations on cretinism (q.v.), descriptions of institutions for mental defectives, and claims for the curability of mental retardation. The journal came to an end after its third issue, because Rösch, the moving spirit behind the enterprise, emigrated to the United States following the political upheavals of 1848 in Germany.
Bibliography: Kanner, L. 1964. *A history of the care of the mentally retarded.*

BERDACHE. A term once used by the Sioux Indians of North America to describe a particular sexual role assigned by the medicine man, or shaman (q.v.), to a male adolescent who has revealed significant dreams. He dresses like a woman and is excused military activities, but, in spite of his sexual indifference to women, he is not necessarily a homosexual.

Bibliography: Erikson, E. H. 1939. Observations on Sioux education. *J. Psychol.* 7: 101-56.

BERENGARIO DA CARPI, JACOPO (1470-1550). An Italian surgeon, born in Carpi, near Modena. He studied medicine in Pavia and Bologna. He was accused of vivisection, but, in fact, his writings were based on observation of the human body during surgical operations. He wrote several books on anatomy, and his sketches of the anatomy of the brain illustrated the lateral ventricles and the formation of the choroid plexus, thus improving knowledge and correcting past mistakes. Benvenuto Cellini (q.v.) was under his care.
Bibliography: Castiglioni, A. 1946. *A history of medicine*, trans. and ed. E. B. Krumbhaar.

BERGASSE, NICOLAS (1750-1832). A French lawyer. He was a disciple of Franz Mesmer (q.v.) and edited those works of his that were published in France. He defended Mesmer from many attacks but finally quarrelled with him when Mesmer objected to Bergasse revealing ideas on animal magnetism (q.v.) in a treatise.
Bibliography: Tinterow, M. M. 1970. *Foundations of hypnosis: from Mesmer to Freud.*

BERGER, HANS (1873-1941). A German psychiatrist. He became an assistant to Otto Binswanger (q.v.) and eventually succeeded him in the chair of psychiatry (q.v.) at the University of Jena. He was the first to devise a method of measuring the electric activity of the brain in man. The first electroencephalogram (q.v.) was obtained by him in 1924, and the technique was announced in a paper published in 1929. Until the final result, he kept his research secret, and its importance was not realized until many years later. He was also interested in telepathy (q.v.) on which he often lectured. The rise of nazism in Germany depressed him intensely, and he eventually committed suicide by hanging.
Bibliography: Haymaker, W., and Schiller, F. 1970. *The founders of neurology.* 2d ed.

BERGGASSE 19. The Viennese residence of Sigmund Freud (q.v.). It was used as an ordinary apartment until it was restored as a memorial to Freud and as a center of information, education, and research in psychoanalysis (q.v.). It was officially opened as a memorial in June 1971.
Bibliography: Freud, E., Freud, L., and Grubrich-Simitis, I. 1978. *Sigmund Freud.*

BERGIER, WILLIAM LE (*or* PASTOUREL) (?-1431). A young French shepherd who was used to stimulate enthusiasm in the French army in the same way as Joan of Arc (q.v.) did. He was said to have the stigmata (q.v.) of Saint Francis on his hands and feet and to experience visions during which

God advised him. Captured by the English, he was thrown into the Seine with his hands and feet tied. The chroniclers of his time wrote that he was insane.
Bibliography: Ireland, W. W. 1885. *The blot upon the brain: studies in history and psychology.*

BERGMANN, GUSTAV VON (1878-1955). A German physician. He believed that emotional illness was responsible for most duodenal ulcers.
Bibliography: Bergmann, G. von 1913. Ulcus duodeni und vegetatives Nervensystem. *Berliner Klinische Wchnschr.*, 50: 2374.

BERGSON, HENRI(1859-1941). A French philosopher. He studied the understanding of change in time and how the individual is conscious of the indivisible continuity of change. According to him, memory (q.v.) was not stored in the brain but was a psychical function. He thought that evolution and transmitted variations were dependent on the original impulse of life connected with psychological factors. In 1913 he was elected president of the London Society for Psychical Research.
Bibliography: Hanna, T., ed. 1962. *The Bergsonian heritage.*

BERIBERI. A disorder caused by vitamin B deficiency. It produces some mental symptoms, the most prominent of which are lassitude and depression. The term *beriberi* does in fact mean "I cannot." Its aetiology was not discovered until the twentieth century, and it is likely that some abnormal mental behavior in primitive cultures and antiquity was caused by it.
Bibliography: Goldenson, R. M. 1970. *The encyclopedia of human behavior.*

BERKELEY, GEORGE (1685-1753). A philosopher, born in Ireland of an English family. He matriculated from Trinity College in Dublin at the age of fifteen and fulfilled his early promise by becoming a brilliant philosopher. In 1705 he founded with friends a society for the discussion of the new philosophy of Robert Boyle (1627-1691), Isaac Newton (1642-1727), and John Locke (1632-1704). When he was still in his twenties, he developed a new principle, which he called subjective idealism. He presented it in his book *Essay towards a New Theory of Vision* (1709). In it he concluded that all knowledge is derived through the senses, a limited and subjective experience that does not give a true picture of the world. An unexpected inheritance from Esther Vanhomrigh, Swift's (q.v.) *Vanessa*, whom he had met only once, may have contributed to the more orthodox outlook of his later life. He traveled to England, France, and Italy. He planned a university in Bermuda for Indians, and after many delays he was granted a charter for it by George II. In 1734 he was made Bishop of Cloyne in County Cork, Ireland, but his longing for an academic life led him to Oxford where he died a year after his arrival.

Bibliography: Luce, A. A., and Jessop, T. E., eds. 1948-1951. *The works of George Berkeley.* 9 vols.

BERLIN, RUDOLF (1833-1897). A German ophthalmologist. In 1887 he described word blindness, which he termed *dyslexia* (q.v.).
Bibliography: Schmidt, J. E. 1959. *Medical discoveries: who and when.*

BERLIOZ, LOUIS HECTOR (1803-1869). A French composer, son of a physician. He was sent to Paris to study medicine, but anatomical dissections so repelled him that he abandoned the idea and turned to music as a profession. Following an unhappy love affair, he attempted suicide by taking a large dose of opium (q.v.). His love for the actress Harriet Smithson, whom he married in 1833, and his later disillusionment with her inspired the *Symphonie Fantastique*, subtitled *Episode in the Life of an Artist.* He invented the musical idée fixe (q.v.), a theme that is repeated in all movements of a composition and reflects almost an obsession (q.v.) with a given musical expression. Berlioz was as unconventional in musical composition as in his own behavior; he was moody and oversensitive; his life was punctuated with dramatic love affairs. At the height of some of them he would plan murder and suicide but was then content with less drastic solutions. His last years were sad and lonely, especially after the death of his only beloved son, Louis.
Bibliography: Harzun, J. 1951. *Berlioz and the romantic century.* 2 vols.

BERMANN, GREGORIO (1896-1972). An Argentinian psychiatrist. In the 1920s he introduced psychoanalytic techniques into Latin America. His interest in psychoanalysis (q.v.) led him to travel to Vienna to visit Sigmund Freud (q.v.). However, later in his clinical career he abandoned psychoanalysis. He wrote on paranoia (q.v.) and obsessive (*see* OBSESSION) states. In 1936 he founded the journal *Psicoterapia* and in 1950 was one of the founders of the Associacion Psiquiatrica de la America Latina, which brought together fourteen national psychiatric societies in Latin America.
Bibliography: Leon, C.A., and Rosselli, H. 1975. Latin America. In *World history of psychiatry*, ed. J. G. Howells.

BERNADETTE, SAINT (1844-1879). Born Bernadette Soubirous in Lourdes, France. She was the eldest child of a poor miller. She was undersized, sickly, and slow-witted. Her visions at the age of fourteen gave rise to the shrine of the Virgin Mary at Lourdes (q.v.). Her claims that she could see and hear the Virgin Mary caused an epidemic of visionaries in the region and led to her admission to a convent to shelter her from publicity. A lifelong asthmatic, she would remark that she was "getting on with the job of being ill." She was canonized in 1933 for her simple and humble faith rather than for her visions.

Bibliography: Trochu, Francis. 1957. *Saint Bernadette Soubirous 1844-1879*, trans. J. Joyce.

BERNARD, CLAUDE (1813-1878). A French physiologist. He investigated chemical phenomena of the body and the function of the sympathetic nervous system and won the grand prize of the Academie des Sciences (q.v.) three times. He considered organisms and environment integrated in a global environment, thus anticipating the transactional approach. Alfred Adler (q.v.) was influenced by his ideas. *Introduction to the Study of Experimental Medicine*, published in 1865, is regarded as his main work. Bernard was the first scientist to be honored by a state funeral in France.
Bibliography: Zilboorg, G. 1941. *A history of medical psychology.*

BERNARD, PRUDENCE. A natural somnambulist (*see* SOMNAMBULISM) born in France. August Lassaigne (q.v.) saw her perform when she was eighteen years old. He was so impressed that he became converted to magnetism (q.v.) and married her. He said of her that "in waking state she is a woman, in somnambulism she is an angel"; he also compared her to Joan of Arc (q.v.), believing that her mission in life was to bring France back to the true faith. Despite her angelic qualities, her husband found it difficult to hypnotize her if they had quarrelled.
Bibliography: Lassaigne, A. 1851. *Mémoirs d'un magnétiseur, contenant la biographie de la somnambule Prudence Bernard.*

BERNFELD, SIEGFRIED (1892-1953). A pioneer of psychoanalysis (q.v.) born in Austria. Even as a student he was interested in psychological phenomena. He once hypnotized his younger brother and was terrified when he could not bring him back from the trance state. He employed scientific methods in the study of children's writings, and then wrote on education, behavior problems, Jewish culture, and the community life of young people. He also applied psychoanalytic theory to problems concerning child psychiatry (q.v.), especially in the educational field. In 1926, he settled in Berlin and worked at the Berlin Institute for Psychoanalysis. He was deeply interested in political issues and felt restless as a new social order spread through Europe. He left Germany for Austria, then went to France, and finally settled in the United States with his third wife, who was also his coworker. He regarded Sigmund Freud's (q.v.) work as final and wrote several papers tracing the origin of Freud's theories. He was the author of several books.
Bibliography: Alexander, F.; Eisenstein, S.; and Grotjahn, M., eds. 1966. *Psychoanalytic pioneers.*

BERNHEIM, HIPPOLYTE-MARIE (1837-1919). A French physician. He became interested in hypnosis (*see* HYPNOTISM) when he failed to cure a

patient of sciatica, and a country doctor, Ambroise-August Liébeault (q.v.), succeeded, using hypnosis. He became Liébeault's pupil in 1882, the same year in which Jean Martin Charcot (q.v.) convinced the Académie des Sciences (q.v.) that hypnosis was an hysterical (*see* HYSTERIA) manifestation. Bernheim disagreed with Charcot and believed that hypnosis could be induced in most people and used in therapy. He emphasized the role of suggestion. His ideas were accepted by the Nancy School (q.v.) and hypnotism became a recognized form of treatment for the neuroses (*see* NEUROSIS). His experiments with post-hypnotic suggestion and his work in general greatly influenced Sigmund Freud (q.v.). The term "psychobiology" (q.v.) was first used by Bernheim.
Bibliography: Ellenberger, H. F. 1970. *The discovery of the unconscious.*

BERNINI, GIANLORENZO (1598-1680). An Italian sculptor, painter, and architect of the Baroque period. His work shows a forceful psychological content that is especially noticeable in his marble group *The Rapture of St. Theresa*, which depicts a woman in a trancelike state of ecstasy (q.v.).
Bibliography: Hibbard, H. 1965. *Bernini.*

BERRYMAN, JOHN (1914-1972). An American poet. He was an alcoholic (*see* ALCOHOLISM), unstable and depressed, who, in his own words, "felt rotten about myself" in spite of his recognition and success. In 1970 he underwent a religious conversion to Catholicism, which seems to have added to his feelings of despair and his obsession that life was a series of delusions. His poems project an intense loneliness and despair, sometimes thinly covered by bravado. His father, whom he mourned throughout his life, shot himself when the poet was still a child. He, in turn, committed suicide (q.v.) by jumping from a bridge over the Mississippi. His last book of poems, *Delusions etc., of John Berryman*, appeared posthumously and reflects his turbulent emotional state.
Bibliography: Berryman, J. 1972. *Delusions, etc.*

BERSERK. A term of uncertain etymology; possibly from the Icelandic, meaning a strong and ferocious Norse warrior fighting in a frenzied rage. It may refer quite literally to the bear coat he wore. It sometimes is explained as a derivative of *baresark*, or bare shirt, alluding to one so enraged and careless of his own safety that he fights without armor.
Bibliography: 1970. *Oxford English dictionary.*

BERTALANFFY, LUDWIG VON (1901-1972). An Austrian biologist. In 1945, he proposed a general systems theory that was concerned with elucidating the basic general elements of a system that are applicable to all systems. He gave special attention to living systems, including psychiatry. In 1949 Bertalanffy emigrated to the United States, where he was professor

of theoretical biology at State University of New York at Buffalo. He was a founder member of the Center for Advanced Study in Theoretical Psychology and contributed to the field of psychiatry with many of his works. *General Systems Theory* (1968) was the last of his thirteen books, most of which have been translated into eight languages.
Bibliography: Bertalanffy, L. von. 1968. *General systems theory: foundation, development, applications.*

BERTRAND, ALEXANDRE. A French physicist. In the early nineteenth century he undertook an objective and systematic investigation of mesmerism (q.v.). He related facts about the first magnetizers. According to him, they experienced severe shocks from an electric discharger. Shocks that are now considered very mild so affected some of them that they had to spend two days in bed. Other physicists performed experiments so dangerous that they occasionally caused death.
Bibliography: Bertrand, A. 1832. *Traité du somnambulisme et des différentes modifications qu'il présente.*

BERTRUCCIO, NICCOLŎ (?-1347). An Italian physician. He developed a simple classification of personality based on three qualities: imagination, or fancy, judgment, or thinking power, and memory or recollection. He was the author of a compendium and of commentaries on Hippocrates (q.v.) and Galen (q.v.). He used human dissections to describe the brain.
Bibliography: Whitwell, J. R. 1936. *Historical notes on psychiatry.*

BERYL. A precious stone. It was treasured during the Middle Ages (q.v.) and the Renaissance when it was believed to possess the power of protection against peril and the ability to quicken a man's intellect.
See also PRECIOUS STONES.
Bibliography: Evans, J. 1922. *Magical jewels.*

BESS O' BEDLAM. An Elizabethan term used to indicate a female mendicant posing as an inmate of Bethlem Royal Hospital (q.v.). It was a popular character in contemporary plays and literature.
See also TOM O' BEDLAM.
Bibliography: O'Donoghue, E. G. 1914. *The story of Bethlehem Hospital.*

BETA TESTS. A series of tests developed in the United States during World War I to assess the intelligence of illiterate recruits, who could not use the alpha tests (q.v.). The tests revealed 46,000 men of such low intelligence that they were considered untrainable and were discharged.
Bibliography: Yerkes, R. M., ed. 1921. Psychological examining in the United States Army. *Mem. Nat. Acad. Sci.* 15.

BETEL. The popular name of *Areca catechu* which is a masticatory stimulant, popular in the East since ancient times. It is made from the betel nut, betel leaves, lime, and other ingredients that vary from culture to culture.
Bibliography: Emboden, W. 1972. *Narcotic plants*.

BETHE, ALBRECHT (1872-1931). A German psychologist who suggested that the stereotyped behavior of such social insects as ants and bees indicated that they were robots. In 1898, he published the results of his research, querying whether psychic qualities should be ascribed to these insects whose actions he regarded as purely mechanistic. With Jacques Loeb (q.v.) he was one of the leaders of the mechanistic movement (*see* MECHANISTIC THEORIES) in psychology (q.v.).
Bibliography: Boring, E. G. 1950. *A history of experimental psychology*.

BETHEL COLONY FOR EPILEPTICS. A colony for epileptics (*see* EPILEPSY) established in 1867 near Bielefeld, Germany. It was organized to resemble as much as possible an ordinary community. It provided occupational and recreational activities for the patients, who were encouraged to live normal lives. Beginning as a small community, it grew into a large one consisting of many thousands of patients. The colony's success was observed with interest throughout the world and stimulated the foundation of many other similar institutions.
Bibliography: 1937-1940. Institutions for treatment and care of epilepsy in the different countries of the world. *Epilepsia*. 2d ser. 1: 105-13.

BETHEL HOSPITAL. The oldest standing mental hospital in England. It was founded in 1713 by Mary Chapman (q.v.) in the parish of Saint Peter Mancroft in the city of Norwich, England. In 1648 a house had stood on the same grounds and had been used by the Roundheads who ruled the city. During a Royalist attack ninety-six barrels of gunpowder stored within the buildings had exploded, wrecking it. On the same spot Bethel Hospital was built for "persons afflicted with lunacy or madness (nor such as are fools or idiots from their birth)." It remained under Mary Chapman's control until her death. At that time, trustees were appointed under the terms of her will and received "the sole power of appointing and ordering of Doctors, Apothecaries, and other persons whom they shall judge necessary to be employed in this Charity." In 1765 a charter of incorporation was granted to the trustees by George III (q.v.). The maximum number of patients ever housed in Bethel Hospital was seventy-five. From its beginnings, the hospital enjoyed a good reputation for using modern methods. Later, in keeping with its reputation, it accepted patients on payments scaled to their circumstances. It survives to this day as an annex to one of the regional mental hospitals.
Bibliography: Bateman, F., and Rye, W. 1906. *The history of the Bethel Hospital at Norwich*.

BETHLEHEMITES. A religious order of hospitallers. The order founded many hospitals throughout Europe in the thirteenth century. They were pledged to offer, in the words of Pope Innocent IV (q.v.), "shelter to the poor, the stranger, the pilgrim, and to Christians in any other afflictions." Bethlehemites looked after the sick and the insane in Bethlem Royal Hospital (q.v.). They wore a red star with a dark blue center on their habit, which suggests a connection with the red cross of the crusaders and the star of Bethlehem.
Bibliography: O'Donoghue, E. G. 1914. *The story of Bethlehem Hospital.*

BETHLEM ROYAL HOSPITAL. The first mental hospital in England. In 1247, Simon FitzMary donated land at Bishopsgate in London for the foundation of a priory, so that masses could be celebrated for the salvation of his soul. The priory also was to provide a place for the bishop and clergy of Bethlehem to stay when visiting London. (A wall plaque commemorates the fact that the original priory stood where Liverpool Street Railway Station is now.) It was functioning as a hospital in 1330. In 1346 the priory passed from the protection of the bishop to the protection of the City of London. In 1402, following complaints of misappropriation of funds, it was inspected, and it emerged that of its fourteen patients, six were *mente capti*, insane. In 1547 it was incorporated as a royal foundation, called the Hospital of St. Mary of Bethlehem, which was shortened to Bethlehem Hospital or Bethlem Hospital, for the care of lunatics. Its name, corrupted to Bedlam (q.v.), became synonymous with madhouse, and it is often mentioned in the plays and literature of the time, including the plays of William Shakespeare (q.v.). After the Great Fire of London in 1666, the hospital was moved in 1676 to a new building in Moorfields that had been designed by Robert Hooke (q.v.), a physician and architect. It was regarded as the most magnificent hospital building in Europe; its entrance was adorned with two sculptures by Caius Gabriel Cibber (q.v.) representing melancholy and raving madness. Visiting Bedlam became an accepted form of entertainment. Samuel Pepys, John Evelyn, Jonathan Swift, Samuel Johnson, and James Boswell (qq.v.) were among some of the visitors who went through the famous "Penny Gates" (q.v.). Edward Tyson (q.v.) was appointed as the first physician of the new hospital. In his time, 1,294 patients were treated there. Richard Hale (q.v.) followed him and was succeeded by James Monro (q.v.) and other members of the same family for about a century. At the beginning of the nineteenth century the hospital building was found to have deteriorated. It was surrounded by buildings rather than the open fields of two centuries ago. A new move became necessary and was accomplished in 1815, when the hospital moved to Lambeth Road in St. George's Field, Southwark. The new building was designed by J. Lewis. The porch with Ionic columns and the dome were designed by Sydney Smirke (1781-1867) in 1830. Many important advances in psychiatry (q.v.) were made at Bethlem, notwith-

standing its earlier reputation for patient ill-treatment. In 1920 that part of the building that still survived became the Imperial War Museum, and Bethlem was once more moved to new premises, which it still occupies, in Monks Orchard, Eden Park, Beckenham. It amalgamated with Maudsley Hospital in 1948 to form a single postgraduate teaching hospital. The London University institute of psychiatry is associated with it.
Bibliography: O'Donoghue, E. G. 1914. *The story of Bethlehem Hospital.*

BETHNAL HOUSE. A private madhouse in Bethnal Green, London. It housed several hundred pauper patients. Due to overcrowding and lack of proper supervision, conditions in the private asylums (q.v.) of the early nineteenth century deteriorated to the point where they were publicly denounced. The ensuing scandal forced the College of Physicians to take inspections more seriously and also led to the formation of the Metropolitan Commissioners in Lunacy in 1828. By 1844 Bethnal House, whose degradation had been directly instrumental in making these changes, had so improved that it was praised for the comfortable conditions it offered to its patients.
Bibliography: Gordon, S. and Cocks, T.G.B. 1952. The case of the White House at Bethnal Green. In *A people's conscience.*

BETONY. A plant that was recommended for preventing "monstrous nocturnal visions and . . . frightful visions and dreams" in the herbal of Apuleius Platonicus, which dates from the fifth century. It was also mentioned in the *Great Herbal*, published in England in 1526. It is listed there as beneficial for anxiety, and a mixture made of powdered betony and warm water and wine is suggested.
Bibliography: Rohde, E.S. 1974. *The old English herbals.*

BEXLEY HOSPITAL. A mental hospital in Kent, England, opened in 1898. Previously, Sir Hiram Maxin had lived in a house there and it was on the ground around it that he built, in 1894, a large flying machine, driven by steam, which achieved a limited powered flight some nine years before the Wright Brothers.

BEZOAR STONE. A calculous concretion found in the stomachs of certain ruminants. It was much used in medieval medicine in Europe. Robert Burton (q.v.) in his *Anatomy of Melancholy* (q.v.) claimed that it was taken from the "belly of little beast in the East Indies" and brought to England by merchants. According to him, the bezoar "hath special virtue against all melancholy affections" and that it takes away sadness, and makes him merry that useth it." The stone is still used in Malaya, where it is called *batu gulliga.*
Bibliography: Haggard, H. W. 1976. *Devils, drugs, and doctors.*

BHAGAVAD-GITA. A Sanskrit poem of 700 verses inset in the Mahabharata epic and written sometime between the sixth and fourth century B.C. In the *Gita* the mind is conceived of as a field containing opposing drives. Mental functions are divided into *jnana* (cognition), *karma* (conation) and *bhakti* (affect). Methods for attaining mental calmness are described as well as personality types and what could be called psychotherapy (q.v.). Depression and anxiety are described in the early parts of the Gita.
Bibliography: Venkoba Rao, A. 1975. India. In *World history of psychiatry*, ed. J. G. Howells.

BHANG. The Indian name for Cannabis sativa (q.v.), Indian hemp, or marijuana.
Bibliography: *Everyman's encyclopedia*. 1978. Ed. Girling, D.A.

BIANCHI, LEONARDO (1848-1927). An Italian psychiatrist and neurologist. He reorganized psychiatric services in Naples. His work included research in the semiology of the nervous system, hemiplegia, and cerebral localization of brain diseases. In 1920, his experiments on monkeys demonstrated that the bilateral destruction of the frontal lobes causes character changes.
Bibliography: Mora, G. 1975. Italy. In *World history of psychiatry*, ed. J. G. Howells.

BIATHANATOS. A work by John Donne (q.v.) posthumously published in 1644. It deals with suicide (q.v.) and is subtitled *A Declaration of that Paradoxe or Thesis that Self-Homicide is not so Naturally Sinne that It may Never be Otherwise.* Donne argued that not all those who die by their own hands are terrible sinners, condemned to eternal damnation, but rather people who, at the time of their suicide, have a "propensnesse" for it and are emotionally sick. He warned that "many and severe laws against an offence" do not necessarily indicate the enormity of an unlawful act.
Bibliography: Donne, John. 1644. Reprint. 1930. *Biathanatos.*

BIBLE. The Bible contains numerous examples of interest to psychiatry. The Hebrews regarded insanity as a manifestation of possession (q.v.) by evil spirits, or as a sign of God's will: "On that day, says the Lord, I will strike every horse with panic and its rider with madness" (Zech. 12:4), or "he shall smite thee with madness, and blindness and astonishment of heart" (Deut. 28:28). In the Old Testament Saul, David, and Nebuchadnezzar (qq.v.) serve as examples of abnormal personalities. There are still more references to abnormal behavior and hysteria (q.v.) in the New Testament: tormented (Matt. 4:24), hysterical paralysis (Matt. 9:2); hysterical mutism for eight days (Luke 1:20,64); hysterical mutism (Matt. 9:32); hysterical blindness and mutism (Matt. 12:22); and madness or possession by devils (Matt. 8:28 and Mark 9:17). Treatment was by exorcism (q.v.): Jesus cast out the devil from two possessed men and transformed the spirits that tormented them into pigs that madly rushed over the cliffs into a lake and destroyed themselves (Matt. 8:28; Mark 5:1-13; Luke 8:26-33). A form of music therapy (q.v.) is also mentioned: David playing the lyre for Saul. There are at least two references to mechanical restraint (q.v.): Jeremiah (29:26) and Mark (5:2-4). Epilepsy (q.v.) is referred to in the Old Testament: the son of Beor (Num. 24:4, et seq.) fell into a trance, saw visions, and heard the words of God. In the New Testament (Acts 9:3) there is the case of Saul, who, on the road to Damascus, had a fit with a visual aura, loss of consciousness, hallucinations (q.v.) and postepileptic stupor. Another patient, a child, was apt to fall into fire or water as a consequence of his epilepsy (Matt. 27:15). The cases of two other children are reported in Luke (9:38) and Mark (9:17). Other psychological symptoms or effects that can be found in the Bible include: hyperemotionalism (Gen. 27:34); emotional disorder causing repression or temporary impotence (Gen. 20:1-18); hydrophobia (Lev. 26:22); psychopathological graying of hair (Lev. 48:1-2); effects of good news (Gen. 48:1-2); epilepsy (Gen. 17:3); stuttering (Ex. 4:10, 6:12); hallucinations (q.v.) (Lev. 26:36-37); and glossolalia (q.v.) (Acts 2:1-4). Pharaoh's dream (q.v.) (Gen. 41) has provided a great deal of interesting material for psychoanalysts and dream interpreters. In the Old Testament there are five instances of suicide (q.v.): Saul, his armor bearer, Achithophel, Zimri (q.v.), and Samson (q.v.). The one instance of suicide in the New Testament is Judas Iscariot (q.v.). (For specific information concerning individuals in the Bible, look under the name of the individual.) Bibliography: Wise, C. A. 1956. *Psychiatry in the Bible*.

BIBLIOMANIA. An obsessive (*see* OBSESSION) and unreasonable love of collecting books. One bibliomane, a Spanish scholar by the name of Don Vicente, even committed murder to obtain a book he wanted. John Ferriar (q.v.), in a poem entitled *Bibliomania* (1809) wrote:

What wild desire, what restless torments seize
The hapless man, who feels the book-disease.
Bibliography: Hunter R., and Macalpine, I. 1963. *Three hundred years of psychiatry, 1535-1860*. 1963.

BIBLIOTHERAPY. Celsus (q.v.) was one of the earlier authors to suggest reading as therapy for mental patients. Books, he said, could be read correctly or incorrectly, if the latter the patient will benefit from correcting his method. Recitation was recommended, as well as the memorization of passages, which was thought to fix the patients' attention on a subject. Shakespeare thought that books could "beguile sorrow" (*Titus Andronicus*, 4, i).

In the late eighteenth century, Benjamin Rush (q.v.) advocated bibliotherapy for mental patients, and in the nineteenth century John M. Galt (q.v.) wrote about it in his textbook on the treatment of insanity, making theoretical and practical suggestions for its use in asylums.

Bibliography: Schneck, J. M. 1950. Bibliotherapy in neuropsychiatry. In *Occupational therapy*, ed. W. R. Dunton, Jr., and S. Licht.

BICÊTRE. A French institution for the mentally ill located in Paris. The name is a corruption of Wicestre, which in turn originates from the bishop of Winchester, Jean de Pontoise, who in 1285 built a castle on the spot where the hospital is now. The castle became the property of the king in 1346 and was burned down during the uprising of 1411. The ruins became a place of evil repute. Louis III rebuilt it as an institution for invalid soldiers and considerably enlarged it. In 1656 Louis XIV, the Sun King, transformed it into a general hospital. It became a combination of hospital and prison, housing beggars, criminals, youths of debauched habits (who were regularly fumigated [*see* FUMIGATION] for their syphilis [q.v.]), the chronically ill, and old people with nowhere to go. By 1792 it was more or less exclusively used as a custodial institution for male lunatics, while females lunatics were kept at Salpêtrière (q.v.). The inmates were subjected to a repressive regimen: they were heavily chained and shackled by irons to the wall or the floor. The attendants, who were often convicts, kept them in order by brute force and did not hesitate to use the whip on them. As a result of this treatment, the inmates often rebelled and occasionally even murdered their keepers. The word *Bicêtre* came to mean misfortune or one diabolically wicked. By 1793, when Philippe Pinel (q.v.) was appointed as physician in charge, the institution had the reputation of being one of the worst in the world. Pinel decided to change its dreadful image. He unchained fifty-three patients and reduced all mechanical restraint (q.v.) to a minimum. Daily rounds and clinical observation of the patients replaced the old methods. Victor Hugo (q.v.) referred to the institution in *Les Misérables*.

Bibliography: Semelaigne, R. 1930-1932. *Les pionniers de la psychiatrie Française avant et après Pinel*, vol. 1 and 2.

BICHAT, MARIE FRANÇOIS XAVIER (1771-1802). A French anatomist and physiologist born in Thoriette, France. He was one of the founders of the Society of Medicine, which began in 1799. A pioneer in scientific histology, he identified without the benefit of a microscope twenty-one types of tissue. In fact, he introduced the term *tissue* to describe living matter. According to him, the body had two systems, the vegetative and the animal. The vegetative system dealt with assimilation and growth; the animal system dealt with the body's relations with its environment. He stated that the two systems "are in inverse ratio of development in ontogenetic evolution — the greater the development of the vegetative system, the less developed is

the system of relation," which is now known as the Law of Bichat. He suggested that perception, memory (q.v.), and intellect were located in the brain and the emotions in the viscera.
Bibliography: Boring, E. G. 1950. *A history of experimental psychology.*

BIEDL, ARTHUR (1869-1933). A German physician. He described in detail a syndrome that combines obesity, sexual underdevelopment, retinitis pigmentosa, mental deficiency, and other abnormalities. It had been described previously by John Zachariah Laurence (1830-1874) and R.C. Moon. Thus, it is referred to as the Laurence, Moon, Biedl syndrome.
Bibliography: Schmidt, J. E. 1959. *Medical discoveries: who and when.*

BIELSCHOWSKY, MAX (1869-1940). A German neurologist. He discovered silver impregnation of nerve fibers and published his findings on the cytoarchitecture of the cerebral cortex as well as various studies on neurological disorders.
Bibliography: Haymaker, W., and Schiller, F. 1970. *The founders of neurology.* 2d ed.

BIENVILLE, M.D.T. DE (1726-1813). A French physician who lived and worked in Holland. He believed that the uterus (q.v.) was genetically significant in mental disorders and that repressed, unsatisfied, and excessive sexual needs led to depression and then to mania. The treatment he suggested included bleeding (q.v.) and a diet (q.v.) that excluded rich foods and beverages. In 1771 he published a book, *La nymphomanie, ou traité de la fureur utérine,* in which he presented his ideas on the link between "immoderate cupidity" and mental disorders. The book, which was popular, was translated into a number of languages. Dr. Edmond S. Wilmot translated it into English in 1785.
Bibliography: Hunter, R., and Macalpine, I. 1963. *Three hundred years of psychiatry.*

BILE. A humor (q.v.) of the body.
See also BLACK CHOLER.

BILFINGER, GEORG BERNHARD (1693-1750). A German philosopher, mathematician, and physicist. Unlike Gottfried W. Leibniz (q.v.) he thought that monads, Leibniz's units of force, are not both spiritual and physical, but either one or the other. He believed that the term "divine harmony" refers only to the relationship between soul and body, rather than to harmony within the universe.
Bibliography: 1971. *Encyclopedia Brittanica.*

BILO. A term used in Madagascar to cover a therapeutic rite. The patient exhibits symptoms of restlessness and overanxiety; his treatment consists of prolonged festivities, sometimes lasting over two weeks, during which he is treated as a king and great deference is shown to him. At the end of the period the patient drinks the blood of an ox that has been sacrificed to him. At this point, the ego boosting he has received from the festivities is supposed to have cured him; an added incentive to be cured is the fact that if he is not cured, he is badly regarded by the community, which may even expel him.

Bibliography: Ellenberger, H. F. 1970. *The discovery of the unconscious.*

BINET, ALFRED (1857-1911). A French psychologist, born in Nice. In 1889, he founded the first French psychological laboratory at the Sorbonne, and from 1894 until his death he was its director. Binet's early studies on hypnotism (q.v.) were published in his first book *The Psychology of Reasoning* (1886), which is an exposition of abnormal psychology (q.v.). He later investigated a wider field that included studies on sensibility, optical illusion, arithmetical prodigies, famous chess (q.v.) players, changes in personalities, intellectual weariness, and suggestibility. He used his two daughters as subjects for experimentation in mental testing. He promoted interest in human intellectual capacities and stressed individual differences. With Theodore Simon (q.v.) he developed the well-known Binet-Simon scale (q.v.). He was one of the founders of *L'année Psychologique* (q.v.), the first French periodical on psychology. His best-known works include *Studies in Psychology* (1888); *Changes in Personality* (1892); and *Thoughts about Children* (1900).

Bibliography: Watson, R. I. 1965. *The great psychologists.*

BINET-SIMON SCALE. A series of graded tests of intelligence. In 1904 the French minister of public instruction asked Alfred Binet (q.v.) to devise a test that would differentiate between normal and subnormal children. Between 1905 and 1911 in collaboration with Theodore Simon (q.v.), Binet developed three scales by which judgment, ability to abstract, comprehension, and reasoning could be assessed and correlated to age levels. The tests have been accepted throughout the world and translated into many languages.

Bibliography: Binet, A., and Simon, T. 1915. *A method of measuring the development of the intelligence of young children,* trans. C. H. Town.

BINGGELI, JOHANNES. The Swiss founder of a nineteenth-century sect called Forest Brotherhood. His religion advocated sexual intercourse, especially with Binggeli, as the prescribed treatment for all illnesses. He distributed his own urine among his followers, who used it medicinally. In 1896 he was tried for incest (q.v.) after his own daughter became pregnant following the treatment he had administered. His sentence was served in an asylum because it was found that his actions were the consequence of a disordered mind.

Bibliography: Camp, J. 1973. *Magic and myth in medicine.*

BINSWANGER, OTTO (1852-1929). A German psychiatrist and professor at Jena University. He contributed important histological studies to the field of brain anatomy and devised new methods of examining pathological changes in brain diseases. He also conducted research in neurosis (q.v.), progressive paralysis, and epilepsy (q.v.). Hans Berger (q.v.) was one of his assistants and succeeded him as professor.
Bibliography: Haymaker, W., and Schiller, F. 1970. *The founders of neurology.* 2d ed.

BION, WILFRED RUPRECHT (1897-1979). A psychoanalyst born in India of British parents. His psychiatric training in England was influenced by the work of Sigmund Freud (q.v.) and Carl G. Jung (q.v.). He completed his training by studying psychoanalysis (q.v.) with Melanie Klein (q.v.). He became an authority in group relations, and his work in this field, described in his book *Experience in Groups,* which now is regarded as a classic, has played an important part in the training of psychotherapists. He was director of the London Clinic of Psycho-Analysis and president of the British Psycho-Analytical Association.
Bibliography: Bion, W. R. 1961. *Experience in groups.*

BIRCH, JOHN (1745?-1815). A British surgeon at Saint Thomas Hospital in London, where he founded an electric department. He used electricity (q.v.) in the treatment of depressed patients. A special apparatus was made for him by George Adams, a famous instrument maker, and using this, Birch applied electric currents to the heads of his patients and "passed shocks through the brain." His success was somewhat variable, but his reports, included in Adams' book, provide the earliest accounts of depression treated by direct application of electricity to the head.
Bibliography: Adams, George. 1799. *An essay on electricity, explaining the principles of that useful science; and describing the instruments.* 5th ed.

BIRCHER-BENNER, MAXIMILIAN OSKAR (1867-1939). A Swiss physician, dietitian, and psychotherapist. He opened a private sanitorium in Zurich, where he held lectures on physical and mental health, drawing on his experience with psychotherapy (q.v.). One of his most famous cases was that of Ikara (q.v.).
Bibliography: Ellenberger, H. H. 1970. *The discovery of the unconscious.*

BIRCH TREE. A tree that was believed in antiquity to give protection against witches (*see* WITCHCRAFT) and drive away evil spirits. Because of this belief, lunatics (q.v.) were sometimes birched.
Bibliography: Cooper, J. C. 1978. *An illustrated encyclopaedia of traditional symbols.*

BIRTH TRAUMA. A theory developed by Otto Rank (q.v.). He believed that every individual's life is affected by the terrifying experience of birth, which, if not overcome, may lead to neurosis (q.v.).
Bibliography: Rank, O. 1924. *The trauma of birth.*

BLACKBURN, I. W. An American physician, born in Philadelphia. In 1884 he was appointed special pathologist to the Government Hospital for the Insane in Washington, D.C. (now known as Elizabeth's Hospital [q.v.]), thus becoming the first full-time pathologist in an American mental hospital. He was particularly interested in the relationship between the brain and insanity and his studies reflected the new impetus given to research on the anatomy and functions of the nervous system.
Bibliography: Deutsch, A. 1949. *The mentally ill in America.*

BLACK CHOLER (*or* **BLACK BILE**). One of the humors (q.v.). It was linked with melancholia (q.v.) and suicidal (*see* SUICIDE) thoughts, but early medical writers could not decide whether black choler was the cause of depression or whether depression caused an excess of black choler. Democritus (q.v.) agreed with Hippocrates (q.v.) that it indirectly caused madness as a carrier of warmth and cold. If the black choler were too warm, it would cause fury; if too cold, stupor and melancholia.
Bibliography: Zilboorg, G. and Henry, G.W. 1941. *A history of medical psychology.*

BLACK COMEDY. Drama purporting to be comedy but introducing a somber, despairing, or painful view of the world. Black comedy attempts to create a reaction in its audience by laughing at pain and suffering. The term is derived from the work of Jean Anouilh (1910-   ). The term *dark comedy*, which was coined by the critic J. L. Styan in 1962, usually is applied to the form of drama in which laughter and despair are inextricably mixed as in Anton Chekhov's (q.v.) plays.
Bibliography: Styan, J. L. 1968. *The dark comedy.*

BLACKMORE, SIR RICHARD (1653?-1729). An English physician and composer of indifferent poetry. He wrote on hypochondria (q.v.) and hysteria (q.v.). He was one of the first medical authors to use the term melancholy (*see* MELANCHOLIA) to indicate depression rather than madness. He distinguished between mild and severe depression, diagnosing the latter if his patients complained of "marks of a design upon their lives." He recommended the use of opium (q.v.) for anxiety but warned that the dosage should be carefully assessed to prevent the patient from becoming addicted to it. Blackmore became a fashionable London practitioner and accumulated a wealthy clientele, who regarded him as a kind of oracle. Eventually he was appointed physician to William III (1650-1702) and Queen Anne (1665-

1714). He was less successful as a poet; Samuel Johnson (q.v.) seems to have been the only one who praised his verses.
Bibliography: Blackmore, R. 1725. *A treatise of the spleen and vapours.*

BLACK SPOTS. Black spots on the nails or on other parts of the body were believed to be due to black choler (q.v.), especially if they appeared over the spleen. They were considered premonitions of depression or disaster. Robert Burton (q.v.) reported that such spots were supposed to reappear over fixed time periods concomitant with humoral (*see* HUMORAL THEORY) changes.
Bibliography: Burton, R. 1621. Reprint. 1964 *Anatomy of melancholy.*

BLACKSTONE, SIR WILLIAM (1723-1780). A famous English jurist, professor of English law at Oxford University, and member of Parliament. He was the author of *Commentaries on the Laws of England* (1765-1769), the best-known history of the doctrines of English law. He defined the concepts of legal responsibility for idiots (q.v.) and lunatics (q.v.) and described how the crown offered protection to their interests and properties. His writings greatly influenced the jurisprudence of the United States.
Bibliography: Hunter, R., and Macalpine, I. 1963. *Three hundred years of psychiatry.*

BLAKE, ANDREW (1785-1842). A British physician. After obtaining his degree in Glasgow, he became a surgeon with the British army and served in the West Indies. On his return to England in 1832, he became physician to the Nottingham Asylum. His work on delirium tremens (q.v.) divided the course of the disease into three "distinct stages," each with its own different treatment. In November 1841, he was chairman of the first annual meeting of the newly formed Association of Medical Officers of Asylums and Hospitals for the Insane (q.v.) which eventually became the Royal College of Psychiatrists.
Bibliography: Blake, A. 1840. *A practical essay on . . . delirium tremens. . . .*

BLAKE, WILLIAM (1757-1827). An English poet and artist born in London, the son of a hosier from the Soho district. He left school at the age of ten to join a drawing school and when he was fourteen became an apprentice to an engraver. A solitary child, he was a voracious reader and began to write poetry when he was only twelve years old. Even as a child he had hallucinations (q.v.) and visions of angels. Strong, intelligent, and confident, he did not hesitate to use his imagination in all his productions, which were so unconventional that they were rejected by many of his contemporaries. When he was twenty-five years old, he married the daughter of a market gardener, an uneducated girl who learned to paint and draw to help her husband. Blake had a strong attachment to his young brother Robert whom he nursed during his last illness, going without sleep for two weeks. At the

moment of Robert's death, Blake had a vision of his released spirit and for the rest of his life claimed that he was in communication with his brother and received strength and advice from him. Henry Fuseli (1761-1825) (q.v.) was a friend and admirer of Blake. Both his engravings and his poems show a mystical approach to life, often dramatically expressed in an identification of ideas with terrifying symbols, which make his works of special interest to psychiatry (q.v.). He died singing.
Bibliography: Wilson, M. 1971. *The life of William Blake.*

BLANDFORD, G. FIELDING. An English physician. He followed the nineteenth-century fashion of overclassification. In *Insanity and Its Treatment* (1871), he established twenty groups of mental disease.
Bibliography: Blandford, G. F. 1871. *Insanity and its treatment.*

BLAVATSKY, HELENA PETROVNA (1831-1891). A Russian theosophist born at Ekaterinoslav. She traveled widely in Tibet and India. Her interest in spiritism and the occult sciences led to the establishment of the Theosophical Society in 1875. Her so-called miracles were later found to be fraudulent, but at the time of her death she had 100,000 followers all over the world. She wrote several works on theosophy, including *Isis Unveiled* (1877) and *The Key to Theosophy* (1889).
Bibliography: Symonds, J. 1959. *Madame Blavatsky.*

BLEEDING. Due to the humoral theory (q.v.), bleeding was frequently prescribed for mental disorders, on the principle that insanity was caused by too much hot blood. After William Harvey's (q.v.) discovery of the circulation of the blood, every disorder was believed to be connected to the blood, and all remedies tended tò concentrate on it. Bleeding in spring and autumn was ordered for patients in all mental hospitals throughout Europe. In 1845 Jean Esquirol (q.v.) condemned the excesses of this practice and quoted a case of an insane man bled thirteen times in forty-eight hours. Philippe Pinel (q.v.) was another authority who spoke against this abuse.
Bibliography: Esquirol, J. E. D. 1845. Reprint. 1965 *Mental maladies: a treatise on insanity.*

BLEULER, EUGEN (1857-1939). A Swiss psychiatrist, born of farming stock in the village of Zollikon, Zurich. As a schoolboy Bleuler was touched by the plight of the local residents in Burghölzli Hospital (q.v.), who, because they spoke the local dialect, could not be understood by the more formal German-speaking professors and the directors at the hospital. He decided to become a psychiatrist in order to help these mental patients. After qualifying, he studied with Jean Martin Charcot (q.v.) and Victor Magnon (1835-1912) in Paris before joining August Forel's (q.v.) staff at the Burghölzli. In 1886 he became director of the mental hospital at Rheinau, which was then the most backward of the Swiss hospitals. Bleuler undertook the task of rehabilitating the hospital with enthusiasm and devotion. His close contact with the patients became the basis for his work on schizophrenia (q.v.) and his theory of psychiatry (q.v.). In 1896 he became director of the Burghölzli, succeeding Forel. He now had ample opportunities for teaching what he had learned during his years at Rheinau, and among his students was Carl G. Jung (q.v.). Bleuler's greatest contribution to psychiatry was his study of schizophrenia (q.v.), a term he coined as a substitute for dementia praecox (q.v.). He saw schizophrenia as a split in psychic functioning due to unknown causes, some primary, or physiogenic, and some secondary, or psychogenic. He called the simultaneous presence of opposed tendencies ambivalence (q.v.). He worked closely with Sigmund Freud (q.v.), but in 1910 broke his association with him, thus starting the split between academic psychiatry and psychoanalysis (q.v.).

Bibliography: Bleuler, E. 1924. *Textbook of psychiatry*, trans. A. A. Brill.
———. 1950. *Dementia praecox or the group of schizophrenias*, trans. J. Zinkin.

BLOCKHEAD. The wooden dummy used by a wigmaker. It has come to mean a brainless, stupid individual.

> Nay, your wit will not so soon out as another man's will—'tis strongly wedged up in a blockhead.
>
> Shakespeare, *Coriolanus*, 2. 3.

Bibliography: 1978. *Brewer's dictionary of phrase and fable*.

BLOCQ, PAUL OSCAR (1860-1896). A French physician. In 1888 he described a psychogenic condition (now known as Blocq's disease) in which the patient is unable to stand or walk, although there is no organic lesion or paralysis.

See also APHEMIA.

Bibliography: Schmidt, J. E. 1959. *Medical discoveries: who and when*.

BLOFOT, RICHARD. A murderer who provides an early example of the plea of diminished responsibility in the English courts. In 1270 he was tried at Norwich jail for the murder of his wife and children whom he had killed in a frenzy. The court concluded that he was not fully responsible and committed him to prison. Six years later his case was reviewed, and his release was opposed as it was said that although his condition had improved he was still dangerous to himself and to others, especially in hot weather.

Bibliography: Talbot, C. H. 1967. *Medicine in mediaeval England*.

BLOOD TRANSFUSION. The first recorded example of blood transfusion used in psychiatric treatment was that undertaken by the French physician Jean Baptiste Denis (q.v.) in 1667. The patient was a young man whose melancholy (*see* MELANCHOLIA) was attributed to an unsuccessful love affair, and the donor was a calf. Similar attempts to cure psychiatric disorders by blood transfusions were undertaken in England and Germany. In England, the subject of the experiment was a patient from Bethlem Royal Hospital (q.v.), and the donor was a sheep. The operation was conducted in the presence of Royal Society (q.v.) members on November 23, 1667. Samuel Pepys (q.v.) recorded the event in his diary.
Bibliography: Hunter, R., and Macalpine, I. 1963. *Three hundred years of psychiatry.*

BLOOMFIELD, ROBERT (1766-1823). An English poet, born in Honington, Suffolk. He was educated by his mother, who was the local schoolmistress. In his youth he was apprenticed to his brother, a shoemaker, and his first poem *Farmer's Boy* (1800) was written in a room where half a dozen men were at work. Later in life he suffered from hallucinations (q.v.) that took the form of scenes that he previously had described in his verses. In spite of some literary success and the help of patrons, he died a poverty-stricken mental wreck, afflicted with blindness. His circumstances have been compared with those of John Clare (q.v.).
Bibliography: Ward, A. C. 1968. *Illustrated history of English literature,* vol. 3.

BLOOMINGDALE ASYLUM. The October 25, 1774, minutes of the Society of the New York Hospital state that the building committee was granted permission "to appropriate the cellar part of the North wing [of the projected general hospital] . . . for wards or cells for the reception of lunatics [q.v.]." The mental patients remained in this basement until a new building, the New York Lunatic Asylum, was erected in 1808. This building, due to the efforts of Thomas Eddy (q.v.) in the years 1817 to 1821, was in its turn transformed into an establishment that was built and conducted on the principles introduced by William Tuke (q.v.) at the Retreat in England. It contained the first authorized, formal psychiatric library in the United States, which later was incorporated in the Oskar Diethelm Library (q.v.). The hospital continues today as the Westchester division of the New York Hospital in White Plains.
Bibliography: Deutsch, A. 1944. *The mentally ill in America.*

BLUMENBACH, JOHANN FRIEDRICH (1752-1840). A German physiologist. Using his large collection of skulls he devised a classification of the human race. He thought that the skulls of cretins (*see* CRETINISM) had particular characteristics and wrote a book on this subject in 1783 entitled *In Cretinismo Capitis Formatio Singularis.*
Bibliography: Kanner, L. 1964. *A history of the care and study of the mentally retarded.*

BLY, NELLIE (1867-1922). Under this pseudonym the American journalist Elizabeth Seaman (*née* Cochrane) wrote a story entitled "Ten Days in a Mad House." It was serialized in the New York *World* in 1887. To get her material she had feigned insanity, and was admitted to the New York City Lunatic Asylum on Blackwell's Island. It was a dramatic exposé subtitled "Feigning insanity in order to reveal asylum horrors; the trying ordeal of the New York *World's* girl correspondent." It was later published as a book.
See also NEW YORK EARLY ASYLUMS.
Bibliography: Rittenhouse, M. 1956. *The amazing Nellie Bly.*

BLYTON, ENID (1897-1968). An English writer of children's books, creator of "Noddy." Her parents separated when she was twelve years old, and her childhood was lonely and traumatic. Her first marriage ended in divorce after she had driven her husband to find consolation in alcohol and another woman. At the same time she found the same consolation first in the protective friendship of the midwife who had attended her in childbirth and then in the love of a middle-aged surgeon, whom she married as soon as she was free. In spite of her apparent interest in children, she was cold and calculating. Her second marriage too was stormy at times, and the storms interfered with her busy working life. She produced some twenty books a year. During the latter part of her life her memory (q.v.) deteriorated and she lived in a fantasy world.
Bibliography: Stoney, B. 1974. *Enid Blyton: a biography.*

BOARDING-OUT OF MENTAL PATIENTS. In 1856 Sir John Bucknill (q.v.), superintendent of Devon County Lunatic Asylum, instituted a scheme of boarding-out patients on the model of the Gheel Colony (q.v.) in Belgium. The boarding-out of mental patients was also popular in Scotland; toward the end of the nineteenth century, about one-fifth of the Scottish insane were cared for by families in private dwellings.
See also COTTAGE SYSTEM, FAMILY CARE, and LIERNEUX.
Bibliography: Letchworth, W. P. 1889. *The insane in foreign countries.*

BOCCACCIO, GIOVANNI (1313-1375). Italian writer, known as the father of Italian prose. His best known work is the *Decameron*, which vividly depicts the society of his time. He was one of the first humanists; his works mark a return to realistic thinking about man and his earthy instincts, which medieval romance had ignored. Later in life, he became a misogynist. His way of life became even more austere after a saintly Carthusian monk on his death-bed exhorted Boccaccio to renounce his worldly studies. Many of his writings provided source material for Geoffrey Chaucer (q.v.) and William Shakespeare (q.v.).
Bibliography: MacManus, F. 1947. *Boccaccio.*

BODIN, JEAN (1530-1596). A French lawyer, best known for his works on political economy and for his position as secretary and counsellor to the Duke of Alençon during the latter's unsuccessful courtship of Queen Elizabeth I. In 1580 he wrote a book, *De la Démonomanie des Sorciers*, that embodied all the old ideas on witchcraft (q.v.) and included refutations of the enlightened views of Johann Weyer (q.v.). He asserted that what may be untrue in nature, may be true in law. This legal differentiation remained for centuries and was preserved in European and American legal codes, which suggested that a man could be legally sane, although in a physician's opinion he was insane.
Bibliography: Franklin, J. H. 1973. *Jean Bodin and the rise of absolutist theory*.

BODY IMAGE. Representation of his or her body held by that person. The concept of body image was developed by Paul F. Schilder (q.v.), who based his approach to the psychology (q.v.) of human personality on it.
Bibliography: Schilder, P. F. 1935. *The image and appearance of the human body*.

BOË, FRANZ DE LE (1614-1672). Also known as Franciscus Sylvius. A Prussian physician, anatomist, and inventor of gin (q.v.). He wrote on convulsions and observed that some mental symptoms disappear during severe physical illness.

BOEOTIA. A region of ancient Greece. Farmers were the principal inhabitants of the region and were regarded as unintelligent and rough; thus, it became renowned for its fools.

BOERHAAVE, HERMANN (1668-1738). A Dutch physician, the son of a clergyman. He was born near Leiden in the Netherlands, where he studied and later taught medicine. He emphasized the importance of returning to Hippocratic (*see* HIPPOCRATES) teaching, including humoral theory (q.v.) and direct observation of patients. One of the most famous practitioners of his time, he had a faithful following of students, who translated his lectures into many languages. His methods of psychiatric diagnosis and treatment remained standard until the end of the eighteenth century. He thought that melancholy (*see* MELANCHOLIA) was caused by black choler (q.v.) and remarked that mania and melancholy might be different phases of the same disorder. He advised bleeding (q.v.), purging (q.v.), ice-cold dousing, and other means of shocking the patient. He invented a spinning chair (q.v.) to make patients unconscious. His many medical works include *Aphorisms, Concerning the Knowledge and Care of Diseases* (1709), which became a standard work throughout Europe. In it he remarkably anticipated malaria therapy (q.v.) by writing that tertian or quartan agues had sometimes cured general paresis.
Bibliography: Lindeboom, G. A. 1968. *Hermann Boerhaave: the man and his work*.

BOISSIER, DE SAUVAGES FRANÇOIS (1706-1767). A French physician, follower of Georg E. Stahl (q.v.). He wrote *Nosologia Methodica* (1768), in which he described more than 2,000 diseases, broken into 10 classes with sub-divisions, like botanical species, as the fashion of the times dictated. His eighth class was dedicated to *folies* and described in a systematic way every aspect of nervous disorders known to him. He divided insanity (*see* INSANIA) into three orders: *morbi deliri, morbi imaginarii,* and *morbi morosi.* He considered the body a mechanism activated by the soul.
Bibliography: Lewis, A. 1967. *The state of psychiatry.*

BOLEYN, GEORGE, VISCOUNT ROCHFORD (?-1536). The brother of Anne Boleyn (1507-1536), the second queen of Henry VIII. In 1529, she obtained for her brother the governorship of Bethlem Royal Hospital (q.v.). He was master of it until 1536, when he was beheaded in the Tower of London, two days before his sister, having been found guilty of high treason and incest (q.v.) with her.
Bibliography: O'Donoghue, E. G. 1914. *The story of Bethlehem Hospital.*

BOMBELLES, COUNT. An Austrian minister to Switzerland. In 1860 he paid an official visit to Abendberg Institution (q.v.). His report to the Austrian government led to its formation of special provisions for the care of idiots.
Bibliography: Kanner, L. 1964. *A history of the care and study of the mentally retarded.*

BOMOR. A Malaysian term for a healer who has become possessed (*see* POSSESSION) during the ritual involved in the examination of the patient. In a state of trance brought about by music and head twirling, he encourages the patient to act out his problems. In the case of psychological illness, the healer limits his treatment to conversation and good advice—a form of psychotherapy (q.v.).
Bibliography: Kramer, B. H. 1970. Psychotherapeutic implications of a traditional healing ceremony: Malaysian main puteri. *Transcultural Psychiatric Research Review.*

BONAPARTE, LOUIS(1778-1846). The favorite brother of Napoleon (q.v.), who made him king of Holland. After one attack of venereal disease when he was twenty, Louis became a hypochondriac (*see* HYPOCHONDRIA). He traveled from spa to spa in search of cure and used his ill health as an excuse to resist or decline the duties and offices his brother imposed upon him. His marriage, also imposed upon him by Napoleon, was a failure, and he separated from his wife. It was rumored that he had homosexual (*see* HOMO-SEXUALITY) tendencies. He abdicated in favor of his son—at Napoleon's insistence—and retired to Graz in 1810. Louis' blind love for his brother eventually turned to suspicion and hatred, which was reversed only after Napoleon's death. At that point Louis identified with him to the point of feeling a paranoid (*see* PARANOIA) delusion of persecution and a continuous need to defend his brother and himself.

Bibliography: Jones, E. 1913. Reprint. 1951. The case of Louis Bonaparte, king of Holland. In *Essays in Applied Psychoanalysis*.

BONET, THÉOPHILE (1620-1689). A French physician, a pioneer in pathological anatomy. He compiled a collection of all the well-known post-mortems up to 1679. This work, entitled *Sepulchretum*, includes descriptions of hypochondria (q.v.) and depression with gastric complaints, which were believed to be caused by animal spirits (q.v.). The same cause was attributed to the emotional instability, moodiness, and depression observed in people in love (q.v.). He reported a case of mania (q.v.) in a young and beautiful woman, who was bled (*see* BLEEDING) thirty times in ten days. She died. Bonet, who conducted the postmortem, did not discover the cause of her mania, nor did he comment on the fatal result of the treatment. He translated into Latin, using the title of *Zodiacus medico-gallicus*, the first vernacular medical journal *Nouvelles Découvertes sur Toutes les Parties de la Médicine*.

Bibliography: Zilboorg, G. 1941. *A history of medical psychology*.

BONHOEFFER, KARL (1868-1948). A German psychiatrist and neurologist, born in Württemberg. He worked with Carl Wernicke (q.v.) and later became director of the famous psychiatric and neurological clinic of Charité (q.v.) in Berlin. In 1924 Bonhoeffer succeeded Emil Kraepelin (q.v.) at the University of Munich. His classification of psychiatric disorders was his main contribution to psychiatry (q.v.). He divided syndromes into *exogenous*, due to a known pathological cause, and *endogenous*, due to a congenital cause. His work included investigations on the symptomatic psychoses, mental disorders in alcoholism (q.v.), chorea, and acute exogenous reactions. He was regarded as an outstanding scientist and a great physician, who managed to retain a balanced and happy view of life in spite of many tragic events. His sons and sons-in-law were victims of the Nazis during World War II. His son, Dietrich Bonhoeffer (1906-1945), is regarded as one of the greatest theologians of today.

Bibliography: Zutt, J.; Straus, E; and Scheller, H., eds. 1969. *Karl Bonhoeffer— Zum Hundertsten Geburtstag am 31. Maerz 1968*.

BONNATERRE, SICARD. A French abbé, professor of natural history at the Central School of Aveyron. The wild boy of Aveyron (q.v.) was taken to him after his capture in 1798. The abbé turned him over to Jean Itard (q.v.), as he realized that the child offered a unique opportunity for

the observation and study of a human being who had developed alone in a state of natural existence.
Bibliography: Itard, J. M. G. 1806. Reprint. 1932. *The wild boy of Aveyron.*

BONNET, CHARLES (1720-1793). A Swiss naturalist, best known for his *Traité d'insectologie* (1745) in which he described the behavior of insects. He accepted Étienne Condilac's (q.v.) doctrine of sensationalism and added to it his own physiological hypotheses. The commonsense psychology of nineteenth-century France owes much to his empiricism, which is best expressed in his book *Essai analytique sur les facultés de l'âme*, published in 1760.
Bibliography: Boring, E. G. 1950. *A history of experimental psychology.*

BOORDE, ANDREW (1490?-1549). An English physician, born near Cuckfield in Sussex and brought up at Oxford. Before reaching the age of majority he was ordained as a monk in the Carthusian order and later became Suffragan bishop of Chichester. After twenty years of religious life he could no longer stand the rigorous discipline of the order, which demanded vegetarianism and fasting, and asked to be released. He went abroad to study medicine, visiting Europe, North Africa, and the Near East. On his return to England he established himself as a practitioner. Thomas Cromwell (1485-1540), one of his patients, sent him on a journey through Europe to report on the feelings there toward Henry VIII. He spent some years at Montpellier from where he wrote the first handbook on Europe to be printed and two medical books, *The Breviary of Health* (q.v.) and *The Dietary of Health* (1542). These were written for the Duke of Norfolk and were probably the first modern works on hygiene. When he again returned to England, he resumed the Carthusian rules and wore a hair shirt, but at the same time he was accused of keeping three loose women in his chamber. He was next heard of in 1549 in the Fleet Prison, London, where he made his will. His *Breviary of Health* contains several references to mental disorders; he said of insanity (*see* INSANIA), "there be four kyndes of madness, Mania [q.v.], Melancholia [q.v.], Frenesis and Demoniachus. This latter doth passe all manner of sicknesses and disease."
Bibliography: Poole, H. E. 1936. *The wisdom of Andrew Boorde.*

BOOSENING. *See* BOWSSENING.

BOOTHAM PARK. *See* YORK LUNATIC ASYLUM.

BORAGE. According to Pliny the Elder (q.v.) and, later, John Gerard (q.v.), this herb "maketh a man merry and joyful." John Evelyn (q.v.) thought that it "chear the hard student," and in Robert Burton's *Anatomy* *of Melancholy* (q.v.) borage is represented in one of the ten scenes on the title page:

> Borage and Hellebore fill two scenes
> Sovereign plants to purge the veins
> Of melancholy, and cheer the heart
> Of those black fumes which make it smart.
>
> Robert Burton, *Anatomy of Melancholy.*

BORELLI, GIOVANNI ALPHONSO (1608-1679). An Italian physicist and astronomer. He was the author of *De Motu Animalium* (1680-1681), a work in which he applied the mathematical principles of statics to animal movement and balance. He believed that nervous action was based on impulses in a fluid column that followed along the whole length of the nerves.
Bibliography: Sigerist, H. E. 1933. *Great doctors.*

BORING, EDWIN GARRIGUES (1886-1968). An American psychologist born in Philadelphia. His father, a druggist, belonged to the Moravian Church, and the predominantly female household was strictly religious. He was not sent to school until he was nine years old, as he was thought to be too "excitable." Eventually he went to Cornell University to study electrical engineering, but his fascination with the teaching of Edward B. Titchener (q.v.) turned his mind towards psychology (q.v.). For twenty-five years he was director of the psychological laboratory (q.v.) at Clark University. He is best remembered for his comprehensive and classic work *A History of Experimental Psychology*, first published in 1929 and subsequently enlarged. He dedicated the book to Titchener.
Bibliography: Stevens, S. S. 1968. Edwin Garrigues Boring. *Am. J. Psychol.* 81: 589-606.

BORIS GODOUNOV. An opera by the Russian composer Modest Petrovitch Mussorgsky (q.v.). Boris' demoniac power, agony of mind, and terrible remorse, which affect him to the point of hysteria (q.v.) with hallucinations (q.v.), are depicted against a background of mass emotion. Mental retardation is also represented by an idiot (q.v.) prophesying woe.
Bibliography: Harewood, Earl of, ed. 1969. *Kobbe's complete opera book.*

BORROMINI, FRANCESCO (1599-1667). An Italian baroque architect. He suffered from fits of depression, which he tried to cure by traveling. His depression would become so great that he would shut himself up in his house for weeks. Eventually he had to be kept under continuous surveillance. He committed suicide (q.v.) in a fit of fury by throwing himself upon a sword that had been carelessly left on a table in his room. Some see signs of psychosis in his work.
Bibliography: Wittkower, R., and Wittkower, M. 1963. *Born under Saturn.*

BORROW, GEORGE(1803-1881). An English author, educated in Edinburgh, Scotland. He studied law but abandoned it to learn several languages and travel through Europe, Russia, and Morocco. He became fascinated by gypsies and their lore and lived with them and offered them hospitality on his estate. He suffered from deep depression. The descriptions of screaming horrors and delirium (q.v.) occurring in his partly autobiographical novel *Romany Rye* (1857), which deals with gypsy life, are said to be taken from personal experience.
Bibliography: Collie, M. 1982. *George Borrow: eccentric.*

BORSTAL SYSTEM. A term applied to the system of institutional care given to adolescent offenders. The name is taken from the name of a village in Kent, England, where the experiment began in 1902.
Bibliography: Bottoms, A.E., and McClintock, F. H. 1973. *Criminals coming of age.*

BOSCH, HIERONYMUS (c.1450-1516). A Flemish painter. The mystical symbols and allegories appearing in his work were comprehensible to his contemporaries, although they now are obscure. He painted fantastic representations of hostile demons, witches (*see* WITCHCRAFT), monsters, and gruesome creatures. He seems to have been obsessed (*see* OBSESSION) with fears of metamorphosis, as a recurrent theme in his works is the transformation of human beings into animals or vegetable forms. Other themes that reflect abnormal preoccupations are perverted sexual acts and the birth of monstrous creatures, which led to the suggestion that he was a member of the Adamites (q.v.). His paintings have an hallucinatory (*see* HALLUCINATIONS) quality that has led to speculations about his mental health, even though preoccupation with the supernatural and sin, guilt, and retribution was common in his time. He overtly represented insanity (*see* INSANIA) in *The Ship of Fools* (q.v.) and in *The Cure of Folly.* The latter painting depicts the cutting of the stone of madness (q.v.) from the head of a man. His extravagant symbolism and strange images have found an echo in Surrealism (q.v.).
Bibliography: Baldass, L. von. 1960. *Hieronymus Bosch.*

BOSE, KATRICK. An Indian scientist. In 1931, with Ganneth Sen (q.v.) he described the use of *Rauwolfia serpentina* (q.v.) in the treatment of psychosis (q.v.), which led to a renewed interest in the drugs derived from it.
Bibliography: Alexander, F. G. and Selesnick, S. T. 1966. *The history of psychiatry.*

BOSQUILLONNER. A word coined by French medical students. It refered to the reckless use of bleeding (q.v.) by Edouard François Marie Bosquillon (1744-1816).
Bibliography: Semelaigne, R. 1912. *Aliénistes et philanthropes.*

BOST, JEAN (1817-1881). A French musician, horseman, and soldier. In 1844 he abandoned the secular life and became a theologian with a special

interest in orphaned children. In 1854 he founded a home, La Famille Évangélique, for them at Laforce. One day he found an idiot (q.v.) child abandoned on his doorstep. As the child's condition made her unsuitable for the existing orphanage, he took her into his own home and eventually founded two special asylums (q.v.) for the mentally retarded. The Bathesda, for girls, opened its doors to five patients in 1855 and was followed three years later by Shiloh, a home for boys. Bost also founded two homes for epileptic (*see* EPILEPSY) children.
Bibliography: Kanner, L. 1967. *A history of the care and study of the mentally retarded.*

BOSTON ALMS HOUSE. Probably the first almshouse established in New England. It was founded in 1662 in Boston. Its inmates included an indiscriminate mixture of the poor, vagrants, the sick in body or mind, and criminals of all ages.
Bibliography: Deutsch, A. 1949. *The mentally ill in America.*

BOSTON LUNATIC HOSPITAL. Boston Lunatic Hospital came into existence in 1839, following a legislative statute of 1836 that directed the counties of Massachusetts to establish "a suitable and convenient appartment or receptacle for idiots [q.v.] and lunatics [q.v.], or persons not furiously mad." Its first superintendent was Dr. John Butler (q.v.). The hospital was in fact an adaptation of the Suffolk County Institution. The hospital was one of the few American institutions that Charles Dickens (q.v.) praised in his *American Notes for General Circulation* (1842).
Bibliography: Deutsch, A. 1949. *The mentally ill in America.*

BOSWELL, JAMES (1740-1795). A Scottish biographer and diarist well known for his *Life of Samuel Johnson* (1791). He was born in Edinburgh, the son of a Scottish judge, Alexander Boswell, Lord Auchinleck; his mother was a Bruce, which sustained Boswell's claim that he was a cousin of George III (q.v.). As a child he was often ill. He was afraid of ghosts and the dark; he was often depressed; and at the age of seventeen he became ill for a long period, perhaps suffering from a nervous breakdown. His recovery brought about a great change: his disposition became outgoing, his health good, and his shyness gave way to a gregarious search for pleasure in writing verses and running after actresses. Having thoroughly angered his father, he ran away to London and became a Roman Catholic. His conversion, kept secret until his death, was not taken seriously by him, and he continued to lead the life of a libertine. He remained inwardly, however, insecure, anxious, and depressed. An entry in his London journal, for July 22, 1763, tells of his relief in confiding his depression to Samuel Johnson (q.v.) and learning that Johnson too was melancholic (*see* MELANCHOLIA). Johnson advised him to keep his mind occupied, exercise, and live moderately, adding that

"melancholy people are apt to fly to intemperance, which gives a momentary relief but sinks the soul much lower in misery." Later Edmund Malone's (1741-1812) support and encouragement enabled Boswell to complete his *Life of Samuel Johnson.* In his last year he was a broken and worried man in poor physical and mental health. His brother John (q.v.) was insane and his own daughter, Euphemia, was mentally deranged.
Bibliography: Pottle, F. A., ed. 1950. *Boswell's London journal.*

BOSWELL, JOHN (1743-1798). Younger brother of the famous diarist James Boswell (q.v.). He suffered from periods of insanity (*see* INSANIA) and was treated by Dr. John Hall (q.v.) at St. Luke's House (q.v.). He was invalided out of the Army because of his mental state. James Boswell described his condition in his writings, noting his "silent state," his "gentle torpor," alternating with periods of excitement.
Bibliography: Boswell, J. 1928-1930. Private Papers of James Boswell from Malahide Castle. *The Isham collection,* ed. G. Scott and F. A. Pottle.

BOTANICAL LUNATIC ASYLUM. Edward Augustus Bowles (1865-1954), a great English gardener, regarded plants as individuals. If any of them were misfits or oddities, he would banish them to his lunatic asylum, presided over by a magnolia that he regarded as sane.
Bibliography: Allan, M. 1973. *E.A. Bowles and his garden at Myddelton House.*

BOTHWELL, JAMES HEPBURN, EARL OF. *See* HEPBURN, JAMES, EARL OF BOTHWELL.

BOTTELL, WILLIAM (1875-1956). An English mnemonist. His memory (q.v.) was so phenomenal that he was able to make a living by it. In 1901 he started a stage career in London at the Palace Theatre, where he appeared every night to answer questions from the audience. He had an enormous memory storage of dates, details of past events, and the lives of famous people. He became well known as "Datas, the Memory Man."
Bibliography: Yates, F. 1966. *The art of memory.*

BOUCHUT, JEAN ANTOINE EUGÈNE (1818-1891). A French physician who introduced the intubation of the larynx in croup. He became interested in neurotic (*see* NEUROSIS) phenomena and described neurasthenia (q.v.) in a book entitled *Du Nervosisme,* published in 1860. He is also remembered for his valuable history of medicine.
Bibliography: Garrison, F. H. 1929. *An introduction to the history of medicine.*

BOUDHI. Intelligence in Hindu medical psychology (q.v.). Boudhi is one of the endowments of the soul, together with *ohankara,* or consciousness.
Bibliography: Zilboorg, G. and Henry, G. W. 1941. *A history of medical psychology.*

BOUILLAUD, JEAN BAPTISTE (1796-1881). A French physician, born at Garat. He was author of several medical works. After studying inflammation of the brain, he suggested that definite cerebral areas were connected with particular functions, thus delimiting motor, perceptual, and intellectual activity. He was the first to localize the speech center in 1825. He was a great admirer of Franz Gall (q.v.) and equated his phrenology (q.v.) to scientific psychology (q.v.). In clinical practice, he was one of the last believers in the beneficial use of copious bleeding (q.v.).
Bibliography: Boring, E. G. 1950. *A history of experimental psychology.*
Bouillaud, J. B. 1825. *Traité clinique et physiologique de l'encéphalite ou inflammation du cerveau et de ses suites.*

BOURNE, ANSEL (1826-?). An American carpenter who lost his sight, voice, and hearing after declaring that he would rather go without these faculties than go to church. They were restored to him when he announced his conversion. Thirty years later he suddenly developed a different personality with the name of Albert Brown and moved to another area. One day, however, he woke up in his former personality of Ansel Bourne and was disoriented in his new surroundings about which he remembered nothing. He became a patient of William James (q.v.), who explored his experiences under hypnosis (*see* HYPNOTISM).
Bibliography: Hodgson, R. 1891-1892. A case of double consciousness. *Proceedings of the Society of Psychical Research.* 7: 221-55.

BOURNEVILLE, DÉSIRÉ-MAGLOIRE (1840-1909). A French neurologist. In 1883 he was elected deputy from Paris and while a deputy voted the first national funds for the care of retarded children and epileptics (*see* EPILEPSY). Working with others, he demonstrated that certain forms of mental deficiency are associated with specific structural anomalies in the brain. In 1880 he described a condition of convulsions, sebaceous adenoma, and mental deficiency, which is usually referred to as tuberous sclerosis (q.v.), or Bourneville's disease. In 1898, he outlined a program of special teaching and classes for retarded children.
Bibliography: Kanner, L. 1964. *A history of the care and study of the mentally retarded.*

BOVARISM. A term meaning the failure to differentiate between reality and fantasy. It is derived from the novel *Madame Bovary* by Gustave Flaubert (q.v.). The novel describes the life of a young woman whose aspirations do not coincide with her mode of life, hence her need to substitute the perceptual world with daydreams.
Bibliography: Flaubert, G. *Madame Bovary.* 1959. Trans. by Hopkins, P.

BOVEY, JAMES (1622-?). A citizen of London, merchant, legal expert, traveler, and writer. John Aubrey (q.v.) included him in his *Brief Lives.*

Aubrey portrayed him as a rather meticulous, obsessional (*see* OBSESSION) person forever engaged in lawsuits, one of which lasted for eighteen years. Not surprisingly, he had "a weake stomach, which proceeded from the agitation of the braine." Among his works, Aubrey listed one entitled *The Causes of Diseases of the Mind* and another on *The Cures of the Mind, viz. Passions, Diseases, Vices, Errours, Defects.*
Bibliography: Dick, O. L., ed. 1949. *Aubrey's Brief Lives.*

BOVINUS BAMBERGENSIS. The name given by Carolus Linnaeus (q.v.) to a feral child (q.v.) discovered among herds of oxen in Bamberg, Germany.
Bibliography: Barr, M. W. 1904. *Mental defectives.*

BOWSSENING. A Celtic term meaning "to immerse in a holy well." This type of immersion was practiced throughout the United Kingdom until the twentieth century. Among the wells that were used were Saint Nun's in Altarnum, Cornwall, Saint Fillan's in Scotland, Saint Winifred's in Flintshire, and Saint Ronan's in Scotland (qq.v.). The process of the well-cure for mental illness was as follows:

The frantic person was placed on the wall with his back to the water; without being permitted to know what was going to be done he was knocked backwards into the water by a violent blow on the chest, when he was tumbled about in a most unmerciful manner until fatigue had subdued the rage which unmerited violence had occasioned. Reduced by ill-usage to a degree of weakness which ignorance mistook for returning sanity, the patient was conveyed to church with much solemnity, where certain masses were said over him.

See also IMMERSION.
Bibliography: Mackenzie, D. 1927. *The infancy of medicine.*

BOYINGTON, HORATIO. An American judge who as a member of the Massachusetts House of Representatives in 1846 instituted a committee to inquire into the number, condition, and possibility of treatment of idiots. The inspiration behind this move came from Dr. Samuel Gridley Howe (q.v.), who became chairman of the committee and wrote the report. The government provided funds for the committee for a period of three years, and at the Perkins Institution the first school for severely retarded children was opened in Massachusetts in 1848, as an experiment.
Bibliography: 1848. *Report made to the legislature of Massachusetts on idiocy.*

BOYLE, HELEN (1869-1957). An English physician. In 1905 she founded Lady Chichester Hospital (q.v.) in Brighton, England. It was the first hospital to provide inpatient treatment for early neurotic disorders. It is now located in Hove, Sussex.

BOZZOLO, CAMILLO (1845-1920). Italian physician. Lethargic encephalitis, later known as Bozzolo's disease, was described by him in 1895.
Bibliography: Schmidt, J. E. 1959. *Medical discoveries: who and when.*

BRACTON, HENRY DE (?-1268). An English ecclesiastic and judge. Between 1235 and 1259, he wrote the first complete and systematic treatise on
the laws of England in the Middle Ages (q.v.) entitled *De Legibus et Con-
suetudinibus Angliae.* He held that a madman could not be considered responsible for his actions.
Bibliography: Zilboorg, G. and Henry, G. W. 1941. *A history of medical psychology.*

BRAHMS, JOHANNES (1833-1897). A German composer, born in the
slums of Hamburg. His mother, who was seventeen years older than his
father, was a bad-tempered woman, notorious for her ugliness. His father
gave him his first music lessons, and by the time he was nine years old, he
1974): 45-54; Howard,was playing in the local taverns and brothels, where
the prostitutes petted him. As an adult, he found that only from them could
he gain sexual satisfaction. He developed a hopeless passion for Clara Schumann (1819-1896), who was fourteen years his senior and the wife of Robert
Schumann (1810-1856). He later became fond of three other women, each
a mezzo-soprano, but he never married. The enigma of why Brahms resisted
marriage has been discussed by Edward Hitschmann (q.v.) in an essay entitled "Johannes Brahms and Women" (1933). Even after attaining fame,
Brahms remained of simple tastes and habits, his only addiction being to
very strong coffee.
Bibliography: Gal, H. 1963. *Brahms: his work and personality.*

BRAID, JAMES (c.1795-1860). A surgeon and hypnotist, born in Scotland.
After attending a performance by Charles Lafontaine (q.v.), he became
interested in magnetism (q.v.) and set out to demonstrate that it had nothing
to do with magnetic fluid. He failed to recognize the psychological element
in hypnosis (*see* HYPNOTISM) and believed that the trance was merely a
physical phenomenon, which was the product of muscle fatigue due to
prolonged concentration that in turn led to exhaustion and to what he called
nervous sleep (q.v.). He invented the term *neurypnology* (q.v.) from which
"hypnosis" is derived. Braid expounded his theories in 1843 in a work
entitled *Neurypnology, or the Rationale of Nervous Sleep.*
Bibliography: Ellenberger, H. F. 1970. *The discovery of the unconscious.*

BRAIDISM. A term coined in 1860 by Joseph P. Durand de Gros (q.v.).
It was a substitute for hypnotism (q.v.), which emphasized sleep rather than
suggestion, and was derived from James Braid (q.v.).
Bibliography: Tinterow, M. M. 1970. *Foundations of hypnosis.*

BRAIN. A British journal dedicated to neuropathology (q.v.). It was founded in 1878 by Sir James Crichton-Browne (q.v.), who was coeditor of it for the first eight years of its publication.

BRAIN, CONCEPTS OF. Hippocrates (q.v.) believed that pleasure and sorrow arose from the brain, but he did not ascribe to it any psychological qualities. Diseases of the brain, according to him, were due to an imbalance of humors (q.v.). Aristotle (q.v.) regarded the function of the brain as subordinate to the heart; the heart was the sensorium and produced vapors that were then cooled and condensed in the brain. Galen (q.v.) was unclear about the brain; he located psychic functions in the brain and believed that feelings and movement originated through the brain when it was struck by stimuli. In the Middle Ages (q.v.) and the Renaissance the brain was supposed to be divided into three ventricles. Thomas Vicary (q.v.) wrote that "in the foremost ventricle are five wits: also the fancy and the imagination. In the second or middle ventricle is thought. In the third ventricle is the Memory." This was the concept of the brain held by William Shakespeare (q.v.). After William Harvey's (q.v.) discovery of the circulation of the blood, it was again believed that vapors rising to the brain caused mental disorders. Neurotic (*see* NEUROSIS) states were called "the vapors" (q.v.). Réne Descartes (q.v.) thought that the pineal gland was the location of the soul. Later psychologists regarded the brain as the organ through which stimuli were transformed into feelings, thoughts, and behavior after they had been perceived by the all important sense organs. Franz J. Gall (q.v.) reduced psychology (q.v.) to cerebral localization; each area was related to a special psychological function. The physicians of the nineteenth century concentrated their investigations of mental disorders on the pathology of the brain. They were, of course, unable to correlate cerebral lesions with emotional symptoms.
Bibliography: 1959. *The history and philosophy of knowledge of the brain and its functions.* Anglo-American Symposium. Sponsored by Wellcome Historical Medical Library.

BRAMWELL, BYRON (1847-1931). A British physician. His books now are considered classics in the field of neurology (q.v.); among them are *The Disease of the Spinal Cord* (1882) and *Intracranial Tumours* (1888). He described the functions of the hypothalamus and emphasized its importance.
Bibliography: Haymaker, W., and Schiller, F. 1970. *The founders of neurology.* 2d ed.

BRANDIN, ABEL. A French physician of the nineteenth century. Beginning in 1820, he practiced for about twenty years in Latin America. He was perhaps the first in Latin America to organize psychiatry (q.v.) on the lines then current in Europe. He wrote extensively on various aspects of psy-

chiatry, including legal problems connected with mental disorders. He advocated the introduction of occupational therapy (q.v.) and, somewhat contradictorily, the use of tranquilizing devices then popular in Europe, such as the spinning chair (q.v.) devised by Benjamin Rush (q.v.).
Bibliography: Leon, C.A., and Rosselli, H. 1975. Latin America. In *World history of psychiatry*, ed. J. G. Howells.

BRANKS. An instrument of punishment consisting of a headpiece of iron or leather with a gag for the mouth. It sometimes was termed a "scold's bridle" or "witch's bridle." It was in use in Scotland from at least the sixteenth century.
Bibliography: Andrews, W. 1890. *Old time punishments.*

BRANT, SEBASTIAN (1457?-1521). *See* NARRENSCHIFF.

BRASS BANDS. In the nineteenth century most mental hospitals in England had a brass band. The musicians were drawn from the staff or the patients, or both. Accounts of their activities are to be found in many hospitals' records. Downshire Hospital (q.v.) records reveal that the band played an important role in the opening of the hospital. Dr. William Henry Parsey (1851-1884), the superintendent of Hatton Asylum (q.v.), in Warwickshire, usually was met at the gate by the hospital band when he returned from leave; he was then played up the drive to the tune of "See the Conquering Hero Comes." The brass bands provided music for various occasions, including dances, another feature of social life in nineteenth century asylums (q.v.). Sir Edward Elgar (q.v.) began his professional life as a bandmaster in a mental hospital.
Bibliography: Howells, J. G., and Osborn, M. L. 1975. Great Britain. In *World history of psychiatry*, ed. J. G. Howells.

BRATTLE, THOMAS (1658-1713). An American merchant and religious reformer in Cambridge, Massachusetts. In 1692 he witnessed the witchcraft (q.v.) trials at Salem (q.v.). He condemned the proceedings, even though he too believed in witches and evil spirits, because he realized that some of the accused were mentally ill and needed treatment rather than punishment. In a letter to a friend he wrote:

They are deluded, imposed upon, and under the influence of some evil spirits; and therefore unfitt to be evidences either against themselves, or any one else. These confessours (as they are called) do very often contradict themselves, as inconsistently as is usual for any crazed, distempered person to do.
Bibliography: Deutsch, A. 1937. *The mentally ill in America.*

BREATH HOLDING. A means of suicide (q.v.). When afflicted by unbearable melancholia (q.v.), some members of primitive tribes in the Niger Valley have committed suicide by literally holding their breath.
Bibliography: Fedden, H. R. 1938. *Suicide.*

BRENTANO, CLEMENS MARIA (1778-1842). A German writer and poet, uncle of Franz Brentano (q.v.). He was a restless, unbalanced individual. His one period of happiness was during his brief first marriage to Sophia Mereau, which lasted for three years and ended with her death. His second marrige failed, and he was left in a state of emotional collapse. He went to Dülmen, Germany, where he spent six years recording the revelations of Anna Katharina Emmerich (q.v.). In his later years he dabbled in astrology (q.v.), alchemy (q.v.), and other pseudo-sciences, eventually becoming totally deranged.
Bibliography: Seidel, I. 1944. *Clemens Brentano.*

BRENTANO, FRANZ (1838-1917). A priest and philosopher born in Marienberg, Germany, from an old Italian family. Opposing the church's position on the infallibility of the pope, he resigned from the priesthood and the chair of philosophy at Würzburg and became professor of philosophy at Vienna. Here Sigmund Freud (q.v.) attended his lectures. Brentano again had to resign his position when he fell in love with a Catholic, whom under Austrian law he could not marry because he had been a priest. He changed his citizenship to Saxon and got married, but fourteen years later his wife died. Disheartened, ill, and nearly blind, he left Austria and went to Switzerland and then to Florence in Italy. As a pacifist, however, he found no peace there, as Italy entered World War I in 1915. He moved to Zürich where he died. His work is of great importance in the history of experimental psychology (q.v.). "Experience alone influences me as a mistress," he wrote, and he accepted nothing that he could not prove. He believed that psychology (q.v.) is not the content of mind, but the act (hence the term, *act psychology* [q.v.]), and that persons or experiences should be related to the environment. His best known work is *Psychologie vom empirischen Standpunkte* (1874), which represents his movement away from dogma and toward experience.
See also AUSTRIAN SCHOOL.
Bibliography: Rancurollo, Anton C. 1968. *A Study of Franz Brentano: his psychological standpoint and his significance in the history of psychology.*

BRENTRY CERTIFIED INEBRIATE REFORMATORY. An institution for the care of alcoholics (*see* ALCOHOLISM) of both sexes who were considered to be in moral danger. It was established in Bristol, England, toward the end of the nineteenth century. It was managed by the Reverend Harold Nelson Burden (q.v.) and his wife, who previously had worked in a small

house for alcoholic women, the Institution for Inebriates. The Burdens had been influenced by the ideas of Octavia Hill (q.v.) and had helped her in her work with the poor of London.
Bibliography: Jancar, J. 1972. Fifty years at Brentry Hospital, 1922-1972. *Bristol Med.-Chir.J.* 87: 23-30.

BRETHREN OF THE FREE SPIRIT. An heretical fraternity developed in the Middle Ages (q.v.). They believed that they could achieve a permanent union with God and become holier than the saints, thus making the church and the sacraments superfluous. As they assumed that their souls were incapable of sin, they allowed all kinds of license, including sexual orgies and incest (q.v.) without any feeling of guilt.
Bibliography: Churchill, W. 1956. *A history of the English-speaking peoples.*

BRETON, ANDRÉ (1896-1966). A French poet. He was introduced to the theories of Sigmund Freud (q.v.) when he was a medical student, and the more extreme tenets of psychoanalysis (q.v.) found fertile ground in his imagination. His poetry often deals with what he termed induced hallucination (q.v.), free image, and objective magic (q.v.). Breton formed a group of Dadaists (q.v.) and in 1924 founded the Surrealism (q.v.) movement. He was a communist and an adherent of Leon Trotsky (1879-1940).
Bibliography: Browder, C. 1967. *André Breton: arbiter of Surrealism.*

BRETON, NICHOLAS (1545?-?1626). An English writer of prose and verse. He was a melancholy (*see* MELANCHOLIA) man, who considered himself on the verge of insanity. In his poem written in 1584 *Forte of Fancie* he described conditions in a hospital for the insane and presented sketches of the patients that were based on factual observation at Bethlem Royal Hospital (q.v.). His *A Post with a Packet of Mad Letters* was very popular and frequently reprinted in the seventeenth century.
Bibliography: Breton, N. 1893. *A bower of delights: verse and prose,* ed. A. B. Grosart.

BREUER, JOSEPH (1842-1925). A physician and psychologist born in Vienna, Austria. His father was a teacher of religion; his mother died when he was still a child. He was a brilliant student and an unassuming and selfless man. He became *privat dozent* and was offered the title of extraordinary professor, but he resigned the first and refused the second in order to devote himself completely to his patients. Although his practice was financially rewarding and allowed him to travel and live well, he was never avaricious and would not charge those who were too poor to pay. Breuer was a cultured man, well versed in literature, poetry, art, and music. Among his scientific achievements are the discovery of the function of the semicircular canals in 1875. Breuer believed that the body's energy regulates psychic activity. He

used hypnosis (*see* HYPNOTISM) in his medical practice and found that hysterical (*see* HYSTERIA) patients could recall and discuss harmful events under hypnosis. Using this method, Breuer was able to lead his patients to discussions of memories and emotions that had been suppressed because they were too hurtful. He produced some spectacular cures, the most famous of which is that of Anna O. (q.v.). He treated her from 1881 until 1882, and the theoretical assumptions derived from her case led him and Sigmund Freud (q.v.), his friend and collaborator, to the development of cathartic hypnosis and formed the basis on which Freud built psychoanalysis (q.v.). Breuer discontinued his therapeutic sessions with Anna O. and fled from Vienna, when he found that transference was causing his patient to fall in love with him. In 1895 he and Freud resumed working together and published *Studies in Hysteria* in which they formulated their ideas about catharsis (q.v.) and its use in therapy. Even in his old age, Breuer was a kindly, simple, and warm person, who retained his brilliant faculties and the affection and respect of those around him.
Bibliography: Oberndorf, C. P. 1953. Autobiography of Joseph Breuer. *Int. J. Psychoanal.* 34: 64.

BREVIARY OF HEALTH, THE. A work written in 1547 by an English Carthusian monk and physician named Andrew Boorde (q.v.). It contains several references to mental disorders, their causes and treatment. The following quotation from it implies Boorde's awareness of the existence of psychosis (q.v.) and neurosis (q.v.) as two separate clinical categories: "This impediment may come by nature and kynde, and then it is uncurable, or else it may come by a greate feare or a greate study."
Bibliography: Poole, H. E. 1936. *The wisdom of Andrew Boorde.*

BRICKNER, RICHARD MAX (1896-   ). An American neurologist. While operating for the removal of a tumor, he excised parts of the frontal lobe. He noticed that after the operation the patient seemed less anxious yet showed no intellectual deterioration. Brickner's observations stimulated interest in psychosurgery (q.v.).
Bibliography: Alexander, F. G., and Selesnick, S. T. 1966. *The history of psychiatry.*

BRIDEWELL. Originally a palace of King John (c.1167-1216), located in Blackfriars, London. It derived its name from a well within its grounds dedicated to Saint Bride. Cardinal Thomas Wolsey (q.v.) rebuilt it and gave it to Henry VIII. Shakespeare located there the third act of *Henry VIII*. In 1553, Edward VI gave it to the city of London to be used as a royal hospital (one of five) for the correction of vagrants. Political and religious offenders were imprisoned and tortured there. In 1557, Bridewell was made responsible for the administration of Bethlem Royal Hospital (q.v.). This arrangement lasted nearly eighty years and was greatly resented by Bethlem Royal

Hospital because, among other disadvantages, it was obliged to receive patients from Bridewell without payment. Most of Bridewell's buildings were destroyed by the Great Fire of London in 1666, but those parts that survived continued to be used as a penitentiary for vagrants and unruly apprentices. It was demolished in 1863.
Bibliography: O'Donoghue, E. G. 1923. *Bridewell Hospital.*

BRIERRE DE BOISMONT, ALEXANDRE (1798-1881). A French physician who became interested in mental disorders and dedicated himself to their study. He observed the relationship between suicide (q.v.) and homicide, and wrote papers on the influence of civilization on mental illness and on patients' writings. His main work was a successful volume on hallucinations (q.v.), which was published in three editions. He was a frequent contributor to the *Annales Médico-psychologiques* (q.v.) and became secretary-general of the Société médico-psychologique.
Bibliography: Brierre de Boismont, A. 1859. *On Hallucinations,* trans. R. T. Hulme.

BRIGGS, L. VERNON (1863-1941). An American psychiatrist, born in Boston, Massachusetts. He was the author of a Massachusetts law adopted in 1921 which provided for routine mental examination before a trial. It is called Brigg's law in his honor.
Bibliography: Deutsch, A. 1937. *The mentally ill in America.*

BRIGHAM, AMARIAH (1798-1849). An American physician, born in New Marlboro, Massachusetts. After practicing general medicine for some years, he became professor of anatomy in New York. In 1840 he was superintendent of the Hartford Retreat (q.v.) and three years later became superintendent of the Utica State Hospital (q.v.) in New York, which had just opened and was still uncompleted. As the patients poured in and the accommodations proved inadequate for them, Brigham undertook the supervision of structural changes, as well as a program of training for the staff and the inauguration of new approaches to treatment. He felt that custodial care was not enough and that the hospital should have the more positive aim of improving the clinical state of the patients. He was a firm believer in occupational therapy (q.v.) and instituted various activities to keep the patients busy. In 1844, at his own expense, he founded the *American Journal of Insanity,* which he edited and had printed in the hospital. The journal later became the *American Journal of Psychiatry* (q.v.). It was devised by him as a tool for communication with the public. He hoped to dispel the superstition still enveloping mental disorders and to obtain support for further expansion and improvement. He was one of the original thirteen founders of the American Psychiatric Association (q.v.). Brigham wrote on many subjects, including cholera, religion, clinical psychiatry (q.v.) , and neurology (q.v.). His most successful book was *Remarks on the Influence of*

Mental Cultivation upon Health, which was widely read in the United States and Europe.

Bibliography: Deutsch, A. 1937. *The mentally ill in America.*

BRIGHT, TIMOTHY (c.1550-1615). An English physician, born in Cambridge. He studied medicine at Trinity College in Cambridge and in Paris, where he witnessed the St. Bartholomew's Day massacre in 1572. He was a cultured, if erratic, man, who was versed in music, languages, and literature. His first book, published in 1580, was *The Sufficiencie of English Medicines*, in which he praised the qualities of medical remedies made from native herbs. This work was followed by two more volumes, which were based on his lectures on medicine delivered at Cambridge. In 1585 he was appointed physician to St. Bartholomew's Hospital in London. There he wrote *A Treatise of Melancholie* (q.v.), the first book on mental disorders to be written in English. It was quoted by Robert Burton (q.v.) and was said to have inspired William Shakespeare (q.v.). Bright then turned his efforts toward devising a system of shorthand, which he dedicated to Queen Elizabeth, who granted him exclusive teaching and publishing rights. The neglect of his clinical duties led to his dismissal in 1591. He became more involved in religious activities and through influential friends obtained a living at Methley, in the West Riding of Yorkshire. But, even there he did not settle and moved on to a living at Barwick-in-Elmet. Once more complaints of neglected duties were brought against him. He ended his days near his brother at Shrewsbury.

Bibliography: Keynes, G. 1962. *Dr. Timothie Bright (1550-1615): a survey of his life with a bibliography of his writings.*

BRILL, ABRAHAM ARDEN (1874-1948). An American psychiatrist, born in Austria. At the age of fifteen he left Austria for the United States. He arrived penniless, having been robbed during the journey, and could not speak a word of English. He worked in a saloon, where he was allowed to sleep on the floor, and later earned his living by teaching English, billiards, and the mandolin. By sheer determination, he acquired an education and a degree in medicine. He worked in a mental hospital and qualified as a neuropathologist. Once established, he went first to France to study at the Bicêtre (q.v.) and then to Zürich, where he became a member of a group that studied Sigmund Freud's (q.v.) concepts and their application under Eugen Bleuler (q.v.) at the Burghölzli Hospital (q.v.). Brill quickly grasped the theoretical and clinical importance of Freud's work in the field of psychopathology (q.v.). He became a courageous and active supporter of psychoanalysis (q.v.) as a form of treatment for the neuroses (*see* NEUROSIS) and enthusiastically introduced it in the United States. He translated Freud's writings into English and published them in a series of monographs. He also translated Carl G. Jung's (q.v.) work. He was a warm person, a devoted husband, father, and grandfather, and he enjoyed the company of children. He was interested in music, literature, sports, and ornithology, and, despite a busy clinical practice, teaching and writing.

Bibliography: Alexander, F.; Eisenstein, S.; and Grotjahn, M., eds. 1966. *Psychoanalytic pioneers*.

BRINVILLIERS, MARIE MADALEINE D'AUBRAY, MARQUISE DE (1630?-1676). French noblewoman notorious for her depraved life. A typical psychopath, she felt no compunction in destroying those who stood in her way. She poisoned her father, her two brothers and many others. She was discovered and hanged, but the formula of her secret poison defied all effort of identification.

Bibliography: Stokes, H. 1912. *Madame de Brinvilliers and her times, 1630-1676*. 2d. ed.

BRIQUET, PAUL (1796-1881). A French physician. In 1859 he became the first to describe *ataxia analgica hysterica*, a condition in which the patient shows anesthesia (q.v.) of the skin and muscles of the leg.

Bibliography: Schmidt, J.E. 1959. *Medical discoveries: who and when*.

BRISLINGTON HOUSE. The first purpose-built private asylum opened near Bristol, England, in 1804. It was owned and directed by Dr. Edward Long Fox (q.v.). In 1814 it was inspected by Edward Wakefield (q.v.), who later contributed to government's inquiry into madhouses. He wrote that the house was well kept, clean, and orderly. Each patient had his own bedroom and was encouraged to do some kind of work about the house or the garden. It was, however, difficult to find suitable work for "gentlemen" who were unused to manual work. One famous patient there was John Thomas Perceval (q.v.).

Bibliography: Macalpine, I., and Hunter, R. 1969. *George III and the mad-business*.

BRISSAUD, EDOUARD (1852-1909). A French neurologist, born at Besançon, France. After teaching pathological anatomy for a number of years, he became professor of neurological pathology in 1894. For one year in 1893 he was in charge of Jean-Martin Charcot's (q.v) course on the diseases of the nervous system, which was held at the Salpêtrière (q.v.). He wrote several books on neurology (q.v.) and edited, with Henri Bouchard and Charcot, a six volume work, *Traité de Medicine* (1891-94). The *Neurological Review* was founded by him. He classified various kinds of mental degeneration and described spasms and tics of the face. Brissaud became an expert on injuries linked with conversion hysteria (q.v.) and his advice was often sought in medico-legal cases.

Bibliography: Haymaker, W., and Schiller, F. 1970. *The founders of neurology*. 2d. ed.

BRISTOL LUNATIC ASYLUM. A mental hospital opened in Bristol, England in 1861 to replace St. Peter's Hospital (q.v.). During World War I most of its male staff was called into the armed services, and the hospital was taken over by the War Office. The mental patients were transferred to other hospitals, or boarded out. It reopened in 1920 and in 1921 changed its name to Bristol Mental Hospital. Since 1960 it has been called Glenside Hospital.

BRITISH JOURNAL OF PSYCHIATRY. See ASYLUM JOURNAL.

BRITISH JOURNAL OF PSYCHOLOGY. The official organ of the British Psychological Society (q.v.). It was founded in 1904, and the first editors were William H. Rivers (q.v.) and Charles S. Myers (q.v.).
Bibliography: Boring, E. G. 1950. *A history of experimental psychology.*

BRITISH PSYCHOLOGICAL SOCIETY. The official body of British psychologists. It was founded in 1901 at University College in London. The first meeting was summoned by Professor James Sully (q.v.). In 1919 it extended its membership to anyone interested in psychology (q.v.).
Bibliography: Hearnshaw, L. S. 1964. *A short history of British psychology.*

BROADGATE HOSPITAL. An English mental hospital built in Beverley, Yorkshire, in 1871. It took its name from Broadgate Farm, which had previously owned the land. The towns in the area vied with each other to have the hospital within their boundaries. The first one hundred patients were transferred to it by train from the Clifton Asylum at York. The Beverly *Guardian*, reporting their arrival and their passage through the town in buses and cabs, stated that "they appeared to take a lively interest in what was going on in the streets." In the evening a ball was given at the hospital, and the patients danced for three hours to the strains of a string band. Dancing seems to have been a popular recreation, as it is recorded that in the following year, 1872, the staff formed a brass band (q.v.), which played at the patients' weekly dances.
Bibliography: Kavanagh, B. T. 1971. *Broadgate Hospital.*

BROADMOOR HOSPITAL. An institution in Crowthorne, Berkshire, England, founded in 1863 as a criminal lunatic asylum under the management and control of the Home Office. In 1960 it was taken over by the Ministry of Health as a special hospital under special security conditions for the treatment of dangerous, violent, or criminal patients. The hospital deals with mentally ill patients who are within the normal range of intelligence. Although the patients are subject to compulsory detention, within the requirements of security psychotherapy (q.v.) and group thereapy (q.v.) are carried out. Until the construction of Broadmoor, dangerous lunatics (q.v.)

had been confined at Bethlem Royal Hospital's (q.v.) criminal department. Broadmoor was spacious and comfortable in comparison with Bethlem's criminal department; so much so that in 1927 an old man knocked at the front gate of Broadmoor begging for admission. He was recognized by the oldest warden as a James Kelly who had escaped thirty-nine years earlier. He declared he had never been so content as when he had been in the hospital, and was readmitted.
Bibliography: McGrath, P. G. 1966. Hospital care of the mentally abnormal offender. *Proc. Roy. Soc. Med.*, 59: 699-700.

BROCA, PAUL (1824-1880). A French psychiatrist, neurologist, and anthropologist. He is considered the founder of modern brain surgery as well as one of the greatest names in modern anthropology. He originated craniometry, a method of determining the ratio of brain and skull dimensions, and devised various instruments for taking these measurements. In 1859 he founded the Anthropological Society of Paris. While at Bicêtre (q.v.) he had under his care a patient who, although he was intelligent and had no apparent muscular paralysis, had been unable to speak for thirty years. Broca's autopsy, after the patient's death, uncovered a lesion of the third frontal convolution of the left cerebral hemisphere. From this lesion, Broca was able to localize the center for speech (Broca's area). He presented the brain, preserved in alcohol, to the Anthropological Society of Paris and published his findings in 1861. This date now marks the first scientific discovery of the precise localization of mental functions.
See also APHEMIA.
Bibliography: Haymaker, W., and Schiller, F. 1970. *The founders of neurology*. 2d. ed.

BRODIE, SIR BENJAMIN COLLINS (1783-1862). An English surgeon, professor of comparative anatomy and physiology, physician to George IV, sergeant-surgeon to William IV and Queen Victoria. He was interested in diseases of the joints, and it was while observing a young woman suffering from unspecified pains in the knee that he came to the conclusion that the majority of upper class women who complained of pain in the joints were hysterics (*see* HYSTERIA). He postulated that certain paralyses were of hysterical origin and not caused by pathology of either the brain or the spinal cord. He also regarded certain gastrointestinal disorders the result of nervous affections. He thought that the hysterical patient unconsciously simulated symptoms and that therapy therefore demanded desuggestion, rather than suggestion.
Bibliography: Brodie, B. C. 1837. *Lectures illustrative of certain nervous affections*.

BRODIE, WILLIAM (?-1788). A cabinetmaker, deacon of the Incorporation of Edinburgh Wrights and Masons. By day he ran a respectable business, and by night he was the head of a gang of burglars that operated in Edinburgh. He fled Scotland but was captured in Amsterdam, shipped back to Scotland, and condemned to death. He laughed his way to the gallows whose efficient deadly drop he had himself designed. Robert Louis Stevenson (q.v.), in collaboration with W. E. Henley, wrote a play about him, entitled *Deacon Brodie, or the Double Life* and remarked that Brodie, like Dr. Jekyll and Mr. Hyde (q.v.), could not resist evil for its own sake.

BRODMANN, KORBINIAN (1868-1918). A German neurologist, born at Liggersdorf. He worked with Oskar Vogt (q.v.) and Alois Alzheimer (q.v.) at the Berlin Neuro-biological Institute and later became professor at Tübingen, in 1913. He postulated that the cortex is organized anatomically along the same principles in all mammals. He classified cortical types according to the morphogenesis of the cortex. His most famous work is *Foundation of Comparative Localization of the Cerebral Cortex*, published in 1909.
Bibliography: Haymaker, W., and Schiller, F. 1970. *The founders of neurology.* 2d. ed.

BROMIDES. Compounds of bromide discovered in 1826 by Antoine Balard (1802-1876), a French chemist. Twenty years later, bromides were widely used in psychiatry (q.v.). As depressants they produce sedation, thus reducing anxiety and symptoms of disturbed behavior. In the early part of the twentieth century they were so fashionable in the United States that twenty percent of all prescriptions were for bromides. They are less popular now because of modern substitutes and because of their tendency to cause a subdelirious state known as *bromism.*
Bibliography: Alexander, F. G. and Selesnick, S. T. 1966. *The history of psychiatry.*

BRONTË. The name of a remarkable English family of writers who flourished in the nineteenth century. Their father was a Methodist clergyman; their mother died after bearing six children in seven years. The first two daughters died of tuberculosis in childhood. An aunt, Elizabeth Branwell, looked after the family but was incapable of warmth. The children, however, received some measure of affection from a kindly servant, a Yorkshire woman who remained with the family for thirty years. **Maria** (1813-1825) the eldest, was pushed into premature maturity by her father, who entrusted to her the proof-reading of his manuscripts when she was only six years old. By the time she was seven, she could absorb the contents of newspapers, give a condensed version to her brother and sisters, and discuss the events with her father. She mothered the only male child in the family, **Branwell** (1817-1848), with devotion, until her death in 1825 when eleven years old. All the children wrote complicated stories and lived in a world of fantasy populated by their imagination. Branwell, probably the most unstable of them, was prone to violent temper tantrums, which the family believed were the result

of an uncauterized mad dog's bite. Maria's death affected him even more deeply than the rest of the family; she had been a great stabilizing influence in his life. An extremely clever child, he liked to demonstrate how he could write with both hands at the same time, writing in Latin with one hand and in Greek with the other. His ambitions to be a painter came to nothing as he became an alcoholic (*see* ALCOHOLISM) and an opium (q.v.) addict. His early death seems to have precipitated the death of **Emily** (1818-1848) who died three months after him. **Anne**'s (1820-1849) was the third death the Brontës had to bear within a few months. **Charlotte** (1816-1855), the most famous of the sisters, was exceptionally shy, but passionate; she tasted fame too late to really enjoy it. Despair and bitterness mark many of her writings. In 1854, she married, without great enthusiasm, her father's curate, the Reverend Arthur Bell Nicholls and died of pregnancy toxemia a year later. The father survived and was devotedly cared for by Charlotte's husband. The best known books by the sisters are: *Jane Eyre* (1847), *Shirley* (1849), and *Villette* (1853) by Charlotte, *Wuthering Heights* (1848) by Emily, who also wrote poems with Charlotte, and *Agnes Grey* (1848) by Anne.
Bibliography: Lane, M. 1953. *The Brontë story.*

BROOKE HOUSE. A house in London in which Dr. John Monro (q.v.) and later Dr. Henry Monro (q.v.) ran a private institution for mental patients. The building itself included parts of the Manor House of Clapton, dating from the Elizabethan period; it was destroyed by bombs during World War II.
Bibliography: Parry-Jones, W. Ll. 1972. *The trade in lunacy.*

BROOKS, MARY POTTER. The wife of Adolph Meyer (q.v.). She became interested in her husband's work and undertook visits to his patients' homes to learn more about their lives by direct observation. She is considered the first American social worker.
Bibliography: Alexander, F. G. and Selesnick, S. T. 1966. *The history of psychiatry.*

BROSIUS, C. M. (1825-1910). A German psychiatrist who successfully advocated the introduction of the nonrestraint policy into German asylums (q.v.).
Bibliography: Zilboorg, G. 1941. *A history of medical psychology.*

BROSSIER, MARTHA. A French woman accused of being a witch (*see* WITCHCRAFT) possessed by the devil. Jean Riolan (q.v.) and Louis Duret (q.v.), two sixteenth-century physicians, were among those who examined her. Their opinion was "nihil a demone; multa ficta, a morbo pauca" [nothing from the devil; many things feigned, few things from disease]. An example of early enlightened views of abnormal behavior in an hysterical (*see* HYSTERIA) woman.

Bibliography: Trevor-Roper, H. R. 1969. *The European witch-craze of the sixteenth and seventeenth centuries.*

BROTHERS, RICHARD (1757-1824). An English sailor. He was a religious fanatic, who claimed to be a nephew of God sent to earth to preach a new religion. He founded a sect called the Anglo-Israelites, which attracted a number of influential people. He accurately predicted the deaths of Louis XVI and Gustavus III, king of Sweden, but went too far when he announced that George III (q.v.) would soon die and he would take his place on the throne. He was sent to prison and then to an asylum (q.v.).

Bibliography: 1973. *Folklore, myths and legends of Britain.* Ed. Readers Digest Association Ltd., London.

BROTHERS KARAMAZOV, THE. One of the greatest novels in European literature, written by Fyodor Dostoevsky (q.v.). It represents Dostoevsky's faith in the spiritual values of mankind and is a masterful psychological study of family interactions. It also reflects the author's preoccupation with parricide and his own guilt about his relationship with his father. The Karamazov father is depicted as a sensual, irrational, and depraved individual; his sons, like himself, are tormented, guilty, and sorrowing.

Bibliography: Dostoevsky, F. M. 1979. *The brothers Karamazov*, trans. C. Garnett.

BROTHERS OF MERCY. A religious order, also called Hospitallers of St. John of God, founded by João de Deus (q.v.) in the sixteenth century. The brothers were dedicated particularly to the mentally ill. The mental hospital of Santa Maria della Pietà (q.v.) in Rome was established by them.

Bibliography: McMahon, N. 1959. *The story of the hospitallers of Saint John of God.*

BROUSSAIS, FRANÇOIS JOSEPH VICTOR (1772-1838). A French physician born at Saint-Malo. He was a surgeon in the army and in the navy during the French Revolution. In 1831 he was appointed professor of general pathology at the University of Paris. He was an acrimonious opposer of the work of Philippe Pinel (q.v.) and found few followers of his own theory of irritation, which emphasized the importance of the stomach. He believed that gastrointestinal irritation was the cause of most diseases and that treatment should consist of appropriate diets (q.v.), purges (*see* PURGING), and bleeding (q.v.). In addition to works on physiology, he wrote *De l'irritation et de la folie* (1828) in which he extended his theory of irritation to the aetiology of insanity. The epidemic of cholera that decimated the population of Paris in 1832 was partially responsible for the refutation of his views.

Bibliography: Zilboorg, G. 1941. *A history of medical psychology.*

BROWN, JOHN (1735-1788). A physician, born in Scotland. His father was a laborer of modest means, but Brown was able to study medicine

thanks to the generosity of two professors at Edinburgh University, Donald Monro and William Cullen (q.v.). In spite of his gratitude to them, he vigorously attacked their teachings, including the bleeding (q.v.) that they advocated. Because of the antagonism his attacks aroused, he left Edinburgh and qualified from St. Andrew's University. His medical reforms were based on his theory of excesses and deficiencies (Brunonian theory). According to this theory, a "sthenic" state was produced by overstimulation, while "asthenia," a state of nervous weakness, was caused by lack of stimulation. He treated asthenia with huge doses of stimulants, which often resulted in the death of the patient. He thought that insanity was due to violent passions of the mind and that the apathy of depression was caused by a lack of stimulation. In keeping with this belief, his treatment consisted of rousing the patient at all costs, even by brutal and cruel means. Psychiatry (q.v.) suffered a long setback because of these ideas, which were readily accepted. In 1786, he moved to London, where he acquired a large practice. He presented his theories in *Elementa Medicinae* (1780), a book that made him famous. He died suddenly of apoplexy.
Bibliography: Guthrie, D. 1958. *A history of medicine.*

BROWN, THOMAS (1778-1820). A Scottish philosopher and physician. He was only twenty years old when he published a criticism of Erasmus Darwin's (q.v.) *Zoonomia.* He was a disciple of Dugald Stewart (q.v.), and from 1810 to 1820, both men simultaneously occupied the chair of moral philosophy at the University of Edinburgh. Brown's lectures were extremely popular and were so polished that after his death they were published in their original form. He explained the functions of the mind through the principle of suggestion and believed that perception is given unity and significance by muscular sensation. He was the first to consider in detail the secondary laws of association (*see* ASSOCIATIONISM). He was also a poet with several volumes of verses to his credit.
Bibliography: Brown, Thomas. 1820. *Lectures on the philosophy of the human mind.*

BROWNE, SIR THOMAS (1605-1682). An English physician, born in London, the son of a wealthy mercer. He studied medicine at Oxford University as well as at the universities of Montpellier, Padua and Leyden. A taciturn and solitary man, he said of himself, "I am no way facetious, nor disposed for the mirth and galliardize of company." He attributed this to having been born "in the planetary hour of Saturn." In 1637, he settled in Norwich, married four years later, and produced a family of twelve children. *Religio Medici* (q.v.), his best known work, was written in 1635, but published in 1643. It was followed by other volumes on medicine, on antiquarianism, and on religion. In *Religio Medici* Browne discussed two orders of truth: one arrived at by reasoning and the other accepted by faith or intuition. Thus, in this discussion he exposed the contradictions of the

human mind and showed a grasp of psychological motivation. Although erudite and tolerant, he seems to have believed in witches and was instrumental in convicting women accused of witchcraft (q.v.). He was knighted in 1671 in recognition of his unwavering support for the royalist cause.
Bibliography: Finch, J. S. 1950. *Sir Thomas Browne.*

BROWNE, WILLIAM ALEXANDER FRANCIS (1805-1885). A Scottish psychiatrist, born in Stirling. As a student, he came under the influence of George Combe (q.v.) and his brother Andrew, both of whom were fervent exponents of phrenology (q.v.). This helped to develop Browne's interest in psychiatry (q.v.), and he traveled abroad to study under Jean Esquirol (q.v.). After some years in general practice he was appointed medical superintendent of Montrose Asylum (q.v.). His lectures to the managers of the hospital were published in 1837, under the title *What Asylums Were, Are and Ought to be* (q.v.). The title clearly indicates his indignation at the way in which the insane were treated, and the work so impressed Elizabeth Crichton that she asked him to be resident medical officer at the hospital she was founding, the Crichton Royal Hospital (q.v.). He accepted and held the position for eighteen years, bringing about many reforms. Visitors were encouraged, restraint (q.v.) abolished, social and recreational activities introduced, and precise and detailed clinical records kept on each patient. In 1854 he was the first to institute formal lectures in the training of the nursing staff; he also advocated that women should volunteer for work in asylums (q.v.) as a religious duty. In 1837, after a new Scottish lunacy act was passed, he became senior medical commissioner in lunacy, and again his enlightened attitude made itself felt in the reforms instituted in asylums throughout Scotland. He resigned his post as commissioner in 1870 because he was becoming increasingly blind.
Bibliography: Browne, W. A. F. 1837. *What asylums were, are, and ought to be.*

BROWNING, ELIZABETH BARRETT (1806-1861). An English poet. Her father treated his twelve children like slaves, believing that they should obey him without question. She began writing verses and prose at the age of ten, and her poems were published when she was seventeen. The psychological shock of seeing her favorite brother drowned and physical ill health confined her to a darkened room, where she lived as an invalid and a recluse, jealously guarded by her tyrannical father. Her poems came to the notice of Robert Browning (q.v.), who fell in love with her and persuaded her to elope with him to Italy. Browning worked hard to overcome her addiction to laudanum. Her father never forgave her for eloping, but she was ideally happy and recovered her health.
Bibliography: Taplan, G. B. 1957. *Life of Elizabeth Barrett Browning.*

BROWNING, ROBERT (1812-1889). An English poet and playwright. After his marriage to Elizabeth Barrett (*see* Browning, Elizabeth Barrett),

they lived in seclusion in Italy for fifteen years. Among his best works is *Dramatis Personae*, a collection of psychological monologues. His interest in psychological problems is also shown in his poem "Mesmerism" (1855), in which a woman is compelled by a mesmerizer (*see* MESMERISM) to come to him on a rainy night; he is appalled by his new-found power and prays that he will be given the strength to not abuse it.
Bibliography: Ward, M. 1968-1969. *Robert Browning and his world*. 2 vols.

BROWNRIGG, ELIZABETH (?-1767). The wife of an English house-painter. She practiced midwifery, a profession little suited to her psychopathic (*see* PSYCHOPATHY) personality. She murdered her apprentice, Mary Clifford, in a most barbarous way and was hanged for her crime.
Bibliography: Bayley, C. 1800. *A full and particular account of the life of Elizabeth Brownrigg*.

BROWN-SEQUARD, CHARLES ÉDOUARD (1817?-1894). A French physiologist and physician who practiced and taught in France and England. He was the first to demonstrate that epilepsy (q.v.) could be induced in guinea pigs. He described a syndrome in which the patient is paralyzed on one side of the body and has loss of sensation on the other side. It is caused by a lesion on one side of the spinal cord.
Bibliography: Haymaker, W., and Schiller, F. 1970. *The founders of neurology*. 2d. ed.

BROWN STUDY. An expression meaning vacuity of mind under the appearance of thought. The French *sombre rêverie* describes it better; *sombre* means gloomy, sad, or dull. *Brun*, translated as brown, has the same meaning.
Bibliography: *Brewer's Dictionary of Phrase and Fable*. 1978. Ed. I. H. Evans.

BRÜCKE, ERNST WILHELM VON (1819-1892). A German physician and leading physiologist. He believed that the functioning of the living organism was dependent only on the principles of physics and chemistry rather than a vital force or substance. Sigmund Freud (q.v.) studied with Brücke for six years and learned from him the strict scientific approach that he was to apply to his own work. He often acknowledged that Brücke had had a great intellectual influence on him.
Bibliography: Alexander, F. G., and Selesnick, S. T. 1966. *The history of psychiatry*.

BRUEGHEL (*or* BREUGHEL) PIETER (c.1525-1569). A Flemish painter. In his earlier paintings he vividly depicted fear and horror in a manner similar to Hieronymus Bosch (q.v.), but less dreamlike and showing an element of rationalization within the religious concepts of his time. His misshapen creatures seem to be the product of haunting fantasies, and the sexual aberrations appearing in many of his works are presented in such a way that they arouse disgust rather than erotic feelings. His series of paintings entitled

Vices and *Virtues* illustrate his pessimistic view of the world. These emphasize the negative aspects of inner life, greed, envy, and jealousy, as stronger than the positive aspects, justice, fortitude, and industry. The *Temptation of St. Anthony* has an hallucinatory quality that was later adopted by the followers of Surrealism (q.v.). In 1564, Brueghel settled in Brussels, where he married the daughter of his teacher Pieter Coeck. She must have had a beneficial influence on his life as he no longer painted demons and horrifying subjects but instead turned to religious themes and the representation of people in more normal situations. He depicted them with compassion and with unusual insight into the limitations of human nature. On his deathbed he instructed his wife to destroy the more explicit of his drawings, probably because he felt guilty about them. Of his two sons, Pieter (c.1564-1637) specialized in painting infernal beings, evil people, and flames, and therefore was called "Hell" Brueghel; in contrast, the younger son, Jean (1568-1625), was called "Velvet" because of his gentle still-lifes.

Bibliography: Brueghel, P. 1973. *Complete edition of the paintings.*
Glück, G. 1953. *The large Bruegel book.*

BRUELE (*or* **BRANT**) **GUALTHERIUS** (fl.1585). A Dutch physician. He wrote *Praxis Medicinae Theorica et Emperica Familiarissima* in which, beginning at the head and going to the foot, he described diseases, their prognosis, course, and treatment. His classification of mental disorders appears to have been influenced by Jean Fernel (q.v.) because he combines humoral theory (q.v.) with a topographical outlook.

Bibliography: *Wellcome Catalogue of Printed Books*, vol.1. 1962. Ed. Poynter, F.N.L.

BRUNS, LUDWIG (1858-1916). A German psychiatrist and neuropathologist, born in Hanover. He was the first to describe paroxymal headache with vertigo and vomiting when the position of the head is altered. It is now known as Bruns's syndrome.

Bibliography: Jablonski, S. 1969. *Eponymic syndromes and diseases and their synonyms.*

BRUNSWICK. The capital of a free state in northern Germany in the thirteenth century. It provided care for the mentally ill as early as 1224. The hospital was dedicated to the Virgin Mary and called the Jungfrau Maria Hospital.

Bibliography: Whitwell, J. R. 1936. *Historical notes on psychiatry.*

BRUSQUET (?-1563). A fool (q.v.) at the court of King Francis I of France. He attained such fame that he was listed in several encyclopedias until the nineteenth century.

Bibliography: Kanner, L. 1964. *A history of the care and study of the mentally retarded.*

BRUTUS, MARCUS JUNIUS (86-42 B.C.). One of the murderers of Julius Caesar. As a young man he wrote poetry and philosophical treatises. In one of his essays he condemned suicide (q.v.), but nevertheless, after his defeat near Philippi, he took his own life by running on his sword.
Bibliography: Fedden, H. R. 1938. *Suicide.*

BUCHANAN, JOSEPH (1785-1829). An American physician, born in Washington County, Virginia; he spent his childhood in poor circumstances. His extraordinary intelligence was apparent from his early years, and he gained a reputation as a genius when still at school. He invented machines, studied medicine and became professor of the Institutes of Medicine at Transylvania University, wrote and edited books, established a school based on Johann Pestalozzi's (q.v.) system, studied law and lectured on it, and wrote on sciences, history, and philosophy. His work *The Philosophy of Human Nature* (1812) was in advance of the time; it presents a materialistic explanation of spiritual experiences. It subordinated the mind to the body and defined it as "nothing more than a repetition of the sensorial action, which formed an integral part of the prior perception." Buchanan applied the principles of association (*see* ASSOCIATIONISM) to feelings, beliefs, and volition. His contemporaries did not approve of his philosophy, especially the clergy, who regarded him as an atheist and refused to accept his original contributions to psychology.
Bibliography: Adams, J. F., and Hoberman, A. A. 1969. Joseph Buchanan, 1785-1829: pioneer American psychologist. *J. Hist. Behav. Sci.* 5: 340-48.

BUCHAREST CENTRAL HOSPITAL FOR MENTAL AND NERVOUS DISORDERS. A Rumanian mental hospital founded by Alexandru Obregia (q.v.). The construction began in 1906, but, because of World War I, it was not completed until 1923. It contained pavilions with over 2000 beds and annex buildings for special therapies. Because many patients came from rural areas, special emphasis was given to farm work as a part of occupational therapy (q.v.).
Bibliography: Predescu, V., and Christodorescu, D. 1975. Rumania. In *World history of psychiatry*, ed. J. G. Howells.

BUCK, PEARL S. (1892-1973). An American novelist. Her parents and her husband were missionaries in China, where she was brought up. Her novel *The Good Earth* vividly described peasant life in China, and won for her the Nobel Prize for Literature in 1938. Her eldest daughter was mentally retarded, and she described the child's disability and care in *The Child Who Never Grew Up* (1950). Her other works dealing with mental retardation are *The Gifts They Bring: Our Debt to the Mentally Retarded* and *The Time is Noon*. Pearl Buck was also active in providing adoptive homes for illegitimate Amerasian children.
Bibliography: Harris, T. F. 1969. *Pearl S. Buck: a biography.*

BUCKLE, RICHARD MAURICE (1837-1902). A Canadian psychiatrist, born in England. He was a descendant of Sir Robert Walpole, the English prime minister. He led an adventurous life, worked as a laborer and a miner. When he was twenty years old, he suffered severe exposure in a snowstorm. Frostbite damage to his feet caused one foot to be amputated and left the other permanently damaged. After this experience, he decided to study medicine and, after qualifying, spent some years in Europe before returning to Canada. He became superintendent of the London Psychiatric Hospital, in Ontario, Canada, in 1877. He at first believed that mechanical restraint (q.v.) was necessary for the good of the patients, but he later abolished it together with sedative drugs. He advocated employment for most insane patients and introduced female nurses in male wards. His philosophy was that the life of every patient could be made more tolerable by a process of humanization. He suggested the introduction of colonies for certain groups of patients seventy years before they were actually inaugurated.
Bibliography: Greenland, G. 1972. The complete psychiatrist. *Can. Psychiat. Assn. J.* 17: 71.

BUCKNILL, SIR JOHN CHARLES (1817-1897). An English physician. He was the first superintendent of the Devon Asylum, a position that he held from 1844 to 1862. His methods of treatment were original and insightful. He used a psychological approach, abolished restraint (q.v.), and inaugurated a system of boarding-out of mental patients (q.v.) in seaside cottages, where they could enjoy a holiday away from the asylum. He was the first editor of the *Asylum Journal* (q.v.) and coeditor of *Brain* (q.v.). In 1860 he became the president of the Association of Medical Officers of Asylums and Hospitals for the Insane (q.v.) (now the Royal College of Psychiatrists) and the first honorary member of its sister association of the same name in America (now the American Psychiatric Association [q.v.]). In 1862 he became Lord Chancellor's Visitor in Lunacy, a position that gave him the opportunity to propagate his views on nonrestraint. His interest in literature led to his book *The Psychology of Shakespeare*, published in 1859. With Daniel H. Tuke (q.v.) he wrote *A Manual of Psychological Medicine* (1858), which was considered a standard work for many years and influenced the practice of psychiatry in both England and the United States; their classification of mental disorders was based on the main symptom presented in each category. A lesser-known activity of Bucknill was his organization of a corps of volunteer part-time soldiers to defend the coast line of Exeter and South Devon from the French in 1852. It was the forerunner of the Territorial Army.
Bibliography: Bucknill, J. C., and Tuke, D. H. 1858. Reprint. 1968. *A manual of psychological medicine.*

BUDDHA (SAKYAMUNI, GAUTAMA, *or* **SIDDARTHA)** (563?-?483 B.C.). An Indian philosopher and sage, son of the king of Kapilavastu in

Nepal. His name means "the Enlightened." When he was about thirty years old, he tired of luxuries, left his palace, and went wandering through India. He found penance and asceticism (*see* ASCETICS) futile. Through long meditations he evolved his own religion, which was based on the belief that suffering and existence are inseparable, sufferings are caused by desire, and therefore, the suppression of desire is desirable. His final aim became the extinction of individual existence and the emancipation of the spirit. He taught and founded many monasteries in the Ganges Valley. His doctrines, which attracted many disciples, developed into the great Asiatic religion Buddhism.
Bibliography: Humphreys, T. C. 1962. *Buddhism*.

BUDGEL, EUSTACE (1686-1737). An English writer. He lived in an era when suicide (q.v.) was regarded as a tiresome act, neither condemned nor glorified. He killed himself by jumping into the river Thames after loading his pockets with stones. Alluding to *Cato*, a play by his cousin Joseph Addison (1672-1719), he left a note saying, "What Cato did and Addison approved cannot be wrong."
Bibliography: Alvarez, A. 1971. *The savage god*.

BUFFON, GEORGES LOUIS LECLERC DE (1707-1788). A French naturalist and author of several works. In his natural history he tried to evolve a classification embracing all facts of nature. He discussed evolution and its limitation and anticipated some genetic theories, which influenced psychiatry. His *Histoire Naturelle* was published in forty-four volumes between 1749 and 1804.
Bibliography: Heim, R., ed. 1952. *Les grands naturalists français*.

BUGLOSS (BUGLE). A weed growing in meadows and fields. In the *Great Herbal* (1526), it is recommended for its ability to "preserve the mynde" if eaten often. Modern herbalists advise a decoction made with this herb to prevent nightmares (q.v.) and cure delirium tremens (q.v.).
Bibliography: Law, D. 1969. *Herb growing for health*.

BUHLER, KARL (1879-1963). A Viennese psychologist. He introduced the concept of functional pleasure, which postulated that autonomous body activities at times are used solely as a source of pleasure and have no other purpose. This concept advanced the understanding of the psychology of play and led to a revision of the theory of instincts.
Bibliography: Waelder, R. 1933. The psychoanalytic theory of play. *Psychoanal. Quart.* 2: 208-24.

BUKHT YISHU. A term meaning "servants of Christ." It was the name of a medical family who fled Constantinople in the eighth century because of religious strife. They settled in Baghdad, and their services were much appreciated by the caliph. They treated mental disorders by frightening their patients and reproaching them for their behavior. These methods were used by one of them to cure the insane wife of Harun-al-Rashid (q.v.) (763-809), the idealized caliph of the *Arabian Nights*.

Bibliography: Elgood, C. 1951. *A medical history of Persia and the eastern caliphate.*

BUMKE, OSWALD (1877-1950). A German psychiatrist and neurologist, born in Stolp, Pomerania. He studied the alterations occurring in the pupil in some mental diseases. He was the first to describe the peculiar dilation of the pupil that is the result of certain psychic stimuli. Is is now known as Bumke's pupil. He published several works on psychiatry (q.v.) and neurology (q.v.) and was the editor of the *Handbuch der Geisteskrankheiten* (1928-33), and of the *Handbuch der Neurologie* (1935-37). He was one of Nicholai Lenin's (q.v.) physicians in Moscow.

BUNYAN, JOHN (1628-1688). An English author and preacher, the son of a tinsmith, born near Bedford, England. After briefly attending the village school, he took up his father's trade until the age of sixteen when he enlisted in the army to escape his stepmother. Later, moved by the religious books left to him by his dead wife, he became a preacher, and his first writing was against the Quakers (q.v.). He was sentenced to twelve years in prison for preaching without a licence. During this period he wrote *Grace Abounding to the Chief of Sinners* (1666), an autobiographical work relating the frightening visions he experienced as a child, his violent adolescence, and his overwhelming feelings of guilt. Depression and religious mania (q.v.) racked him, agitation exhausted him, and he incessantly searched the Bible (q.v.) for a word of hope that his soul might be saved. After his release from prison in 1672, Bunyan resumed his pastoral work but again was imprisoned and began his masterpiece, *The Pilgrim's Progress from This World to That Which Is to Come* (1678).

Bibliography: Lindsay, J. 1937. *John Bunyan.*

BURDEN, HAROLD NELSON (1859-1930). A British clergyman. With his wife, he undertook missionary work among the Ojibway Indians in Canada. The death of his two children and his own poor health forced him to return to Britain, where his wife became involved in prison visiting. In 1889, following their experience with prisoners, they founded for alcoholic women the Institution for Inebriates. This institution was modified later to care for mentally retarded patients. They went on to found the Brentry Certified Inebriate Reformatory (q.v.). In 1902, Burden founded the National Institution for Persons Requiring Care and Control; this was followed by Stoke Park Hospital (q.v.) for mental defectives in 1909. His sound financial acumen and good management allowed these enterprises to run efficiently and expand when necessary. His life and financial resources were completely dedicated to the cause of the mentally retarded. He not only provided for their care but also stimulated and financed research in the causes, treatment, and prevention of mental retardation.

Bibliography: Jancar, J. 1969. Sixty years at Stoke Park Hospital (1909-1969). *Bristol Med.-Chir. J.* 87:23-30.

BURDETT, HENRY CHARLES (1847-1920). A British hospital administrator. He was secretary and general superintendent of the Queen's Hospital in Birmingham, and the founder of the Home Hospital Association for Paying Patients. He wrote several books about hospitals, the most important of which was *Hospitals and asylums of the world* (q.v.). Burdett built a model hospital at Claybury, near London.

Bibliography: Burdett, H. C. 1891. *Hospitals and asylums of the world.*

BURGHÖLZLI HOSPITAL. The psychiatric clinic and mental hospital of the University of Zürich in Switzerland. The hospital is for patients with acute and prognostically hopeful illnesses. Originally the mental hospital for the Canton of Zürich was in Rheinau, a beautiful island on the Rhine. The building previously had been a monastery and could accommodate over 600 patients. In 1860 it was found to be inadequate and a new hospital was built. Wilhelm Griesinger (q.v.), the professor of medicine in Zürich, was its first director. Auguste Forel, Eugen Bleuler, and Carl Jung (qq.v.) were among those who contributed to the significant role that the Burghölzli played in the history of psychiatry (q.v.).

Bibliography: Lewis, A. 1967. *The state of psychiatry.*

BURGLARY. A nonpunishable offense in the seventeenth-century law of England if committed by a child under fourteen or by "poore persons that upon hunger shall enter a house for victuall under the value of twelve pence; nor in naturall fooles, or other persons that bee non compos mentis. . . ."

Bibliography: Dalton, M. 1618. Reprint. 1727. *The country justice, conteyning the practise of the justices of the peace out of their sessions.*

BURKMAR, LUCIUS. A young American student who was used by Phineas Quimby (q.v.) in experiments involving magnetism (q.v.). In a trance Burkmar could diagnose diseases and suggest the appropriate treatment with outstanding results. Quimby gradually came to realise that it was not magnetism, clairvoyance, or any other mysterious quality, but people's faith in them that brought about the cures.

Bibliography: Alexander, F. G., and Selesnick, S. T. 1966. *The history of psychiatry.*

BURNS, ROBERT (1759-1796). A Scottish poet, famous for his passionate, vivacious, and at times despairing verses. His reckless merriment and drink-

ing often masked a troubled mind. He was an irritable man, a hypochondriac (*see* HYPOCHONDRIA) and on his own admission given to "incurable melancholy." He loved wine and women too well.
Bibliography: Lindsay, M. 1954. *Robert Burns.*

BURROW, N. TRIGANT (1875-1950). An American phylobiologist and psychiatrist. He began as a follower of Sigmund Freud (q.v.) but then developed his own form of analysis, phyloanalysis, which investigated how human behavior is modified by adjusting the internal tension pattern. When these tensions are distorted by anxiety, neurosis results. Therapy consists in reducing and correcting distortions of perception of events.
Bibliography: Burrow, N. T. 1953. *Science and man's behavior.*

BURROWS, GEORGE MAN (1771-1846). An English physician who practiced in London, having started his medical career at the age of sixteen as a surgeon's apprentice. The Apothecaries Act of 1815 was brought about by his persistence. The act gave to medical practitioners medical and legal status as well as an examination run by their own association. Burrows left general practice to dedicate himself exclusively to psychiatry (q.v.), having established a private asylum (q.v.) of his own, the Clapham Retreat (q.v.). He was offended by the French claim that insanity (*see* INSANIA) and suicide (q.v.) were more common in England than elsewhere and tried to prove that France had the greater number of insane and Paris had more suicides than London. In his publication *An Inquiry into Certain Errors Relative to Insanity* (1820), he postulated that insanity was highly curable and claimed that he, himself, had cured 81 percent of all mental patients in his private asylum. He claimed a recovery rate of 91 percent for those who had been ill less than a year. The figures were accepted in spite of his small sample, and his practice was greatly increased. In 1828, his *Commentaries on Causes, Forms, Symptoms and Treatment of Insanity* was published. Again he showed great optimism about the therapy of mental disorders but suggested no new approaches to treatment. The volume appeared ten years after it had been announced, because, according to the author, he had lost the briefcase containing his original notes. The work opened with the words "Insanity is the scourge brought down on sinful men by the wrath of the Almighty," an almost medieval concept. Yet, Burrows was one of the first to recognize that general paralysis of the insane (q.v.) was a newly discovered disease, which organically affected the brain. His recognition of this fact opened the way to a pathology of insanity and put psychiatry on the same level with scientific medicine.
Bibliography: Hunter, R., and Macalpine, I. 1963. *Three hundred years of psychiatry.*

BURT, CYRIL LODOWIC (1883-1971). A British psychologist. He translated the Binet Simon (q.v.) tests from French for use in England. He was especially interested in educational problems and juvenile delinquency and was the author of several volumes on a variety of subjects. After his death some of his findings on intelligence were seriously questioned.

Bibliography: Burt, C. L. 1925. *The young delinquent.*

————. 1952. *The causes and treatment of backwardness.*

Hearnshaw, L. S. 1979. *Cyril Burt, psychologist.*

BURTON, ROBERT (1577-1640). An English divine, born at Lindley Hall in Leicestershire. His childhood was unhappy and he lacked parental affection. He did not enjoy his school days, which he later compared to slavery. He studied divinity at Oxford and remained there as a don for the rest of his life, which was, in his own words, "silent, sedentary, solitary, and private." His interest in geography and maps may indicate a suppressed longing for travel. His best friends were his books. Burton's interest in medicine may have been fostered by his mother, who had a reputation for possessing "excellent skill in chirurgery, sore eyes and aches." The *Anatomy of Melancholy* (q.v.) was written in an attempt to ease his own depression and reflects much of the author's personal experience of life. His sarcasm marks a dissatisfaction with the world and a bitterness at his solitude, which he had not the strength to break. He was, as he said, "a drinker of water." A bachelor's fascination with love and sex is disclosed in his book, a third of which he dedicated to love-melancholy. Like most of his contemporaries, he believed in witches (*see* WITCHCRAFT) and thought that "they can cure and cause most diseases. . .melancholy amongst the rest." In many things he was in advance of his time. He could see the relation between mental disorder and social environment, and he advocated socialized medicine, special hospitals, free housing for the poor, and pensions for the old. He never escaped his own melancholy (*see* MELANCHOLIA), and John Aubrey (q.v.), wrote in his *Brief Lives*: "tis wispered that, non obstante all his ostrologie and his booke of Melancholie, he ended his dayes in that chamber by hanging him selfe."

Bibliography: Evans, B., and Mohr, G. J. 1944. *The psychiatry of Robert Burton.*

Aubrey's brief lives. 1949. ed. Dick, O. L.

BUTHAVIDYA. The fourth part of the Ayurvetic system of ancient Hindu medicine. The writings in the Buthavidya deal with mental disorders, which usually were attributed to possession (q.v.) by evil spirits.

Bibliography: Zimmer, H. 1948. *Hindu medicine.*

BUTLER, JOHN (1803-1890). An American psychiatrist. He was the first superintendent of the Boston Lunatic Hospital (q.v.). In 1843, he moved to the Retreat for the Insane at Hartford, Connecticut, where he remained for nearly thirty years and exercised a progressive influence. He was one of the original thirteen founders of the American Psychiatric Association (q.v.).

He was also an expert on the legal aspects of insanity and the courts often asked his opinion in difficult cases involving the plea of insanity. He retired to private practice in 1873.

Bibliography: Deutsch, A. 1949. *The mentally ill in America.*

BUTLER, SAMUEL (1612-1680). An English poet famous for his satire in three cantos, *Hudibras*, in which he ridiculed Presbyterians and Independents. He was a court favorite, but died in poverty. Agrippa (q.v.) was satirized by him together with his dog, believed by the church to be a demon. Butler thought that only external phenomena could be observed and that "we cannot reason with our cells, for they know so much more than we do that they cannot understand us."

Bibliography: Holt, L. E. 1964. *Samuel Butler.*
Veldkamp, J. 1924. *Samuel Butler.*

BUTTERCUP. A yellow-flowered ranunculus. In the Greco-Roman period it symbolized madness.

Bibliography: Cooper, J. C. 1978. *An illustrated encyclopaedia of traditional symbols.*

BYRON, GEORGE GORDON, LORD (1788-1824). An English poet, born in London. He was born with a clubfoot and epilepsy (q.v.). His first epileptic fit occurred at birth, followed by others in later life. His father "Mad Jack" Byron, an officer in the Guards, died when he was three years old, and he spent his childhood in Aberdeen, Scotland, with his mother, who alternately spoiled and abused him, taunting him about his deformed foot. He was unpopular at school and showed signs of anxiety by continuously biting his nails. Excitement was said to precipitate epilepsy in him. He is a good example of organ inferiority, as postulated by Alfred Adler (q.v.), inasmuch that he was deeply embarrassed by his lame foot. Poetry was initially rejected by him as something repelling. He had his first love affair at fifteen, missing a whole school term because of it. At University, in Cambridge, he kept several bulldogs and a bear, causing comment by his fellow students. In 1815, he married an heiress, Anne Isabella Milbanke, by whom he had a daughter, Augusta Ada. The marriage lasted one year, at the end of which his wife obtained a separation, claiming that he was insane. During this period he drank heavily and took laudanum (q.v.). There were rumors that he had an incestuous (*see* INCEST) relationship with his half sister, Augusta Leigh, and he was known to be bisexual. In consequence of the scandal, he left England and lived in Italy, where he formed a passionate relationship with the Countess Teresa Guiccioli (1801?-1873). His poetry attacked hypocrisy in politics, religion, and morals, and although critics assailed its immorality it remained popular.

Bibliography: Maurois, A. 1930. Reprint. 1963. *Byron*.

BYZANTIUM. Ancient Istanbul. A mental hospital, or morotrophium (q.v.) existed in this city as early as A.D. c. 300.

Bibliography: Whitwell, J. R. 1936. *Historical notes on psychiatry*.

C

CABANIS, PIERRE JEAN GEORGE (1757-1808). A French physician, revolutionary, and philosopher. Because he did not do well at school as a child, his father sent him to Paris, telling him to look after himself. He educated himself, studied medicine, and became the personal physician and friend of Hornoré Mirabeau (q.v.) a leader of the French Revolution. Cabanis became a member of the legislative Committee of Five Hundred. He was interested in psychological phenomena and believed in the existence of a whole personality as opposed to an organic predisposition. He studied consciousness and investigated whether or not the victims of the guillotine remained conscious after beheading. He concluded that they did not and that consciousness depends on the brain. His findings then were collected in a volume entitled *Rapports du Physique et du Moral de l'Homme*. (1802). He believed that every man had a right to work and was a passionate opponent of the death sentence. Cabanis supported materialism and, because of his views, is considered the founder of physiological psychology.
Bibliography: Ackerknecht, E. H. 1966. *Medicine in the Paris hospital 1794-1848*.

CACODEMONOMANIA. A term coined by Jean Esquirol (q.v.) to indicate that class of insane who believe that they are in communication with God, who inspires them to preach and convert mankind.
Bibliography: Esquirol, J. E. D. 1845. Reprint. 1965. *Mental maladies: a treatise on insanity*.

CADIVA INSANIA. An obsolete Latin term for epilepsy (q.v.), literally meaning "falling insanity."

CADUCA PASSIO *or* CADUCUS MORBUS. An obsolete Latin term for epilepsy (q.v.), meaning "falling disease."

CADUCEUS. An emblem of medicine, a staff encircled by two snakes. Originally it was depicted as the staff of Aesculapius (q.v.) with only one snake coiled around it. The staff with two serpents was carried by Hermes, the messenger of the Greek Gods, and it was said to induce sleep when used as a wand. In the sixteenth century Hans Holbein the Younger (q.v.) designed a title page device using two serpents curled around the staff for Johann Froben, a publisher of medical books. Holbein again used the emblem for the arms of such famous English physicians as John Caius (q.v.) and William Harvey (q.v.). From then on the double snake was believed wrongly to be a symbol of medicine itself and was adopted as such.
Bibliography: Schouten, J. 1967. *The rod and serpent of Asklepios.*

CAELIUS AURELIANUS. A Roman physician of the fifth century A.D. His writings, which are derived from those of Soranus (q.v.), contain many interesting cases of mental disorder. He regarded insanity as a medical problem resulting from bodily disorders. He wrote at length about "incubi" (*see* INCUBUS), which he believed to be the cause of insomnia and night terrors. He thought that insanity was more common in men than in women. Aurelianus insisted that diagnosis should be based on a total picture of the individual rather than on isolated single symptoms. He was against the harsh methods of handling the insane and advocated humane treatment, including sunbathing for chronic afflictions. He emphatically condemned the practice of castrating epileptics (*see* EPILEPSY), a common form of treatment in his day.
Bibliography: Drabkin, I. E., ed. and trans. 1950. *Caelius Aurelianus, on acute diseases and on chronic diseases.*

CAESAR, JULIUS (100?-44 B.C.). Roman statesman and military commander. The Roman historian Suetonius (70-140 A.D.) described him as a tall, strong man, dark-eyed and full-faced, enjoying excellent health until the last few years of his life when he became prone to episodes of fainting and nightmares (q.v.). Suetonius also reported that Caesar on two occasions had suffered epileptic (*see* EPILEPSY) fits in public places. William Shakespeare (q.v.) gave a dramatic account of Caesar's epilepsy:

> He fell down in the market-place and, foam'd at mouth, and was speechless.
> [Julius Caesar, 1. 2]

Bibliography: Muccini, P. 1973. *Julius Caesar.*

CAGLIOSTRO, ALESSANDRO DI. *See* BALSAMO, GIUSEPPE.

CAGOTS. A tribe of people found in southern France afflicted with cretinism (q.v.). They may have been Pyreneans or Basques or Goths driven

out of Spain. Because of prejudice, they were obliged to live in isolation and wear distinguishing badges. Their name may have derived from "Canis Gothus," Goth dog, denoting the contempt in which they were held. Their community was self-supporting, thus it is unlikely that all of them were cretins. Prejudice against them was so strong that in the eleventh century they were sold as slaves, forced to enter a church by a separate door, and could only use holy water that had been set aside specifically for them. In 1460 it was suggested that they should not be allowed to walk barefooted, in case they spread their "infection." They were used for all the more humiliating and dangerous jobs, such as fire fighting. In the middle of the eighteenth century legal decrees, which forbade people to abuse them and extended to them the privileges of ordinary citizens, were enforced for their protection. Jean Esquirol (q.v.) still referred to them in 1845, but he added that they were then rarely met.
Bibliography: Kanner, L. 1964. *A history of the care and study of the mentally retarded.*

CAIRO LUNATIC ASYLUMS. The earliest known hospital in Cairo caring for the insane was that founded by Ahmed ibn Túlún about A.D. 873. Túlún was in the habit of visiting his hospital daily. One day a lunatic (q.v.) begged a pomegranate from him and then threw it at him. He never visited the hospital again. By the fifteenth century there are accounts of five hospitals with chambers or cells set aside for lunatics. The finest was the Al-Mansur Hospital (q.v.).
See also ASYLUMS, EGYPT, and KALAWOUN HOSPITAL.
Bibliography: Browne, E. G. 1921. *Arabian medicine.*

CAIUS, JOHN (1510-1573). An English physician, scholar, and author of scientific and antiquarian books. His name was a latinization of Keys or Kayes. He was president of the College of Physicians nine times. In 1557 he elevated Gonville Hall to the status of a college and gave it the name of Gonville and Caius College. The figure of Dr. Caius in William Shakespeare's (q.v.) *Merry Wives of Windsor* is said to be based on him. Samuel Pepys (q.v.) reported in his diary that Thomas Muffet, the author of a book entitled *Health's Improvement, or Rules for Preparing All Sorts of Food* (1655), wrote about Dr. Caius "being very old, and living only at that time upon woman's milk, he, while he fed upon the milk of an angry, fretful woman, was so himself; and then, being advised to take it of a good-natured, patient woman, he did become so, beyond the common temper of his age."
Bibliography: Ven, J. 1901. *Caius College.*

CAJAL, SANTIAGO RAMÓN Y (1852-1934). A Spanish histologist. As a child, he had been considered a dullard, his artistic talents had been regarded as poor, and even the shoemaker and the barber to whom he was apprenticed had a poor opinion of his ability. He struggled to gain a medical degree and, later, to make his discoveries known. Cajal undertook extensive research in the structure and physiology of nerve cells, and in 1889 he established that each neuron is separated from other neurons by a gap, or synapse. He also devised a new staining method for histological research on nerve tissues. In 1906, in conjunction with Camillo Golgi (q.v.), he received the Nobel Prize for medicine. He was also interested in psychology and studied, for example, the psychology of Quixotism. He wrote on love and women and concluded his musing by stating, "It is good to adapt things to our sensibilities but it is much healthier to adapt our sensibilities to things." Bibliography: Craigie, E. H., and Gibson, W. C., 1968. *The world of Ramón y Cajal.* Cajal, S. R., 1937. *Recollections of my life.*

CALAMINT. *Satureja Calamintha*, a small plant growing in chalky soil. An infusion of its tiny blue flowers was believed to be efficacious in the treatment of brain disorders.
Bibliography: Law, D. 1969. *Herb growing for health.*

CALANUS (?-323 B.C.). An Hindu philosopher of the Gymnosophist (q.v.) sect. When he became ill, he regarded his sickness as a state of impurity and asked to be burned alive on a funeral pyre.
Bibliography: Akhilananda, S. 1946. *Hindu psychology.*

CALCAR, JAN STEVENSZOON VAN (1499?-?1550). A pupil of Titian (1477-1576) and friend of Andreas Vesalius (q.v.). He illustrated Vesalius' *De Humani Corporis Fabrica* with magnificent plates of the bones and the nervous system in particular. The text and his illustrations were based on direct observation and revolutionized the study of the human body.

CALENTURA. A Spanish term for the morbid compulsion to jump into the sea that assailed sailors on long voyages. Jean Pierre Falret (q.v.) studied it closely and associated it with delirium (q.v.).
Bibliography: Falret, J. 1839. Délire. In *Dictionnaire des études médicales.*

CALIGULA (A.D. 12-41). A Roman emperor, son of Germanicus Caesar and Agrippina the Elder (q.v.). His real name was Gaius Caesar, but he was nicknamed Caligula because of the military shoes (*caligae*) that he wore. He showed moderation during the first period of his reign, but around 38 A.D. he suffered a severe illness, which completely changed his character. He became extremely cruel and enjoyed watching men being tortured and killed. He committed innumerable crimes, including incest (q.v.). His behavior indicates that he was probably psychotic (*see* PSYCHOSIS). He made his horse a consul. His excesses outraged the people and led to his assassination. In *Lives of the Caesars*, Suetonius (70-140 A.D.) wrote of him:

He had neither health of body nor of mind. As a boy, he was troubled with epilepsy [q.v.], and when he arrived at the years of manhood, though he could endure fatigue, he was sometimes seized with a sudden faintness, so that he could scarcely move, stand, or collect himself. He was himself sensible of the weakness of his mind, and had thoughts of retiring in order to clear his brain. He was believed to have got a philtre from his wife Caesonia which threw him into a frenzy. He was much disquieted by want of sleep, not resting at night more than three hours, and even then his sleep was broken and troubled by strange images; among other things the ocean seemed to come and speak with him, so during a great part of the night he would sit down at table, or wander through the vast galleries of his house, wishing for the approach of day. To this weakness of mind may be attributed two vices of an opposite character—great confidence and an excessive timidity.

Bibliography: Ireland, W. W. 1885. *The blot upon the brain: studies in history and psychology.*
Suetonius. *Lives of the Caesars.*

CALLIPEDIA. A term derived from the Greek and meaning "the desire to produce a beautiful child." It was believed that an expectant mother should look on beautiful objects and images of beautiful children in order to produce a beautiful child. The belief is associated with magic (q.v.) and primitive beliefs designed to protect mother and fetus from bad and ugly influences.

CALMEIL, LOUIS FLORENTIN (1798-1895). French physician and pioneer in psychiatric research. With Antoine Bayle (q.v.) he demonstrated that paralysis was frequent among the insane, that it was caused by pathological brain changes, and that the mental disorders occuring in such patients were a consequence of these changes. He called the disease general paralysis of the insane (q.v.) and concretely correlated its clinical manifestations to organic changes, although he did not discover that syphilis (q.v.) was the causative agent.

Bibliography: Calmeil, J. L. 1826. *De la paralysie chez les aliénés.*

CALONNE, ERNEST DE (1822-1887). A French writer. To assuage his craving for fame, he pretended to have discovered a new comedy by Molière (q.v.), *Le Docteur Amoureux*, which in fact he had written. To make his deception more credible, he forged a manuscript with old paper and faded ink. He is an excellent example of *pseudologia fantastica* (q.v.).

Bibliography: Harvey, P., and Heseltine, J. E. 1959. *Oxford companion to French literature.*

CALVAERT, DENYS (1540-1619). A Flemish painter. He was melancholy (*see* MELANCHOLIA), shy, at times paranoid (*see* PARANOIA), and given to angry outbursts. His miserly way of life enabled him to leave a large fortune on his death.

Bibliography: Wittkower, R., and Wittkower, M. 1963. *Born under Saturn.*

CALVIN, JOHN (1509-1564). A Swiss theologian and reformer, who was born in France. Destined for the church from childhood, he studied theology and law. He met many brilliant thinkers in Paris and was influenced by the new Christian humanism. He abandoned the Catholic church and organized a new, reformed religious movement that became known as Calvinism. After he was banished from Paris, Calvin took refuge in Geneva and became a kind of dictator. His reforms brought about changes in the law, the police, trade and industry, and sanitary regulations. He was a severe and irritable man who suffered from chronic illness. He dressed simply and ate sparingly. Calvin had an unusually retentive memory (q.v.) and was able to rise to great intellectual efforts. His brand of religion, which amounted to fanaticism, left little room for pleasure. Sin was ever present and ever clamoring for expiation. Thus, he is associated with the psychopathology (q.v.) of guilt and sin. He believed that mental defectives were filled with Satan. His main work was *Institutes of the Christian Religion* (1536), which was written in Latin.
Bibliography: Parker, T. H. L. 1975. *John Calvin: a biography.*

CAMBYSES I (fl.580 B.C.). Father of Cyrus, king of Persia. He was said to be epileptic (*see* EPILEPSY), and his "sacred disease" was blamed for his insane behavior. Many Persians, on the other hand, believed that he had been driven mad by excessive drinking.
Bibliography: Brothwell, D., and Sandison, A. T. 1967. *Disease in antiquity.*

CAMERON, DONALD EWEN (1901-1967). British psychiatrist. He became professor of psychiatry at McGill University in Montreal in 1943 and was the first president of the World Psychiatric Association (q.v.). Insulin treatment for schizophrenia (q.v.) was introduced in North America by him.
Bibliography: Cameron, D. E. 1968. *Psychotherapy in action.*

CAMISARDS. The eighteenth-century name for the French protestant peasants of the Cévennes. It was derived from the white shirt, or *chemise*, that they wore. They were given to religious exaltation, prophesies, and ecstatic (*see* ECSTASY) phenomena, which was often imitated even by their children. They believed themselves to be guided by encouraging voices and lights in the sky. Their preachers usually spoke while in a trance, going through four stages of ecstasy, which were characterized by what they called the warning, the whisper of inspiration, the prophesy, and the gift. Benjamin Franklin (q.v.) reported that his first employer, a Huguenot printer, was one "of the French Prophets," who "could act their enthusiastic agitations."
Bibliography: Rosen, G. 1968. *Madness in society.*

CAMISOLE. In nineteenth-century asylums, a shirt made of strong canvas, used to restrain (*see* RESTRAINT) violent mental patients. Its long sleeves allowed for the patient's arms to be folded, and the extra length then was tied at the back. A variation was a square of material that bound the arms to the body and fastened at the back.
Bibliography: Gilman, S. L. 1981. *Seeing the insane.*

CAMPANELLA, TOMMASO (1568-1639). An Italian philosopher and poet. He became a Dominican brother in adolescence. He opposed the philosophy of Aristotle (q.v.) because he believed that all knowledge should depend on observation rather than on deduction. He, therefore, evolved a philosophy based on the senses, which he described in his *Philosophia Sensibus Demonstrata* published in Naples in 1591. In 1599 he was arrested, accused of plotting against the Spanish rulers of Naples, and imprisoned. He was subjected to torture and sleep deprivation (q.v.), which led to mental confusion, disorientation, and, not surprisingly, persecution mania (q.v.) . After two years in prison, his mental state was such that physicians were consulted to establish whether he was insane or was feigning insanity to escape punishment. Their opinions were divided, and he remained in prison, where he was allowed to write many philosophical and poetic works. He finally was released in 1629 and allowed to spend the rest of his life in a Dominican monastery in France. He wrote over eighty books, including *De Sensu Rerum et Magia* (1620); *Civitas Solis* (1623), a description of an Utopian state, and *Philosophia rationalis* (1637).
Bibliography: Bonansea, B. M. 1969. *Campanella.*

CAMPBELL, ALFRED WALTER (1868-1937). An Australian physician. He studied in Edinburgh, Vienna, and Prague and was an assistant to Richard von Krafft-Ebing (q.v.). He wrote his doctoral thesis on "The Pathology of Alcoholic Insanity." As resident medical officer at Rainhill Asylum, near Liverpool, he directed the laboratory of pathology and conducted valuable research in neurology (q.v.) with the encouragement of Sir Charles Sherrington (q.v.). In 1905, having published his main work, *Histological Studies on the Localization of Cerebral Function*, he returned to Australia and dedicated himself to neurology and psychiatry. His style of writing and lecturing was renowned for its clarity and precision, and his map of the brain is considered a classic.
Bibliography: Haymaker, W., and Schiller, F. 1970. *The founders of neurology.* 2d. ed.

CAMPBELL CLARK, A. (1852-1907). A British physician. He was the medical superintendent of Bothwell Asylum in Lanarkshire, England. In

1880 he pioneered the training of mental nurses and instituted a successful course for them. His recommendations resulted in the establishment of the mental nursing certificate of the Royal Medico-Psychological Association (q.v.).
Bibliography: Walk, A. 1961. The history of mental nursing. *J. Ment. Sci.* 107: 1-17.

CAMPTOCORMIA. A term introduced by Alexander Achille Souques (1860-1944) during World War I to indicate a forward bending of the trunk of the body. It was found in soldiers suffering from traumatic neurosis (q.v.).

CAMUS, ALBERT (1913-1960). An Algerian-born French writer and philosopher. He became famous with his nihilistic novel *L'Etranger* (1942) and his essay, *Le Mythe de Sisyphe* (1942) on suicide (q.v.). His work, which is psychologically interesting, deals with the plight of man whose efforts in a world full of absurd situations and disasters are futile.
Bibliography: McCarthy, P. 1982. *Albert Camus: a critical study.*

CANARY ISLANDS. According to Jean Esquirol (q.v.), in antiquity inhabitants of these islands threw themselves into an abyss in honor of their gods. They believed that such a death would bring them eternal happiness.
Bibliography: Esquirol, J. E. D. 1845. Reprint. 1965. *Mental maladies: a treatise on insanity.*

CANDLE IN THE DARK, A. A book written in England in 1656 by Thomas Ady. In it he attacked the belief in witchcraft (q.v.), using the Bible (q.v.) as his reference. He argued that nowhere in the Bible was the word "witchcraft" used with the same meaning that his contemporaries gave to it. He went on to argue that there were no proofs of witchcraft in the Scriptures.
Bibliography: Ady, T. 1656. *A candle in the dark.*

CANISTRIS, OPICINUS DE (c. 1296-1350). An Italian cleric, born in Pavia. From the time of an unspecified illness at the age of thirty-eight, he suffered hallucinations (q.v.), partial loss of memory (q.v.), hysterical (*see* HYSTERIA) loss of function in his right hand, and temporary impairment of speech. After the use of his right hand had been "miraculously" restored, he executed large drawings for the Holy See, and it is in these drawings and the autobiographical notes written on the same sheets that signs of mental disorders can be found. The drawings and the notes reveal guilt and obsessional (*see* OBSESSION) self-accusations.
Bibliography: Kris, E. 1952. *Psychoanalytic explorations in art.*

CANN, SIR WILLIAM (fl. 1740). A town clerk of Bristol, England. In 1746 he became insane and his deputy and clerk were also affected—a clear case of *folie à trois* (*see* FOLIE À DEUX). Sir William cut his own throat; the other two were sent to Mason's Madhouse (q.v.).
Bibliography: Evans, J. 1824. *A chronological outline of the history of Bristol, and the stranger's guide through its streets and neighbourhood.*

CANNABIS SATIVA. Commonly called Indian hemp, an annual plant native to western and central Asia. All parts of it are intoxicating. In small doses it causes exhilaration and may act as an aphrodisiac. Larger doses produce mental exaltation, intoxication, and double consciousness, ending in loss of memory (q.v.) and gloominess. Addiction to it causes indigestion, depression, impotence, and body waste. In Eastern medicine it is used in many forms for various disorders.
Bibliography: Gamage, J. R., and Zerkin, E. 1969. *A comprehensive guide to the English-language literature on Cannabis.*

CANNIBALISM. The eating of human flesh. There are many legends about cannibalism. The Greeks, for example, believed that the god Cronus had devoured his children as a defense against the prophesy that they would dethrone him. Aristotle (q.v.) noted in his *Ethics* that very primitive people and the mentally ill have been known to eat human flesh. He cited the case of a young man who killed and ate his mother. During the Middle Ages (q.v.), witches (*see* WITCHCRAFT) were believed to eat children. In primitive cultures cannibalism is often a ritual practice. The term is derived from the tribal name of the Carib Indians.
Bibliography: Tannahil, R. 1975. *Flesh and blood: history of the cannibal complex.*

CANNON, WALTER BRADFORD (1871-1945). An American physiologist. His investigations on the relationship between the emotions and the vegetative nervous system led to new theories about the effects of rage and fear on the body. He demonstrated that emotional states can trigger physiological functions that allow the organism to cope with certain situations, such as the fight-flight reaction of the body in response to stress. His theories have been applied to studies of the effects of emotional stress in chronic organic disorders and have contributed to the advancement of psychosomatic medicine (q.v.).
Bibliography: Cannon, W. B. 1929. *Bodily changes in pain, hunger, fear and rage.*

CANTERBURY CATHEDRAL. The seat of the archbishop and primate of England. It was the scene of the martyrdom of Saint Thomas à Becket (1118?-1170) in 1170. A thirteenth-century window in the Trinity Chapel

depicts a bound maniac, being beaten with birch rods and dragged to the shrine of Saint Thomas, where he is cured and gives thanks to the saint. See also HENRY OF FORDWICH.
Bibliography: Bonser, W. 1963. *Medical background to Anglo-Saxon England.*

CANTERBURY TALES, THE. The great work of Geoffrey Chaucer (q.v.). It presents a vivid picture of life in the Middle Ages (q.v.). One of the characters is a wandering friar, who begs alms for a hospital that cares for the "possessed" (*see* POSSESSION). He offers exorcism (q.v.) as treatment, but he is challenged with the affirmation that charms against the devil and fumigation (q.v.) are more efficacious.
Bibliography: Chaucer, G. 1952. *The Canterbury tales,* trans. N. Coghill.

CANTHARIS VESICATORIA. *See* SPANISH FLY.

CAPGRAS, JEAN MARIE JOSEPH (1873-1950). A French psychiatrist who first described a psychotic (*see* PSYCHOSIS) state, which he termed *illusion des sosies* (illusion of doubles), whereby a patient is unable to identify a person whom he recognizes as being familiar. He explains this by insisting that individuals are being impersonated by impostors or doubles. It is known now as Capgras syndrome.
Bibliography: Enoch, M. D. and Trethowan, W. H. 1979. *Uncommon psychiatric syndromes.*

CAPITAL. The English translation of *Das Kapital.* Karl Marx (q.v.) wrote this work in the British Museum, after settling down in London in 1849. It was published in Berlin in three volumes between 1867 and 1895. As well as economic topics, it discussed the sociological aspects of mankind. Marx believed man was alienated from himself because society was divided into struggling classes. He went on to say that it was not enough to explain society; the need was to change it. Some of Sigmund Freud's (q.v.) concepts paralleled Marx's. Alfred Adler's (q.v.) basic thinking was influenced by Marxism.
Bibliography: Marx, K. 1867. Reprint, 1957. *Capital,* trans. E. Paul and C. Paul.

CAPPE, CATHERINE (*née* **HARRISON**) (1743-1821). A British woman, wife of Newcombe Cappe, dissenting minister of York, and stepmother of Dr. Robert Cappe, physician to The Retreat (q.v.) at York. She was a philanthropist who worked to improve the conditions of mental hospitals. With a group of women, she regularly visited the insane in The Retreat at York and in other hospitals in the area and then reported on the nursing standards and conditions in the wards. She corresponded with Benjamin Rush (q.v.), who thought highly of her. In 1816, she wrote a guide for female visitors entitled *On the Desirability and Utility of Ladies Visiting the Female Wards of Hospitals and Lunatic Asylums.*
Bibliography: Hunter, R., and Macalpine, I. 1963. *Three hundred years of psychiatry.*

CAPPELLINO, GIOVANNI DOMENICO (1580-1651). An Italian painter who was obsessional (*see* OBSESSION) and solitary to a marked degree. The biographer of Genoese artists, Raffaele Soprani, writing in 1674, described how Cappellino's pupils were ordered to walk slowly when in his room in order not to raise dust, to keep objects in an exact position, and to wash carefully anything touched by visitors. Cappellino would not handle coins. He measured his steps geometrically when out walking, and any companion had to follow his example. Once when his mother fell in the mud, he would not go near her for days. He changed houses because he thought that the sun, reflecting off a wall near his room, was causing his headaches, but he then complained that the new house smelt badly. He died alone and neglected because he would not allow anyone in to care for him.
Bibliography: Wittkower, R., and Wittkower, M. 1963. *Born under Saturn.*

CARACALLA (A.D. 188-217). A Roman emperor whose real name was Marcus Aurelius Antoninus. He is famous for his extravagances, cruelty, and treachery. He assassinated his brother in order to become the sole ruler of the empire and, according to tradition, had 20,000 of his relatives and friends murdered. His aggression and love of destruction led to the burning of Aristotle's (q.v.) books. He was said to have practiced witchcraft (q.v.), to have associated with sorcerers, and to have offered human sacrifices to the devil. He was murdered at the instigation of Macrinus (A.D. 164-218), who succeeded him.
Bibliography: Boak, A. 1955. *A history of Rome.*

CARAVAGGIO, MICHELANGIOLO MERISI DA (*or* **AMERIGI DA CARAVAGGIO**) (1573-1610). An Italian painter. His works show a dramatic and often violent approach to his subject matter. His own life was no less wild and passionate. He attracted the hatred of his contemporaries in spite of his recognized genius. He was often in trouble for brawling, fighting, and stealing. Caravaggio's vicious temper on one occasion led to homicide and his banishment from Rome. He traveled to Naples and thence to Malta, where he was well received until he offended a state dignitary and again was banished. His wanderings and adventures continued until he died of a violent fever while trying to return to Rome.
Bibliography: Hinks, R. 1953. *Michelangelo Merisi da Caravaggio.*
Kitson, M. 1968. *The complete paintings of Caravaggio.*

CARBON DIOXIDE THERAPY. A form of treatment for neurotic (*see* NEUROSIS) patients introduced in 1946 by Ladislas Joseph von Meduna (q.v.). Carbon dioxide is inhaled to the point of coma.
Bibliography: Goldenson, R. M. 1970. *The encyclopedia of human behavior.*

CARDANO, GIROLAMO (1501-1576). Italian mathematician, astrologer, and physician of great brilliance. His father, a lawyer who believed in the occult, could not marry his mother because of her social inferiority. He was not loved by either parent, and his illegitimacy prevented him from joining the Milan college of physicians, although he had a medical diploma. Cardano gambled heavily and was so improvident that at one point he lived in an almshouse with his wife and son. He wrote a treatise on how to bring up children, but his own two sons were criminals and drunkards (one of them poisoned his wife and was beheaded), and his daughter stooped to every conceivable vice. He became famous as a mathematician, but he was said to have stolen from Nicolo Tartaglia the solution of the cubic equation that he then published as his own. He was well known throughout Europe as a doctor. The Archbishop of Scotland, John Hamilton, was one of his patients, whom he cured of asthma. In his *De Utilitate ex Adversis Capienda* he wrote that psychopathy (q.v.) was "nothing but a disorder of the mind" and added that the psychopaths were not insane but were able to exercise some choice. He understood that a doctor often owes his success to the faith of his patients. Despite his brilliance and genuine power of scientific reasoning, he was incredibly superstitious and believed in demons, astrology (q.v.), and chiromancy. In 1570 he was imprisoned for heresy, having praised Nero's (q.v.) persecutions of the Christians and having dared to cast Jesus Christ's horoscope. He died at seventy-five in Rome, poor and alone.
Bibliography: Cardan, J. 1575. Reprint. 1962. *The book of my life*, trans. J. Stoner.

CARGO ANXIETY. A form of anxiety found in New Guinea and Melanesia. It is linked with the cargo cult, which is based on the belief that some great event is about to take place. The event usually is described as the arrival of ancestral spirits bringing highly valued cargo. A prophet announces the coming event, and all existing stores of food are destroyed, as it is believed that they will be replaced by new and better supplies. The cult and its delusional (*see* DELUSION) and paranoid (*see* PARANOIA) manifestations stem from insecurity and dissatisfaction with the existing way of life.
Bibliography: Worsley, P. 1970. *The trumpet shall sound: study of "cargo" cults in Melanesia.*

CARGO CULT. *See* CARGO ANXIETY.

CARKESSE, JAMES (fl. 1652-1679). English writer of verses and clerk in Samuel Pepys' (q.v.) office at the Admiralty. He became deranged and was admitted first to Finnesbury Madhouse, then owned by Dr. Thomas Allen (q.v.), and subsequently to Bethlem Royal Hospital (q.v.). He wrote about

his experiences in both places in a book of poems printed in 1679 and entitled *Lucida Intervalla*.
Bibliography: Hunter, R., and Macalpine, I. 1963. *Three hundred years of psychiatry*.

CARLO ALBERTO (CHARLES ALBERT) (1798-1849). King of Sardinia and prince of Savoy and Piedmont. He was a strong supporter of Italian unity and in 1848 declared war on Austria. In his attempt to reorganize his kingdom and to introduce many new regulations, he appointed a committee of physicians, chemists, and geologists to study cretinism (q.v.) in the mountainous parts of his lands. His insistence on soil analysis is an indication of the then common belief that cretinism was related to chemicals in the soil. The report of the commission, which was published in 1848, suggested that provisions for the mentally deficient should be based on those at the Abendberg Institution (q.v.). In the last year of his life, Carlo Alberto abdicated and went in exile to a monastery in Oporto, Portugal, where he became progressively more depressed.
Bibliography: Cappelletti, L. 1891. *Storia di Carlo Alberto*.
Omodeo, A. 1941. *La leggenda di Carlo Alberto nella recente storeografia*.

CARLOS, DON (CARLOS OF AUSTRIA) (1545-1568). The son of the consanguineous marriage of Philip II (q.v.) of Spain and Maria of Portugal. He was said to have inherited his grandmother's (Joanna of Castile [q.v.]) insanity, but his environment was also highly abnormal. He was brought up by his aunt, Juana of Portugal, a gloomy and bigoted woman. He showed signs of abnormal behavior in childhood. As an adolescent, he fell down a dark staircase and injured his head; he became delirious and as a last resort, after many remedies had been tried, the mummified body of a holy friar, a hundred years dead, was put next to him in the bed. Don Carlos recovered but became prone to religious mania (q.v.) and appalling rages, during which he would attack those around him. He was often confined to bed by his own gluttony. He was intensely jealous of his father, who married Elizabeth of Valois, after having Carlos' betrothal to her annulled. When he confided to his confessor that he wanted to kill his father, he was imprisoned. In prison he poured icy water on the floor and walked on it, called for ice and snow to be put in his bed, and drank gallons of icy water, refusing food for days on end. When he died, it was rumored that he had been murdered by a slow poison in his food. His mysterious death has been the subject of many dramas by such writers as Thomas Otway (1652-1685), Johann Schiller (q.v.), and Vittorio Alfieri (q.v.) and of an opera by Guiseppe Verdi (1813-1901).
Bibliography: Crankshaw, E. 1971. *The Habsburgs*.

CARLOTA. *See* CHARLOTTE.

CARLSON, ANTON J. (1875-1956). A physiologist. He was born in Sweden and emigrated to the United States as an adolescent. His research

covered a wide field and included work on the physiology of hunger. He considered appetite a sensory reaction, distinct from that of hunger.
Bibliography: Flugel, J. C. 1945. *A hundred years of psychology.*

CARLYLE, THOMAS (1795-1881). A writer and historian, born in Dumfriesshire, Scotland, son of a mason. He began to write when he was still quite young and became particularly interested in German literature. In 1843, he turned his attention to social problems and politics. Carlyle believed that the rule of the strongest, as in medieval times, was best. He was a lifelong sufferer of insomnia, depression, and dyspepsia. His wife, Jane Welsh (q.v.), died in 1866, after a marriage of forty years. From her diary he learned what a miserable life she had led because of his neglect and his unrelenting preoccupation with his own affairs. Among his best known works are *French Revolution* (1837); *Past and Present* (1843) and the *History of Frederick the Great* (1865), on which he spent fourteen years.
Bibliography: Campbell, I. M. 1974. *Thomas Carlyle.*

CARNEGIE, SUSAN (*née* **SCOTT**) (1744-1821). A Scottish philanthropist. She married George Carnegie, a rich merchant, who had served under Bonnie Prince Charlie, had escaped to Sweden, and had made a large fortune there. She used her position to start an appeal for funds to build a hospital for the mentally ill and the sick poor. Montrose Royal Mental Hospital (q.v.) came into being in 1781, financed in the greatest part by members of the Carnegie family. Susan Carnegie is regarded as the pioneer of mental care in Scotland. Her contributions to the promotion of social welfare were enormous, even though she had many family commitments, including nine children of her own and a foster child. The managers of the asylum invited her to sit for her portrait in 1815, but she was too modest to accept.
Bibliography: Henderson, D. K. 1964. *The evolution of psychiatry in Scotland.*

CAROLINE MATILDA (1751-1775). Queen of Denmark and sister of George III (q.v.). When she was fifteen years old, she married King Christian VII (q.v.), but the marriage was an extremely unhappy one. The King was cold, brutal, and already on the brink of madness. She was often so deeply depressed that she prayed for death. She was treated for depression by the court physician, Johann Struensee, and fell in love with him. Because of his influence on the king, he became the virtual ruler of Denmark, until his arrest and execution for treason and adultery. Caroline then was divorced and exiled to the Castle of Celle in Hanover, where she died in her twenty-fourth year. It was rumored that she had been poisoned, but recent work by Macalpine and Hunter leads to the conclusion that she was a victim of porphyria (q.v.).

Bibliography: Chapman, H. W. 1971. *Caroline Matilda: queen of Denmark*.
Macalpine, I. and Hunter, R. 1969. *George III and the mad-business*.

CARPENTER, MARY (1807-1877). An English philanthropist who trained as a teacher. Her interest in the problems of children led to her work in the field of juvenile delinquency. Her book *Juvenile Delinquents: Their condition and treatment* (1853) contributed to the passage of the Juvenile Offenders Act of 1854. She founded a school for neglected children, reformatories for girls, and industrial schools. She undertook several trips to India to advise on female education and prison management. As well as treatises on education and criminal reform, she wrote verses and her memoirs.

Bibliography: Carpenter, M. 1851. *Reformatory schools for the children of the perishing and dangerous classes and for juvenile offenders*.

CARPHOLOGY. A Galenic (*see* GALEN) term indicating the aimless plucking of clothes and bedcovers by patients in delirious (*see* DELIRIUM) states or with senile psychiatric disorders. William Shakespeare (q.v.) describes this behavior in relation to Falstaff's death:

I saw him fumble with the sheets.

[Henry V, 2. 3]

Bibliography: Temkin, O. 1973. *Galenism*.

CARR, HARVEY A. (1873-1954). An American psychologist. He began his studies in the field of mathematics and teaching, but switched to psychology because of his admiration for the instructor in that subject. He worked in the fields of comparative psychology, visual space perception, and educational theory. His writings contributed to the field of functional psychology. He questioned whether or not certain aspects of the mind could be scientifically investigated and believed that developmental history could be more important than experimental methods.

Bibliography: Murchison, C., ed. 1936. *A history of psycholoy in autobiography*, vol. 3.

CARRACCI, ANNIBAL (1560-1609). An Italian painter. After completing the beautiful paintings in the Palazzo Farnese in Rome, he became progressively more depressed and unable to work. A contemporary physician, Giulio Mancini wrote that "he was taken ill with a fatuity of mind and memory [q.v.] so that speech and memory failed him and he was in danger of instantaneous death." After a brief recovery he died. His contemporaries were sure that melancholy (*see* MELANCHOLIA) had caused his death, but

treatment may have been an accelerating factor, as it consisted of bleeding (q.v.) him.
Bibliography: Wittkower, R., and Wittkower, M. 1963. *Born under Saturn.*

CARRIAGE-DRIVING. A form of diversion therapy. In the nineteenth century depressed patients were encouraged to take up this activity. Vittorio Alfieri (q.v.) is said to have been able to bear his deep melancholy (*see* MELANCHOLIA) by this means. Prosperous Englishmen took the place of their coachmen and drove through the streets of London.
Bibliography: Esquirol, J. E. D. 1845. Reprint. 1965. *Mental maladies: a treatise on insanity.*

CARROLL, LEWIS. *See* DODGSON, CHARLES LUTWIDGE.

CARUS, CARL GUSTAV (1789-1869). A German physician, philosopher, and painter. After specializing in obstetrics, he became interested in psychology. He defined psychology as the science of the soul's development from the unconscious (q.v.) to the conscious; and equated the unconscious with the creative force. He divided human life into three periods: preembryonic when man is only a cell; embryonic when the unconscious develops; and postnatal when the unconscious directs growth and function. According to him, consciousness developed gradually after birth, but the individual remained dominated by the unconscious and returned to it in dreams (q.v.). His book *Psyche* (1846) anticipated the teachings of dynamic psychiatry and contained many ideas in advance of his time, as well as some outdated concepts. Carus' theories were a close approach to psychoanalysis (q.v.), and he is regarded as a predecessor of Carl Jung (q.v.), but his lack of first hand experience with the behavior of mentally disordered patients led him to speculations rather than to factual conclusions. He studied physiognomy and tried to elevate it to the level of science in his book *Symbolism of the Human Figure* (1853).
Bibliography: Ellenberger, H. F. 1970. *The discovery of the unconscious.*

CASANOVA DE SEINGALT, GIOVANNI GIACOMO (1725-1798). An Italian adventurer, born in Venice. He was illegitimate, and his grandmother, whom he loved very much, raised him. When he was nine years old, his mother boarded him out in Padua. In his memoirs he remarks "thus she got rid of me." His memoirs also record his first childhood recollection: a nosebleed which was treated by an old woman, who locked him in a chest, blew smoke round him, and then recited incantations (q.v.). As a twelve-year-old he wanted to study medicine, but, to please his protectors, he began the study of law. He graduated when he was seventeen years old and in the same year experienced the first of his many amorous adventures by seducing two sisters in the same night. His turbulent life took him all over

Europe, and he met popes, kings and great literary figures. His temperament was full of contrasts: he could be brutal and tender, brilliant and stupid, honest and treacherous. He was a priest, a lawyer, a soldier, an author, a musician, a gambler, a poor man, and a very rich one, but in his restlessness he remained essentially lonely. Many of the women he seduced were physically abnormal and he was also believed to be a homosexual. His interest in the occult led to his meeting with Madam la Marquise d'Urfé, who was similarly interested. The marquise wanted a change of sex, and Casanova relieved her of large sums of money by promising that he could arrange it. In his old age he became librarian to Count Waldestein, in Bohemia. At seventy-two he began his famous *Story of My Life* (1826-1838). He said he was writing it "to prevent despair from devouring my poor existence or making me lose my reason." He also stated "I can truly say I have lived."
Bibliography: Masters, J. 1969. *Casanova*.

CASPER, JOHANN LUDWIG (1796-1864). A Prussian physician. He was interested in the field of legal medicine as it related to psychiatry, a subject much in vogue in the nineteenth century. He became an authority on criminal responsibility and was the first to use statistics in the study of suicide (q.v.). His book *A Handbook of the Practice of Forensic Medicine* was considered a standard work and was translated into several languages. In England it was translated by Dr. George Balfour and published by the Sydenham Society in 1845.
Bibliography: Goshen, C. E. 1967. *Documentary history of psychiatry*.

CASSANDRA. In Greek mythology, the beautiful daughter of Priam of Troy. Apollo (q.v.) gave her the gift of prophecy, but, because she had refused his advances, he ordered that she should not be believed. She is a tragic figure, aware of disasters to come and yet helpless in her unheeded warnings. The name Cassandra has come to mean "a prophet of doom."
Bibliography: 1959. *Larousse encyclopedia of mythology*.

CASSEL HOSPITAL. A hospital for the psychoanalysis (q.v.) of neurosis (q.v.) at Ham Common in London. It was founded in 1920 as the last of Sir Ernest Cassel's foundations. It is unique among English hospitals because all the physicians are psychoanalytically trained and because it contains a unit for the admission of whole families, one of the finest such units in the world.

CASSIANUS, JOHANNES (360?-?435). A hermit, also known as Cassian, Johannes Massiliensis, and Johannes Eremita. He probably was born in Provence and became a monk, as well as a theologian. He spent some years in isolation in the Egyptian deserts and later founded several monasteries in

France. In his writings he described *acedia* (q.v.), a condition of sorrow and melancholy (*see* MELANCHOLIA) that often afflicted monks.
Bibliography: Wenzel, S. 1967. *The sin of sloth: acedia in medieval thought and literataure.*

CASSIODORUS, FLAVIUS MAGNUS AURELIANUS (c.490-c.585).
A Roman philosopher, statesman, and physician. In his later years he became a monk and founded a monastery where he taught his brethren to transcribe manuscripts from the Greek and to care for the sick. He emphasized the need to study Hippocrates (q.v.) and Galen (q.v.). He wrote on mathematics, history, art, and philosophy. His treatise *De Anima* deals with spiritual problems and speculates on the nature of the soul.
Bibliography: Alexander, F. G., and Selesnick, S. T. 1966. *The history of psychiatry.*

CASTLEREAGH, ROBERT STEWARD, VISCOUNT (1769-1822). An
Irish politician, member of the Irish Parliament, and later a member of the British Parliament. He was a powerful, tenacious, and ruthless man, obsessed with work and remarkably successful in controlling his emotions. Some months before his death, his personality is said to have changed: he became oversensitive, emotional, forgetful, and suspicious. He lost his self-confidence, became depressed and agitated, and prone to severe headaches, insomnia, and periods of confusion. He retired to his country home with his wife and personal physician and remained under constant supervision, which he managed to avoid once. He cut his throat with a penknife and died almost instantly. His depression, which led to his suicide (q.v.), was said to have been precipitated by anonymous letters accusing him of homosexuality (q.v.).
Bibliography: Hyde, M. H. 1967. *The strange death of Lord Castlereagh.*

CASTOREUM (*or* CASTOR). A musky, glandular secretion of the beaver.
Indians and Europeans used it as a medicine for colic, epilepsy (q.v.), frostbite, and hysteria (q.v.).

CATALENTIA. A term for epilepsy (q.v.) coined by Paracelsus (q.v.).

CATATONIA. A term first used in 1874 by Karl Ludwig Kahlbaum (q.v.).
In his monograph *Die Katatonie oder das Spannungsirresein* (1874), he described catatonia as a condition in which the patient takes up peculiar postures and remains in them in a stuporous state.
See also BARTLEBY THE SCRIVENER.
Bibliography: Kahlbaum, K. L. 1874. Reprint. 1973. *Catatonia*, trans. Y. Levij and T. Pridan.

CATERHAM ASYLUM. An asylum (q.v.) situated near London, opened
in 1870. It was designed to accommodate fifteen hundred patients and con-

sisted of three floors, each of which formed an enormous common ward. It was meant for poor patients who, according to the law, were either chronic harmless lunatics (q.v.), or idiots, or imbeciles (q.v.). But, because of exigency, mental patients of every category were sent there. For the first two years children, as well as adults, were kept at Caterham. It was later renamed Saint Lawrence Hospital.

See also LEAVESDEN ASYLUM.

Bibliography: Ayers, G. M. 1971. *England's first state hospitals and the metropolitan asylums board.*

CATHARS. An heretical Christian sect that flourished in Europe in the twelfth and thirteenth centuries. One of their ascetic (q.v.) practices, called *endura*, allowed a sick person to commit suicide (q.v.) by refusing food, thus ensuring that he entered heaven in a guiltless state. Other means of suicide used by them were poison or bleeding to death.

Bibliography: Runciman, S. 1947. *The medieval Manichee.*

CATHARSIS. A Greek term used by Aristotle (q.v.) in the *Poetics* to indicate the emotional and spiritual cleansing of an audience during the performance of great tragedies. He believed that it was brought about by feelings of terror and pity. In psychiatry (q.v.) the term refers to the discharge of emotions occurring in patients under hypnosis (*see* HYPNOTISM). It was first used by Joseph Breuer (q.v.) in connection with the case of Anna O. (q.v.). The paper discussing the cathartic method was written by Breuer in collaboration with Sigmund Freud (q.v.) in 1893 and was entitled *On the Psychical Mechanisms of Hysterical Phenomena.* Breuer believed, as did Freud at first, that the release of the emotion attached to the symptom by recollecting the first time the symptom had occurred caused the symptom to disappear. This corresponded with Freud's belief that neurosis (q.v.) had its origin in trauma alone. Freud later changed his view to allow for the possibility of symptoms also arising out of conflict and thus developed his new therapy of free association of which the cathartic method was only a part.

CATHERINE OF SIENA, SAINT (c.1347-1380). An Italian religious writer, the twenty-fifth child of a dyer. She was given to ecstatic (*see* EC-STASY) visions of Christ and subjected to terrible temptations even in early childhood. Four hundred of her letters have survived. In them she writes of her experiences and revelations. Her visions were recorded by her confessor, Father Raimondo of Capua. She converted many sinners and prevailed on Pope Gregory XI to return to Rome. She is a patron saint of Italy.

Bibliography: Kellison, M., and Falconer, J. 1973. *Life of Saint Catherine.*

CATHERINE THE GREAT (1729-1796). Empress of Russia. She was one of five children, only two of whom reached adulthood. Her father was

ineffectual, and her mother was highly neurotic (*see* NEUROSIS) and unable to feel any affection for her daughter. At sixteen she married the heir to the Russian throne, Peter III (q.v.), a weak, dim-witted, uneducated youth. The strain of her marriage and her failure to produce an heir left her prone to headaches, sleeplessness, and general poor health. When she did become pregnant it was rumored that it was with the help of a chamberlain. After two miscarriages she produced a son, Paul (q.v.), who was immediately taken over by her mother-in-law, the powerful Empress Elizabeth. On the death of Elizabeth, Catherine deposed her husband, who shortly after was strangled, and took command herself. She was strong and hardworking, but a nymphomaniac (*see* NYMPHOMANIA) even in her old age. She founded one of the earliest foundling hospitals to discourage abortion and infanticide (q.v.).
Bibliography: Oldenburg, Z. 1965. *Catherine the Great.*

CATHISOPHOBIA. A term derived from the Greek meaning "a morbid fear of sitting down or of remaining sitting still."

CATOCHUS. A term included by D. H. Tuke (q.v.) in his *Dictionary of Psychological Medicine* (q.v.). He defined it as "an old term for catalepsy, but it has been more especially applied to that phase of ecstasy [q.v.] or trance in which the patient is conscious, but cannot move or speak. Under this head would be comprised those cases in which persons have been laid out as dead and even buried, without being able to arouse themselves or show signs of life."
Bibliography: Tuke, D. H. 1892. *A dictionary of psychological medicine.*

CATON, RICHARD (1842-1926). An English surgeon. In 1875 he became the first to record the action currents in the brains of animals, thus paving the way to the development of the electroencephalogram.
See also HANS BERGER.
Bibliography: Schmidt, J. E. 1959. *Medical discoveries: who and when.*

CATTELL, JAMES McKEEN (1860-1944). An American psychologist. He studied at Lafayette College in Pennsylvania and later worked at Leipzig under Wilhelm Wund (q.v.), who related how Cattell simply had presented himself to him saying "Herr Professor, you need an assistant, and I will be your assistant!" Cattell returned to the United States and established a psychological laboratory (q.v.) at the University of Pennsylvania in 1888. In 1891 he established another laboratory at Columbia University. He remained at Columbia until his dismissal in 1917 because of his pacifist attitude toward America's entry into World War I. In 1890 he pioneered and developed techniques for mental testing; the term "mental test" was invented by him and the Psychological Corporation (q.v.) was founded by him in 1921. He

was a prolific author and the editor of several psychological and scientific journals. With James Baldwin (q.v.) he founded the *Psychological Review* (q.v.). His work covered reaction time, reading and perception, association, psychophysics, the "order of merit" method, and individual differences.
Bibliography: Poffenberger, A. T. 1947. *James McKeen Cattell: man of science.*

CATTELL, RAYMOND BERNARD (1905-). An English psychologist, now a naturalized American citizen. His work has been in the field of personality and motivation evaluation. He has devised a culture-free, nonverbal intelligence test (q.v.).
Bibliography: Cattell, R. B., and Kline, P. 1977. *Scientific analysis of personality and motivation.*

CAUTERIZATION. A term derived from the Greek meaning "to burn." Cauterization of the head was practised usually on women in magic (q.v.) rituals during the Neolithic period. In medieval times it was common treatment for epilepsy (q.v.) and insanity. It was performed by means of corroding chemicals or heated instruments. The inhabitants of Dageston, on the Caspian Sea, believed that cauterization of the vertex would prevent illness. This practice may have given rise to the tonsure prescribed by religious orders. In the nineteenth century cauterization, sometimes by means of moxa (q.v.), was still used extensively as a form of therapy for mental and nervous disorders.
Bibliography: Brothwell, D., and Sandison, A. T. 1967. *Diseases in antiquity.*

CELLINI, BENVENUTO (1500-1571). Italian sculptor and goldsmith, pupil of Michelangelo (q.v.) and protégé of kings and popes. He was a creative psychopath. He began his memoirs by claiming that his ancestry went back to Julius Caesar (q.v.). Cellini was extremely selfish; modesty was a quality unknown to him and he tended to exaggerate all he reported. He was a difficult man, given to irascibility and letting his temper lead him into all sorts of brawls. He was once imprisoned for homicide. He was arrogant and passionate. Paranoia (q.v.) never left him; he complained of plots against him and, in his old age, believed that his food was being poisoned. His autobiography, first published in 1730, is a vivid but exaggerated record of events during the High Renaissance in Italy.
Bibliography: Cellini, B. 1968. *Autobiography*, trans. A. Macdonell.

CELSUS, AULUS CORNELIUS (25 B.C.-A.D. 50). A Roman nobleman who wrote on medicine. He was not a physician because it was a profession considered beneath his social standing, but he wrote on medical subjects, drawing his material from seventy-two medical authors. *De Re Medicina*, written in elegant Latin, was neglected in antiquity and in the Middle Ages (q.v.), but was rediscovered in the fifteenth century. In 1478 it became one

of the first medical books to be printed, and it was greatly valued and quoted. The work consists of eight books; the third book is devoted to mental diseases. Celsus presented mental disorder as a disease affecting the whole personality. He classified mental disorders into: 1) Phrenitis (q.v.), delirium (q.v.) with fever; 2) Melancholia (q.v.), depression; 3) one due to false images and disordered judgment, presumably schizophrenia(q.v.); 4) Delirium due to fear; 5) Lethargus, coma; and 6) Morbus comitialis, epilepsy (q.v.), which he asserted may be cured in boys by the first coitus and in girls by the first menstruation. The term *insania* (q.v.), insanity, was first used by him. The methods of treatment suggested by him included bleeding (q.v.), frightening the patient, emetics, enemas, total darkness, and decoctions of poppy (q.v.) or henbane (q.v.), as well as more pleasant ones such as music (*see* MUSIC THERAPY), travel, sport, reading aloud, and massage. He was aware of the importance of the doctor-patient relationship. His nonmedical works on agriculture, law, military science. and philosophy have been lost.
Bibliography: Spences, W. G., trans. 1935. *Celsus: De medicina.*

CENOSPUDIA. A term derived from the Greek meaning "a zealous study of frivolities." Another term for this type of mental preoccupation is brown study (q.v.).
Bibliography: Tuke, D. H. 1892. *A dictionary of psychological medicine.*

CENTURY OF THE CHILD. A book by the Swedish author Ellen Key, originally published in 1889. In it she predicted that the twentieth century would be more concerned with the physical and psychological welfare of children, as well as their education and their rights, than the previous century had been.
Bibliography: Key, Ellen. 1909. *The century of the child.*

CEREBRAL HYPERAEMIA. A condition described in 1878 by William A. Hammond (q.v.). According to him, "a person considered to be suffering from what is called nervous prostration or exhaustion, is simply the subject of emotional disturbance and a consequent condition of cerebral hyperaemia." Although he quoted extensive data to support his theory, he could not prove the existence of cerebral hyperaemia, and it did not replace the fashionable neurasthenia (q.v.).
Bibliography: Hammond, W. A. 1883. *A treatise on insanity in its medical aspects.*

CEREBRI ANATOME. The title of a by Thomas Willis (q.v.). It was an important work that greatly advanced the knowledge of the brain. Richard Lower, the most famous physician in London at that time, prepared model dissections of the brain for it, and the plates are said to have been drawn by Sir Christopher Wren (q.v.), the architect of St. Paul's Cathedral.

Bibliography: Scherz, B., ed. 1969. *Historical aspects of brain research in the seventeenth century.*

CEREBRO-CARDIAC NEUROPATHIA. A term coined by Maurice Krishaber (q.v.) to describe the condition later called anxiety neurosis (q.v.).
Bibliography: Krishaber, M. 1873. *De la névropathie cérébro-cardiaque.*

CEREBROPATHIA PSYCHICA TOXEMICA. A disease first described and named by Sergei Korsakov (q.v.) in 1887. It is associated with polyneuritis, and it is now known as Korsakov's Syndrome (q.v.).
Bibliography: Korsakov, S. S. 1890. Eine psych. Störung combiniert mit multipler Neuritis. *Allg. Zeitschr. f. Psych*, 46.

CEREBROTONIA. A term derived from the Greek meaning "a stretching of the brain." In W. H. Sheldon's (q.v.) classification, cerebrotonic is a personality type associated with the ectomorphic physical type. Individuals in this group find pleasure in the exercise of cognitive activities.
Bibliography: Shelden, W. H. 1940. *The varieties of human physique.*

CERISE, LAURENT (1807-1869). A French physician. He formulated a theory that tried to take account of the contribution of language to the development of behavior and tried to determine the role played by language in the pathogenesis of mental disorders. He thought that language and social institutions were inseparable. His concept of "the goal of activity" included teaching man to direct his ideas and feelings, and giving society a collective purpose. Most of his work was incorporated in a volume entitled *De Fonctions et des Maladies Nerveuses* published in 1842. Cerise was one of the first editors of *Annales Médico-Psychologiques* (q.v.).
Bibliography: Starobinski, J. 1974. The role of language in psychiatric treatment in the French romantic age. A note on Dr. Laurent Cerise. *Psychol. Med.* 4: 360-63.

CERLETTI, UGO (1877-1963). Italian neuropsychiatrist, originator of the electroconvulsive method of treatment. While living and working in Rome, he noticed that pigs in the city slaughterhouse were stupefied by electric current before they were slaughtered. He began working on the field of electroconvulsive therapy, and eventually he and Lucio Bini (1908), another Italian neuropsychiatrist, administered the first electroshock treatment to a schizophrenic (*see* SCHIZOPHRENIA) patient on April 15, 1938. His scientific papers were presented to the Menninger Foundation's (q.v.) museum and archives by his widow in 1972.
Bibliography: Cerletti, U. 1950. Old and new information about electroshock. *Am. J. Psychiat.* 107: 87-94.

CERQUOZZI, MICHELANGELO (1602-1660). An Italian painter. His paintings usually depicted beggars, paupers, and other characters of low life.

These subjects became fashionable, and he became wealthy. But, he became a miser, afraid to spend his earnings, always fearful of robbery, unable to sleep through anxiety, and continually devising new hiding places for his money. His biographer Giambattista Passeri (1610-1679) wrote that "he never married because he preferred to endure an incommodious life than put up with the company of a wife whose continuous expenses frightened him."
Bibliography: Wittkower, R., and Wittkower, M. 1963. *Born under Saturn.*

CERVANTES SAAVEDRA, MIGUEL DE (1547-1616). A Spanish novelist, poet, and playwright who had an unusual deep understanding of the psychology (q.v.) of mental illness. His father was a surgeon-apothecary. In 1569, a warrant was issued for Cervantes' arrest on the grounds of wounding a man in Madrid; the sentence awaiting him was ten years in exile and the loss of his right hand. He escaped but lost his left hand, two years later, fighting against the Turks. He was captured by the Turks and taken as a slave to Algiers. Ransomed, he returned to Spain and resumed a restless life, marred by debts, excommunication, prison sentences, and escapes. In 1604 he returned to Valladolid (q.v.), where he had spent his early childhood. An asylum (q.v.) had existed there since 1436, and Cervantes, who knew it well, acquired from it his knowledge of abnormal behavior, which he used in his masterpiece *Don Quixote* (q.v.). After its publication in 1605, he became famous, but fame did not prevent him from becoming embroiled in more litigation. A spurious sequel to his *Don Quixote* appeared in 1614 with a stinging preface that attributed to Cervantes physical and mental abnormalities. He retaliated by rushing to print his own sequel with some bitter remarks about the whole episode. He died reconciled with his church, leaving a wife and one much loved illegitimate daughter.
Bibliography: Predmore, R. L. 1973. *Cervantes.*

CÉZANNE, PAUL (1839-1906). A French painter. As a child he was obstinate and given to temper tantrums, culminating in hysterical rage (*see* HYSTERIA). He was shy, subject to frequent mood changes, anxious, and unsociable. The initial rejection of his paintings greatly added to his self-doubt. He was so insecure that at one point, when François Auguste Rodin (1840-1917) greeted him, he was overwhelmed and burst into tears. He fled when Claude Monet (1840-1926) complimented him, fearing that he was being mocked. He was deeply hurt by the lack of understanding his paintings received, and he retired more and more into a solitary life, becoming almost a hermit in Aix-en-Provence, the town of his birth. Until his death his reputation as a great painter rested with the young avant-garde artists.
Bibliography: Perruchot, H. 1961. *Cézanne.*

CHAMBRE ARDENTE (BURNING COURT). A special court instituted in Paris in the sixteenth century. It dealt with cases of heresy and special

aspects of other crimes, such as poisoning. The room where it operated was covered completely with black draperies and lit by torches even in daytime. In 1677 the chambre ardente investigated the case against La Voisin, Catherine Deshayes Monvoisin, a woman accused of plotting the death of the king and dauphin. She was found guilty of selling poisons and charms and burnt alive; many high-ranking people were implicated by her. The whole affair was sparked off by the quasi-hysterical phobia (*see* PHOBIA) of witchcraft (q.v.).
Bibliography: Robins, R. H. 1970. *The encyclopedia of witchcraft and demonology.*

CHAMOMILE. An herb recommended as a sedative in the ancient herbals. Infusions of chamomile also were used in cases of hysteria (q.v.). It was one of the sacred herbs of the Saxons. Persian medical works referred to its odor, which was supposed to induce sleep.
Bibliography: Le Strange, R. 1977. *A history of herbal plants.*

CHANCERY LUNATICS. An English legal term applied to those persons found to be insane after their relatives had petitioned the Lord Chancellor to institute an inquisition into their state. Relatives usually petitioned to prevent the mentally ill from dissipating their estates, which could then be supervised by the crown. The procedure originated in the eighteenth century.
Bibliography: Parry-Jones, W. Ll. 1972. *The trade in lunacy.*

CHANGELING. In the pre-Christian superstition of Celto-Germanic origin, a child substituted for another, an elf. An abnormal child was believed to be a changeling, especially if the child was mentally retarded, a cretin (*see* CRETINISM), or hydrocephalic. The main cause for comment was the appearance of the child and the fact that he would not talk or laugh, but screamed continuously. A child's irresponsiveness, his inability to talk or laugh, was a sign that he was not human but had been substituted for the stolen child by the fairies, or elves. If he could be made to talk or smile, the spell would be broken and the original child would reappear. The reason for the elves stealing a child of man was their envy for the human soul; they were also believed to marry the stolen child to one of their own race to better their stock. Newborn babies and very young children were guarded constantly. They were protected by amulets (q.v.) worn around the neck and by placing near them objects that would keep the elves away. Once a parent found that the cradle contained a changeling, two contradictory remedies were available: The child could be treated so kindly that he would smile and break the spell, or he could be ill-treated so cruelly that the elf-parent would rescue him out of pity.
Bibliography: Forbes, T. R. 1966. *The midwife and the witch.*

CHANGELING, THE. A tragedy by Thomas Middleton (1570?-1627) and William Rowley (1585?-?1642) first performed in 1623. The subplot concerns

a keeper of a madhouse, an obvious reference to Bethlem Royal Hospital (q.v.). He is an old man who keeps his young wife shut up with the patients. Her lover, to gain access to her, pretends to be insane and is admitted into the hospital.
Bibliography: O'Donoghue, E. G. 1914. *The story of Bethlehem hospital.*

CHANGE OF SEX. Delusions (q.v.) about changes of sex sometimes occur in psychotic (*see* PSYCHOSIS) patients. Primitive people believe that children will not reach manhood by a process of development but rather through magic (q.v.) ceremonies of initiation.
Bibliography: Storch, A. 1924. *The primitive archaic forms in schizophrenia,* trans. C. Willard.

CH'AO IUANGFANG. A seventh-century Chinese philosopher. In 610 he wrote *General Treatise of the Causes and Symptoms of Diseases* in which he described nearly sixty nervous and mental disorders, including hysteria (q.v.), various kinds of paralysis, and speech disorders.
Bibliography: Kiev, Ari. 1968. *Psychiatry in the Communist world.*

CHAPMAN, MARY (1647-1724). An Englishwoman, born in Norwich. She married the rector of Thorpe, a small Norfolk town. When he died in 1713, she followed his wishes and built a hospital for "persons afflicted with lunacy [*see* LUNATIC] or madness (nor such as are fools or idiots [q.v.] from their birth." This was Bethel Hospital (q.v.), the second oldest mental hospital in England and the oldest still in its original building. Mrs. Chapman took up residence in the hospital on the day it opened and remained there until her death. By her will, her estate was settled on the trustees for the continuance of the hospital. A marble slab in Thorpe Church, where she is buried, reminds posterity of her philanthropy.
Bibliography: Bateman, F., and Rye, W. 1906. *The history of the Bethel Hospital at Norwich.*

CHAPTAL. A young student, the first patient of Philippe Pinel (q.v.). They were both students at the University of Montpellier. Chaptal became depressed and anxious when he felt that too much was demanded of him. Pinel, realizing his friend's state of mind, asked him to visit his house every day in order to read the classics together, thus offering him what amounted to psychotherapy (q.v.).
Bibliography: Semelaigne, R. 1891. *Les grands aliénistes Français.*

CHARACTEROLOGY. A pseudoscientific way of assessing personality by the study of gestures, painting, or handwriting, graphology (q.v.).

CHARAKA. An Hindu writer on medical matters in the first century A.D. His name means "the wanderer." He believed that health was the result of a balance between air, mucus, and bile; disease was the work of evil spirits. He accurately described many disorders, including insanity, epilepsy (q.v.), and idiocy (*see* IDIOT). He was aware of the importance of emotions and passions in the aetiology of mental disorders. The plant Nardus root (q.v.) (Nardostachys Jatamonsi) was used by him in the treatment of mental patients needing sedation.

Bibliography: Venkoba Rao, A. 1975. India. In *World history of psychiatry*, ed. J. G. Howells.

CHARCOT, JEAN-MARTIN (1825-1893). French neurologist and psychiatrist, second son of a carriage builder; his mother was not yet seventeen when he was born. At school he showed talent in drawing, especially caricatures, and for a time thought of becoming a painter. By the time he was twenty-three years old, he had completed his medical education, and he became an intern at the Hôpitaux de Paris and at the Salpêtrière (q.v.). His doctoral thesis, written in 1853, dealt with rheumatoid arthritis and established him as a talented clinical investigator. His interest turned to degenerative diseases of the nervous system and to clinical neurology (q.v.). In 1862 he was appointed physician-in-charge at Salpêtrière. His reputation as a neurologist gave weight to his studies on hysteria (q.v.), which he believed to be an organic disorder of the nervous system. In his studies, he retained some of the ancient belief that hysteria was associated with the uterus (q v.) by relating the convulsive crises of the hysteric to the ovaries. His lectures on hysterical paralysis were enlivened by his dramatic mimic demonstrations of the various gaits and postures of patients and by photographs, which were used for the first time in medical teaching. Once his reputation was established, he openly showed his interest in hypnosis (*see* HYPNOTISM). He regarded the ability to be hypnotized as a symptom of hysteria and therefore within the field of pathological phenomena. Because of his interest and beliefs hypnosis became more acceptable to medical circles and The Académie des Sciences (q.v.), which had rejected mesmerism (q.v.). Thus he paved the way for the discoveries of Sigmund Freud (q.v.), who was for a time his student and admirer. Charcot was accused not only of being cold to his patients but also of arranging his clinical demonstrations as a show for a public that included not only physicians and students, but also actresses, journalists, and the merely curious. His patients were hypnotized by assistants, no patient was ever hypnotised by him. He dismissed any malingering apparent in these sessions as a peccadillo of the sick and remained unaware that some performances were induced by financial gain and that others were of iatrogenic origin, suggestion playing an important part.

He was a colorful character, who enjoyed a considerable social life. His wife was very wealthy and they entertained interesting authors, politicians and artists in their lavishly furnished neo-Gothic house, which abounded in stained-glass windows and objets d'art. He found relaxation in painting

and collected items that combined artistic interest with psychiatric significance. He collaborated with Paul Richer on a monograph entitled *Les Demoniaques dans l'Art* (1887). In later life he became more aware of the criticism aimed at his theories and set about revising them, but death cut short his efforts.
Bibliography: Guillaim, G. 1959. *J-M. Charcot, 1825-1893: his life—his work*, trans. and ed. Pearce Bailey.

CHARENTON. A mental hospital near the Park of Vincennes in Paris. It was founded in 1642, continuing the work of the monks of St. Jean de Dieu, who originally built it as a monastery, where the mentally ill were cared for. It was destroyed and rebuilt several times before it was finally restored under Louis Philippe (1773-1850) in 1830. Jean Esquirol (q.v.) was one of the distinguished physicians who worked there. Calling anyone a "pensionnaire de Charenton" remains the equivalent of saying "you are mad."
Bibliography: Letchworth, W. P. 1889. *The insane in foreign countries.*

CHARISMA. A term derived from the Greek *charis*, meaning "grace." The Charites, or Graces, were goddesses personifying charm and grace. In early Christian times, the term was used to describe special miraculous gifts of prophesy, healing, and such like. In psychiatric jargon, charismatic people are individuals who are regarded as leaders, set apart from their followers, emotionally uninvolved, but presenting a humanistic facade and empathic understanding of the needs of their followers.
Bibliography: Caldwell, J. M. 1972. Notes on Charisma. In *The psychiatric forum*, ed. G. Usdin.

CHARITÉ (GERMANY). A Berlin hospital with a famous psychiatric and neurological clinic. Karl Ideler, Wilhelm Griesinger, and Karl Bonhoeffer (qq.v.) were among its directors.

CHARITÉ DE CHÂTEAU-THIERRY. An eighteenth-century French institution for the mentally ill. Like many hospitals of its time, it was also used as a house of correction.
Bibliography: Rosen, G. 1968. *Madness in society.*

CHARLES I (1600-1649). King of Great Britain and Ireland. In order to raise money for war with Scotland, he tried to ingratiate the citizens of London by renewing their ancient privileges. One of these measures in 1638 granted a charter to the city of London that confirmed it as the government of Bethlem Royal Hospital (q.v.) and granted to it the possession of Bethlem's estates.
Bibliography: O'Donoghue, E. G. 1914. *The Story of Bethlehem Hospital.*

CHARLES II (1661-1700). King of Spain. His father was fifty-six years old when he was born and died four years later. From infancy, Charles was weak, deformed, and mentally retarded. It was obvious that he was incapable of fulfilling his role as king, but political interests and intrigues kept him on the throne. In an effort to secure the succession, he was married twice, first to a French princess and then to an Austrian one, but both marriages were without issue. The Spanish court would not admit his impotence and preferred to believe that he was the victim of Austria's witch-craft (q.v.). All kinds of bizarre superstitions grew around him.
Bibliography: Nada, J. 1960. *Carlos the bewitched.*

CHARLES V (1500-1558). Holy Roman emperor and king of Spain. Both his mother Joanna of Castile (q.v.) and his great-grandmother Isabella of Portugal (q.v.) were insane. His father died when he was six years old. He was brought up by his aunt, Margaret of Austria, a capable woman who loved and guided him. Her influence, rather than his genetic heredity, is apparent in his life. While not a genius, he was certainly devoted to his family and to his country. He suffered from gout, which made him irritable, but he obstinately refused Andreas Vesalius' (q.v.) advice to diet. His re-action to anxiety and stress was to overeat, thus exacerbating his illness. He spent the last three years of his life in retirement, studying astronomy and astrology (q.v.) and indulging his passion for clocks. A few months before his death he became extremely depressed and fearful about the salvation of his soul. He ordered that his obsequies should be celebrated and a tomb erected. At the funeral service he was solemnly shrouded and laid in his coffin. After the ceremony, he rose and retired to his apartments and gave himself up to more awful meditations.
Bibliography: Brandi, K. 1965. *The Emperor Charles V.*

CHARLES VI (1368-1422). King of France. He was said to have become insane after exposure to the sun for a long period while hunting, or while engaged in military exercises.
Bibliography: d'Avout, J. 1943. *La querelle des Armagnacs et des Bourguignons.*

CHARLESWORTH, EDWARD PARKER (1783-1853). An English physician who practiced in Lincoln. In 1820 he was appointed visiting physician to the Lincoln Asylum (q.v.). He introduced many innovations there, in-cluding classification of the patients, proper exercise, and the abolition of the more severe forms of restraint (q.v.). John Conolly (q.v.) was greatly influenced by his views. Charlesworth was so passionately convinced of his nonrestraint policy that it is said he challenged Dr. Corsellis, a physician of opposed views, to a duel. Corsellis elected to fight with the pen on the

pages of the *Lancet*, but when the fight on the printed pages took place, his adversary was not Corsellis but R. G. Hill (q.v.).
Bibliography: Hunter, R., and Macalpine, I. 1963. *Three hundred years of psychiatry.*

CHARLOTTE (CARLOTA) (1840-1927). Empress of Mexico, the only daughter of Leopold I of Belgium. She married Maximilian, archduke of Austria in 1857 and accompanied him to Mexico when he was made emperor of it in 1864. She was subject to acute depression and periods of hysterical (*see* HYSTERIA) religious fervor. In Mexico she isolated herself from the world and spent much of her time in brooding silence, bemoaning her childless state. Her strange delusions (q.v.) and obsessions (q.v.) were attributed sometimes to poisoning from hallucinogenic mushrooms. After Maximilian's position in Mexico became untenable, she fled to Europe to seek help from the pope and Napoleon III. There, she became paranoid (*see* PARANOIA) and her already clouded state of mind ended in insanity. The final crisis occurred in Rome when late one night she insisted upon taking refuge in the Vatican, to the consternation of pope Pius IX, who had to make hasty arrangements for transforming the library into a bedchamber for her and her lady-in-waiting. She became so afraid of poison that she had all her food cooked in her presence and would only drink the water she herself had collected from street fountains in the city. Joseph von Riedel (q.v.), the director of the Vienna Lunatic Asylum, attended her. Eventually she was confined to the castle of Bouchout near Brussels and spent the remaining forty-eight years of her life there.
Bibliography: Haslip, J. 1971. *Imperial adventurer: Emperor Maximilian of Mexico and his empress.*

CHATEAUBRIAND, FRANÇOIS RENÉ, VICOMTE DE (1768-1848). French author and statesman. His mother suffered from religious mania (q.v.), and his father was such a solitary man that he avoided company whenever possible. Chateaubriand's early childhood was spent in his family's castle. His only companion was his sister Lucille, a strange child given to periods of intense depression and paranoia (q.v.). She became insane and killed herself. Chateaubriand was himself melancholy (*see* MELANCHOLIA), for he wrote, "I was acquainted with suffering from my earliest childhood: I bore a germ of suffering within me. . . .A strange poison mingled itself with all my feelings." He tried to commit suicide (q.v.), but the gun he used misfired. After the death of his mother and his sister he turned to religion, not so much as a form of truth but as something beautiful and poetic. Of his many works, two are at least partially autobiographical, *René* (1805) and *Mémoirs d'Outre-Tombe* (1850).
Bibliography: Sieburg, F. 1961. *Chateaubriand.*

CHATIN, GASPARD ADOLPH (1813-1901). A French physician. In 1850 he demonstrated that iodine could be used in the prophylaxis of endemic goitre and cretinism (q.v.).
Bibliography: Schmidt, J. E. 1959. *Medical discoveries: who and when.*

CHATTERTON, THOMAS (1752-1770). An English poet. His father, who died before Thomas' birth, was a dissipated individual who meddled in magic (q.v.); his mother was a nonentity who was incapable of a warm relationship; and his sister suffered periods of derangement. He compensated for his lonely childhood with self-deceptions and illusions of importance. He was only ten years old when he wrote his first poem, which was published in the local paper. Many of his verses were morbid, dealing with death, suicide (q.v.), and bodily corruption. Despite his own ability, he sheltered an elaborate fraud by fabricating a romance in prose and verse that purported to be the work of a fifteenth-century monk by the name of Thomas Rowley. He also tried to pass a treatise on painting as a work written in 1469. Yet, some of his own poems and his burlesque opera *The Revenge* (1769) were quite successful. He lived in a state of continuous depression, and his extreme poverty added to his feeling of despair. He was only seventeen years old when he committed suicide by taking arsenic.
Bibliography: Meyerstein, E. H. W. 1930. *A life of Thomas Chatterton.*

CHAUCER, GEOFFREY (c.1340-1400). An English poet. His first poem *The Boke of the Duchesse* is a lament on the death of John of Gaunt's first wife, Blanche of Lancaster. In the poem Chaucer gives a fine description of melancholy (*see* MELANCHOLIA). It has been said that he was describing his own melancholy. His greatest work, the *Canterbury Tales* (q.v.), also contains references to emotional and mental disorders.
Bibliography: Brewer, D. 1978. *Chaucer and his world.*

CHAULIAC, GUY DE (c.1300-1368). French surgeon and physician to three popes in Avignon. His treatise, translated in French with the title *Grande Chirurgie*, was printed in 1592 and became a standard manual for physicians for three hundred years. In it he dealt with trepanation (q.v.), advising that the operation should never be done when the moon is full.
Bibliography: Garrison, F. H. 1968. *An introduction to the history of medicine.*

CHEADLE ROYAL HOSPITAL. See MANCHESTER LUNATIC HOSPITAL.

CHEKHOV, ANTON PAVLOVICH (1860-1904). Russian dramatist and author. He grew up in an overly religious household with an overly strict father, who whipped him every day. As a child, Chekhov found it difficult to believe that not all children were beaten by their parents. In turn he rejected religion and was brutal to his own children. He qualified as a doctor and practiced briefly before turning to writing. His works portray family life in Russia and show considerable insight into human behavior and emotional problems. In addition to his short stories, his most famous works are

the plays *Uncle Vanya* (1900), *The Three Sisters* (1901), and *The Cherry Orchard* (1903).
Bibliography: Hingley, R. F. 1976. *A new life of Anton Chekhov.*

CHEROMANIA. An obsolete term derived from the Greek and meaning a "morbid impulse to cheerfulness." In the Middle Ages (q.v.) it was commonly observed as a reaction to the insecurity arising from epidemics and other life-threatening disasters. In psychosis (q.v.) it is present in manic-depressive patients in a state of elation. *Cherophobia* indicates the opposite phenomenon, a morbid fear of gaiety.
Bibliography: Hecker, J. F. K. 1846. *The epidemics of the Middle Ages*, trans. B. G. Babington.

CHERVIL. A fragrant plant whose name comes from the Greek term meaning "to rejoice." Herbalists believed it to be beneficial in nervous disorders, the treatment of depression, and the treatment of poor memory (q.v.).
Bibliography: de Baïracli Levy, J. 1974. *The illustrated herbal handbook.*

CHESS. A game that, according to Indian tradition, was invented by Buddhist priests as a substitute for war, which they regarded as sinful. Other cultures have different beliefs about its origin, but it seems to have been used as a form of displacement of affects. In medieval times it was very popular until the church condemned it. Fines were imposed on chess players, and the game was blamed for arousing "violent passions."
Bibliography: Jones, E. 1951. *Essays in applied psychoanalysis.*

CHEVIGNÉ. A French soldier dismissed from the army of the French Revolution. Becoming drunk one evening, he passed himself off as a general and found himself in Bicêtre (q.v.), where he was kept for ten years. Philippe Pinel (q.v.) freed him of his chains and made him his bodyguard. Chevigné, a giant of a man, saved the life of his benefactor by fighting off a crowd that wanted to lynch Pinel on the suspicion that he harbored priests and spies in the hospital.
Bibliography: Semelaigne, R. 1891. *Les grands aliénistes Français.*

CHEVREUL-PENDULUM. A contraption consisting of a weight suspended by a piece of string about fifteen inches long; the weight was made to sway over a white chart on which two lines were drawn intersecting at right angles. It was devised by Michel Chevreul in about 1833 as an aid to suggestibility, or as a test for concentration. He believed that the pendulum was directed by the subject's unconscious (q.v.) thinking.
Bibliography: Ellenberger, H. F. 1970. *The discovery of the unconscious.*

CHEYNE, GEORGE (1671-1743). A British physician, educated in Scotland, who practiced in Edinburgh, London, and Bath. He was a student of

Hermann Boerhaave (q.v.). He believed that neurosis (q.v.) was common among the English and was the explanation for the high frequency of suicide (q.v.). To him the "English malady" was depression and other emotional disorders. In his book *The English Malady: or a Treatise of Spleen, Vapours, Lowness of Spirits, Hypochondriacal and Hysterical Distempers* (1733), he discussed the causes, nature, and treatment of neurotic behavior. He thought that luxurious living, humid climate, sedentary occupations, and town life promoted neurosis by causing "a siziness or viscidity in the fluids" and a loss of tone in the nerves. According to him, material progress, as well as freedom in politics and religion, was another cause of mental instability, which afflicted mostly intelligent people, sparing "fools, weak or stupid persons" with "dull souls." Low diet, emetics, and purging (q.v.) were the remedies he recommended. The book contained one exceptional feature: it was illustrated by the author's own case history to demonstrate that neurosis is nothing to be ashamed of, as it is an illness like any other. Cheyne's disease is listed in medical dictionaries as hypochondria (q.v.).
Bibliography: Hunter, R., and Macalpine, I. 1963. *Three hundred years of psychiatry.*

CHIARUGI, VINCENZO (1759-1820). An Italian physician who specialized in the treatment of skin disorders and mental illness. After he was appointed to the Hospital of Bonifazio (q.v.) in Florence in 1789, he introduced many reforms. Mental patients were housed in separate wards, restraint (q.v.) was mitigated, nurses were specially trained, and active treatment was instituted. He believed that insanity was caused by the deterioration of the brain. His classification of mental diseases and his methods of treatment closely resembled those of Philippe Pinel (q.v.). He gave new impetus to the use of opium (q.v.) in treatment by administering it as an ointment to be rubbed on the skin, rather than as a drug to be taken by mouth. Chiarugi wrote many works on pellagra (q.v.), venereal diseases, hermaphrodism, and insanity.
Bibliography: Mora, G. 1975. Italy. In *World history of psychiatry*, ed. J. G. Howells.

CHIAVARI. A town in northwestern Italy, near Genoa. The first Italian asylum (q.v.) for the mentally retarded was established there in 1889 by Antonio Gonnelli-Cioni. It was later moved to Vercurago.
Bibliography: Barr, M. W. 1904. *Mental defectives.*

CHILD GUIDANCE CLINICS. Clinics that emerged in the nineteenth century in response to investigations into psychopathic (*see* PSYCHOPATHY) behavior in young people. They were viewed originally as a means of preventing juvenile delinquency. Eventually these clinics began to deal with more subtle behavior problems. William Healy's (q.v.) work with delinquents in the juvenile courts of Cook County in 1909 was continued in the founding of the Judge Baker Clinic in Boston in 1912. This was followed by the experimental clinics of the National Committee for Mental Hygiene and led to the establishment of many clinics in the United States. Alfred Adler (q.v.) founded the first child guidance clinic in Vienna in 1919. The child guidance movement was imported into the United Kingdom in the 1920s. In 1927 the first English child guidance clinic was established. It was the East London Child Guidance Clinic, begun as a voluntary effort by the Jewish Health Organization. In 1928 the Child Guidance Council was organized. The first demonstration clinic was established with the help of the Commonwealth Fund at Islington in 1929 and became known as the London Child Guidance Clinic. By 1932 the movement had spread outside London, and a clinic under a local education authority had been established in Birmingham. In 1944 there were ninety-five child guidance clinics, half of which were organized by local authorities, twenty-two were staffed by mental hospitals, and nine were voluntary. During the same period the movement extended into Europe.

Bibliography: Howells, J. G. and Osborn, M. L. 1980-81. The History of Child Psychiatry in the United Kingdom. *Acta Paedopsychiat.* 46: 193-202.

Schneck, J. M. 1975. United States of America. In *World history of psychiatry*, ed. J. G. Howells.

CHILD PSYCHIATRY. A subspecialty of psychiatry concerned with psychiatric disorders in children. The term was coined by Marcel Manheimer when he used it as a subtitle of his monograph on *Les Troubles Menteux de l'Enfance"* in 1899. Psychiatric disorders in children attracted little attention in early medical writers. Some pediatricians in the fifteenth century, such as Cornelius Roelans (q.v.), referred to children's sleep disorders. Thomas Phaire (q.v.), in the sixteenth century, added epilepsy (q.v.) and enuresis to the discussion of children's mental disorders. His contemporary, Sebastianus Austrius (q.v.), stressed the importance of psychological remedies for psychological disorders in childhood. Cases of mass hysteria (q.v.), possessions (q.v.), and fits were usually recorded during this period in the literature concerning demoniacal possessions. In the eighteenth century, the French physician Brouzet (?-?1772) wrote about infantile jealousy and sibling rivalry in his *Education Medicinale des Enfants* (1754), and Johann Greding (q.v.) described a child who was "raving mad" at birth and so strong that four women had difficulty in restraining him. With the advent of the nineteenth century, the increase in interest in psychiatric disorders gradually embraced children's disorders as well, especially psychosis (q.v.) and mental retardation. Wilhelm Griesinger (q.v.) included hypochondria (q.v.), anxiety, and suicidal (*see* SUICIDE) states in his list and stressed the importance of psychological factors in the aetiology. Jean Esquirol (q.v.) reported cases of children with homicidal impulses. Other authors discussed "moral insanity" (q.v.) in children. Henry Maudsley (q.v.) classified childhood mental disorders under the same headings used for adult disorders but devoted several pages of his *Physiology and Pathology of the Mind* (1867) to "insanity in early life." In 1887, Hermann Emminghaus (q.v.) wrote *Psychic Disturbances in Childhood*, which is one of the earliest systematic presentations of childhood psychiatry. He was followed by Paul Moreau de Tours and Marcel Manheimer in France, and William Ireland (q.v.), in England. More contributions on infantile psychosis, came from Emil Kraepelin (q.v.), Theodore Heller (*see* Heller Disease) and Sante De Sanctis (q.v.). The first classic work in the field, *Child Psychiatry* (1935) by Leo Kanner (q.v.), marked the new era.

CHILD PSYCHOLOGY. Toward the end of the nineteenth century, the systematic study of child development became fashionable, and a number of authors made careful, detailed observations on the development of behavior in young children. There is, for example, the unpublished work of Amos Bronson Alcott (q.v.), as well as the "Biographical Sketch of an Infant," written in 1876 by Charles R. Darwin (q.v.). The first journal on child psychology, the *Pedagogical Seminary* (q.v.), was founded in America in 1891, by Granville Stanley Hall (q.v.). Two years later in 1893 the British Association of Child Study was established in England, while in Germany the Berlin Association for Child Psychology was founded by Carl Stumpf (q.v.). Sigmund Freud's (q.v.) theories gave an immense impetus to studies in child psychology in the twentieth century.
See also PSYCHOLOGY.

CHILDREN'S BUREAU. An organization established in the United States in 1912 by a federal act under President William Howard Taft (1857-1930). It was formed to investigate and report on all matters of child welfare. Its first director was Julia C. Lathrop (q.v.), a social worker with progressive ideas in child care. Its publications are for parents, as well as workers in child welfare; they reflect the current knowledge in child care and cover the physical and psychological aspects of it.
Bibliography: Rosen, G. 1968. *Madness in society.*

CHILD STUDY ASSOCIATION. In 1886 a group of American women, aware of their responsibility to their children and of the importance of their children's mental health, organized the Society for the Study of Child Nature in New York. The idea spread, and eventually the many groups united to form the Federation for Child Study Association of America in 1924. It has had an important influence on child health in the United States.
Bibliography: Rosen, G. 1968. *Madness in society.*

CHILD WELFARE LEAGUE OF AMERICA. An organization founded in 1930. With other child welfare, social, and educational bodies, the league has made important contributions in public health programs by introducing

mental health concepts to professional health workers, who are in direct contact with children.
Bibliography: Rosen, G. 1968. *Madness in society.*

CHINA. In ancient China, mental disorders were treated with some forms of faith healing. Possession (q.v.) by spirits and demons was a commonly held belief, and institutions for the insane were in existence a millennium before Christ. By about 300 B.C. special institutions for the insane were opened in Peking. The *Yellow Emperor's Classic of Internal Medicine* (c.1000 B.C.) discusses psychiatric disorders. The Nei Ching (q.v.), or canon of medicine, dating from the last period of the Chou dynasty, about 249 B.C., believed the brain to be composed of the same material as the marrow of the bones. The skull served as the main reservoir of the marrow. When the marrow was in abundance, the individual would have a general feeling of well-being. The Nei Ching also described in full detail the complex doctrine of the pulse, and it stated that in cases of insanity a "superficial" and "overflowing" pulse is a good omen, but a "deep" and "quick" one is unfavorable. Confucius (q.v.) only referred to madness once, when he told of a madman who followed him about singing and crying out "O Fang! O Fang!" It is suggested that this was a case of feigned insanity (q.v.). Hypnosis (*see* HYPNOTISM) was practiced from early times; exorcism (q.v.) charms, and other supernatural practices were used in therapy. In the nineteenth century medical missionaries introduced Western methods of treatment.
Bibliography: Koran, L. M. 1972. Psychiatry in Mainland China: History and Recent Status. *Am. J. Psychiat.* 128: 84-91.

CH'IN HUANG-TI. Chinese emperor of the second century B.C., builder of the Great Wall. He ordered the burning of many philosophical works and caused the suicide (q.v.) of about five hundred philosophers who were unwilling to survive without their books and therefore threw themselves into the sea.
Bibliography: Fedden, H. R. 1938. *Suicide.*

CHIROMANCY. The art of palmistry, or the prophesying of future events in an individual's life by the study of his palms. It has been practiced since early times in every part of the world. The early religious books of India and China (q.v.) refer to it; and it was widely practiced in the Middle Ages (q.v.) in Europe, where it was associated with witchcraft (q.v.) and astrology (q.v.). Areas of the hands were described by the names of the planets then known and by references to the sun and the moon. In England, Henry III condemned chiromancy and made it illegal by an act of Parliament. In 1735 the English laws forbidding witchcraft (q.v.) again declared chiromancy illegal, and these laws were not repealed until 1951. Chiromancy was popular

in the sixteenth century among all classes of people. Girolamo Cardano (q.v.) wrote an unpublished treatise on it.
Bibliography: Penrose, L. S. 1973. Fingerprints and Palmistry. *Lancet*. 1: 1239-42.

CHIROMANIA. A term derived from the Greek. It implies a relationship between masturbation (q.v.) and insanity, a common belief in the nineteenth century.
Bibliography: Tuke, D.H. 1892. *A dictionary of psychological medicine.*

CHOLER. The concept of the four humors (q.v.) developed in antiquity remained in use until the seventeenth century. They consisted of blood, phlegm, yellow bile (or yellow choler), which was hot and dry, and black bile (or black choler [q.v.]), which was cold and dry. Black choler was said to be the cause of melancholy (*see* MELANCHOLIA) which often was undifferentiated from insanity. Hermann Boerhaave (q.v.) in *Aphorisms: Concerning the Knowledge and Cure of Diseases* (1709), wrote that melancholy "arises from that Malignancy of the Blood and Humors, which the Antients have called Black Choler: and again, though this Disease doth begin in what is called the Mind, it yet doth render the choler black in the Body very soon."
Bibliography: Temkin, O. 1973. *Galenism.*

CHOREA DEMONOMANIA. Another term for choromania (q.v.), the frenzied dancing, at times accompanied by other hysterical (*see* HYSTERIA) behavior, which was observed in the Middle Ages (q.v.) and later. Those affected were believed to be possessed (*see* POSSESSION) by the devil. The phenomenon, which often reached the size of an epidemic, was spread by mass suggestion and imitation. Small communities, living in conditions of seclusion and repression, were particularly prone to it. In a French convent, for example, a nun who mewed like a cat began an epidemic of mewing among the other nuns, and in a German convent an epidemic of biting was reported.
Bibliography: Hecker, J. F. C. 1846. *The epidemics of the Middle Ages*, trans. B. G. Babington.

CHOREA LASCIVA. A term for Saint Vitus' dance (q.v.), or chorea, suggested by Paracelsus (q.v.), who objected to attaching the names of saints or devils to a disease. The adjective *lasciva*, which implies the sexual nature of hysteria (q.v.), somewhat anticipates the psychoanalytic findings of a much later period.
Bibliography: Pachter, H. M. 1951. *Paracelsus.*

CHOROMANIA. A term derived from the Greek. It is used to describe a condition in which the patient is unable to resist a hysterical (*see* HYSTERIA)

impulse to dance or to make rhythmic movements. It was common in the Middle Ages (q.v.). It is more popularly known as dancing mania (q.v.).
Bibliography: Tuke, D. H. 1842. *A dictionary of psychological medicine.*

CHRISTIAN II (1481-1559). King of Denmark, Norway, and Sweden. He was called Christian the Cruel and "the Nero of the North" because of his harshness, especially against the nobility. His life was punctuated by acts of extreme cruelty; his psychopathic (*see* PSYCHOPATHY) personality also revealed itself in his private life. His mistress was the daughter of an innkeeper. Her mother exerted such great influence over Christian and was so hated by the nobles that her sudden death was said to have been caused by poison. Christian was deposed, driven out of the country, and finally imprisoned for the rest of his life.
Bibliography: Oakley, S. 1972. *Story of Denmark.*

CHRISTIAN VII (1749-1808). King of Denmark and Norway. As a child, he was deprived of love and subjected to the harsh control of his tutor, who completely brutalized him. He grew up a depraved drunkard and a misogynist. He was married to Caroline Matilda (q.v.) but divorced her in 1772. He became insane and in 1784 was forced to relinquish the crown to Frederick VI.
Bibliography: Nors, P. 1928. *The court of Christian VII of Denmark.*

CHRISTIAN SCIENCE. A religious movement founded in 1866 by Mary Baker Eddy (q.v.). It believes that pain and illness are illusions and that belief in the power of God is all that is needed to achieve healing.
Bibliography: John, DeWitt. 1971. *The Christian Science way of life.*

CHURCH CROSSES AND PILLARS. Stone monuments, often commemorative. In the Middle Ages (q.v.) lunatics (q.v.) were sometimes bound to them overnight as a means of curing them. The following lines from *The Monarchie* by Sir David Lyndsay (1490-1555), refer to the cross at New Barthwick, southeast of Edinburgh:

> They bryng mad men on fuit and horsse,
> and byndes them to Saint Mangose Crosse.

Bibliography: Tuke, D. H. 1882. *History of the insane in the British Isles.*

CHURINGA. Stones or pieces of wood that the Australian aborigines believe to have magical (*see* MAGIC) qualities. They represent the souls or the minds of the owners and are carefully hidden in secret places.
Bibliography: Drever, J. 1952. *A dictionary of psychology.*

CIBBER, CAIUS GABRIEL (1630-1700). A Danish sculptor who worked in England. He provided the two statues representing melancholy and raving madness that embellished the entrance to Bethlem Royal Hospital (q.v.) when it was rebuilt in 1676. They were considered by many to be his best work, but the English poet Alexander Pope (1688-1744) referred to them as "great Cibber's brazen, brainless brothers." When the hospital moved to St. George's Fields in 1815, they were put in the new entrance hall, but, because they were naked figures, they were covered up to prevent them from offending the public. On committee days they were uncovered for the benefit of the Governors. In 1858 they were removed from the hospital but eventually returned to it and are now in its museum.
Bibliography: O'Donoghue, E. G. 1914. *The story of Bethlehem Hospital.*

CICERO, MARCUS TULLIUS (106-43 B.C.). Roman politician, orator, and stoic (*see* STOICISM) philosopher. Although he was not a physician, he wrote about medicine. He objected to the Hippocratic (*see* HIPPOCRATES) theory of black choler (q.v.) as a cause of melancholy and believed that it was caused by psychological factors, such as fear, anger, and pain. He asserted that emotions can affect the body and produce physical disorders. In his *Tusculanae Disputationes* (q.v.), Cicero differentiated between insanity and emotional illness, or melancholy. Thus, he objected to the Greeks calling frenzy, what the Romans called melancholia (q.v.). He believed that the soul could be healed just as the body could be healed, not by the gods, but by men skilled in the specific art of healing.
Bibliography: Birkholz, A. M. 1806. *Cicero medicus.*

CINQUEFOIL. A plant found on wasteland. Its botanical name *Potentilla canadensis* derives from the word *potens*, powerful, a reference to its use in folk medicine as a powerful sedative. It is also a valued treatment for epilepsy (q.v.) and hysterical (*see* HYSTERIA) disorders.
Bibliography: de Baïracli Levy, J. 1974. *The illustrated herbal handbook.*

CIPHER METHOD. A method referred to by Sigmund Freud (q.v.) in his discussion of the interpretation of dreams (q.v.), which are, as it were, coded messages needing a known key to be understood.
Bibliography: Freud, S. 1933. *The interpretation of dreams*, trans. A.A. Brill.

CIRCE. In Homeric (*see* HOMER) legend she was a sorceress skilled in the use of magic (q.v.) and venomous potions, which she made from herbs gathered on her island. She changed Ulysses' (q.v.) companions into swine, but he forced her to restore them. The Pontine marshes in southern Italy have been identified with Circe's island, and it is possible that the malaria then rife in those regions produced the hallucinations (q.v.) that gave rise to the legend of magic transformations.
Bibliography: Murray, A.T. 1925. *Homer. The Odyssey.*

CIRCULATING SWING. A machine that could rotate a patient seated on it as many times as one hundred gyrations a minute. It caused vomiting, purging (q.v.), and often fainting. This type of machine enjoyed a certain popularity among the medical profession during the latter part of the eighteenth century and into the beginning of the nineteenth century. They were useless as well as potentially dangerous, and were eventually abandoned.
Bibliography: Morison, A. 1828. *Cases of mental disease, with practical observations.*

CIRILLO, DOMENICO (1739-1799). An Italian physician who worked in his native city of Naples. He used music to treat a woman who had been admitted to hospital for insanity. Noticing that she made slight rhythmical movements, he suspected that she was a victim of tarantism (q.v.) and called in a band of musicians to play dance music. According to his report, she got out of bed and danced violently; for the next three days she improved, but on the third day she suddenly died. He wrote a paper, "Some account of the tarantula," which was published in 1770 in the *Philosophical Transactions* (q.v.) in London.
Bibliography: Mora, G. 1971. 1970 Anniversaries. *Am. J. Psychiat.* 127: 78.

CITERROCHEN. A fish that is naturally charged with electricity (q.v.). Pedanius Dioscorides (q.v.) in his *Materia Medica* wrote that these fish had been used in the treatment of headache and other disorders of psychosomatic origin. They were applied to the patient's head as a kind of shocking device.
Bibliography: Kallaway, P. 1946. The part played by electric fish in the early history of bioelectricity and electrotherapy. *Bull. Hist. Med.* 20: 112-37.

CLAIRVOYANCE. The ability to anticipate future events. In antiquity and even in more recent times, in some communities it has been thought that the insane have special powers that enabled them to foresee future events. The Stoics (*see* STOICISM) were among those who held this belief.
Bibliography: Hall, A. and King, F. 1975. *Mysteries of prediction.*

CLAPARÈDE, ÉDOUARD (1873-1940). A Swiss psychologist. He believed that consciousness is a biological function at the service of the organism; he called this the "law of momentary interest," whereby an individual becomes conscious of a need only when it is not biologically satisfied and demands gratification. He was interested in many psychological problems and studied sleep and hysteria (q.v.), as well as conducting experiments on hypnosis (*see* HYPNOTISM) in animals. He succeeded in hypnotizing pigs and goats. His approach to the study of child psychology (q.v.) was functional. He had a laboratory in Geneva and founded the Rousseau Institute for educational psychology in that city.
Bibliography: Flugel, J. C. 1945. *A hundred years of psychology.*

CLAPHAM RETREAT. A private asylum (q.v.) in London, England. It was owned by Dr. George M. Burrows (q.v.) until 1843.
Bibliography: Parry-Jones, W. Ll. 1972. *The trade in lunacy.*

CLARE, JOHN (1793-1864). An English poet. His father was a laborer, and he himself worked as a farmhand and herdsman. At times he wandered the countryside with gypsies in search of casual work. Several of his poems were published between 1820 and 1835. In 1837 he became insane and was admitted to a private madhouse run by Dr. Matthew Allen (q.v.). He escaped in 1841, but his freedom was short-lived, and he was soon within the walls of the Northampton General Lunatic Asylum (q.v.), where he remained until his death. The verses he wrote while a mental patient were published after his death, as was an autobiography of his early years. He described himself as "a half mad melancholy dog"; in a vivid phrase he pointed to the aetiology of his condition, "homeless at home." His last poem, *I am! Yet what I am who cares, or knows?* is included in the *Oxford Book of Verse.*
Bibliography: Tibble, J. W., and Tibble, A. 1956. *Clare: his life and poetry.*

CLARKE, JACOB AUGUSTUS LOCKHART (1817-1880). An English neurologist. After qualifying in medicine, he entered general practice but still found time to conduct anatomical and histological investigations of the nervous system. He illustrated these with his own excellent drawings. The presence of the nucleus dorsalis (column of Clarke) was established by him. In 1869, after several honors had been bestowed on him for his scientific contributions, he dedicated himself completely to neurology (q.v.).
Bibliography: Haymaker, W. and Schiller, F. 1970. *The founders of neurology.* 2d. ed.

CLARKE, JEREMIAH (1673-1707). British composer and organist at St. Paul's Cathedral. He was the composer of the "Trumpet Voluntary," which was wrongly attributed to Henry Purcell (q.v.). As a rejected suitor, he became depressed and eventually committed suicide (q.v.) by shooting himself in the head in his house at St. Paul's Churchyard in London.
Bibliography: Scholes, P. A. 1967. *The Oxford companion to music.*

CLAUDIUS II (MARCUS AURELIUS CLAUDIUS) (A.D. 214-270). A Roman emperor. He was interested in the occult arts and under his reign people began to study and practice alchemy (q.v.). He was so obsessed (*see* OBSESSION) with abnormal phenomena that he erected a statue to a magician.

CLEANTHES (301-225 B.C.). Greek Stoic (*see* STOICISM) philosopher. He committed suicide (q.v.) by starving himself to death, thus proving that he could practice his school's precept of acceptance of pain.
Bibliography: Rosen, G. 1971. History in the study of suicide. *Psychol. Med.* 1: 267-85.

CLEOMENES I (c. 519-487 B.C.). Spartan king. According to Herodotus (q.v.), his behavior became increasingly peculiar after succeeding to the throne. He began, for example, striking Spartans in the face with his sceptre. Found unfit to reign, he was imprisoned with his feet in stocks. Ultimately he succeeded in borrowing a knife and committed suicide (q.v.) by multiple lacerations of his body. It was said that Cleomenes lost his reason as a consequence of drinking his wine neat. Herodotus advanced the theory that his madness was divine punishment for having deposed Demaratus, the previous king of Sparta.
Bibliography: Brothwell, D., and Sandison, A. T. 1967. *Diseases in antiquity.*

CLEOPATRA VII (69-30 B.C.). Queen of Egypt. She married her brother Ptolemy XII and ruled with him until he drove her out. On his death she married her younger brother Ptolemy XIII and allowed him to rule, while she became Julius Caesar's (q.v.) mistress. She eventually murdered him to advance her son by Caesar. After Caesar's death, Antony, captivated by her beauty, became her lover, and they had twin children. When Octavian came to power, she committed suicide (q.v.), possibly through poison or the bite of an asp. She was notorious for her greed, cruelty, and ruthlessness, as well as for intelligence and beauty.
Bibliography: Lindsay, J. 1971. *Cleopatra.*

CLÉRAMBAULT, GAÉTAN DE (1872-1934). A French psychiatrist. His approach was mainly organic, and his work included research on the symptomatology of delirium (q.v.) caused by ether (q.v.), chloral, or hashish (q.v.). He studied the causes and course of chronic hallucinatory (*see* HALLUCINATION) psychoses (*see* PSYCHOSIS) and described patients who believed that their minds were controlled by outside influences (now known as the Clérambault-Kadinsky complex). Erotomania (q.v.) was described by him. He committed suicide (q.v.).
Bibliography: Pelicier, Y. France. 1975. In *World History of Psychiatry*, ed. J. G. Howells.

CLEVENGER, SHOBAL VAIL (1843-1920). A neurologist born in Italy, but brought up and educated in the United States. He was the first to describe the *inferior temporal sulcus* of the cerebral hemisphere. He wrote on comparative physiology and psychology, spinal concussion, and the legal aspects of insanity.
Bibliography: Clevenger, S. V. 1903. *The evolution of man and his mind.*

CLEVER HANS (DER KLUGE HANS). The name of a horse trained by Von Osten in Germany in 1901. It was the first of several horses trained to carry out arithmetical operations of considerable complexity. The experiment provided material of great interest in the study of animal psychology (q.v.) and ethology.
Bibliography: Rosenthal, R., ed. 1965. *Clever Hans, the horse of Mr. Von Osten by Oskar Pfungst.*

CLIMATE. Climate was often blamed for insanity. Jean Esquirol (q.v.) thought that warm climates produced less insanity than cold ones. He regarded marshy districts as particularly bad, producing dementia and imbecility (*see* IMBECILE). Both Timothie Bright (q.v.) and Robert Burton (q.v.) had held similar beliefs earlier. As Bethlem Royal Hospital (q.v.) was located originally near a marshy area, the idea may have originated from associating its inmates with their surroundings.

CLITORIS. Surgical removal or cauterization (q.v.) of the clitoris was used in the nineteenth century as treatment for hysteria (q.v.).
Bibliography: Cesbron, H. 1909. *Histoire critique de l'hystérie.*

CLIVE, ROBERT, BARON CLIVE OF PLASSEY (1725-1774). English general, statesman, and founder of the British empire in India. When he was two and a half years old, he was sent to live with an aunt and uncle who so spoiled him during a serious illness that he completely dominated them and had to be bribed to allow them a little freedom. The entire town where he went to school pleaded with his headmaster to remove him because of his bad influence on other children. The tradesmen dreaded him; he once lay in the gutter in front of a shop and dammed the water until it flooded the premises. After the death of his aunt, he was moved to other schools and finally his father in despair sent him to India "to die of a fever for all it mattered." In India, he was so lonely and depressed that he unsuccessfully tried to shoot himself. Later, however, he found his vocation in the army. His turbulent but brilliant career as a soldier and a diplomat led to his virtual rule of Bengal and the founding of the British Indian Empire. He returned to England in 1767 and was met with a storm of abuse that ended in a parliamentary inquiry. His health was shattered, and he relapsed in the deep depression that had often shadowed his life. He turned to opium (q.v.) for relief but eventually reached the limit of endurance and committed suicide (q.v.).
Bibliography: Bence-Jones, M. 1974. *Clive of India.*

CLOETTA, MAX (1868-1940). A Swiss pharmacologist. Cloetta's mixture is a combination of drugs, usually administered per rectum, used in sleep treatment (q.v.).

CLOTEN. A character in William Shakespeare's (q.v.) play, *Cymbeline*. He is the best description of mental retardation in Shakespeare's plays. He is called an ass and a fool, and other characters express surprise that he is the son of an intelligent woman. Shakespeare made a clear distinction between mental retardation and insanity in his line: "Fools are not mad folks" (*Cymbeline*, 3. 3).

CLOUSTON, SIR THOMAS SMITH (1840-1915). A British psychiatrist and neurologist, born in Scotland. He was physician superintendent of Morningside, one of the royal asylums (q.v.) . He was the first to study juvenile general paralysis and to demonstrate its relationship to congenital syphilis (q.v.). In 1877 he reported a case of general paresis in a sixteen-year-old boy, and his findings were later confirmed by a postmortem on this patient. He also initiated a movement for better training of mental nurses. His book *Clinical Lectures on Mental Disease*, published in 1883, has remained a standard work for twenty-five years.
Bibliography: Clouston, T. S. 1883. *Clinical lectures on mental diseases.*

CLOVIS II (633-656). Merovingian king of the Franks. He was said to have been struck with madness as punishment for uncovering the body of Saint Denis.
Bibliography: Burton, R. 1621. Reprint. 1968. *The anatomy of melancholy.*

CLUB DES HASCHICHINS. A club existing in Paris in the nineteenth century. Its members, who were mostly eccentric men of letters, met at the Hôtel Pimodan, where they gathered round a table on which was a bowl containing a mixture of honey, pistachio nuts, and cannabis sativa (q.v.). Théophile Gautier (q.v.) and Charles Baudelaire (q.v.) were among its members.
Bibliography: Todd, J. 1968. Drug addiction and artistic genius. *Practitioner.* 201: 513-23.

CLYSTER. The injection of liquids per rectum. From antiquity and into the nineteenth century, it was considered the appropriate treatment for mental disorders; the aim was to wash out devils, black choler (q.v.), or physical impurities that were thought to cause insanity.
Bibliography: Esquirol, J. E. D. 1845. Reprint. 1965. *Mental Maladies: a treatise on insanity.*

CLYTEMNESTRA. A character in Greek drama. She murders her husband Agamemnon after taking his cousin Aegisthus for a lover. She is troubled

by ominous dreams, which are fulfilled as her son Orestes (q.v.), torn by loyalty to both parents, goes mad and kills her. In Homer's (q.v.) *Iliad* she is described as a weak woman, but she is more often represented as a forceful character tormented by pathological jealousy, fury, and grief. The Clytemnestra complex refers to a woman who destroys her husband to enjoy one of his male relatives.
Bibliography: Simon, B. 1978. *Mind and madness in ancient Greece.*

CNIDUS. One of the schools of medicine in ancient Greece. Such schools as Cnidus, Cos (q.v.) and Rhodes were based on temples of healing and often were located near medicinal springs. Each school gave particular emphasis to at least one aspect of medical practice. Cnidus was renowned for the importance it attached to diagnosis. The mentally ill were accepted for treatment on the same basis as patients suffering from physical disorders.
Bibliography: Phillips, E. D. 1973. *Greek medicine.*

COBHAM, ELEANOR (?-?1446). An English noblewoman. She married her lover, the Duke of Gloucester, after his first marriage had been annulled. In 1441 she was accused of practicing witchcraft (q.v.). It was said she had made a wax image of Henry VI (q.v.) and exposed it to the fire so that the king would likewise waste away. She was ordered to walk barefoot and dressed as a penitent through London for three days and then was imprisoned for the rest of her life.
Bibliography: Churchill, W. 1956. *A history of the English-speaking peoples,* vol. 2.

COCA. A South American shrub, also found in Java. The natives chew coca leaves in order to withstand extreme fatigue and hunger. Nicholas Monades (1493-1588), a Spanish physician, introduced it to Europe in 1569, and in the late nineteenth century an infusion of coca leaves was popularized in France as a stimulant. The drug cocaine (q.v.) is obtained from its leaves.
Bibliography: Morton, J. F. 1977. *Major medicinal plants.*

COCAINE. An alkaloid of coca (q.v.). It was isolated by Albert Niemann in 1859. Sigmund Freud (q.v.) was interested in its action as a local anaesthetic and suggested this possibility to his friends, Leopold Köningstein and Carl Koller (q.v.), who were ophthalmologists. Cocaine was first used as an anaesthetic by Carl Koller, who reported his findings to a medical congress in Heidelberg in 1884. Freud was unaware of the addictive qualities of cocaine. He used it himself with no ill effects and then employed it to treat the morphine withdrawal symptoms in his friend Ernst von Fleischl-Marxow (q.v.), who became a severe cocaine addict.
Bibliography: Morton, J. F. 1977. *Major medicinal plants.*

COCKATRICE. A legendary monster, also called basilisk (q.v.), popularly accepted as a fact until the seventeenth century. Pliny the Elder (q.v.) mentioned it in his natural history, *Historia Naturalis*. It was said to originate from a cock's egg hatched by a serpent and was supposed to have the power to kill by its glance. The superstitious belief in the evil eye (q.v.) is probably connected with it. Geoffrey Chaucer, Edmund Spenser, and William Shakespeare (qq.v.) are among those who mention it:

A cockatrice hast thou hatch'd to the world,
Whose unavoided eye is murderous.

[*Richard III*, 4. 1]

Bibliography: Borges, J.L. 1970. *Imaginary beings.*

COCKTON, HENRY (1807-1853). An English writer. In his novel *The Life and Adventures of Valentine Vox, the Ventriloquist*, published in 1840, he denounced the way in which private asylums (q.v.) were conducted and described the horrors endured by the patients. He argued that some had been declared insane wrongly and had been confined in madhouses by greedy relatives. He wrote that on the occasion of visits by the Commissioners in Lunacy (q.v.), patients were "goaded to madness" by being tickled with feathers while chained to their beds, thus they would appear raving and irrational at the time of inspection.
Bibliography: Parry-Jones, W.Ll. 1972. *The trade in lunacy.*

COCTEAU, JEAN (1889-1963). French poet, writer, and film director of great versatility. He was a leader of the avantgarde in the period between the two world wars. His psychological approach is most evident in *Les Enfants Terrible* (1929) and *Les Parents Terrible* (1938). He underwent treatment for addiction to opium (q.v.) and described his experiences in *Opium* (1930), a diary in which the pleasant time of intoxication is contrasted with the depression and miseries of treatment and withdrawal. He was reluctant to admit that opium was harmful and asserted that he owed to it his "most perfect hours."
Bibliography: Todd, J. 1968. Drug addiction and artistic genius. *Practitioner.* 201: 513-23.

CODEX THEODOSIANUS. A collection of constitutions issued by the emperor Theodosius II (401-450). In 429 the codex prohibited magic (q.v.) on the grounds that it was a bad practice. Magicians were regarded as criminals by the judicial authorities thus paving the way for the prosecution of witches (*see* WITCHCRAFT) and the so-called possessed (*see* POSSESSION).
Bibliography: Zilboorg, G. A. 1941. *A history of medical psychology.*

COGGESHALL. A locality in Essex, England, where the inhabitants were reputed to be extremely foolish. It is said that on one occasion they put

hurdles in the bed of a stream to divert it, and on another they chained a wheelbarrow in a shed fearing that it "would go mad" after a mad dog had bitten it. "A Coggeshall job" came to mean something silly.
Bibliography: 1978. *Brewer's dictionary of phrase and fable.*

COGHILL, GEORGE ELLETT (1872-1941). An American neuroanatomist. He conducted important research into the embryology of behavior, correlating the growth of the nervous system with changing patterns of behavior. He used salamanders as his subject of study and later experimented with opossums. His work led to modifications in the theory of development of behavior and encouraged fresh research in biology and psychology.
Bibliography: Herrick, C. J. 1949. *George Ellett Coghill: naturalist and philosopher.*

COITER, VOLCHER (1534-1600). An anatomist, born in Groningen, Netherlands. He studied under Gabriele Fallopie (1523-1562) in Padua, and Ulisse Aldrovandi (1522-1605) and Giulio Cesare Aranzio (1530-1589) in Bologna. His knowledge of the central nervous system was far superior to that of his contemporaries. He performed vivisections on dogs, goats, lambs, and birds, which he trephined to observe the pulsating brain. Through his work, he demonstrated that speech, respiration, sensation, and motion are maintained even after removal of substantial portions of the brain.
Bibliography: Herrlinger, R. 1952. *Volcher Coiter.*

COKE, SIR EDWARD (1552-1634). An English judge and writer of legal books. His work *Institutes of the Laws of England,* published between 1628 and 1644, contains passages concerning criminal responsibility. He wrote that the execution of a madman is "a miserable spectacle, both against the law and of extreme inhumanity and cruelty, and can be no example to others." He listed four classes of people whose responsibility for their acts should be considered in passing sentence: 1) idiots (q.v.), 2) those who have lost their memory (q.v.) and understanding because of sickness, grief, or other accident, 3) lunatics (q.v.), even if they have lucid intervals, and 4) those who are deprived of memory and understanding by their "own vicious acts," for example, drunkards. He regarded the last group as unworthy of legal privileges because their affliction was self-inflicted. He exempted the others from responsibility.
Bibliography: Tuke, D. H. 1892. *A dictionary of psychological medicine.*

COLBERT, JEAN BAPTISTE (1619-1683). A French statesman who served under Louis XIV. At Colbert's instigation the king abolished the death sentence for those found guilty of witchcraft (q.v.) and sorcery.
Bibliography: Zilboorg, G. 1941. *A history of medical psychology.*

COLBURN, ZERAH (1804-1840). American Methodist preacher and professor of languages. He was a child prodigy who was able to do complicated

calculations in a few seconds. While doing them, his body would twist into contortions. His father exhibited him in Britain and in France, but he lost his remarkable ability as he grew into adulthood and could never explain the mental process that brought the answers into his mind so rapidly.
Bibliography: Colburn, Z. 1883. Reprint. 1977. *A memoir of Zerah Colburn written by himself.*

COLD. Jean Esquirol (q.v.) believed that excess of cold could cause insanity. As an example he quoted the experiences of the French soldiers who were seized with what was called phrenetic delirium (q.v.) and mania (q.v.) during Napoleon's disastrous retreat from Russia in 1812. Cold was also held responsible for prolonged depressions.
Bibliography: Esquirol, J. E. D. 1845. Reprint. 1965. *Mental maladies: a treatise on insanity.*

COLDITZ CASTLE. A castle twenty miles southeast of Leipzig in Germany. It was a mental hospital before World War II, but during the war it was used as a prisoner of war camp. It became famous for its prisoners' escape attempts. It has now reverted to a mental hospital.
Bibliography: Reid, P. R. 1975. *Colditz story.*

COLERIDGE, SAMUEL TAYLOR (1772-1834). English poet and philosopher. He began to take laudanum (q.v.) at a very early age to assuage the pain of rheumatism; by the time he was in his thirties he was consuming enormous quantities of it daily. Thomas De Quincey (q.v.) thought that Coleridge's addiction stimulated his philosophical works but destroyed the poet in him. However, *Kubla Khan* (q.v.) one of his best poems, was written under the influence of opium (q.v.). In 1795 he married Sara Fricker, the sister-in-law of Robert Southey (q.v.). In 1808 he left her and his family to depend on the generosity of Southey and the small annuity given to him by Thomas Wedgwood (1771-1805). He went to stay with various friends, a habit he had long cultivated, and his dependence on opium increased. His feelings are described in *Fears of Solitude* and *Dejection* (1802) in which he described dejection as:

> A grief without a pang, void, dark and drear,
> A stifled, drowsy, unimpassion'd grief
> Which finds no natural outlet, no relief
> In word, or sigh, or tear.

Jean Martin Charcot (q.v.) adopted a saying of this sad poet as his favorite maxim: "the best inspirer of hope is the best physician."
Bibliography: Lafebure, M. 1974. *Samuel Taylor Coleridge—a bondage of opium.*

COLLEGIUM INSANORUM. A private asylum (q.v.) in St. Albans, Hertfordshire, England, also known simply as The College. It was opened

by Dr. Nathaniel Cotton (q.v.) around 1745, and one of his patients was William Cowper (q.v.). His charges were from three to five guineas per week. College Street in St. Albans is named after it.
Bibliography: Parry-Jones, W. Ll. 1972. *The trade in lunacy.*

COLLIER, JAMES STANFIELD (1870-1935). A British physician. His interest in neuropathology resulted in valuable clinical descriptions of many neurological conditions, including cerebral diplegia, epilepsy (q.v.), aphasia, agnosia, and intracranial aneurysm.
Bibliography: Haymaker, W., and Schiller, F. 1970. *The founders of neurology.* 2d. ed.

COLLIN, MICHEL (1905-1974). A French priest. He was ordained in 1933. Two years later he promoted himself to bishop and founded a sect called the Apostles of Infinite Love. His odd behavior led to his defrocking, but the Vatican's displeasure did not deter him from calling himself Pope Clement XV after a variety of hallucinatory (*see* HALLUCINATION) experiences.

COLLINS, WILLIAM (1721-1759). English poet, son of a Chichester hatter. He studied at Magdalene College, Oxford, and published verses while still a student. From Oxford he moved to London, where his poverty limited his activities until an uncle left him a large sum of money. He was a great planner but so irresolute that his projects seldom came to fruition. He is best remembered for his *Odes*, especially the longest of them, *Ode On the Popular Superstitions of the Highlands.* Samuel Johnson (q.v.) wrote of him in his *Lives of the Poets*: "He languished some years under that depression of mind which enchains the faculties without destroying them, and leaves reason the knowledge of right without the power of pursuing it."

Although Collins tried to fight his depression by drinking and by traveling abroad, he eventually had to be admitted to an asylum (q.v.); later, his sister cared for him until his death. Most references describe him as insane, but Johnson categorically stated: "His disorder was not alienation of mind, but general laxity and feebleness, a deficiency rather of his vital than intellectual powers."
Bibliography: Johnson, S. 1779. Reprint. 1967. *The Lives of the English Poets.*

COLLINS, WILLIAM WILKIE (1824-1889). An English novelist. He was addicted to opium (q.v.), and the plot of one of his novels, *The Moonstone* (1886), is woven around the effect of opium on the protagonist, who remembers nothing of his actions of the previous night once his intoxication is ended. Collins was a friend of Charles Dickens (q.v.), who probably relied on his advice as well as direct observation in describing the effects of opium in *The Mystery of Edwin Drood.*
Bibliography: Robinson, K. 1974. *Wilkie Collins: a biography.*

COLNEY HATCH ASYLUM. An asylum opened in London in 1851. It was built to accommodate over 1,000 patients and later was enlarged to handle twice as many. The medical staff expected to manage such a large establishment originally consisted of two alienists, who were expected to diagnose, classify, and treat all the patients. The admission records reflect the Victorian (q.v.) attitude toward deviations in behavior: "addiction to socialism" and "erroneous religious beliefs" were considered sufficient aetiological descriptions of insanity. An ex-sergeant of the Guards was kept busy drilling partially paralyzed patients, who were marched up and down to the sound of military music. In 1937 the asylum's name was changed to Friern Hospital.
Bibliography: Hunter, R., and Macalpine, I. 1974. *Psychiatry for the poor. 1851 Colney Hatch Asylum, Friern Hospital 1973.*

COLOMBIER, JEAN (1736-1789). A French physician. He was in charge of the Hôtel-Dieu (q.v.) in Paris and became one of the pioneers of French psychiatry. The king became interested in his ideas and ordered him to publish a report that would give instructions for those working with the mentally ill and regulations for the proper construction and management of asylums (q.v.). Colombier was appalled at the indifference of the public toward the insane and disturbed by the number of mentally ill people who had nowhere to go or, when institutionalized, received no treatment. He advocated segregating the patients according to the type and degree of their disorder and recommended that each patient should have a bed to himself, rather than four to a bed, as was then usual. Philippe Pinel (q.v.) read his report and was greatly impressed by it.
Bibliography: Semelaigne, R. 1930. *Les pioneers de la psychiatrie française.*

COLOMBO, MATTEO REALDO (1516?-?1559). An Italian physician, born in Cremona. He was a pupil of Andreas Vesalius (q.v.). His book *De Re Anatomica* (1558) included anatomy and the physiology of the brain, which he regarded as the seat and origin of all sensation, motion, and intellect. Colombo performed vivisections, but rather than using the commonly preferred dog, he used pigs. His work on the circulation of the blood was quoted by William Harvey (q.v.) and began the trend away from Galenism (*see* GALEN) toward scientific physiology.
Bibliography: Symposium. 1959. *The history and philosophy of the brain and its functions.*

COMATA. One of the four orders, under class two, neuroses, in William Cullen's (q.v.) classification.
Bibliography: Hunter, R. and Macalpine, I. 1963. *Three hundred years of psychiatry.*

COMBE, ANDREW (1797-1847). A Scottish physician. Despite continuous poor health, he became a surgeon. His interest in mental disorders was first aroused when he attended lectures by Johann Spurzheim (q.v.) and by Jean Esquirol (q.v.) in Paris. He was particularly impressed by phrenology (q.v.) and became a leader in its application to mental disorders. He stressed the importance of assessing individual differences before proceeding to treatment and his concepts initiated the development of systematic psychotherapy (q.v.). With his brother George (q.v.) he founded and edited the *Phrenological Journal* (q.v.) to which both contributed extensively. His two main works on phrenology were *Observations on Mental Derangement: Being an Application of the Principles of Phrenology to the Elucidation of the Causes, Symptoms, Nature and Treatment of Insanity* (1831) and *Outlines of Phrenology* (1838).
Bibliography: Goshen, C. E. 1967. *Documentary history of psychiatry.*

COMBE, GEORGE (1788-1858). A Scottish barrister, son of an Edinburgh brewer and brother of Andrew Combe (q.v.). He abandoned his legal career when he became an ardent believer in phrenology (q.v.) and a follower of Franz Gall (q.v.) and Johann Spurzheim (q.v.). He lectured on phrenology in the United States to spread the doctrine. In 1820, he founded the Phrenological Society. In 1823, in collaboration with his brother, he began the *Phrenological Journal* (q.v.). His reputation was such that in 1846 Prince Albert asked him to assess the phrenological development of the royal children. He wrote in defense of phrenology as well as on education and social ethics and admonished that the "moral and intellectual organs" should be strengthened by spiritual guidance and hygiene. He founded an annual lecture on psychology at Edinburgh University.
Bibliography: Combe, G. 1847. Reprint. 1970. *Constitution of man considered in relation to external objects.*

COMENIUS (or KOMENSKY), JOHN AMOS (1592-1670). A Czech educator and theologian. He could be considered the first educational psychologist. Religious and political unrest drove him to Poland, then to Sweden, and finally to Holland. His methods of teaching made him famous. He devised the first illustrated textbook for children, *Orbis Sensualium Pictus*. It was published in Latin in 1654 and translated into Hungarian four years later. He advocated a gradual education that would cover manners, diction, and general knowledge of the environment.
See also EDUCATIONAL PSYCHOLOGY.
Bibliography: Kanner, L. 1964. *A history of the care and study of the mentally ill.*

COMITALIS MORBUS. Another Latin term for epilepsy (q.v.), derived from *comitia*, Roman constitutional groups presided over by a magistrate.

It was customary to adjourn the meeting if someone suffered an epileptic attack.

Bibliography: Brothwell, D. and Sandison, A.T. 1967. *Diseases in antiquity.*

COMMERCIAL HOSPITAL AND LUNATIC ASYLUM. An American institution in Cincinnati, Ohio. The hospital itself was inaugurated in 1823, and the asylum (q.v.) opened in 1827. It acommodated 160 patients in a three-storey building. Treatment was nonexistent. Restraint (q.v.) was widely used, and the patients were kept in cells and prevented from communicating with each other. The basement was used as a poorhouse and an orphanage.

Bibliography: Ford, H. A. and Ford, K. B. 1881. *History of Cincinnati, Ohio.*

COMMISSIONERS IN LUNACY. A committee of fifteen people created by the secretary of state in England in 1845. They replaced the Metropolitan Commissioners in Lunacy created in 1828 who had replaced the five medical commissioners of the College of Physicians, who had been established in 1774. They were empowered to inspect madhouses and to refuse or to revoke licenses. They had jurisdiction over the whole of England and Wales, not just the area of metropolitan London.

See also INSPECTION OF MADHOUSES.

Bibliography: Hunter, R., and Macalpine, I. 1963. *Three hundred years of psychiatry.*

COMMIUS JODOCUS (c.1500-1564). A Dutch physician. He differentiated between delirium (q.v.) and phrenitis (q.v.), considering the first to be an acute general fever with mental symptoms and the second to be an inflammation of the brain or its membranes. He linked furor (q.v.) and melancholia (q.v.), but claimed the presence of rage distinguished furor from melancholia. According to him, melancholia flatuosa was a special form of melancholia resulting from affections of the spleen and liver.

Bibliography: Whitwell, J. R. 1936. *Historical notes on psychiatry.*

COMMODUS, LUCIUS AELIUS AURELIUS (A.D. 161-192). Roman emperor also known as Marcus Antonius. It is said that an attempt upon his life so disordered his brain that he became extremely cruel and extravagant. He demanded divine worship from his subjects, kept three hundred concubines and as many boys, offered human sacrifices to the gods, fought with wild beasts in the arena, and sent thousands to their deaths on the slightest pretext. One of his favorite amusements was to bleed men with a surgical lancet. A typical psychopath, he had no sense of shame and ordered that his most infamous actions should be included in the public records. Eventually his concubine Marcia and the prefect of the praetorian guard arranged his murder by poison and strangulation.

Bibliography: Hyslop, T. B. 1925. *The great abnormals.*

COMPARATIVE PSYCHOLOGY. George Romanes' (q.v.) work on animal behavior is responsible for the term and the systematization of this branch of psychology (q.v.). In 1876, Herbert Spencer (q.v.) entitled one of his essays *Comparative Psychology* and in 1889 a laboratory for this discipline was established in Paris at the Sorbonne. Systematic observation and experimentation made comparative studies of behavior more scientific, and in 1914 John Watson (q.v.) published a book entitled *Behavior: An Introduction to Comparative Psychology.*
Bibliography: Flugel, J. C. 1945. *A hundred years of psychology.*

COMPASS TEST. A test devised by Ernst Weber (q.v.) to determine at what distance two simultaneous touches on the skin are felt as two. Primitive people, women, and young children have a lower threshold for perceiving two touches with a smaller distance between them.
Bibliography: Flugel, J. C. 1945. *A hundred years of psychology.*

COMPENSATION NEUROSES. Certain neuroses (*see* NEUROSIS), which, according to a theory formulated by Alfred Adler (q.v.) in 1907, are a compensation for a feeling of social or physical inferiority. Overcompensation may result in aggression. In more recent times the expression also has been used to indicate emotional reactions that are dependent on financial compensation for injury.
See also INFERIORITY COMPLEX.
Bibliography: Adler, A. 1917. *Organ inferiority and its psychical compensation.*

COMPLETION TESTS. Psychological tests that require the completion of a story or a sentence. They were first devised by Hermann Ebbinghaus (q.v.) in 1897 for testing mental capacities in school children.
Bibliography: Rabin, A. J., and Haworth, M. R. 1960. *Projective techniques with children.*

COMPLEX. An unconscious or half-conscious cluster of thoughts that are emotionally tinged and in conflict with accepted ideas. The concept was first introduced by Carl G. Jung (q.v.).
Bibliography: Ellenberger, H. F. 1970. *The discovery of the unconscious.*

COMPLICATION FUSION. A term denoting two kinds of interaction between ideas: complication when ideas belong to different sense departments (for instance hearing and vision), fusion when they belong to the same sense departments. It was first used by Johan F. Herbart (q.v.).
Bibliography: Flugel, J. C. 1945. *A hundred years of psychology.*

COMPOS MENTIS. A Latin expression meaning "in full possession of mental faculties." The expression comes from Tacitus, *Annals*, II, 27.

COMTE, AUGUSTE (1798-1857). French philosopher and mathematician, founder of sociology, and the originator of the positivist philosophy. He coined the term *positivism* (q.v.), by which he meant that which is immediately observable, basic, and undebatable, as opposed to that which is speculative or inferential. He disputed the validity of introspection and tried to improve the human race by sociological ethics and a religion of humanity, whose patron saint was the woman he loved, Madam Clotilde de Vaux. He devised a classification of the sciences in which he gave psychology a special place. He was an arrogant and intolerant man, who believed that his friends should support him. Comte planned his books without notes and wrote the final versions of them completely from memory. In 1828 he suffered a mental breakdown and toward the end of his life became insane.
Bibliography: Marvin, F. S. 1965. *Comte, the founder of sociology.*

CONARIUM. A term in the philosophy of René Descartes (q.v.) referring to the point of contact between mind and body. Sigmund Freud (q.v.) called it the id (q.v.).
Bibliography: Hinsie, L. E. 1948. *Understable psychiatry.*

CONCILIATOR DIFFERENTIARUM. A work by Pietro d'Abano (q.v.), which was published posthumously in 1476. In it d'Abano asserted that mental disorders could be ameliorated by suggestion, if the therapist was a person of authority with a kindly disposition. He also advocated the explanation of dreams (q.v.), provided that the personality of the patient was taken into consideration.
Bibliography: Mora, G. 1975. Italy. In *World history of psychiatry*, ed. J. G. Howells.

CONDIE, DAVID FRANCIS (fl. 1844). A nineteenth-century American physician who practiced in Philadelphia. He was a pioneer in recognizing the importance of emotional influences on infants. In 1844, he wrote a treatise on the diseases of childhood and included a discussion on "moral treatment," or the correct psychological handling of young children. He warned parents against harshness and advised them to exercise great care in choosing a nurse for their children.
Bibliography: Condie, D. R. 1844. *A practical treatise on the diseases of childhood.*

CONDILLAC, ÉTIENNE BONNOT DE (1715-1780). French philosopher, ecclesiastic, and intellectual. He was a friend of Denis Diderot and Jean Rousseau (q.v.). His empiricism was based on the doctrine of sensationalism, which he derived from the philosophy of John Locke (q.v.), whose work was introduced to France by him. Condillac explained the mind as a mosaic of sensations that were accumulated by a mechanical process. According to him, knowledge, judgment, and volition were derived from elementary sensations. Working from this thesis, he claimed that a statue

endowed with a single sense could through experience acquire all the main intellectual capacities. His writings on philosophy, psychology, politics, history, and economics are noteworthy for their clarity, logical exposition, and elegance of style. His most important work is the *Traité des sensations*, published in 1754.
Bibliography: Boring, E. G. 1950. *A history of experimental psychology.*

CONDITIONALISM. A term introduced by Carl G. Jung (q.v.). He derived it from the physiologist and philosopher Max Verworn (1863-1921). Jung maintained that given certain conditions, certain dreams (q.v.) could occur and therefore conditionalism endeavored "to conceive strict causality by means of interplay of conditions, to enlarge the simple significance of the relations between effects."
Bibliography: Jung, C. G. 1938-1939. *Seminar on children's dreams.*

CONDITIONED REFLEX. A term first used by Ivan P. Pavlov (q.v.) to indicate a neural response acquired through a stimulus or a combination of stimuli.
Bibliography: Pavlov, I. P. 1928. *Lectures on conditioned reflexes*, trans. W. H. Gantt.

CONFESSIONS. The title of Jean Jacques Rousseau's (q.v.) biography. It is a candid work of self-revelation. Thoughts and incidents are honestly described, even when they are mean and discreditable. In the latter part of the *Confessions* Rousseau may have been influenced by his deep suspicion of people, but much of the hostility against him was real, and it was only natural that it should affect his life and thoughts.
Bibliography: Rousseau, J. J. 1970. *Confessions*, trans. J. M. Cohen.

CONFESSIONS OF AN ENGLISH OPIUM-EATER. A book by Thomas De Quincey (q.v.), first published in 1821 in the *London Magazine*. The work was largely autobiographical. De Quincey related how he began to take opium (q.v.) to relieve facial neuralgia and later became addicted to it, consuming large quantities of laudanum (q.v.), a tincture of opium. He wrote that opium "proved to be the sole agent equal to the task of tranquillising the miseries left behind by the youthful privations." He also described visions and fearful withdrawal symptoms, but the book ended with the hopeful if short-lived assumption that the addiction had been conquered.
Bibliography: De Quincey, T. 1822. Reprint. 1960. *Confessions of an English opium eater*, ed. J. E. Jordan.

CONFUCIUS (*or* **K'UNG FU-TZU**) (550 or 551-478 B.C.). A Chinese philosopher from an impoverished noble family. He was chiefly a teacher; his ethical principles embraced all aspects of family and social life on a

temporal level, rather than a supernatural religious level. His sayings greatly influenced the character of the Chinese people. The basic rule of his philosophy was, "Do not unto others what you would not wish done unto yourself." The Chinese tolerance toward the mentally afflicted is a direct reflection of Confucius' teachings, and his book on family sayings contained a reference to hospitals for the insane in China.
Bibliography: Smith, D. H. 1974. *Confucius.*

CONGRESS OF PSYCHOLOGY. The First International Congress of Psychology met in Paris, France, in 1889 under the presidency of Jean Martin Charcot (q.v.) and Theodule Ribot (q.v.). It was attended by 203 delegates from twenty countries. Since 1951 the international congresses of psychology have been organized by a body of psychologists known as the International Union of Scientific Psychology. This organization came into existence during the thirteenth congress in Stockholm, Sweden.
Bibliography: Misiak, H. and Sexton, V. S. 1966. *History of psychology.*

CONNECTICUT STATE HOSPITAL FOR THE INSANE. An American mental hospital opened near Middletown, Connecticut in 1868. Dr. A. M. Shew was its first superintendent. It originally housed one hundred patients, but their number soon increased to several thousands.
Bibliography: Deutsch, A. 1949. *The mentally ill in America.*

CONNOR, BERNARD (c. 1666-1698). An Irish physician, medical writer, and historian. In his *Evangelium Medici: Medicina Mystica,* which was published in London in 1697, he attacked miracles and those cures attributed to supernatural forces. In the same work he discussed wolf children (q.v.).
Bibliography: Molson, L. 1972. *Wolf children.*

CONOLLY, JOHN (1794-1866). An English psychiatrist, born at Market Rasen, Lincolnshire. His father, an Irishman, died when he was an infant, and his mother remarried. His stepfather, a Frenchman, taught him French and gave him an appreciation of French literature. After graduating from Edinburgh University, Conolly went to France and was influenced by Philippe Pinel's (q.v.) methods. He practiced in Sussex and at Stratford-upon-Avon. He became an enthusiastic supporter of Shakespearian activities and was twice elected mayor. In 1830, after four years as professor of medicine in London, he returned to general practice in Stratford. He became interested in phrenology (q.v.) and founded a phrenological society. In 1839, he went to Middlesex as resident physician to the Hanwell Asylum (q.v.). It was here that he was able to practice his projected reforms in the treatment of the mentally ill. He abolished mechanical restraint (q.v.) and began a vigorous movement for more humane treatment of the insane. His controversial philosophy had a great impact on American psychiatry (q.v.) and was a

contributing factor in the foundation of the American Psychiatric Association (q.v.) in 1844. Among Conolly's works are *An Inquiry Concerning the Indications of Insanity, with Suggestions for the Better Protection and Care of the Insane* (1830); *The Croonian Lectures* (1849); and *The Treatment of the Insane without the Use of Mechanical Restraints* (1856). He died of a stroke that occurred after he had spent a harrowing hour weeping on the coffin of his favorite granddaughter. Henry Maudsley (q.v.) was his son-in-law.
Bibliography: Hunter, R. and Macalpine, I. 1963. *Three hundred years of psychiatry.*

CONRAD, KLAUS (1905-1961). An Austrian psychiatrist and neurologist. His early training was undertaken under Julius Wagner von Jauregg (q.v.) and Otto Pötzl, and later he was influenced by the work of Henry Head (q.v.) and John Hughlings Jackson (q.v.). In order to study the hereditary and biological aspects of epilepsy (q.v.), he examined 253 sets of twins and published the results in a book entitled *The Constitutional Type as a Genetic Problem*, which was published in 1941. He was interested in the psychophysical organization of the mind and the pathological changes of the brain. Conrad suggested a new classification of psychoses (*see* PYSCHOSIS) based on gestalt (q.v.) principles. Most of his work was published in German.
Bibliography: Hirsch, S. R. and Shepherd, M., eds. 1974. *Themes and variations in European psychiatry.*

CONSCIENTIA. A Latin term employed by Cicero (q.v.) in discussing feelings of guilt and scruples.

CONSENSUS. A Galenic term literally meaning agreement. Galen (q.v.) thought that parts of the body may become disordered by direct affection or "consensus." For example, he considered mania (q.v.) and melancholia (q.v.) as disturbances of the animal spirits directly affecting the brain, but drunkenness affected the brain indirectly, i.e. by consensus, as the warm vapors had first disordered the heart and the liver.
Bibliography: Harkins, P. H., trans. 1963. *Galen: On the passions and errors of the soul.*

CONSTABLE, JOHN (1776-1837). An English painter, renowned for his serene landscapes. The skies in his paintings reflected his moods. After the death of his wife in 1828, he was bitter and troubled. His state of mind so worried his friends that one of them, John Fisher, wrote to him "Whatever you do, Constable, get thee rid of anxiety." In 1835, writing about his feelings and his painting of Stonehenge, he wrote: "Can it be wondered at that I paint continual storms?"
Bibliography: Leslie, C. R. 1951. *Memoirs of the life of John Constable.*

CONSTANCE. The mother of Arthur, the king's nephew, in William Shakespeare's play *King John*. The death of her son greatly disturbs her, and she is accused of being mad. In a remarkable passage Shakespeare had her make a clear distinction between madness and emotional disorder. She claims that she is sane because she is aware of her own identity, is sensitive to emotional hurt, and retains her memory (q.v.) and reason. She ends her speech by stressing that she lacks the cardinal symptom of insanity, the inability to feel:

I am not mad; too well, too well I feel the different plague of each calamity.

[*King John*, 3. 4.]

CONSTANTINE THE AFRICAN (c. 1020-1087). He was a Jew, born in Carthage and converted to Christianity. He traveled to Babylonia, India, Ethiopia, and Egypt, learning the medical sciences of the countries he visited. In search of peace and tranquility, he became a monk at Monte Cassino and spent the remainder of his life translating medical works from Arabic into Latin. These translations made important medical texts available in the West. Among his works is *Liber Melancholiae*, a manuscript of which is preserved in Westminister Abbey in London. Constantine distinguished three kinds of soul: a soul that gives life and is common to all living things, a feeling soul that is found in men and animals, and a rational soul that is unique to human beings. He believed that melancholia (q.v.) is caused by the fumes of black choler (q.v.) rising to the brain and resulting in confusion of thought and insanity. His writings greatly influenced medical practice in the Western world.
Bibliography: Talbot, C. H. 1967. *Medicine in mediaeval England.*

CONSTANTINOPLE. A timarahane, or house of correction, for the insane was founded in Constantinople in the sixteenth century. It was named Suleimanie Asylum (q.v.).
Bibliography: Whitwell, J. R. 1936. *Historical notes on psychiatry.*

CONSTIPATION. From antiquity until the nineteenth century difficulty in evacuating bowels was often regarded as one of the causes of insanity and drastic remedies were employed to combat it. Voltaire (q.v.) claimed that constipation caused depression and that the determinations of the great were often influenced by it.
See also CLYSTERS and PURGING.

Bibliography: Esquirol, J. E. D. 1845. Reprint. 1965. *Mental maladies: a treatise on insanity.*

CONSTRUCTION, ORGANIZATION AND GENERAL ARRANGEMENTS OF HOSPITALS FOR THE INSANE, ON THE. A famous book by Thomas S. Kirkbride (q.v.), published in the United States in 1854. In it the author elaborated on the construction and design principles for hospitals for the insane he had drawn up for the Association of Medical Superintendents. He believed that asylums (q.v.) should be located in the country, constructed with wings round a central administrative block, be easily accessible with pleasant and extensive grounds, house no more than 250 patients with separate wards for different classes of patients, and enjoy proper drainage, ventilation, and heating. The volume became the standard textbook on mental hospital construction in America, and its rules were strenuously defended against modifications. Eventually the Kirkbride plan capitulated to the demand for larger hospitals and changing social needs.
Bibliography: Deutsch, A. 1949. *The mentally ill in America.*

CONTAGION OF THE IMAGINATION. A term used in the seventeenth century by Sir Kenelm Digby (q.v.). It indicated what is now known as *folie à deux* (q.v.). He used as an example a gentlewoman who was so depressed following her husband's death that her behavior became odd, and she was believed to be possessed (*see* POSSESSION) by evil spirits. Her hysteria (q.v.) was transmitted to her young attendants, who were cured by being isolated from her. The lady, however, recovered only after the black humors (q.v.) had been purged (*see* PURGING) away.
Bibliography: Hunter, R., and Macalpine, I. 1963. *Three hundred years of psychiatry.*

CONTINUOUS WORK. The study of continuous work, such as in adding, was pioneered by Emil Kraepelin (q.v.). He devised special forms to record experiments involving adding. His adding sheets have become part of the accepted equipment in psychological laboratories (q.v.).
Bibliography: Flugel, J. C. 1945. *A hundred years of psychology.*

COOLIDGE, EMELYN LINCOLN. An American pediatrician. He was the first to use the term "hospitalism" (q.v.) as a description of apathy and lack of response to treatment observed in infants hospitalized for long periods. He advised mothering by nurses to bring about recovery.
Bibliography: Coolidge, E. L. 1909. Care of infants who must be separated from their mothers because of some especial need on the part of the child. *Papers and discussions of the American Academy of Medicine Conference on Prevention of Infant Mortality.*

COOPER, THOMAS (1759-1839). English natural philosopher, lawyer, and physician. In 1794 his democratic ideas caused him to leave England

and to settle in the United States. He became professor of chemistry in various colleges and wrote manuals of American law, as well as an encyclopedia of sciences. He was influential in establishing the first medical school and the first hospital for the insane in South Carolina.
Bibliography: Cooper, T. ed. 1836-39. *Statutes at large of South Carolina.*

COOVER, JOHN EDGAR (1872-1938). An American psychologist who worked in the field of psychical research. He devised various experiments to demonstrate how correct guesses could be made of apparently inaudible words and how written letters could be guessed even when they were placed far enough away from the subject to be indistinguishable from small dots. He contributed to various works on psychical research.
Bibliography: Flugel, J.C. 1945. *A hundred years of psychology.*

COPHO. A twelfth-century anatomist of the Salerno Medical School (q.v.). He wrote one of the first treatises on anatomy but based his descriptions on the dissection of pigs.
Bibliography: Zilboorg, G. 1941. *A history of medical psychology.*

CORAL. A remedy for asthma and affections of the brain in the seventeenth century and earlier. Robert Burton (q.v.) in his *Anatomy of Melancholy* (q.v.) quoted Liéven Lemnius (q.v.) when he attributed to coral and carbuncle the ability to "drive away childish fears, devils, overcome sorrow, and hung about the neck repress troublesome dreams." Paracelsus (q.v.) recommended it against melancholy (*see* MELANCHOLIA). It is still used in India in the hospital of the state of Hyderabad, which follows the Moslem system of medicine, *Unani,* and employs powdered gems, dried fruit, and indigenous spices in the treatment of various disorders. *See also* PRECIOUS STONES.

CORDELIA. The youngest daughter of Lear, king of Britain. Holinshed's *Chronicles of England, Scotland, and Ireland* (1577) records that she inherited the kingdom after his death but lost it to her nephews, who then took her prisoner. The humiliation of her situation affected her mind and she committed suicide (q.v.).

CORNELIAN. A hard, reddish quartz. The *Dispensatory* of Renodaeus, first published in 1608, attributed the power of resting the mind, assuaging anxiety, and preventing nightmares (q.v.) to the cornelian.
Bibliography: Evans, J. 1922. *Magical jewels.*

CORNELIUS, HANS (1863-1947). A German philosopher. His empirical theories contributed to the psychology of perception. He wrote on the doctrine of form-quality (*Gestaltqualität*), which he regarded as an attribute resulting from an analytic process of attention, rather than a founded content.
Bibliography: Boring, E.G. 1950. *A history of experimental psychology.*

CORNELIUS RUFUS. A Roman of the first century A.D. He wanted to commit suicide (q.v.) but waited throughout the reign of Domitian (q.v.) because he did not wish to die under a tyrant. He nurtured his death wish through the years and once Domitian was dead, Cornelius Rufus killed himself.
Bibliography: Fedden, H.R. 1938. *Suicide*.

CORNELL INDEX TEST. A questionnaire that hoped to reveal psychopathic (*see* PSYCHOPATHY) traits and disorders with psychosomatic aetiology. It was devised by the American psychologist Ethel Letitia Cornell (1892-).

CORPUS JURIS CIVILIS. The main body of Roman law, codified in the reign of Justinian (483-565). It provided specific legal norms concerning the mentally ill. Besides defining the criminal responsibility of the mentally ill, it considered their ability to testify, to make a will, to marry and divorce, and to dispose of their goods. It also took under consideration the influence of drunkenness or strong emotions on criminal behavior.
Bibliography: Jolowicz, H. F. 1972. *Historical instruction to the study of Roman law*.

CORVO, BARON (1860-1913). The assumed name of Frederick William Rolfe, English writer, painter, and schoolmaster. He became a convert to the Roman Catholic faith and wished to become a priest. Denied this, he built up an elaborate fictitious life. It was a form of wish-fulfilment in which he was the central character, arrogant, self-important, and ungrateful. His best work, *Hadrian the Seventh*, is a projection of his own hopes and disappointments. His bitterness and paranoia (q.v.) are reflected in the venomous letters he wrote, the unfortunate recipients of them being addressed with such abuse as "Quite cretinous creature." He died in Venice in the manner in which he lived: lonely and poor. His pockets were found stuffed with compromising notes capable of starting innumerable scandals.
Bibliography: Benkovitz, M. J. 1971. *Frederick Rolfe: Baron Corvo*.

COS. An island in the Aegean sea, the location of one of the Greek schools of medicine; two more were located at Cnidus (q.v.) and Rhodes. The school at Cos gave great importance to prognosis. Hippocrates (q.v.) was trained at Cos.
Bibliography: Zilboorg, G. 1941. *A history of medical psychology*.

COSIN, RICHARD (1549?-1597). An English lawyer. Within the realms of forensic psychiatry, he recognized such mental disorders as: furor (q.v.),

madness; dementia, distracted of wit; insania, foolishness; fatuitas and stultitia (q.v.), idiocy and near-idiocy; lethargie, forgetfulness; and delirium (q.v.), dotage. He considered those suffering from furor or dementia to be legally irresponsible because they were "utterly ignorant of anything done by themselves, or in their presence." The others were considered only partially insane and therefore responsible for their actions. He wrote an account of the trial of William Hacket (q.v.).
Bibliography: Hunter, R., and Macalpine, I. 1963. *Three hundred years of psychiatry.*

COSMAS AND DAMIAN, SAINTS. Arab Christian physicians. They were twin brothers who were martyred by Diocletian (245-313) in A.D. 303. When crucifixion, stoning, and other means miraculously failed to kill them, they were decapitated. The Emperor Justinian (483-565) had a church built in Constantinople in their honor. Those who were sick in body and mind slept in the church and were said to be cured by the saintly brothers, who appeared to them in dreams (q.v.). The apparitions suggested prescriptions or cured illness during sleep in imitation of earlier practices of incubation (q.v.).
Bibliography: Pollak, K. 1968. *The healers: the doctor, then and now.*

COSTA BEN LUCA (864-923). A Christian from Baalbek in Syria. In his writing on the difference between soul and spirit he adhered to the theory of ventricular localization of the functions of the mind. Thus, he introduced a basically Christian idea to classic Arab writers.
Bibliography: 1959. *Symposium: the history and philosophy of the brain and its functions.*

COTARD, JULES (1840-1887). A French neurologist. His name has been given to the psychiatric syndrome first described by him in which the patient denies many or all propositions. Hence the Cotard syndrome is also called the "insanity of negation."
Bibliography: Enoch, M.D. and Trethowan, W.H. 1979. *Uncommon psychiatric syndromes.*

COTON HILL. A small mental hospital at Stafford, England. It is an example of the type of independent institution that emerged in England in the nineteenth century. It was a charitable, nonprofit-making concern that catered to private paying patients and a small number of patients who could not afford payment. The legislation of the time required these hospitals to be registered, thus insuring their conformity to reasonable standards.
Bibliography: Parry-Jones, W.Ll. 1972. *The trade in lunacy.*

COTROBUM. A term cited by Avicenna (q.v.) and used by Arab physicians to denote lycanthropy (q.v.). It referred to a small insect, a water spider or

fly, that hovered on the surface of water, rushing about seemingly without any aim.
Bibliography: Whitwell, J. R. 1936. *Historical notes on psychiatry.*

COTTA (*or* COTTEY), JOHN (1575?-?1650). An English physician who practiced at Northampton. He was interested in the relationship between witchraft (q.v.) and clinical disorders and published two books on the subject, *A Short Discoverie of Unobserved Dangers of Several Sorts of Ignorant and Unconsiderate Practisers of Physicke in England* (1612) and *Triall of Witchcraft* (1616). He believed in witches but felt that too much emphasis was given to so-called devil's marks and trials by water.
Bibliography: Stephen, L., and Lee, S. eds. 1900. *The dictionary of national biography.*

COTTAGE SYSTEM. An old form of care for the mentally ill, whereby patients are housed in the community rather than a hospital. The Gheel colony (q.v.) in Belgium, an example of this method, is over 900 years old. After a period when massive state hospitals were popular toward the end of the nineteenth century the cottage system was revived, and examples of it were to be found both in Europe and in the United States, for instance at Kankakee (q.v.), Illinois.
See also BOARDING-OUT OF MENTAL PATIENTS and FAMILY CARE.
Bibliography: Zilboorg, G. 1941. *A history of medical psychology.*

COTTON, NATHANIEL (1705-1788). English physician and poet. He owned a private asylum (q.v.) in St. Albans, Hertfordshire, England, called the Collegium Insanorum (q.v.) or simply, The College. The patients were treated with kindness and enjoyed a personal relationship with their physician. The poet William Cowper (q.v.) was a patient there for two and a half years; he and Cotton enjoyed each other's company and discussed "things of the spirit." Cotton did not write specifically about mental disorders, but he did alert others to the state of depression that often follows acute fevers and infections.
Bibliography: Hunter, R., and Macalpine, I. 1963. *Three hundred years of psychiatry.*

COTUGNO, DOMENICO (1736-1822). An Italian physician who studied and practiced in Naples. He described the cerebrospinal fluid, the way in which it surrounds the brain, its circulation, and its pathological states. He loved libraries and was deeply interested in art, classical literature, and music; these interests were reflected in his clinical writings, as, for example, when he wrote, "The cochlea is our harpsichord." He is regarded as one of the founders of neurology (q.v.).
Bibliography: Haymaker, W., and Schiller, F. 1970. *The founders of neurology.* 2d. ed.

COUÉ, ÉMILE (1857-1926). A French physician and pharmacist. He became interested in hypnotism (q.v.) and studied under Hippolyte-Marie

Bernheim (q.v.) and Ambroise-August Liébeault (q.v.). In 1910 he founded a free clinic in Nancy, where he practiced psychotherapy (q.v.) according to his own methods of hypnosis and suggestion. He claimed that organic changes could be brought about by suggestion and that diseased organs could be healed by the power of imagination. Autosuggestion (q.v.) was the basis of his technique, and he is said to have used the term first in 1922. He is remembered for his saying, "Every day and in every way I am becoming better and better," which became a formula not only for the sick but also for the gay set of those days and the source of many newspaper cartoons.

Bibliography: Coué, E. 1922. *Self mastery by conscious autosuggestion.*

COUNCIL OF BRAGA. In A.D. 563 the Christian church condemned suicide (q.v.). It was the first official action taken against suicide by the church. Its condemnation was confirmed by the councils of Auxerre in A.D.578 and Antisidor in A.D.590. The Synod of Nimes in A.D. 1284 prohibited burial in consecrated ground to suicides, but usually the prohibition was ignored if the individual was insane or suffering from emotional disorders at the time of his death.

Bibliography: Rosen, G. 1971. History in the Study of Suicide. *Psychol. Med.* 1: 267-85.

COUNCIL OF NICAEA. An assembly of theologians that crystallized Christian dogma in A.D. 325. Its attitude influenced medieval psychology (q.v.) because it retained some of the Platonic (*see* PLATO) philosophy of primary ideas and subjectivism.

Bibliography: Zilboorg, G. 1941. *A history of medical psychology.*

COUNTER-REFORMATION. A reform movement within the Catholic church in the sixteenth century after the establishment of Protestantism. Religious zealots were determined to exterminate heretics. Some mentally ill people were regarded as possessed (*see* POSSESSION) by the devil, subjected to the most appalling tortures, and often condemned to death by burning in an effort to save their souls by destroying their bodies. The *Malleus Maleficarum* (q.v.) replaced medical textbooks. Theologians and monks took over a field that belonged to the physicians.

Bibliography: Zilboorg, G. 1941. *A history of medical psychology.*

COUNTY ASYLUMS. Small institutions for the insane poor in England. Provision was made for their establishment following an act of Parliament in 1808. They provided up to 300 beds each and at first were controlled by a lay master.

See also ASYLUMS, and INSANE POOR, LEGISLATION IN ENGLAND.

Bibliography: Hunter, R., and Macalpine, I. 1963. *Three hundred years of psychiatry.*

COUVADE. An ancient custom, found mostly among primitive peoples. In the couvade the father takes to bed after the birth of his child. It more commonly refers to sympathy pains and discomforts experienced by some men during pregnancy of their wives. The phenomenon has been observed and commented upon by many writers. Francis Bacon (q.v.) wrote in his *Sylva Sylvarum: or a Naturall Historie* (1627): "There is an opinion abroad (whether idle, or no I cannot say) That loving and kinde Husbands have a sense of their Wives breeding Childe by some accident in their own Body." James Primrose, an English physician writing in 1638, attributed such disorders to "simpathy, antipathy, contagion, fascination, and other such trifles. . ." Contemporary psychiatry recognizes the couvade as a syndrome.
Bibliography: Trethowan, W. H. 1972. The Couvade Syndrome. In *Modern perspectives in psycho-obstetrics*, ed. J. G. Howells.

COWLEY, ABRAHAM (1618-1667). An English poet and dramatist. He wrote his first of many epic works at the age of ten. As a Royalist he was involved in diplomatic work, which he abandoned when he began the study of medicine at Oxford. As well as writing on philosophy, he wrote commentaries and essays on contemporary life; in his *Several Discourse* (1668) he described the events of visiting day in an asylum, Bethlem Royal Hospital (q.v.).
Bibliography: O'Donoghue, E. G. 1914. *The story of Bethlehem Hospital.*

COW PARSNIP. A wild herb. John Gerard (q.v.) in his *Herball* (1597) wrote of this herb: "If a phrenticke or melancholicke man's head bee anointed with oile wherein the leaves and roots have been sodden, it helpeth him very much, and such as bee troubled with the sickness called the forgetfull evile."
Bibliography: Rohde, E. S. 1974. *The old English herbals.*

COWPER, WILLIAM (1731-1800). An English poet. His childhood was a sad one: his mother died before he was six years old; of seven children born to her only two survived infancy. He was bullied and tormented at school and this so affected him that he became depressed and began to experience delusions (q.v.). In his loneliness he wrote verses "To keep the silence at bay and cage / His pacing manias in a worldly smile." His first serious attack of depression leading to suicidal thoughts occurred in 1753, but in the following year he was well enough to practice as a barrister in the Middle Temple in London and to contemplate marrying his cousin Theodora Cowper, but her father forbade the marriage because of Cowper's poor health. Cowper then became intensely religious. In 1763 he was offered a clerical post in the House of Lords. He became so anxious over the examination required for the position that he "began to look upon madness as the only chance remaining"; he wished for it and "looked forward to it with impatient expectation," fearing only that he would not become mad in time to avoid the dreaded examination. He made three suicide attempts by taking laudanum (q.v.), by throwing himself into the Thames, and finally by trying to hang himself with his scarlet garters. They broke, and he reported his intense guilt, "I led myself down, howling with horror. . ." Following this episode he was placed in the care of Dr. Nathaniel Cotton (q.v.) at his private asylum (q.v.), the Collegium Insanorum (q.v.). Cowper remained there for two and a half years. On his discharge he lived with the Reverend Morley Unwin, a zealous evangelist, and his wife Mary. He continued to live with her after her husband's death and in 1773 planned to marry her, but again he became hallucinated (*see* HALLUCINATION), suicidal, and convinced that he was damned in the eyes of God. He improved and continued to write poetry and hymns but in 1787 he again became insane and never recovered. His most revealing poem is *The Castaway*, but his state of mind is made painfully clear also in one of his hymns (Hymn IX):

> I hear, but seem to hear in vain,
> Insensible as steel;
> If aught is felt, 'tis only pain,
> To find I cannot feel.

Bibliography: Ryskamp, C. 1959. *William Cowper of the Inner Temple, Esq.*

COWSLIPS. A wild herb. Its flowers were used to make a decoction for the treatment of nervous disabilities, especially chorea and other convulsive disorders. John Gerard (q.v.) quotes a London practitioner "famous for curing the phrensie" as a firm believer in its virtues.
Bibliography: Law, D. 1969. *Herb growing for health*.

COX, JOSEPH MASON (1762-1822). An English physician. He was the first medical man to study and qualify with the aim of practicing psychiatry. His thesis, "De Mania," discussed insanity (*see* INSANIA). In 1788, he assumed control of Fishponds Private Lunatic Asylum (q.v.), which his grandfather had originally established in Stapleton. He believed that insanity and severe physical illness could not occur simultaneously in a person and that a considerable "commotion" in the system would bring about a cure. Hence, among the methods used in his establishment was a swing that caused violent vomiting, vertigo, collapse and, often, loss of consciousness. Some patients were kept in a state of intoxication for several days, and others were deliberately subjected to measures designed to produce physical symptoms. He believed that an excess of blood in the brain was the cause of most mental disorders and wrote that no remedy had any power when paralysis super-

vened—a reference to his observations of general paralysis of the insane (q.v.). Cox learned through direct observation, and this is reflected in his work *Practical Observations on Insanity*, which was published in London in 1804.
Bibliography: Hunter, R., and Macalpine, I. 1963. *Three hundred years of psychiatry.*

COZENS, JOHN ROBERT (1752-1797). English landscape painter of watercolors. His father, Alexander Cozens, was reputed to be a son of Peter the Great of Russia (q.v.). In 1794 he was afflicted by a serious mental disorder and was admitted to an asylum (q.v.) in Smithfield that was managed by Dr. John Monro (q.v.). He remained there until his death.
Bibliography: Osborne, H. 1970. *The Oxford companion to art.*

CRABBE, GEORGE (1754-1832). English poet, surgeon, and clergyman, born in Aldeburgh, Suffolk. His father was an alcoholic (*see* ALCOHOLISM), and the family was frequently destitute. His first published poem was entitled *Inebriety* (1775), and his subsequent works reflect the horrors and appalling hardship of a rural life of poverty. He taught himself botany, pharmacy, and surgery, which he practiced in his native town, before he obtained a succession of positions in the Church. He neglected most of them, preferring to put his efforts into writing. He suffered from bouts of vertigo, possibly Ménière syndrome, for which he was prescribed opium (q.v.). He used it for the last forty years of his life with no apparent ill effects; in fact, his son and biographer attributed his long and healthy life to it. Among his best known works are *The Village* (1783): *The Parish Register* (1807), on which Benjamin Britten's (1913-) opera *Peter Grimes* is based; and *Tales of the Hall* (1819).
Bibliography: New, P. 1976. *George Crabbe's poetry.*

CRAMER, AUGUST (1860-1912). A Swiss psychiatrist, professor of psychiatry at Göttingen in Germany. He founded the Rasemühle sanatorium for nervous diseases and an institution for mentally ill children. Cramer studied the mechanism of hallucinations (q.v.) and believed that compulsive neurotic (*see* NEUROSIS) acts and compulsive talking were disturbances of the muscle sense; he called the syndrome "muscle-sense hallucination of the locomotor apparatus." Cramer was a pioneer of modern mental institutions. Among his works are *Die Halluzinationen in Muskelsinn bein Geisteskranken* (1889) and *Handbuch der Nervenkrankheiten im Kindesalter* (1912).

CRAMP RINGS. Rings made of silver taken from the coffins of the wealthy; sometimes the rings were made of coffin nails or even of pieces of umbilical cord. They were believed to cure epilepsy (q.v.), cramp, rheumatism, and kindred ills. They were linked with the legendary ring of Edward the Confessor (q.v.) who gave his ring to Saint John, when the saint appeared to

him disguised as a beggar. Copper rings and bracelets are still to be seen today: power of suggestion endows them with curative powers.
Bibliography: Radford, E., and Radford, M. 1961. *Encyclopaedia of superstitions.*

CRANIOLOGY. A movement that arose toward the end of the nineteenth century. It claimed to have established a method whereby mental traits could be localized and disorders diagnosed by an examination of the external conformation of the skull.
Bibliography: Flugel, J. C. 1945. *A hundred years of psychology.*

CRANIOTOMY. *See* TREPANATION.

CREATIONISTS. A term applied to early theologians who insisted that God created a new soul every time a child was born. Traducionists believed that the soul was transmitted from parent to child.
Bibliography: Zilboorg, G. 1941. *A history of medical psychology.*

CREECH, THOMAS (1659-1700). English poet and translator of Latin classics. Voltaire (q.v.) claimed that he had written in the margin of his 1682 translation of Lucretius, "N.B. I must remember to hang myself when I have finished my commentary." He postponed the event for another twenty years despite recurring depression. The jury investigating his death brought in a verdict of insanity.
Bibliography: Fedden, Henry R. 1938. *Suicide.*

CRETINISM. A condition of low intelligence associated with goitre. It was common in certain parts of the world, such as the Andes of South America, the Himalayas, and some Pyrenean and Alpine Valleys of Europe. For centuries the physical appearance of the cretin gave rise to many superstitions. He was regarded as particularly favored by the gods in his innocence or as an object of amusement. The Romans, who recognized the condition, bought and kept cretins as curiosities. Felix Plater (q.v.) and Paracelsus (q.v.) described cretinism and established diagnostic criteria. Presently the term is employed to cover a form of mental retardation due to a lack of secretion of the thyroid gland.
Bibliography: Kanner, L. 1964. *A history of the care and study of the mentally retarded.*

CRETIN SKULLS. As early as 1790 a detailed description of cretin (*see* CRETINISM) skulls was given by J. F. Ackermann in his book *Uber die Kretinen, eine besondere Menschenabart in den Alpen* (1790).
Bibliography: Kanner, L. 1964. *A history of the care and study of the mentally retarded.*

CRICHTON, SIR ALEXANDER (1763-1856). An English psychiatrist, pupil of William Cullen (q.v.). He studied medicine in several European

universities and practiced surgery in London before he became a licentiate of the College of Physicians. He was appointed physician to the Westminster Hospital in London in 1795. In 1798 he wrote an important work on psychiatry (q.v.) entitled *An Inquiry into the Nature and Origin of Mental Derangement*. It was the second treatise on psychiatry to be written by a physician to a London teaching hospital (the first was a treatise by Timothie Bright [q.v.]). Crichton introduced several original ideas and a new psychopathological (*see* PSYCHOPATHOLOGY) system; his case histories were mainly borrowed from German authors. He believed that passions affect the nerves through the blood vessels; thus, when vascular activity in the nervous system was inhibited, melancholia (q.v.) resulted. He asserted that the physician must understand his own mind in order to understand his patients'. He was the first physician to write on the legal aspects of mental disorders, citing examples of homicides and suicides (q.v.) taken from German medical literature. He also presented a new understanding of aphasia. He was perhaps the only British psychiatrist who personally had met Philippe Pinel (q.v.). In 1804 he became physician to Czar Alexander I and chief of the Russian medical services. George IV knighted him in 1821.
Bibliography: Leigh, D. 1961. *The historical development of British psychiatry.*

CRICHTON, JAMES (1765-1823). A Scottish physician, born in Sanquhar. After qualifying at the University of Edinburgh, he joined the East India Company and eventually was appointed physician to the governor-general of India. He amassed a considerable fortune by engaging in commerce in India and China. He returned to Scotland and married Elizabeth Grierson. Because they had no children, when he died he left her his fortune with the proviso that she should use some money for a charitable enterprise. She accordingly founded and endowed the Crichton Royal Hospital (q.v.). A church, on cathedral lines, opened in 1897, was erected to the memory of James and Elizabeth Crichton.
Bibliography: Henderson, D. K. 1964. *The evolution of psychiatry in Scotland.*

CRICHTON-BROWNE, SIR JAMES (1840-1938). British psychiatrist, son of William A.F. Browne (q.v.), who added Crichton to his name in honor of the Crichton Royal Hospital (q.v.). He was only nineteen years old when he wrote *The Psychical Diseases of Early Life* (1859). When he was twenty-six years old, he became medical superintendent of the Wakefield Asylum (q.v.). During his tenure there, he established the first neuropathological laboratory and initiated systematic research in mental diseases as part of the hospital's work. In 1871 he founded and edited *West Riding Lunatic Asylum Medical Reports*, which were annual reports that gave statistics, presented unusual cases and described the day to day life of the hospital. He was an author, an orator of wit, and the founder and coeditor of *Brain* (q.v.). He was the lord chancellor's visitor in lunacy from 1875 to

1922; he became a Fellow of the Royal Society (q.v.) in 1883 and was knighted in 1866.
Bibliography: Henderson, D. K. 1964. *The evolution of psychiatry in Scotland.*

CRICHTON ROYAL HOSPITAL. A mental hospital in Dumfries, Scotland. Elizabeth Grieison Crichton used the fortune left to her by her husband, James Crichton (q.v.), to build and endow a lunatic asylum (q.v.) on the outskirts of Dumfries. She intended it to be the best in Europe. It was completed in 1838, and the first patient was admitted in June 1839. Elizabeth Crichton had read *What Asylums Were, Are and Ought to Be* by William A. F. Browne (q.v.) and was so impressed that she appointed him as the first resident medical officer. The institution was all she wanted it to be, and the press described it as "surpassing everything that has yet been established in Europe."
See also ROYAL ASYLUMS.
Bibliography: Henderson, D. K. 1964. *The evolution of psychiatry in Scotland.*

CRITIAS (?-403 B.C.). A Greek orator and politician. He was a pupil of Socrates (q.v.), and Plato (q.v.) introduced him in one of his dialogues. Critias believed that blood was the soul because he believed that sense perception depended on the blood.
Bibliography: Sahakian, W. S. 1968. *History of psychology.*

CROCODILE. The ancient Mayas macerated testicles of crocodiles and mixed them in cold water to make a potion against epilepsy (q.v.).
Bibliography: Von Hagen, V. W. 1970. *El mundo de los Mayas.*

CROOKE, HELKIAH (1576-1635). An English physician, born in Suffolk. He studied medicine at Cambridge and Leyden. He was physician to James I (q.v.) to whom he dedicated his book on anatomy *Mikrokosmographica* in 1616. In 1631 he dedicated the second edition of his book to Charles I (q.v.). In 1619 he was elected "keeper" of Bethlem Royal Hospital (q.v.) and became the first medical man to occupy this position. He petitioned the king for a ruling that Bethlem should be administratively independent of Bridewell (q.v.), saying that Bethlem had not prospered since the union had occurred in 1557. He was a bad and unscrupulous administrator and the governors investigated his affairs in 1625. It seems that he only rarely went to the hospital, which he neglected to the point when Charles I had to investigate the scandal. Crooke, who was dismissed in 1634, was the last of the "keepers" of the hospital. He was one of the first physicians to offer board and treatment to patients in his own home.
Bibliography: O'Donoghue, E. G. 1914. *The story of Bethlehem Hospital.*

CROOKS, WILLIAM (1852-1921). A British politician, Member of Parliament and first Labour mayor of London. At the age of eight he was sent

to the workhouse and later to the Poor Law School of Sutton, Surrey. These experiences influenced the rest of his life and caused him to take a special interest in underprivileged children. He advocated organizing separate courts to deal with young offenders.
Bibliography: Ayers, G. M. 1971. *England's first state hospitals and the Metropolitan Asylum Board.*

CROOKSHANK, FRANCIS GRAHAM (1873-1933). A British physician. He was the author of several medical works, including some in the field of psychological and psychosomatic medicine (q.v.). In 1924, his book *The Mongol in Our Midst* aroused a great deal of public interest and publicity. Crookshank suggested that mongolism (q.v.), now termed Down's syndrome, was an atavistic regression. This idea appealed to the general public, and the work went through three editions.
Bibliography: Crookshank, F. G. 1924. *The Mongol in our midst.*

CROQUE-MITAINE. A fantasy figure, an ogre, or a monster, used by French nurses to frighten children. It is an example of harmful psychological suggestion to induce fear and submission.

CROSSROADS. Suicides (q.v.) and felons were often buried at crossroads to ensure that their spirits would be confused and unable to return to haunt the living. Witches (*see* WITCHCRAFT) and demons were believed to meet at crossroads.
Bibliography: Cooper, J. C. 1978. *An illustrated encyclopaedia of traditional symbols.*

CROUZON, OCTAVE (1874-1912). A French neurologist. He undertook research on hereditary nervous disorders and described craniofacial dysostosis, now known as Crouzon's disease.
Bibliography: Jablonski, S. 1969. *Eponomic syndromes and diseases and their synonyms.*

CROWE, CATHERINE (*née* STEVENS) (1800?-1876). An English writer of an extremely morbid disposition. She was highly neurotic (*see* NEUROSIS), and for a brief period of her life she was believed to be insane. Her best-known work was a collection of stories of the supernatural, entitled *Night-Side of Nature* (1848).
Bibliography: Crowe, C. 1848. *Night-side of nature.*

CROWTHER, BRYAN (1789-1815). A British surgeon, appointed to Bridewell (q.v.) and Bethlem Royal Hospital (q.v.). He was the author of the first book on insanity to be written by a Bethlem surgeon. In it he based his observations on numerous dissections of mental patients' brains, discussed the treatment of the insane, including bleeding (q.v.), and asserted his belief that the insane were not protected from physical illness, thus opposing the theory put forward by Joseph Cox (q.v.). The select committee of the House of Commons, inquiring into the affairs of the hospital in 1815, discovered from the evidence of John Haslam (q.v.), that Crowther had been an alcoholic (*see* ALCOHOLISM), who often had to be restrained with a straitjacket. Haslam suggested that Crowther actually was insane.

Bibliography: Crowther, B. 1811. *Practical remarks on insanity; to which is added a commentary on the dissection of the brains of maniacs; with some account of diseases incident to the insane.*

CRUCHET, JEAN RENÉ (1875-1959). A French physician and neurologist. In April 1917 he was the first to describe epidemic or lethargic encephalitis; a few days later, Constantin von Economo (q.v.) described it in more detail. Cruchet also was interested in neurotic phenomena and in 1951 wrote a book entitled *Le Syndrome Hysterique.*

Bibliography: Schmidt, J. E. 1959. *Medical discoveries: who and when.*

CRUDEN, ALEXANDER (1701-1770). A Scottish bookseller, best remembered for his meticulous and exacting *Complete Concordance to the Holy Scriptures*, published in 1737. He suffered periods of mental derangement from an early age. He had a paranoid (*see* PARANOIA) personality and grandiose ideas. He firmly believed that God had chosen him to reform the nation. His mental state necessitated admission to private asylums (q.v.) on more than one occasion. He described his experiences in these institutions in *The London-Citizen Exceedingly Injured* (1739) and *The Adventures of Alexander the Corrector* (1754). He claimed that he had been wrongly declared mad and had been tricked into confinement in a madhouse.

Bibliography: Oliver, E. 1934. *The eccentric life of Alexander Cruden.*

CRUVEILHIER, JEAN (1791-1874). A French pathologist. He compiled a famous anatomical atlas, which included original illustrations of brain lesions. He was probably the first to describe intracranial epidermoid and disseminated sclerosis.

Bibliography: Haymaker, W., and Schiller, F. 1970. *The founders of neurology.*

CRYSTAL. Transparent quartz or very clear and transparent glass. Ibnu'l Baitar (?-1248), an Arab botanist and herbalist who wrote on the medical virtues of gems, claimed that crystal preserved its wearer from the terrors of the night. *See also* PRECIOUS STONES.

Bibliography: Evans, J. 1922. *Magical jewels.*

CUCKOO. John of Gaddesden (q.v.) in his treatise *Rosa Medicinae*, first printed in Pavia in 1492, recommended the head of a cuckoo hung round the neck to ward off epilepsy (q.v.), because the cuckoo, it was said, also suffered from the complaint.

Bibliography: Whitwell, J. R. 1936. *Historical notes on psychiatry.*

CUEVA VALLEJO, AGUSTIN (1820-1873). A Latin American psychiatrist who pioneered many clinical innovations in Equador. He derived his humanitarian views from the doctrines of Philippe Pinel (q.v.) and Jean Esquirol (q.v.). The school of medicine in Cuenca, Equador, was founded by him.
Bibliography: Leon, C. A., and Rosselli, H. 1975. Latin America. In *World history of psychiatry*, ed. J. G. Howells.

CULLEN, WILLIAM (1710-1790). British physician, founder of the Glasgow Medical School in Scotland. His lectures on physiology at the University of Edinburgh were given in the vernacular instead of Latin, a popular innovation. He evolved a system of classification of diseases based on symptoms, methods of diagnosis, and treatment. His classification of mental diseases was the most comprehensive then attempted and later became the basis of Philippe Pinel's (q.v.) system of nosology. Cullen introduced a physiologic concept of insanity. In his classification, mental diseases came under the class of neuroses (*see* NEUROSIS, a term he introduced) which he defined as disturbed nervous functions due to a deterioration of the intellect or of the voluntary or involuntary nervous system. It could occur without fever or localized pathology. Neuroses were subdivided into four orders: comata (q.v.), adynamias (q.v.), spasms, and vesanias (q.v.) . His treatment was based on the same measures then employed in physiological disorders: diet, purging (q.v.), bleeding (q.v.), vomiting, cold baths, and blistering. But, he also used "moral treatment" for the vapors (q.v.), or low spirits, which he linked with hypochondriasis (q.v.) and dyspepsia. His work greatly influenced the theory and practice of psychiatry in England and in the United States. Benjamin Rush (q.v.), introduced to him by Benjamin Franklin (q.v.), studied under him.
Bibliography: Leigh, D. 1961. *The historical development of British psychiatry.*

CULPEPER, NICHOLAS (1615-1654). English physician, botanist, and astrologer (*see* ASTROLOGY), born in London. In 1649 he translated into English the Latin pharmacopoeia of the College of Physicians of London, of which he was not a member, thus incurring the wrath of the profession. He wrote several popular tracts that combined astrology and herbal remedies in the treatment of physical and mental disorders and translated many Latin medical texts into English for the benefit of lay people. His collection of recipes proved extremely popular and has been reprinted for over 300 years under the title of *Culpeper's Complete Herbal*.
Bibliography: Rohde, E. S. 1974. *The old English herbals.*

CULPIN, MILLAIS (1874-1952). A British surgeon and psychologist. His studies on industrial medical psychology focused attention on the fact that

certain forms of work are particularly trying to unstable people. Following his theories, some occupational diseases have been shown to have a neurotic (*see* NEUROSIS) basis. Among his books are *Psychoneuroses of Peace and War, The Nervous Patient,* and *Medicine and the Man.*
Bibliography: Flugel, J. C. 1945. *A hundred years of psychology.*

CUNNING FOLK. Practitioners of magic (q.v.) in sixteenth-century England. They were highly skilled in the art of suggestion. They were consulted for help in counteracting or preventing the effects of witchcraft (q.v.). Their advice was sought also for help in resolving difficult personal situations, recovering lost property, restoring health, and making important decisions. Some cunning folk attained a high reputation, and the best of them dealt daily with a large number of clients from everywhere in the country. They were seldom persecuted for their deceptions unless their interests clashed with those of the clergy, the medical profession, or other professional groups.
Bibliography: Macfarlane, A. 1970. *Witchcraft in Tudor and Stuart England.*

CURABILITY. Toward the end of the nineteenth century there was a tendency to divide mental diseases into curable and incurable. Emil Kraepelin (q.v.) distinguished between mental disorders that were caused by external conditions and therefore curable and those that were constitutional and therefore incurable. The theory of curability brought an element of predetermination into the assessment of mental disorders and treated curability or incurability as if they were symptoms of different clinical entities.
Bibliography: Zilboorg, G. 1941. *A history of medical psychology.*

CURABILITY OF INSANITY, THE. The title of a book containing the reports of Pliny Earle (q.v.), published in 1887. The author of the book severely criticized the validity of certain hospital statistics on the number of cures in mental hospitals. The book was the result of years of research on American institutions for the insane, and, despite the original antagonism it aroused, it proved a formidable weapon in the destruction of many fallacies. It greatly contributed to the improvement in the methods used in reporting institutional statistics, and it was an influential factor in the establishment of separate hospitals for incurable patients.
Bibliography: Zilboorg, G. 1941. *A history of medical psychology.*

CURANDERISMO. A system of folk medicine of Mexican people. It has its own classification of illnesses, reflecting the cultural pattern. *Curanderos* are folk healers who base their paternalistic treatment on native insight, religion, and culture. They employ elaborate rituals, herbal remedies, and suggestion. *Curanderos* are highly regarded as their healing power is believed to be a divine gift.
Bibliography: Kiev, A. 1968. *Curanderismo: Mexican-American folk psychiatry.*

CURARE. The name given to a group of poisons extracted from plants in South and Central America. The Indians of these regions used it to make their arrows more deadly. It contains several alkaloids that cause muscular paralysis leading to death through respiratory failure. A derivative of curare, d-tubacurarine, is used in experimental research on the reduction of anxiety under aversive stimuli and in studies of feedback and emotion.
Bibliography: Thomas, K. B. 1964. *Curare: its history and usage.*

CUREAU DE LA CHAMBRE, MARIN (1594-1669). French physician to Louis XIV and writer. He believed that animals could reason. He was a student of physiognomy, which he regarded as basic to the understanding of man. He wrote numerous scientific works, including several on the passions, on the function of the soul, on despair, on hate, and on suffering.
Bibliography: Cureau de la Chambre, M. 1640. *Charactères des passions.*

CURLEW RIVER. An opera by the British composer Benjamin Britten (1913-) first produced in 1964. The libretto by William Plomer is an adaptation of an early fifteenth-century miracle play that deals with a demented mother's search for her lost son, kidnapped across the Curlew River. Her sanity is restored when he appears to her in a vision after she has found his grave. In folklore the curlew is associated with evil omens, and in Scotland the bird is connected with ghosts.
Bibliography: 1976. *Kobbe's complete opera Book.*

CURLING, THOMAS BLIZARD (1811-1888). An English surgeon. He may have been the first to give an accurate clinical description of cretinism (q.v.) when, in 1850, he linked thyroid deficiency with "symmetric swelling of fat tissue at the sides of the neck connected with defective cerebral development."
Bibliography: Garrison, F. H. 1929. *An introduction to the history of medicine.*

CURSES. Verbal formulae expressing the wish that evil will befall the person to whom they are directed. Their emotional character contains a strong element of fear that by suggestion often produces the desired results. Both Romans and Greeks had terrifying public curses aimed at enemies, traitors, and offenders against the state. Many examples of curses can be found in history and literature: the curse of Egyptian pharoahs has often been given as the cause of misadventure befalling archeologists; William Shakespeare (q.v.) put a curse on whoever would dare disturb his grave; Rigoletto (q.v.) was terrified by the curse put on him by a noble courtier.

CURZON, GEORGE NATHANIEL (MARQUIS CURZON OF KENDLESTON) (1859-1925). English statesman, viceroy of India, and foreign

secretary. His despotism and attitude of rebellion were frequently criticized. These traits in his character were no doubt the result of the harsh discipline imposed on him as a child by his governess. She devised especially cruel forms of punishment, and he never forgot the pain and humiliation he suffered in his early years. He took his revenge on his masters at Eton with wild acts of insubordination and impertinence, which he continued at Oxford.
Bibliography: Edwardes, M. 1965. *High noon of empire: India under Curzon.*

CUSHING, HARVEY (1869-1939). American surgeon and neurologist, educated at Yale University and Harvard Medical School. His approach to neurophysiology was particularly influenced by Sir Charles Sherrington (q.v.) under whom he worked during a period spent in England. Under Cushing's leadership, neurosurgery became an independent specialty. In addition to medical books, he wrote a literary work, *Life of Sir William Osler*, for which he received the Pulitzer prize in 1926. On his death, his collection of rare historical medical books became the property of the Yale School of Medicine.
Bibliography: Fulton, J. F. 1964. *Harvey Cushing: a biography.*

CUTTER, NEHEMIAH (1787-1859). An American psychiatrist, one of the thirteen founders of the American Psychiatric Association (q.v.). He practiced in Pepperell, Massachusetts, and treated mental patients in his home with such success that new wings had to be built onto his house to accommodate more patients. Eventually their numbers increased to the point where a large hospital had to be built; this was the Pepperell Private Asylum (q.v.), a successful institution despite the prejudice against private mental hospitals. It was burned down in 1853 and not rebuilt, despite Cutter continuing in his career.
Bibliography: Deutsch, A. 1949. *The mentally ill in America.*

CUVIER, G. L. C. F. D. BARON (1769-1832). A French naturalist and holder of numerous governmental positions. He asserted a theory based on the fixity of species. He claimed that the form of an animal could be reconstructed from a single bone and that the relationships between the parts of each animal reflected its adaptation to the environment. His studies earned him the title of founder of comparative anatomy. He was also chairman of a committee appointed to investigate the concepts of phrenology (q.v.) developed by Franz Gall (q.v.).
Bibliography: Boring, E. G. 1950. *A history of experimental psychology.*

CYBERNETICS. The study of communication and control mechanisms common to machines and living organisms. It was established as a science by Norbert Wiener (1894-1964) in his book *Cybernetics* published in 1948. The field of cybernetics has pointed to the similarity between the human nervous system and electronic machines.

Bibliography: Wiener, N. 1965. *Cybernetics: or control and communication in the animal and the machine.* Rev. ed.

CYCLOPHRENIA. A term coined by the Rumanian psychiatrist Alexandru Obregia (q.v.) to indicate periodical manic-depressive psychoses (q.v.).
Bibliography: Predescu, V., and Christodorescu, D. 1975. Rumania. In *World history of psychiatry.* ed. J. G. Howells.

CYCLOTHYMIA. A term introduced by Karl Kahlbaum (q.v.) in his description of cyclic insanity (*see* INSANIA) to indicate a disorder in which the mood of the patient alternates from periods of elation to periods of depression.
Bibliography: Kahlbaum, K. L. 1882. Über zyklisches Irresein. *Irrenfreund,* 10.

CYNANTHROPY. A form of insanity in which the patient believes himself to be a dog.
See also LYCANTHROPY.
Bibliography: Esquirol, J. E. D. 1845. Reprint. 1965. *Mental Maladies: a treatise on insanity.*

CYNICS. Followers of the Greek philosopher Diogenes (412?-323 B.C.), who in turn was influenced by the thinking of his contemporary, Antisthenes. The Cynics preached simplicity, independence, and renunciation of all possessions. Later, from the same doctrine sprang beggar philosophers who wandered all over Greece teaching, preaching, and opposing conventional ways of life. Their philosophy laid the foundation for the development of schools of thought concerned with man, his behavior, and his relationships with other men and his environment.
Bibliography: Dudley, D. R. 1938. *A history of cynicism.*

CYPRESS. A tree associated with sadness and often found in cemeteries. In Giuseppe Verdi's (1813-1901) opera *Ernani,* the dejected hero sings "Viene il mirto a cangiarmi col cipresso" [he comes to change my myrtle with cypress]. Christ's cross was said to have been fashioned from the cypress.
Bibliography: Cooper, J. C. 1978. *An illustrated encyclopaedia of traditional symbols.*

CYPRIAN, SAINT (c.300). Born in Antioch and often confused with Saint Cyprian, bishop of Carthage. According to a fourth-century legend translated from the Greek, he was a famous sorcerer, who could call up evil spirits to help him. When his love potion for a maiden called Justina failed because she was under the protection of the Virgin Mary, he became melancholic (*see* MELANCHOLIA) and called upon the devil for help. The devil told him that he could not help him as the God of the Christians was all powerful. Cyprian became a convert, married Justina, and both were martyred. He is the patron saint of folk healers, especially in Latin America where chapels dedicated to him are often found near their houses.

Bibliography: Dobkin, M. 1969. Folk Curing with a Psychedelic Cactus in the North Coast of Peru. *Int. J. Soc. Psychiat.* 15: 1, 23-32.

CYRENAIC SCHOOL. A Greek school of philosophy founded in 466 B.C. by Aristippus (c.435-c.356 B.C.). Its main tenet was based on the belief that pleasure is the chief end of life; it stressed the importance of sensations. The school engaged in studies of problems relating to human relationships, rather than in studies of abstract discussions of man's place in the universe.
Bibliography: Giannantoni, G. 1958. *I Cirenaici.*

D

DADAISM. An artistic movement resulting from the shock of World War I, and deriving its name from the French term, *dada*, meaning hobbyhorse. It was nihilistic, destructive, and meaningless. It wished to scandalize people and promote anarchy in artistic thought. Its chief exponents were Tristan Tzara (1896-1963), Hans Arp (1887-1966), Marcel Duchamp (1887-1968), André Breton (q.v.), Guillaume Apollinaire (1880-1918), and Max Ernst (1891-1976). The Dadaists were mostly young artists with pacifist views who expressed, often with calculated absurdities, their contempt for the ineffectual establishment that had failed to prevent the war and the mass slaughter of men. The movement began in Zürich, Switzerland, around 1916, spread to most of the large European cities, and burned itself out by 1922. In the United States there was a similar, but independent, movement that had begun in 1913. It merged with the European Dadaism in 1918.
Bibliography: Moverwell, R., ed. 1951. *The Dada painters and poets: an anthology.*

DADD, RICHARD (1817-1886). An English painter, born at Chatham. From adolescence he showed artistic promise, talent, and imagination. When he was twenty-five years old, he accompanied Sir Thomas Phillips (1792-1872) on a tour of the Middle East. His abnormal behavior, then attributed to prolonged exposure to the sun, dates from this tour. Dadd killed his father while under the influence of the so-called fiends that he imagined persecuted him. He escaped to France, but there he was arrested while attempting to kill a man and was committed to an asylum at Clermont. He was returned to England and detained in the Criminal Lunatic Department of the Bethlem Royal Hospital (q.v.), where he was diagnosed as schizophrenic (*see* SCHIZOPHRENIA). He remained there for twenty years. A search of his lodgings after his admission to Bethlem revealed many sketches of his friends. Each sketch illustrated a friend with his throat cut. Also found there were enormous quantities of eggs and ale, the two substances on which he

had lived. He continued painting in the hospital, and his work displays a tendency to overdetail, which is common in psychotic (*see* PYCHOSIS) patients. His canvases are to be found at the Tate Gallery, the Victoria and Albert Museum, and the British Museum. In 1864, Dadd was transferred to Broadmoor (q.v.), where he died of consumption eighteen months later. Two of his brothers and a sister were also insane.
Bibliography: Allderidge, P. 1974. *The late Richard Dadd.*

DAEMONOLOGIE IN FORME OF A DIALOGUE. A book written in 1597 by James I of England and VI of Scotland (q.v.). It was a refutation of *Discoverie of Witchcraft* (q.v.) by Reginald Scot (q.v.) and reflected the anxiety of the period that supernatural phenomena might be mistaken for natural diseases. The book was reprinted in 1603, when James became king of England. In spite of its retrograde views, it brought about a more careful examination of those accused of witchcraft (q.v.) and, possibly for the first time, caused medical evidence to be introduced in trials involving criminal charges.
Bibliography: Hunter, R., and Macalpine, I. 1963. *Three hundred years of psychiatry.*

DAGONET, SIR. King Arthur's fool (q.v.). According to Malory's (d. 1471) *Le Morte d'Arthur* he was knighted by King Arthur.
Bibliography: 1978. *Brewer's dictionary of phrase and fable.*

DAIUNJI. The third daughter of the Japanese emperor Gosanjō, who reigned from 1068 to 1072. When she was eighteen years old, she became extremely melancholy (*see* MELANCHOLIA). Her father spent many days in prayer asking the divinities for advice and was finally inspired to send her to the sacred spring of the temple at Iwakura, near Kyoto. There she drank the holy water and was soon well. Her recovery made the temple so famous that it became a place of pilgrimage for the mentally ill in Japan.
See also IWAKURA HOSPITAL.
Bibliography: Greenland, C. 1963. Family Care of Mental Patients. *Am. J. Psychiat.* 119: 1000.

DALE, SIR HENRY HALLETT (1875-1968). An English physiologist, one of the most influential workers in his field. His discovery of the chemical transmission of nerve impulses was closely allied to his studies of allergy. He was president of the Royal Society (q.v.) from 1940 to 1945, chairman of the Wellcome Trust, and in 1936 received a Nobel Prize with Otto Loewi (q.v.).
Bibliography: Dale, H. 1953. *Adventures in physiology.*

DALI, SALVADOR (1904-   ). A Spanish painter born in Figueras, Spain. He spoke frequently about his personal history and emotional life, which

he described in his autobiography *The Secret Life of Salvador Dalí* (1942). His childhood was characterized by great loneliness and an attempt to fill the void left by his dead brother of the same name. His school experience was unhappy, and his behavior later became attention-seeking and extravagant. He was expelled from the Madrid School of Art. An early association with the little girl Galoutchka influenced his relationship with women and ultimately led to his marriage to Gala, who was the predominant beneficial influence on his adult life. Until his later great canvases, his paintings were dominated by unresolved influences from his childhood. They display turbulence in his attitude toward his father and other people. Aggression, mutilation, and putrefaction are recurring themes. He craved attention both in his paintings and in his behavior. In the middle period of his paintings a number of fetishes (q.v.) recur, for example, insects, rhino horns, crutches, oyster shells, William Tell, and Jean Millet's (1814-1875) *Angelus*. In his later paintings the recurring theme is Gala, and there is rarely a painting without her in some guise or other. Sigmund Freud (q.v.) met Salvador Dalí in 1938, when Dalí was introduced to him by Stefan Zweig (q.v.).
Bibliography: Cowles, F. 1959. *The case of Salvador Dalí.*

DALTON, JOHN (1766-1844). An English physicist. In 1798 he described a red-green color blindness (Daltonism) from which both he and his brother suffered.
Bibliography: Eysenck, H. J. 1972. *Encyclopaedia of psychology.*

DAMEROW, HEINRICH PHILIPP AUGUST (1798-1866). A German psychiatrist. He was fond of traveling and the experience he gathered during visits to foreign mental institutions led to his appointment as an official visitor of mental hospitals in Germany and adviser to the government on psychiatric matters. In 1844, he founded the Nietleben Mental Hospital. He wrote widely in support of the doctrines of psychosomatic medicine (q.v.) and devised a classification of mental disorders that is still used.
Bibliography: Hunter, R., and Macalpine, I. 1963. *Three hundred years of psychiatry.*

DAMIENS, ROBERT FRANÇOIS (1715-1750). A French fanatic. He is an example of someone wrongly accused of criminal insanity. He wanted to warn Louis XV (q.v.) of France to improve his relationship with the French people and chose to do this by slightly wounding the king. He was captured, and the whole of France was encouraged to suggest his punishment. He was horribly tortured with hot irons, boiling oil, and molten lead; his hand was burned off, his tongue torn out, and his body wrenched apart by four horses. The whole procedure was used as a source of entertainment for the court.
Bibliography: Deutsch, A. 1949. *The mentally ill in America.*

DANA, CHARLES LOOMIS (1852-1935). American physician and professor of psychiatry. He was the author of *Textbook of Nervous Diseases*

and Psychiatry (1892) and a number of books linking poetry and medicine. He also wrote a biography of the Seguins of New York, a family of physicians that contributed to science and education.
Bibliography: Dana, C. L. "The Seguins of New York." *Annals of Medical History*, 1924, no. 6, p. 475.

DANCING. In Biblical times dancing, as well as music, was used to produce a frenzy that would lead to a trance during which prophecies, judgments, or messages of special significance were uttered. In primitive societies, dancing is still employed by holy men and native doctors to reach trance states in treatment. It also is employed as a part of the milieu therapies of contemporary mental hospitals.
Bibliography: Sorrell, W. 1967. *The dance through the ages.*

DANCING MANIA. Also termed chorea demonomania (q.v.) or choromania (q.v.). The impulse to dance often was uncontrollable and spread to onlookers through suggestion. Religious fanaticism was also responsible for it. Epidemics of dancing mania occurred in various European cities between the eleventh and the fifteenth century—Bernberg in 1029, Erfurt in 1237, Utrecht in 1278, Aix-la-Chapelle in 1374, Strasbourg in 1418, and Apulia in 1430. It was also called Saint Vitus dance (q.v.) for the procession of dancing patients who went from Strasbourg to the shrine of St. Vitus in Zabern in 1418.
Bibliography: Hecker, J. F. K. 1846. *The epidemics of the Middle Ages*, trans. B. G. Babington.

DANDY, WALTER EDWARD (1886-1946). An American neurosurgeon. In 1918, he introduced diagnostic ventriculography and pneumoencephalography. He devised numerous surgical techniques for the removal of brain tumors and other pathological conditions of the brain.
Bibliography: Haymaker, W., and Schiller, F. 1970. *The founders of neurology.* 2d. ed.

DANTE ALIGHIERI (1265-1321). A great Italian poet whose writings turned the Tuscan dialect into the Italian language. In 1300 he was elected prior of Florence for the guild of physicians and apothecaries, yet it cannot be proved that he was a physician. He may have studied medicine at Bologna and Padua. His writings frequently have clinical observations in them, and they show a deep concern for psychological matters. He may have attended Pietro d'Abano's (q.v.) lectures for his work shows signs of d'Abano's

influence. Dante's philosophy, derived from Aristotle (q.v.), left a permanent mark on Italian thought. His principal works are: *La Vita Nuova* (c. 1292); *Il Convivio* (1304); and *Divina Commedia* (c.1307). *The Divine Comedy* describes a symbolic journey through hell, purgatory, and paradise. He relegated to hell the people he did not like. Jean Martin Charcot (q.v.) often quoted Dante. Giovanni Boccaccio (q.v.) wrote a *Life of Dante*, but even so Dante's life remains obscure.
Bibliography: Giuffre, L. 1925. *Dante e le scienze mediche.*

DAQUIN, JOSEPH (1733-1815). A French psychiatrist. He became director of the department of mental disorders in the hospital of Chambery, and introduced many important humanitarian reforms there. He believed that the insane could be adequately observed only in a hospital and that only from a close study of each patient could a correct diagnosis be made and a plan of treatment evolved. He did not regard mental hospitals as having a purely custodial function. Daquin approached the problem of mental illness with humility and compassion; he wrote, "he who sees a madman without being touched by his state, and who looks at him only to be amused, is a moral monster." Philippe Pinel (q.v.) was his close friend, and Daquin dedicated to him the second edition of his book *Philosophie de la Folie* (q.v.), which outlined the theoretical foundations of the reforms that Pinel practiced. Despite his advanced ideas, Daquin still believed that the moon (q.v.) exercised some influence on mental disorders.
Bibliography: Nyffeler, S. 1961. *Joseph Daquin.*

DARENTH INSTITUTION. An institution in Kent, England, opened in 1878 by the Asylums Board to accommodate mentally subnormal children. It had classrooms and facilities for training 560 children from the ages of five to sixteen. Later, a separate institution accommodating 1,000 adolescents was built beside it to avoid sending the adolescents to adult hospitals. Darenth was the first state institution organized specifically for developing the potentialities of subnormal children. Unfortunately, overcrowding at other asylums meant that Darenth often had to accept hopeless cases. Nevertheless the work of the institution proved to be worthwhile, for its results were encouraging and eventually led to better state facilities for subnormal children. In 1904, an industrial colony was added to it, and the more advanced children were taught a variety of occupations, including engineering, farming, and the production of clothes and domestic equipment. The institution is now known as Darenth Park Hospital.
Bibliography: Ayers, G. M. 1971. *England's first state hospitals and the Metropolitan Asylums Board.*

DARK COMEDY. *See* BLACK COMEDY.

DARRELL, JOHN (c.1562-1602). English exorcist (*see* EXORCISM and itinerant preacher. His first attempt at exorcism took place in 1585, when he tried to free a Catherine Wright from the demon Middlecub. This was followed some years later by more spectacular public performances. The church declared him an impostor, and he was defrocked and imprisoned.
Bibliography: Robbins, R. H. 1970. *The encyclopaedia of witchcraft and demonology.*

DARROW, CLARENCE SEWARD (1857-1938). American lawyer and socialist writer, famous for his defense of several widely publicized trials. He supported the belief that punishment was not an adequate cure for delinquency and that crime could be prevented only by understanding why and how delinquency developed.
Bibliography: Darrow, C. S. 1922. *Crime: its causes and treatment.*

DÁR-UL-MARAFTAN (*or* MARAPHTAN). The term means "Abode of those who require to be chained." It was a mental hospital in Baghdad, founded in approximately 1150. Benjamin of Tudela (d. 1173), a Spanish Jew, mentioned it in his *Travels,* which was a description of his journey though many lands between 1160 and 1173. His book was translated into English by A. Asher in 1840. He found sixty medical institutions in Baghdad. Of the asylum, he wrote:

There is further the large building called the Dár-ul-Maraphtan in which are locked up all those insane persons who are met with during the hot season, everyone of whom is secured by iron chains until his reason returns, when he is allowed to return to his home. For this purpose they are regularly examined once a month by the king's officers appointed for that purpose, and, when they are found to be possessed of reason, they are immediately liberated. All this is done by the king in pure charity towards all who come to Baghdad, either ill or insane, for the king is a pious man and his intention is excellent in this respect.
Bibliography: Elgood, C. 1951. *A medical history of Persia and the Eastern caliphate.*

DARWIN, CHARLES ROBERT (1809-1882). A British naturalist, born in Shrewsbury, England. Throughout his life he suffered from poor health, depression, insomnia, and a host of psychosomatic disorders that allowed him to avoid social engagements and to gain more time for thinking and studying. Other members of his family also suffered from nervous disorders: his grandfather Erasmus Darwin (q.v.) and his uncle Charles stammered badly; his uncle Erasmus committed suicide (q.v.) by drowning in the River Derwent and was said to be insane. His grandmother was an hysteric (*see* HYSTERIA) and an alcoholic (*see* ALCOHOLISM). His wife, Emma Wedgewood, considered him "perfectly sweet tempered"and the "most transparent man" she ever saw. His well-known scientific work permanently joined his name to the theory of evolution of the species through natural selection.

His book *Origin of the Species*, published in 1859, contradicted Biblical doctrine, and he became the target of hostile attacks. His theories, however, had a profound effect on the culture of the whole world and have remained the basis of man's attitude toward himself. Its implication that as there is a physical continuity between man and animal, there is also a continuity of mind affected the development of psychology (q.v.). In 1872 he published *Expression of the Emotion in Man and Animals* (q.v.) in which he discussed behavioral attitudes common to man and animals. His "Biographical Sketch of an Infant" (1877) was a detailed study of the development and behavior of young children that influenced the field of child psychiatry (q.v.).
Bibliography: de Beer, G. 1963. *Charles Darwin: evolution by natural selection.*

DARWIN, ERASMUS (1731-1802). English physician, grandfather of Charles Darwin (q.v.). He was an unorthodox genius, who brought up two illegitimate daughters among his tribe of fourteen children. He formulated a theory of transmutation of the species, which he described in verse. He emphasized the physical basis of thought and emotion and believed that "disordered motions" of the nervous tissues were the cause of all diseases. Based on these beliefs he devised a physiological classification of mental disorders. Jean Esquirol (q.v.) quoted his observations on hallucinations (q.v.). Darwin thought that violent physical measures to shock the system were beneficial in the treatment of insanity and consequently invented machines for spinning patients. George III (q.v.) asked him to be his physician, but he declined. Darwin's works include *The Loves of the Plants* (1789) and *The Temple of Nature, or the Origin of Society*, published in 1803. In 1789 he founded the Philosophical Society of Derby. He was also the founder of the Lunar Society, whose members, all scientists, were called "lunaticks" because they met and dined at full moon to make their journey home easier.
Bibliography: King-Hele, D. 1977. *Doctor of revolution: the life and genius of Erasmus Darwin.*

DASEIN. Existentialist term introduced by Martin Heidegger (q.v.) to mean the field of being that is existence.
Bibliography: Biemel, W. 1977. *Martin Heidegger.*

DAUDET, ALPHONSE (1840-1897). A French novelist of great sensitivity. He contracted tabes dorsalis and was sent by Jean Martin Charcot (q.v.) to Lamelou-les-Bains, where he underwent traction therapy, a form of treatment here that consisted in hanging the patient from a hook for a minute. Daudet described his suffering in his posthumously published diary, which was entitled *La Doulu*, a Provençal term for pain. He was forced to resort to morphine (q.v.) and chloral to combat the pain. His works of psychological interest are *L'Évangelist* (1883), a study of religious mania (q.v.),

Sapho (1884), in which he presented his long liaison with a Frenchwoman, and *L'Immortel* (1888), a social satire of his times, that was met with hostility.
Bibliography: Critchley, M. 1979. *The divine banquet of the brain and other essays.*

DAUL-KULB. An Arabic term coined in the first century A.D. by Najab ud din Unhammed (q.v.). The term describes a state of mania (q.v.) in which destructiveness and gentleness are alternating forms of behavior.
Bibliography: Balfour, J. G. 1878. An Arab physician on insanity. *J. Ment. Sci.* 22.

DAVENPORT, CHARLES BENEDICT (1866-1944). An American physician. As a proponent of eugenics (q.v.), he asserted that the offspring of mentally deficient parents would be mentally deficient themselves and that marriage between feebleminded persons should be forbidden by law. He wrote that defectives could be born to intellectually normal parents only if the parents carried such a heredity from previous generations. He conducted anthropometric studies on drafted troops in World War I.
See also NAM FAMILY.
Bibliography: Davenport, C. B. 1911. *Heredity in relation to eugenics.*

DAVID. A Biblical figure who feigned madness to escape Achish, king of Gath; he "scrabbled on the doors of the gate, and let his spittle fall down upon his beard" (1 Sam. 21: 13). The Bible (q.v.) also records how he played his harp to soothe Saul (q.v.) in his insanity, an early example of music therapy (q.v.).

And whenever the evil spirit from God was upon Saul, David took the lyre and played it with his hands; so Saul was refreshed and was well, and the evil spirit departed from him.

(1 Sam. 16: 23).

Bibliography: Bosch, J. 1965. *David: the biography of a king*, trans. J. Marks.

DAVIES, WILLIAM HENRY (1871-1940). A Welsh poet. He roamed through England and the United States as a peddlar and a beggar and described his experiences in *Autobiography of a Super-tramp* (1908). Among his verses there is a touching poem entitled *The Idiot and the Child.*
Bibliography: Whitwell, J. R. 1946. *Analecta psychiatrica.*

DAVY, ADAM (fl. 1308?). An English poet. He may have been the author of *Alisaunder*, an eleventh-century story in verse of Alexander III (q.v.). He was a fanatic and a visionary; he claimed to have predicted the future, including the destiny of King Edward II in his poem "Five Dreams About Edward II" (c. 1310).
Bibliography: Stephen, L., and Lee, S. 1969. *The dictionary of national biography,* Pt. 1.

DAVY JONES. In nautical superstitions, a spirit of the sea or a devil. His locker is the grave of those who die at sea.
Bibliography: Harvey, P. 1967. *The Oxford companion to English literature.* 1966. 4th ed.

DAWAMESK. A mixture of honey, pistachio nuts, and cannabis indica. Théophile Gautier (q.v.) referred to it as the "green jam" that he, Charles Baudelaire (q.v.), and other artists consumed during drug-taking sessions at the Club des Haschichins (q.v.) in Paris.
Bibliography: Gautier, T. and Thorne, G. 1915. *Charles Baudelaire: his life.*

DAY HOSPITAL. Means by which patients attended hospital for day care programs were first devised in 1947 by Donald Ewen Cameron (q.v.), a Scottish psychiatrist who worked at McGill University in Montreal, Canada. These programs kept patients in touch with society and their families and counteracted the seclusion of mental hospitals.
Bibliography: Goldenson, R. M. 1970. *The encyclopedia of human behavior,* vol. I.

DEAF-MUTISM. The inability to hear or speak. Until the nineteenth century it was considered a form of cretinism (q.v.) because it was believed that the thyroid was a part of the speech apparatus.
Bibliography: Kanner, L. 1963. *A history of the care and study of the mentally retarded.*

DE ANIMA. The title of a book on the human soul and intellect by Aristotle (q.v.).

DE ANIMA BRUTORUM (or TWO DISCOURSES CONCERNING THE SOUL OF BRUTES WHICH IS THAT OF THE VITAL AND SENSITIVE MAN). Possibly the first book on medical psychology, written in 1672 by Thomas Willis (q.v.). In it he discussed melancholy (*see* MELANCHOLIA), which he called "a complicated Distemper of the Brain and Heart," and madness, in which he thought the animal spirits "seem to be all as it were of an open burning or flame." The treatment he advocated included beating, discipline, threats, purges (*see* PURGING) and bleeding (q.v.).
Bibliography: Hunter, R. and Macalpine, I. 1963. *Three hundred years of psychiatry.*

DE ANIMA ET VITA. One of the first works on modern psychology. It was written by Juan Luis Vives (q.v.) in 1538.
Bibliography: *Historical derivations of modern psychiatry* 1967. Ed. J. Goldston.

DEATH INSTINCT. A destructive or self-destructive tendency postulated by Sigmund Freud (q.v.) in 1920 in his *Beyond the Pleasure Principle.* The concept is not accepted by all Freudian analysts.

See also LIFE INSTINCTS.
Bibliography: Fenichel, O. 1945. *The psychoanalytic theory of neurosis.*

DECROLY, OVIDE (1871-1932). A Belgian psychologist. He proposed that children's education should be based on the study of their natural and social environment. Amongst his works are *Evolution de l'affectivité* (1927) and *Developpement du langage* (1930).
Bibliography: Kanner, L. 1964. *A history of the care and study of the mentally retarded.*

DEE, JOHN (1527-1608). A mathematician and astrologer (*see* ASTROLOGY) born in Cambridge, England. He originally acquired a reputation as a magician (*see* MAGIC) because of the stage effects he introduced in a performance of a play by Aristophanes (q.v.). In 1555 Dee was accused of practicing witchcraft (q.v.) against Queen Mary I (q.v.), but he was acquitted. At the court of Rudolf II of Germany, he profitably practiced crystal (q.v.) gazing with Edward Kelley (q.v.) and became the leader of a confraternity dedicated to the search for the philosopher stone (q.v.). His frauds were eventually discovered, and he escaped to England. The shew-stone (show stone) he used in his self-hypnotizing sessions is still preserved in the British Museum. In his *Brief Lives* John Aubrey (q.v.) included a short biography of Dee, in which he mentioned "plates of gold made by projection in the garret of Dr. Dee's lodgings in Prague," an example of the Elizabethan belief in alchemy (q.v.). Queen Elizabeth I trusted him greatly; he was even consulted about the most auspicious day for her coronation. After the Queen's death, he became destitute and possibly senile. He suffered from hallucinations (q.v.), during which he claimed that the Archangel Raphael came to comfort him.
Bibliography: French, P. J. 1972. *John Dee: the world of an Elizabethan magus.*

DE EGAS MONIZ. *See* EGAS MONIZ.

DEFENCE NEUROPSYCHOSIS. Defence neuropsychosis was an expression first used by Sigmund Freud (q.v.) in 1894. Defence dominated Freud's writings and ideas in the 1890s. He published a paper in 1894 entitled "The Defence Neuropsychosis." He saw psychosis, and neurosis arising from the processes set going by the person's need to defend himself against unbearable ideas.
Bibliography: Fine, Reuben. 1979. *A history of psychoanalysis.*

DE FLEURY, MAURICE (1860-1931). A French physician. In addition to studying arthritis, he was particularly interested in emotional problems and in disorders of the nervous system, such as epilepsy (q.v.). Among his works are *Manuel pour l'étude des maladies du système nerveux* (1904) and *L'angoisse humaine* (1925).

DEFOE, DANIEL (1661-1731). An English writer, son of a London butcher. As a writer he used satire against people and ideas that he did not like. He traveled widely in Europe and then returned to England, where he became involved in politics. Fined and imprisoned for his *Shortest Way with Dissenters* (1702), he became a hero of the people. In his later life he became suspicious and paranoid (*see* PARANOIA) and lost his early popularity. He advocated many social reforms, including the construction of a hospital for idiots (q.v.), supervision of madhouses, and regulations for the commitment of patients to asylums (q.v.). In 1706 his journal, *Review*, printed his article "Scheme for the Management of Mad-houses." In the same journal he began a series of articles about a wealthy young woman who, because of hallucinations (q.v.) and very odd behavior, had been diagnosed as insane by Edward Tyson (q.v.) and subsequently admitted to a private madhouse. The paper suggested that she was in fact sane and had been imprisoned because of designs on her money. Defoe wrote about the horrors of private madhouses and recommended that they should be registered. He returned to the subject in 1728, deploring that private asylums were not inspected. He made an impassioned appeal to George II's (q.v.) queen with somewhat wild stories of wives imprisoned in madhouses by their husbands. His interest in mental disorders and in the treatment of the insane is also evident in his comments on Bethlem Royal Hospital (q.v.). He wrote, "I think The Hospital we call Bedlam, to be a Noble Foundation; a visible Instance of the sense our Ancestors had of the greatest Unhappiness which can befal Human kind. . . ." He is best remembered for his book *Robinson Crusoe* (1719), but he was the author of over 250 works.
Bibliography: Moore, J. R. 1958. *Daniel Defoe: citizen of the modern world.*

DEGENERATION. The gradual change to a less healthy state. During the nineteenth century mental disease usually was regarded as a result of hereditary weaknesses. Benedict Augustin Morel (q.v.) was an exponent of this theory, and he developed a method by which signs of mental degeneration could be detected. He believed that certain physical malformations and behavior that was considered deviant from the normal were signs of degeneration. A system of psychiatry based on degeneration evolved from these theories.
Bibliography: Morel, B. A. 1860. *Traité des maladies mentales.*

DÉJÀ VU. An illusionary feeling of having seen something previously. Other illusions of familiarity are *déjà eprouvé*, a feeling of having experienced something before; *déjà pensé*, a new thought that seems familiar; *déjà raconté*, a feeling of having said something before; *déjá voulu*, present desires that seem to coincide with previous desires. Among the early medical practitioners describing the condition are Arthur L. Wigan (1785-1867), in *A New View of Insanity* (1844), John Hughlings Jackson (q.v.), and Pierre

Marie (q.v.). Sir Walter Scott (q.v.) termed the feeling the "sentiment of pre-existence."
Bibliography: Hunter, R. and Malcalpine, I. 1963. *Three hundred years of psychiatry.*

DÉJERINE, JOSEPH JULES (1849-1917). A Swiss neurologist. He studied medicine in Paris and worked at the Bicêtre (q.v.) and at the Salpêtrière (q.v.), where he became professor of psychiatry. He studied the physiology and pathology of sensation and cerebral localization. He evolved his own successful method of psychiatric treatment based on reassurance, sympathy, and suggestion. Déjerine not only realized the importance of the emotional relationship between the patient and the psychotherapist but also realized that emotional factors influenced somatic disorders. He described a form of infantile neuritis (Déjerine's disease) and other diseases, especially those of the thalamus. Throughout his career he had the help and collaboration of his American wife, Augusta Klumpke (1859-1927), a brilliant and charming neurologist.
Bibliography: Boucher, M. 1978. Jules Déjerine. *Hist. Sci. Med.* 12: 357-73.

DE JONG, H. HOLLAND (1895-1956). A Dutch psychiatrist. In his later years he worked in the United States. His work is remembered in connection with the production of mental illness symptoms, especially catatonia (q.v.), in animals.

DEKKER, THOMAS (1570?-?1632). An English dramatist, born in London. Although poverty frequently caused him to be imprisoned for debt, he retained a lovable and kindly nature. His vivid descriptions of life in London show a deep sympathy for the poor and the unfortunate. He used Bethlem Royal Hospital (q.v.) and Bridewell (q.v.) as settings for his satirical play *The Belman of London.*
Bibliography: O'Donoghue, E. G. 1914. *The story of Bethlehem hospital.*

DELAHARA. A disorder that is similar to amok (q.v.) and affects Philippine women. The afflicted person becomes quarrelsome, aggressive, and is exhausted once the attack is over.
Bibliography: Goldenson, R. M. 1970. *The encyclopedia of human behavior.*

DE LA POLE HOSPITAL. An English mental hospital in Willerby, near Hull, so called from the site on which it was built (De la Pole Farm). Originally it was two private asylums (q.v.), the Refuge in Sculcoates, and the Retreat in Summergans, opened in 1814 and 1823 respectively. In 1841 these hospitals merged into the Hull and East Riding Refuge and moved to a new building in Hull. In 1884 the hospital again moved and new buildings were constructed at De La Pole Farm.

DELBOEUF, JOSEPH RÉMY LEOPOLD (1831-1896). A Belgian physician. He became interested in the work of Jean Martin Charcot (q.v.) and traveled to Paris to observe it in person. There he became critical of Charcot's rather careless experiments with hysterical (*see* HYSTERIA) patients because he was aware of the element of suggestion in the symptoms they displayed under hypnosis (*see* HYPNOTISM). His studies contributed to psychophysics and gave rise to a new concept of the sense-distance. He wrote *Éléments de psychophysique* and *Examen critique de la loi psychophisique*, both published in 1883.
Bibliography: Boring, E.G. 1950. *A history of experimental psychology.*

DELEUZE, JOSEPH PHILIP FRANÇOIS (1753-1835). French scholar and scientist, librarian for the French Natural History Society. He was a pupil of Armand-Marie-Jacques Puységur (q.v.), and the revival of magnetism (q.v.) in France is ascribed to him. He approached magnetism from a clinical, scientific point of view. He described various phenomena occurring during somnambulism (q.v.) and pointed out the importance of the magnetizer's will in treatment. He also established the basic principles of posthypnotic phenomena.
Bibliography: Tinterow, M. M. 1970. *Foundations of hypnosis: from Mesmer to Freud.*

DELGADO, HONORIO (1892-1969). Peruvian psychiatrist, professor of psychiatry in Lima. Although he introduced psychoanalysis (q.v.) to South America and was the first Latin American member of the International Psychoanalytic Association, he later abandoned psychoanalysis. He was a prolific writer and his works covered many fields of psychiatry. His influence in academic circles was matched by his work in the national organization of mental health services. In 1938, he founded the Sociedad de Neuropsiquiatria y Medicina Legal del Peru.
Bibliography: Leon, C. A., and Rosselli, H. 1975. Latin America. In *World History of Psychiatry,* ed. J. G. Howells.

DÉLIRE DU TOUCHER. An obsessive (*see* OBSESSION) compulsion to touch objects. Samuel Johnson (q.v.) displayed this symptom.

DELIRIUM. A confused and excited state. In antiquity delirium was synonymous with madness, and the term was used to cover all abnormal behavior. Plato (q.v.) wrote that there were four kinds of delirium, that of the prophets sent by Apollo (q.v.), that of the "initiated" sent by Dionysus (q.v.), that of the poets due to the Muses, and that of lovers caused by Aphrodite and Eros (q.v.). Until the nineteenth century, disorientation with loss of memory and loss of the sense of time and place was considered a sign of mental disease. It eventually was realized that many mental disorders do not display delirium.
Bibliography: Lishman, W. A. 1975. *Organic Psychiatry.*

DELIRIUM TREMENS. A state of agitation, confusion, and tremulousness associated with the withdrawal of alcohol. It was first identified as a separate clinical entity in 1813 by Thomas Sutton (q.v.), who coined the term. It had been observed and described as a toxic state in antiquity. Hippocrates (q.v.) wrote about it and was aware that it was caused by excessive drinking.
Bibliography: Sutton, T. 1813. *Tracts on delirium tremens.*

DELIUS, FREDERICK (1862-1934). An English composer. Although he was born in England of Dutch and German ancestry, he spent most of his life abroad. His parents had an enormous family, and he was one of twelve surviving children. His father was a cruel and punitive man, and his mother was a bitter and unloving woman with no interest in her son and his musical triumphs. She never went to hear his music. In 1890, after failing in the family business and following a stay in the United States, Delius went to live in Paris. He joined a group of artists that included Paul Gauguin (q.v.) and August Strindberg (q.v.), who was already half insane. He shared an interest in the occult with Strindberg. He married Jelka Rosen, a painter. He then formed a close association with Philip Heseltine (q.v.) who lived with him and his wife in their house at Grez-sur-Loing in France. Still in his fifties, Delius gradually became totally paralyzed and blind. His later works were dictated to Eric Fenby, who became his amanuensis in 1928. Fenby and Jelka exercised a great deal of patience in handling Delius, who was a most difficult man. A hypnotist (*see* HYPNOTISM) called Erskine brought about a brief improvement in the condition of the composer, but eventually the pain became so severe that he could bear it only by having someone with him continually, either reading to him or talking with him.
Bibliography: Fenby, E. 1936. *Delius as I knew him.*
Jefferson, A. 1972. *Delius.*

DELPHI. An ancient Greek city, which was believed to be the center of the earth. It was the location of the oracle of Delphi.
See also ORACLES.
Bibliography: Hall, A., and King, F. 1978. *Mysteries of prediction.*

DELUSIONS. Disorders of perception. Delusions were not clearly differentiated from hallucinations (q.v.) until the nineteenth century when Jean Esquirol (q.v.) wrote about them. Asclepiades (q.v.), however, using the term *phantasia* for both hallucinations and delusions, had already divided the phenomena into two classes: those patients who perceive the object they see as something else (now known as delusion) and those patients who see or hear things that are not there (now known as hallucination). The followers of the humoral theory (q.v.) believed that delusions were due to disordered humors.

DELUSIONS, PERSECUTORY. Delusional (see DELUSION) states in which the patient feels that he is being persecuted without reason. They were first accurately described by Karl W. Ideler (q.v.) in a series of clinical case histories published in 1848. Ernest Lasègue (q.v.) described a similar state that he called "persecutory delirium" in 1852. Jean Esquirol (q.v.) included persecutory ideas in the symptomatology of "monomania" (q.v.)

DELVAUX, PAUL (1897-   ). A Belgian surrealist painter. In adolescence he avoided sexual experiences and was afraid of all women, especially his mother. His youthful frustrations are reflected in his paintings of icy maidens, haunted creatures, and statues. His paintings also display an obsession (q.v.) with thoughts of sickness and death.
Bibliography: Haslam, M. 1978. *Real world of the surrealists.*

DEMANDOLX, MADELEINE DE (1593-1670). An emotionally disturbed Provençal girl of noble birth. At the age of twelve she was sent to the Convent of the Ursuline Nuns in Aix-en-Provence (q.v.), but she was soon returned to her family because of her deep depression. She became too fond of her young confessor, Father Gaufridi, and claimed to have been intimate with him. After becoming a nun, she developed symptoms of hysteria (q.v.), including convulsions, loss of speech, and hallucinations (q.v.), which spread to the other nuns. She accused Father Gaufridi of seducing and bewitching her; this led to prolonged ceremonies of exorcism (q.v.) in which the nuns vied with each other in producing spectacular symptoms. Madeleine was said to be possessed by five named demons and 6,661 unnamed ones. The Inquisition (q.v.) condemned Gaufridi to death after horrible tortures. Madeleine was cured temporarily, but later in life she also was accused of witchcraft (q.v.) and spent many years in prison.
Bibliography: Robbins, R. H. 1970. *The encyclopedia of witchcraft and demonology.*

DEMENTIA INFANTILIS. A term introduced by Theodore Heller in 1930 to indicate schizophrenia (q.v.) occurring in children below the age of four. *See also* HELLER DISEASE.
Bibliography: Heller, T. 1969. About Dementia Infantilis, trans. W.C. Hulse. In *Modern perspectives in international child psychiatry*, ed. J. G. Howells.

DEMENTIA PRAECOCISSIMA. A term first used in 1905 by the Italian psychiatrist Sante De Sanctis (q.v.) to describe a psychiatric disorder occurring in very young children. Now it is considered to be childhood schizophrenia (q.v.).
Bibliography: De Sanctis, S. 1969. On Some Varieties of Dementia Praecox, trans. M. L. Osborn. In *Modern perspectives in international child psychiatry*, ed. J. G. Howells.

DEMENTIA PRAECOX. A term coined by Benedict A. Morel (q.v.) in 1852 to indicate those patients who became severely mentally impaired soon after the onset of their illness. It really meant "rapid mental impairment" and not "dementia at an early age," as it was erroneously understood to mean at a later period.
Bibliography: Morel, B. A. 1852. *Etudes cliniques*, vol. 1.

DEMENTIA PRAECOX OR THE GROUP OF SCHIZOPHRENIAS. One of the most authoritative source books on the development and manifestations of schizophrenia (q.v.), a term introduced by its author, Eugen Bleuler (q.v.). It was published in 1911 and was the result of his close personal observations of patients in the asylum of Rheinau and in the Burghölzli Hospital (q.v.).
Bibliography: Bleuler, E. 1950. *Dementia praecox or the group of schizophrenias*, trans. J. Ziskin.

DEMI-VIERGE. A French term, meaning "semivirgin." It was used by the novelist Marcel Prévost (1862-1941) to describe women who feel that they have been deprived of their virginity by nonphysical means. Schizophrenic (*see* SCHIZOPHRENIA) female patients often believe that men have had intercourse with them.
Bibliography: Prévost, M. 1894. *Les demi-vierges*.

DEMOCRITUS (460-370 B.C.). A Greek philosopher, born in Abdera (q.v.). He thought that the human body was composed of constantly moving atoms. He was interested in mental disorders and performed anatomical dissections on animals in search of black choler (q.v.), which he believed to be the cause of madness. He also believed that strong emotions could cause convulsions. Hippocrates (q.v.) attended him when his friends thought that he was insane and prescribed hellebore (q.v.), a remedy readily available in Abdera. Democritus was called "the laughing philosopher" because of his ethical ideal of cheerfulness. Robert Burton (q.v.) described him as "a little wearish old man, very melancholy by nature, averse from company in his latter days, and much given to solitariness." There is a legend that he blinded himself and finally committed suicide (q.v.).
Bibliography: Cole, T. 1967. *Democritus and the sources of Greek anthropology*.

DEMOCRITUS JUNIOR. The pseudonym adopted by Robert Burton (q.v.). He considered his task in *Anatomy of Melancholy* (q.v.) to be similar to that of the Greek philosopher Democritus (q.v.), who had searched for the cause of melancholy (*see* MELANCHOLIA).
Bibliography: Bright, Timothy. 1969. *A treatise of melancholia*.

DEMONIAC POSSESSION. The possession (q.v.) of a human being by a demon. Fear of something that could not be understood created a primitive

belief in a special kind of evil spirit. This superstition played an important part in psychiatry until the end of the seventeenth century. Mental disorders often were ascribed to demoniacal possession, and treatment was designed to expel the devil by various methods ranging from purging (q.v.) and the administration of emetics and sneezing powders to beating and exorcism (q.v.). The *Malleus Maleficarum* (q.v.) only strengthened the medieval belief in devils and witchcraft (q.v.).
Bibliography: Oesterreich, T. K. 1930. *Possession, demoniacal and other.*

DEMONOMANIA. A term used by Jean Esquirol (q.v.) to indicate religious melancholy (*see* MELANCHOLIA) (q.v.). It was derived from the Greek word *demon* meaning divinity, god, or spirit. The term had earlier been used by John B. Erhard (q.v.).
Bibliography: Esquirol, J. E. D. 1845. Reprint. 1965 *Mental Maladies: A treatise on insanity.*

DEMOSTHENES (385?-322 B.C.). The greatest of the Greek orators. He stammered but mastered his disability by willpower. To avoid being taken prisoner when Athens was captured by the Macedonians, he committed suicide (q.v.). The term *Demosthenes complex* means the pathological need to master others with words in order to overcome a feeling of inferiority.
Bibliography: Packard-Cambridge, A. W. 1914. *Demosthenes and the last days of Greek freedom.*

DENDY, MARY (1855-1933). An English philanthropist, active in the field of reforms for the mentally retarded. She not only advocated comprehensive institutional and educational facilities for the mentally subnormal but also founded institutions dedicated to these aims; the best known of these were the Sandelbridge Homes (now Mary Dendy Hospital).

DENDY, WALTER COOPER (1794-1871). A British surgeon. He was interested in mental illness and particularly in phenomena involving altered consciousness, trance, dreams (q.v.), and somnambulism (q.v.). In 1832 he wrote a work entitled *On the Phenomena of Dreams, and Other Transient Illusions.* He studied examples of abnormal mental states mentioned in history and in literature and presented his findings in *The Philosophy of Mystery*, published in 1841. His realization that bodily disorders often had a psychogenic aetiology caused him to advocate psychical methods of treatment, especially in hysterical (*see* HYSTERIA) disorders. He believed that the mind of an emotionally healthy person could influence the mind of a mentally ill patient. He presented these ideas in 1853 in a paper entitled "Psychotherapeia, or the Remedial Influence of the Mind," one of the earliest uses of the term "psychotherapy" (q.v.).
Bibliography: Hunter, R., and Macalpine, I. 1963. *Three hundred years of psychiatry.*

DENHAM, SIR JOHN (1615-1669). English poet and architect. He was unhappily married and was said to have become insane in 1666 as a result of his second wife's faithlessness. Samuel Butler (q.v.) lampooned him for his lunacy (*see* LUNATIC).
Bibliography: Browning, D. C. 1958. *Everyman's dictionary of literary biography.*

DENIS, JEAN BAPTISTE (1643-1704). A French physician, appointed consultant to Louis XIV. He is credited with the first blood transfusion (q.v.), which he performed as treatment for madness. The patient was a thirty-four-year-old man who had arrived naked in Paris with his mind disordered because of an unhappy love affair. He was bled from an arm and the blood that was extracted was replaced with calf's blood. By the following day the patient had become quiet and could think clearly. The operation was acclaimed all over Europe, but the patient did not survive.
Bibliography: Zilboorg, G. 1941. *A history of medical psychology.*

DENMAN, THOMAS (1733-1815). A British physician who practiced obstetrics in London. In his book *An Introduction to the Practice of Midwifery*, he discussed mental disorders that could occur during or soon after childbirth. He thought that these disorders were caused by anxiety and that their duration varied from a few days to several months, but he concluded that the patients were likely to regain their sanity. He advised avoiding the "powerful medicines" usually employed in the treatment of insanity, because the women were already weakened by childbirth.
Bibliography: Hunter, R., and Macalpine, I. 1963. *Three hundred years of psychiatry.*

DE PRAESTIGIIS DAEMONUM. The title of a book by Johann Weyer (q.v.). It was first published in 1563. While maintaining an ambiguous view on the existence of demons, Weyer asserted that witches (*see* WITCHCRAFT) were mentally ill people, who were in need of skilled and humane medical treatment. Weyer's concept that some people will deliberately cause damage to others, while other people may cause harm in their sickness and are not responsible for their actions was new to its time. He believed that those who were evil should be punished and those who were sick should receive medical attention. He considered it the right and the duty of a physician to attend those found to be mentally ill.
Bibliography: Goldenson, R. M. 1970. *The encyclopedia of human behavior.*

DEPTH PSYCHOLOGY. A term coined by Eugen Bleuler (q.v.) at a time when psychoanalysis (q.v.) was equated with the psychology of the unconscious (q.v.).
Bibliography: Bleuler, E. 1924. *Textbook of psychiatry*, trans. A. A. Brill.

DE QUINCEY, THOMAS (1785-1859). An English writer, born in Manchester. His childhood was marked by rejection and death. He was

rejected by his stern and cold mother; his father died when he was seven years old; one of his sisters died of hydrocephalus; and another was killed by a servant. His elder brother William bullied him constantly. His misery continued at school, and he ran away to Wales. He began to take opium (q.v.) at Oxford University to relieve facial neuralgia due to toothache. Later he continued to take it to ease the misery of his life. He described his addiction in *Confessions of an English Opium Eater* (q.v.). He was a friend of Samuel Coleridge (q.v.), who introduced him to William Wordsworth (q.v.) and Robert Southey (q.v.). After his marriage, he had five sons and three daughters, whom he deserted when his wife died. He then went wandering, living in a series of lodgings. Coleridge deplored de Quincey's descriptions of the pleasure of opium intoxication and believed that his followers became opium addicts in imitation of him. Opium was the cause of de Quincey's lack of energy, which often resulted in his abandonment of nearly finished projects. His addiction, however, did not shorten his life, for he lived to be seventy-four. In addition to the *Confessions*, he wrote essays, criticisms, and other literary works. Among them are "On Murder Considered as One of the Fine Arts" (1827), *Autobiographic Sketches* (1834-53), "Suspiria de Profundis" (1845), "Vision of Sudden Death" (1849). The standard edition of his works was published in fourteen volumes between 1889 and 1890 and edited by David Masson (1822 1907)
Bibliography: Lindop, G. 1981. *The opium-eater: a life of Thomas De Quincey.*

DERCUM'S DISEASE. Adiposis dolorosa. It was described in 1892 by Francis Xavier Dercum (1856-1931), an American neurologist. Dercum was the first clinician to use photography to record many of the symptoms of neurological disorders. He was also the first to take photographs of patients in convulsions. He experimented with hypnosis (*see* HYPNOTISM) and was able to produce psychogenic convulsions in hypnotized individuals. Among his works are *The Physiology of Mind* (1925) and *Rest, Suggestion and Other Therapeutic Measures in Nervous and Mental Diseases.*
Bibliography: *A textbook on nervous diseases.* 1895. Ed. Francis X. Dercum.

DEREISTIC THINKING. A form of fantasy thinking, also termed "autistic thinking." Eugen Bleuler (q.v.) described it in 1912 and considered it to be dependent on the emotions of the individual rather than on external realities.
Bibliography: Bleuler, E. 1924. *Textbook of psychiatry*, trans. A. A. Brill.

DERMO-OPTICAL PERCEPTION (DOP). The phenomenon of perception through the skin. Russian scientists were the first to systematically

investigate it in the 1960s, following the examination of a Soviet woman, Rosa Kuleshova (q.v.), who was able to discriminate colors and even read with her fingers. Abnormal sensitivity in the nervous system and the presence of photosensitive substances in the skin may be responsible for DOP. A few cases of skin perception were reported in the nineteenth century.
Bibliography: Goldenson, R. M. 1970. *The encyclopedia of human behavior.*

DERVISHES. A mystic Islamic order. During its rituals, members use songs and dances that result in high religious exaltation.
Bibliography: Brown, J. P. 1927. *The dervishes or Oriental spiritualism.*

DE SANCTIS, SANTE (1862-1935). An Italian physician and professor of psychiatry at the University of Rome. Many important concepts in child psychiatry were anticipated by him. In 1905 at the Fifth International Congress of Psychiatry, held in Rome, he described a form of dementia praecox (q.v.) occurring before puberty, which he called "dementia praecocissima" (q.v.). He was the author of numerous books, including one on dreams entitled *I Sogni* to which Sigmund Freud (q.v.) referred in his own *Interpretation of Dreams*. De Sanctis also wrote on neuropsychiatry, experimental psychology (q.v.), and forensic psychiatry, as well as producing an autobiography, which was published in 1932.
Bibliography: De Sanctis, S. 1969. On Some Varieties of Dementia Praecox, trans. M. L. Osborn. In *Modern Perspectives of International Child Psychiatry*, ed. J. G. Howells.

DESCARTES, RENÉ (1596-1650). French mathematician and philosopher, founder of the Cartesian school of philosophy (from the Latinized form of his name "Cartesius"). It was based upon an almost mechanical view of the universe. According to him, his mother died a few days after his birth, from "a lung disease caused by grief." From his early youth he was in the habit of spending his mornings in bed, thinking. He was educated by the Jesuits and never married, but John Aubrey (q.v.) recorded that he "kept a good conditioned hansome woman that he liked." Descartes claimed that his principles of analytic geometry came to him in a dream. Although he was world famous, he preferred studying to socializing and therefore retired to Holland, where he tried to keep his address secret by living in thirteen towns and twenty-four houses in the space of twenty years. He maintained that at times he was followed by an invisible person. Descartes believed brain function to be independent of brain structures and to be based on animal spirits. He made an analogy between the nervous functions and the harmonic structure of organ music in which the sound depends on the air from the bellows, the distribution of air in the pipes, and the pipes, themselves. In answer to his critics he said "I know myself as a thought, and I positively do not know myself as a brain." He uttered the dictum "Cogito ergo sum"

[I think, therefore I am]. His views in his work *The World* were similar to Galileo's (q.v.) but he held the work back from publication when Galileo was condemned for heresy. In his last book, *Passions of the Soul* (1649), he gave a more experiential and sensualistic interpretation of brain functions and sensory perception. He believed that the seat of the soul was in the pineal gland. He was the first to describe the sensation of pain in phantom limbs. Queen Christina of Sweden asked Descartes to teach her philosophy and sent a warship to fetch him. In the bitter cold of Sweden and before the winter was over, Descartes died of pneumonia. *The World* was eventually published in 1664.

Bibliography: Keeling, S.W. 1968. *Descartes*.

DESCHANEL, PAUL EUGÈNE LOUIS (1856-1922). French writer and tenth president of the French Republic. He was often depressed to the point of suicide (q.v.). On one occasion he threw himself off a moving train, and on another occasion he had to be saved from drowning in a pond. His health finally compelled him to resign the presidency.

Bibliography: L'Etang, H. 1969. *The pathology of leadership*.

DES ESSARTZ, JEAN-LOUIS-CHARLES (1729-1811). A French physician. He believed in the therapeutic value of music in treating mental disorders. His research included work in the field of childhood management and the use of electricity (q.v.) in the treatment of nervous diseases.

See also MUSIC THERAPY.

Bibliography: Des Essartz, J-L-C. 1803. *Reflexions sur la music . . . comme moyen curatif*.

D'ESLON, CHARLES. A French physician, pupil of Franz Mesmer (q.v.), and author of *Observations sur le magnetisme animal* published in Paris, in 1780. He achieved such great success in his practice that Mesmer accused him of stealing his clientele and his secrets. After Mesmer's methods had been rejected by the medical profession, D'Eslon formed a secret organization of laymen, the Society of Harmony, devoted to the promotion of magnetism. With them he put pressure on Louis XVI to appoint a commission to study animal magnetism. The royal commission, appointed from the Académie des Sciences (q.v.) in 1784 and headed by Benjamin Franklin (q.v.), reported that any public magnetic treatment could only have harmful results.

Bibliography: Tinterow, M.M. 1970. *Foundations of hypnosis*.

DESMARETS DE SAINT-SORLIN, JEAN (c.1596-1676). A French dramatist. In his *Comedy of Visionaries* he introduced a number of strange characters who behave in a psychotic (*see* PSYCHOSIS) fashion on stage.

Bibliography: Benét, W. R. 1972. *The reader's encyclopedia*.

DESPINE, ANTOINE. A French general practitioner interested in magnetism (q.v.). He occasionally used it in the treatment of nervous diseases. His detailed description of a case of dual personality in a girl he called Estelle (q.v.) was published in Paris in 1840, and it inspired Pierre Janet (q.v.) to his own research on the same subject.
Bibliography: Ellenberger, H. F. 1970. *The discovery of the unconscious.*

DESPINE, PROSPER. A French magnetizer (*see* MAGNETISM). In 1875 he published *De la Folie au Point de Vue Philosophique ou plus specialement Psychologique*, in which he discussed insanity. He believed that mass hysteria (q.v.) was the result of the "influence which the mind or the emotions exercise on the nervous system."
Bibliography: Ellenberger, H. F. 1970. *The discovery of the unconscious.*

DESSOIR, MAX (1867-1947). A German psychologist and philosopher, considered to be the founder of parapsychology. He believed that for a scientist to be successful in writing, it was important to be well known in university circles, cover a narrow, well-defined field and avoid "popular" writing. Dessoir was particularly interested in the concept of the duality of mind, or dipsychism (q.v.). He expounded this theory in a book entitled *The Double Ego* (1890), which became quite famous. He investigated the sexual instincts of adolescents, emphasizing bisexuality. In 1888, he published a *Bibliography of Modern Hypnotism* covering 801 items from scientific publications only and listing all that was then known on the unconscious (q.v.) mind. He later added a supplement of 382 new titles. He was a historian of psychology. The word psychosophy, meaning the "theology and metaphysics of the soul," was coined by him.
Bibliography: Ellenberger, H. F. 1970. *The discovery of the unconscious.*

DETENTION CENTER. A place for the short-term custody of males between the ages of twelve and twenty-one. It was introduced in England and Wales in 1948 by the Criminal Justice Act. The harsh discipline of the centers was later modified.
Bibliography: Advisory Council on the Penal System. 1974. *England: young adult offenders.*

DETERMINISM. A doctrine that believes human action is determined by external forces. The question of whether or not man is free to choose between good and evil has been the subject of controversy for centuries. Thomas Hobbes (q.v.) wrote that "when will arises, the cause is not the will itself, but something else, not in one's own disposing"; and Baruch Spinoza (q.v.) affirmed that "in the mind there is no absolute or free will, but the mind is determined by another cause, and this lost by another cause and so to infinity." Sigmund Freud (q.v.) believed that free will was not incompatible with the belief in determination.

Bibliography: Hook, S., ed. 1969. *Determinism and freedom in the age of modern science.*

DEUTERONOMY. A book of the Bible (q.v.) in which mental illness is considered a punishment sent by the Lord: "The Lord shall smite thee with madness. . . ." Unlike other references that might be considered metaphorical, this was meant to be accepted literally.
Bibliography: Deut. 28: 28.

DEUTEROPHALLIC. A concept first used by Ernest Jones (q.v.) in his book *The Early Development of Female Sexuality* (1927). He described it as the "dawning suspicion that the world is divided into two classes: not male and female in the proper sense, but penis possessing and castrated."
Bibliography: Jones, Ernest. 1927. *The early development of female sexuality.*

DEUTSCH, FELIX (1884-1964). An Austrian physician and pioneer in psychosomatic medicine (q.v.). He developed a therapeutic technique termed "sector therapy" (q.v.) in which the patient's emotional negative chains of association are broken up and replaced by constructive, positive patterns.
Bibliography: Deutsch, F. 1949. *Applied psychoanalysis: selected objectives of psychotherapy.*

DEUTSCH, HELENE (1886-1982). A German psychoanalyst. She trained under Emil Kraepelin (q.v.) in München. Her early work included research on the role of emotions in memories recalled by association. She became interested in the work of Sigmund Freud (q.v.) and practiced and taught psychoanalysis (q.v.) in England, where she made her home. She was active well into her nineties. Her many works include *The Psychology of Women* (1944-1945).
Bibliography: Deutsch, H. 1973. *Confrontations with myself: an epilogue.*

DE VEGA, CHRISTOPHOROS (?-1573). A Spanish physician, follower of the humoral theory (q.v.) of Galen (q.v.). His studies on mania (q.v.) and melancholia (q.v.) contributed greatly to the understanding of mental and emotional disorders. Of insanity (*see* INSANIA) he wrote:

Insanity is a delirium which has no fever of the hot humour which affects the brain's membranes. It is preceded by certain symptoms which may be considered as antecedents, such as pain and throbbing of the head, terrible insomnia, untimely laughter, rage with no cause and night pollution. After that comes a more violent period, with loquacity, strange fantasies and verbal and bodily aggression. The sick person sometimes throws himself out of the window, tears his clothes, etc. The disease frequently attacks young people.

He also described what later became known as erotomania (q.v.) and suggested that it should be treated by counseling rather than by physical meth-

ods. He was physician to Don Carlos (q.v.), who may have been the model for his description of the symptoms of insanity.
Bibliography: Lopez Ibor, J. J. 1975. Spain and Portugal. In *World history of psychiatry*, ed. J. G. Howells.

DEVELOPMENTAL PSYCHOLOGY. A branch of psychology concerned with the study of changes in behavior through the life span of an individual. It began with the observations of such men as the German philosopher Dietrich Tiedemann (1748-1786), Charles Darwin (q.v.), and Jean Piaget (q.v.).
Bibliography: Klein, D. B. 1970. *A history of scientific psychology.*

DEVIL'S BIT SCABIOUS. The common name of *Scabiosa succisa*, which was popularly believed to have such beneficial medical properties that the Devil bit its root in an effort to destroy it. It was used in the treatment of epilepsy (q.v.) and convulsions in general, as well as for hysterical (*see* HYSTERIA) disorders and as a means of soothing irritable patients.
Bibliography: de Baïracli Levy, J. 1974. *The illustrated herbal handbook.*

DEWEY, JOHN (1859-1952). American philosopher and psychologist. His textbook *Psychology* was published in 1886 when he was twenty-seven years old. It was a sophisticated work despite a certain lack of clarity. In 1894, he became professor of philosophy at the University of Chicago and remained there for ten years. The Chicago school of functional psychology took his work as its organizing principle. Dewey believed in progress and social change. He greatly influenced the development of psychology in the United States and contributed to the advancement of dynamic psychology. James R. Angell (q.v.) said of him "his simplicity of character, originality, and virility of mind brought him the unqualified affection, admiration, and devotion of thousands of students." He wrote numerous books among which are *Critical Theory of Ethics* (1894); *Studies in Logical Theory* (1903); *Logic: The Theory of Inquiry* (1938).
Bibliography: Boring, E. G. 1950. *A history of experimental psychology.*

DIAMOND. A precious stone. According to Girolamo Cardano (q.v.), diamonds have the power to make their wearers unhappy because their brilliance irritates the soul in the same way that strong light irritates the eyes. Conversely, Stephen Batman (d. 1584), writing in 1582, attributed to diamonds the virtues of driving away fear and of helping those who are "lunatike or phrantike". About a century later, Anselmus Boetius de Boot also wrote that diamonds prevented madness and guarded against fear and nightmares (q.v.).
See also PRECIOUS STONES.
Bibliography: Evans, J. 1922. *Magical jewels.*

DIANA. A Roman goddess, identified with the Greek goddess Artemis. She was associated with women, woods, and the moon (q.v.). The high priest of her cult had to be a runaway slave who had murdered his predecessor to claim his position. "Diana's wrath" was another term for lunacy (*see* LUNATIC). "Diana's complex" is the wish of a male to be a female.
Bibliography: Warrington, J. 1961. *Everyman's classical dictionary.*

DIAPHRAGM. The wall of muscles and membranes that separates the thorax from the abdomen. In Greek thought the soul was often sited in the diaphragm. The word *phrenos* originally meant diaphragm and later acquired the added meaning of "mind."
Bibliography: Zilboorg G. 1941. *A history of medical psychology.*

DIAZ DE ISLA, RODRIGO R. (1462-1542). A Spanish surgeon. His work *Tractado contra el mal serpentino*, written in 1510 and published in 1539, contains the first reference to the belief that syphilis (q.v.) was introduced into Spain by Columbus' sailors returning from Haiti in 1493. Diaz de Isla described syphilis as a new disease, never before seen in Barcelona. He was incorrect. He is also credited with treating the sailors before they came ashore.
Bibliography: Garrison, F. H. 1929. *An introduction to the history of medicine.*

DICKENS, CHARLES (1812-1870). An English novelist. His early life was insecure because of his cheerful but feckless father, who was so incapable of providing for his family that he was eventually imprisoned for debt. As a child, Dickens worked in a blacking warehouse and the humiliation of this experience and his father's imprisonment affected him deeply, leaving him with a propensity toward bitterness and depression. Once, writing of himself as a patient, he described his condition as "extreme depression of mind and a disposition to shed tears from morning to night. . . . a dull stupid languor. He has no purpose, power, or object in existence whatever." His married life was unhappy and ended in a much concealed separation, when he became attracted to a young actress, Ellen Ternan, with whom he led a secret life. His novel *David Copperfield* (1850) is partly autobiographical, and the character of Wilkins Micawber (q.v.) is a portrait of his own father. Dickens became a friend of John Elliotson (q.v.), and his interest in mesmerism (q.v.) caused him to try to mesmerize his wife. Phrenology (q.v.) too interested him. He knew most of the progressive psychiatric institutions in Europe, and was a close friend of John Conolly (q.v.). He visited asylums (q.v.) in England and in America and commented on American asylums in his *American Notes* (1842). "A Curious Dance" (1860) is a description of his Christmas visit to St. Luke's Hospital (q.v.) in London, where he was pleased to see nonrestraint policies practiced. "A Curious Dance" was subsequently used by St. Luke's Hospital in an appeal for funds. Dickens'

knowledge of abnormal behavior and his interest in mental and emotional disorders are reflected in many of his writings. His works contain descriptions of senile dementia (Old Chuffey; Mrs. Smallweed; Dr. Manette), schizophrenia (q.v.) (Mr. F.'s aunt), hysteria (q.v.) (Mrs. Clenman; Mr. Merdle; Mrs. Crewler), chronic hypomania (the man over the garden wall who intrigued Mrs. Nickleby), mental retardation (Barnaby Rudge; Mr. Dick; Maggy, Sloppy), and suicide (q.v.) (Jonas; Mr. Merdle). His clinical descriptions of the effects of head injuries were particularly accurate (Mrs. Gargery; Eugene Wraybury), as were his accounts of strokes (Mrs. Skewton; Sir Leicester Dedlock; John Willet). Miss Havisham (q.v.) has given her name to a syndrome. Four of his works (*Sketches by Boz* [1836], *Barnaby Rudge* [1841], *Little Dorrit* [1855-1857], and "No Thoroughfare") are concerned with foundlings and reflect his sympathy for children.
Bibliography: Mackenzie, N., Mackenzie, J. 1979. *Dickens: a life.*

DICKINSON, EMILY (1830-1886). An outstanding American poet. Her life was dominated by her strict father, whose rigid Calvinism she rejected. Following an unhappy love affair, her natural disposition to withdrawal and mysticism became more marked and she completely retired from society, living as a recluse and writing thousands of poems that remained unpublished during her lifetime. On the few occasions when she met people, she appeared dressed completely in white.
Bibliography: Cody, John. 1971. *After great pain: the inner life of Emily Dickinson.*

DICK-READ, GRANTLY (1890-1959). An English physician, born in Beccles, Suffolk, England. He pioneered a technique aimed at producing painless childbirth. His theories were based on explanation and reassurance as well as on physical exercises. He lectured widely and wrote numerous articles and books among which are *Natural Childbirth* (1933) and *Childbirth Without Fear* (1944).

DICTIONARY OF PSYCHOLOGICAL MEDICINE, A. A work compiled by Daniel Hack Tuke (q.v.) and published in 1892 in London. It contains references to all that was then known about insanity and reflected the author's encyclopedic knowledge as well as the assistance of a number of distinguished helpers.
Bibliography: Tuke, D. H. 1892. *A dictionary of psychological medicine.*

DIET. Food substances regularly consumed. For centuries imperfect digestion and certain items of diet were considered to be responsible for mental disorders. In Elizabethan times, Timothie Bright (q.v.) and Robert Burton (q.v.) were among those who discussed diets in the treatment of melancholy (*see* MELANCHOLIA). John Purcell (q.v.) believed that some mental illnesses resulted from poor digestion, which caused food to be changed into "crud-

ities and indigestions." George Cheyne (q.v.) advised a vegetarian diet for his melancholic patients, and John Conolly (q.v.) discussed in detail the dietary arrangements in the ideal asylum (q.v.). He prefaced his remarks with the assurance that the diets were "of course, entirely for pauper patients." In modern times, consideration of a patient's diet is imperative in those mental disorders caused by faulty metabolism. Furthermore, some items of food must be forbidden if a patient is taking a drug that is affected by food or drink.
Bibliography: Tannahill, R. 1973. *Food in history.*

DIFFERENTIAL DIAGNOSIS. A comparison of the symptoms of two different diseases to determine the correct diagnosis. The importance of differential diagnosis in psychiatry (q.v.) has been acknowledged from early times. Aretaeus of Cappadocia (q.v.) carefully distinguished between emotional states and abnormal behavior due to inebriation and between feverish delirium (q.v.) and delirium caused by alcohol. In the thirteeenth century, the *Malleus Maleficarum* (q.v.) differentiated between phenomena connected with witchcraft (q.v.) and natural morbid manifestations.

DIFFERENTIAL PSYCHOLOGY. A branch of psychology that studies individual and group differences in psychological characteristics. It was pioneered by Francis Galton (q.v.).
Bibliography: Anastasi, A. 1958. *Differential psychology.*

DIGBY, SIR KENELM (1603-1665). An English author, diplomat, and naval commander. He was one of the first members of the Royal Society (q.v.). He dabbled in science and became famous for his "sympathetic powder," which he claimed to have learned from a Carmelite monk in Florence. It actually consisted of green vitriol that was dissolved in water and then recrystallized in the sun. Digby claimed that a solution of this powder could be used to soak a bandage saturated in the blood of the patient, and the patient's wound would then heal by "sympathy." He also believed in the magic (q.v.) power of viper's wine to preserve beauty; his wife was said to have died from using it too frequently. He was perhaps the first to describe the clinical syndrome of folie à deux (q.v.) which he termed "contagion of the imagination." Assuefaction (q.v.) was another term used by him to describe what we would now term "conditioning." Digby wrote, among other works, a fantastic and self-praising autobiography entitled *Memoirs*, which was not published until 1827. John Aubrey (q.v.) mentions him in his *Brief Lives*.
Bibliography: Petersson, R. T. 1956. *Sir Kenelm Digby, the ornament of England.*

DIGITUS MEDICINALIS. Also called the leech-finger, or leechman. It was the third finger, next to the little finger, or ring-finger, which in the

Middle Ages (q.v.) was believed to contain a vein that led directly to the heart. Rings worn on this finger were believed to cure illness. In ancient Rome, for example, people suffering from epilepsy (q.v.) were advised to wear a ring enclosing a turquoise-colored jasper (q.v.).
Bibliography: 1978. *Brewer's dictionary of phrase and fable.*

DIGUNA-GUNA. An Indonesian practice in which the medicine man, or *dunkun*, uses a belonging of the victim to effect his bewitching. According to Indonesian belief, the spell will cause a person to fall unwillingly in love with a previously disliked individual, or it will cause an enemy to become physically ill or show signs of madness. The *dunkun* may also induce trances.
Bibliography: Kline, N. S. 1963. Psychiatry in Indonesia. *Am. J. Psychiat.* 119:814.

DIMINISHED RESPONSIBILITY. A plea of diminished responsibility for insane offenders. As early as the thirteenth century, English law provided for such a plea. Several examples of its application are found in history; for example the case of Richard Blofot (q.v.) in 1270 and the Arthurian legend of Lancelot (q.v.). Prior to the thirteenth century insanity was regarded as divine punishment for a sin committed, and insane offenders fared less well. In England it was not until 1843 that the M'Naughten Rules (q.v.) allowed the courts to declare an individual "guilty but insane."
Bibliography: Walker, N. D. 1968. *Crime and insanity in England.*

DINGLETON HOSPITAL. A mental hospital near Melrose, Scotland. The building was begun in 1869, and the first patients were admitted in 1872. It attracted international attention in 1949 when it became the first hospital in the world to adopt a completely open-door policy, due to the enlightened views and pioneer work of its physician superintendent, George MacDonald Bell.
Bibliography: Henderson, D. K. 1964. *The evolution of psychiatry in Scotland.*

DIOGENES (fl. c.460 B.C.). A Greek natural philosopher and physician born in Phrygian Apollonia. He believed that air was the primary substance and the principle of the soul and the intelligence. He wrote anatomical works and was interested in sensation.
Bibliography: Phillips, E. D. 1973. *Greek medicine.*

DIONYSUS (*or* BACCHUS). Thracian fertility god. He represented the irrational element in man. It was believed that he had been born prematurely, when his mother, Semele, was frightened by Zeus (q.v.), who appeared to her in thunder and lightning. He inflicted madness upon those who opposed him. His festivities, the Bacchanalia (q.v.), were marked by mass ecstasy (q.v.) and prophetic delirium (q.v.), which afflicted those possessed by the god.
Bibliography: Simon, B. 1978. *Mind and madness in Ancient Greece.*

DIOSCORIDES PEDANIUS. A Greek physician of the first century A.D. in the service of the Roman emperor Nero (q.v.). His remedies were mostly empirical and related to religious practices. He described some six hundred plants, prescribed mandragora (q.v.) for insomnia, and devised a soporific mixture that promoted deep sleep during surgical operations. His *De Materia Medica* influenced medicine for over fifteen hundred years. It is preserved in a ninth-century illustrated manuscript, now in the Bibliotheque Nationale in Paris and in the Vienna Codex, which was prepared for the Princess Julia Anicia in the sixth century, as well as in other copies and Latin and Arabic translations.
Bibliography: Castiglioni, A. 1946. *A history of medicine*, trans. E. B. Krumbhaar.

DIPPOLDISM. Flogging of school children. The term is derived from Dippold, the name of a German schoolmaster who was convicted of manslaughter. It also means flagellation (q.v.).
Bibliography: Hinsie, L. E., and Campbell, R. J. 1960. *Psychiatric dictionary*.

DIPSOMANIA. Mental disorder arising from alcoholic excesses. The term was introduced by Christoph W. Hufeland (q.v.) at the beginning of the nineteenth century.
See also ALCOHOLISM.

DIPSYCHISM. A model for the study of the human mind that evolved from magnetism (q.v.). It supposed a duality of mind and was refined by Max Dessoir (q.v.) in a book on the double ego.
Bibliography: Dessoir, M. 1890. *Das Doppel-Ich*.

DIRECTED DAYDREAM. A technique in the 1930s devised by the French psychiatrist Robert Desoille. The patient is requested to lie on a couch and then is asked to imagine that he is floating. He reports the thoughts that occur to him, and these are discussed with the therapist.
Bibliography: Desoille, R. 1938. *Exploration de l'effectivité subconsciente par la méthode du rêve éveillé*.

DISCOVERIE OF WITCHCRAFT, THE. A book by Reginald Scot (q.v.), published in 1584. It expressed his enlightened belief, which was supported by his experience as a justice of the peace, that those accused of witchcraft (q.v.), and sometimes the accusers, were mentally ill, rather than possessed by the devil. He realized that his views were too advanced for his times and wrote, "my greatest adversaries are young ignorance and old custome." *Daemonologie in Forme of a Dialogue* (q.v.) was written explicitly to refute his views. The last witch was hanged in England exactly one hundred years after his book was published.
Bibliography: Hunter, R., and Macalpine, I. 1963. *Three hundred years of psychiatry*.

DISEASE OF MELANCHOLY. The title of one of the earliest Arab treatises on psychiatry. It was written in the ninth century by Omran Ibn Ishac.
Bibliography: Baasher, T. 1975. The Arab Countries. In *World history of psychiatry*, ed. J. G. Howells.

DIVINATION. Supernatural means of predicting the future. Most ancient civilizations believed in it. Dreams (q.v.) and their interpretations were a prominent form of divination. They were particularly used in the practice of incubation (q.v.) sleep at health shrines. Possession (q.v.) by a god was also believed to produce prophecies. Other methods of divination were the interpretation of certain natural phenomena, such as earthquakes, thunder, or monstrous births. The practice reflected the anxiety aroused by phenomena that could not be explained and satisfied the need for reassurance by giving an illusion of knowledge.
See also ORACLES.
Bibliography: Lecleraq, A. B. 1975. *History of divination in antiquity.*

DIX, DOROTHEA LYNDE (1802-1887). An American social reformer. She was born in Hampden, Maine, and experienced little love from her father, an unstable, weak, and fanatical itinerant preacher, or from her mother, a depressed, chronic invalid. Her paternal grandfather, Dr. Dix, was the positive influence in her early life. At the age of twelve she escaped from her family and went to live with her grandmother; two years later she began to teach school, and, in spite of poor health, she remained dedicated to that task until she was thirty-nine. Her activities then turned to improving conditions for mental patients housed in almshouses and prisons. Her immense energy and determination brought about changes through Congress and through state legislatures in the United States. She was responsible for the building of no less than thirty state mental hospitals. She traveled to Europe and continued her crusade for better conditions for the pauper insane, bringing about many reforms. Tuberculosis (q.v.), malaria, a number of psychosomatic conditions, and recurrent depression only served to stimulate her activity and her desire to achieve her goals. She died at the age of eighty-five.
Bibliography: Tiffany, F. 1891. *Life of Dorothea Lynde Dix.*

DOBROVSKY, JOSEF (1753-1829). Czech writer and historian. His research into the literary works of his country stimulated a rebirth of literature in Czechoslovakia. Later in life he became mentally ill and was treated by Jan T. Held (q.v.).
Bibliography: Brock, P., and Skilling, H. G. 1970. *The Czech renascence of the nineteenth century.*

DODGSON, CHARLES LUTWIDGE (1832-1898). An English mathematician and writer. His books for children were written under the pseudonym Lewis Carroll. The early death of his mother profoundly affected him. His father was a clergyman, and he himself was ordained in 1861 but seldom preached, possibly because he stammered. His working life was spent at Christ Church, Oxford, where he became a Fellow after taking double honors in classics and mathematics. He could forget his extreme shyness only with little girls to whom he wrote delightful letters. His classic and much quoted work *Alice's Adventures in Wonderland*, published in 1865, originated from the tales he made up to amuse Alice Liddell, the daughter of Henry George Liddell, dean of Christ Church. Dodgson also wrote an unsuccessful novel *Sylvia and Bruno* (1887) in which he introduced supernatural phenomena.
Bibliography: Lennon, F. B. 1962. *The life of Lewis Carroll.*

DODOENS, REMBERT (c.1517-1585). A Dutch botanist. An English translation of his *New Herbal or History of Plants* was available in London in 1586. For melancholia (q.v.) he prescribed borage, tormentil, violets, thyme (qq.v.), winter savorie, and basil.
Bibliography: Arber, A. 1970. *Herbals: their origin and evolution.*

DODS, JOHN BOVEE (1795-1872). An American Universalist minister who was interested in medical problems, especially those of the mind. He believed that the mind worked through an electrical force that resided in the cerebellum. He employed electricity (q.v.) as a form of therapy and was an enthusiastic follower of mesmerism (q.v.), on which he lectured. In 1850 he wrote a book on *The Philosophy of Electrical Psychology.*
Bibliography: Tinterow, M. F. 1970. *Foundations of hypnosis: from Mesmer to Freud.*

DOGIEL, ALEXANDER (1852-1922). A Russian physician who was famous for his neurohistological research. In 1899, he made an important contribution to neurocytology with his classification of the neuron types in the spinal, sympathetic, intestinal, and cardiac ganglia. His lucid and precise writings were illustrated by his own drawings. He continued his work during the Russian revolution and until his death by cerebral hemorrhage.
Bibliography: Haymaker, W., and Schiller, F. 1970. *The founders of neurology.* 2d ed.

DOGMATIST SECT. A sect in Alexandria founded by Thessalus and Draco of Cos, sons of Hippocrates (q.v.). It tried to prevent any further medical research, believing that Hippocrates had recorded all that was essential in medicine. Some followers of Sigmund Freud (q.v.) felt the same about his work, which unfortunately hindered the advancement of psychiatry.
Bibliography: Alexander, F. G. and Selesnick, S. T. 1966. *The history of psychiatry.*

DOG-ROSE. *Rosa canina.* It was so named in antiquity because it was used to treat the bite of a mad dog.
Bibliography: Mayhew, A. 1979. *The rose: myth, folklore and legend.*

DOLCI, CARLO (1616-1686). An Italian painter. His themes were almost invariably religious, displaying an excess of piety, which may have been inculcated in him from childhood by monks. He was obsessional and insecure. On the back of each painting he wrote about his feelings during the work and noted a multitude of other details. When he was thirty-eight years old, he was advised to get married, and a bride was chosen for him. When he could not be found for the ceremony, he was discovered on his knees in a nearby chapel. He subsequently fathered seven daughters. In 1672, he was sent to Innsbruck by Anna de Medici on the occasion of her daughter's marriage to the Emperor Leopold. When Dolci came back, he was markedly depressed and accident prone. Felipo Baldinucci (1624-1696), Dolci's friend and biographer, writing shortly after his death, said:

Poor Carlo began to have so many misfortunes that one cannot count them. These were caused by a pernicious melancholic humour which, due to his pusillanimous, reserved and shy nature, had conquered him so completely that it was no longer possible to exchange a word with him, let alone hold a conversation. He only expressed himself with sighs, the effect, as far as one could see, of a mortal anguish of the heart. His closest friends laboured to draw him away from those thoughts which made him believe that he had by now lost all his ability and was good for nothing. . .

Dolci recovered after a priest ordered him to finish the painting he had begun of the Virgin Mary. Years later, his melancholy (*see* MELANCHOLIA) became worse when he was reproached for his slowness by one of his patrons. Baldinucci again recorded what happened:

He returned home, not at all his usual self, but in a most confused state of mind, to the greatest grief and wonder of his family. From that moment on his thoughts wandered away from art into strange waverings of obscure fantasies.

He never recovered.
Bibliography: Wittkower, R., and Wittkower, M. 1963. *Born under Saturn.*

DOLLHAUS. Early German term meaning "madhouse." As early as 1326 a dollhaus attached to the Georgshospital was erected at Ebing, Germany.
See also ASYLUMS.
Bibliography: Rosen, G. 1968. *Madness in society.*

DOMITIAN, TITUS FLAVIUS (A.D. 51-96). Roman emperor. At first he was a political reorganizer, but he later became unbalanced, suspicious, and embittered, and his reign degenerated into one of vice, persecution, cruelty, and homicide. He was murdered with the connivance of his wife, Domitia.

DONATISM. A form of hypnosis (*see* HYPNOTISM) in which imitation in induction is an important factor. It was so named after Donato, the professional name of Alfred d'Hont (q.v.).
Bibliography: Esquirol, J. E. D. 1865. Reprint 1965. *Mental maladies.*

DONATISTS. A religious Christian sect. It originated in North Africa in the fourth century and finally was annihilated by the Saracens in the seventh century. Donatists were subjected to extremely cruel persecutions, which they welcomed. Their fanaticism often led to frenzy ending in suicide (q.v.).
Bibliography: Alvarez, A. 1971. *The savage god: a study of suicide.*

DONATO. *See* HONT, ALFRED D'.

DONDERS, FRANCISCUS CORNELIUS (1818-1889). Dutch ophthalmologist. His experiments with reaction times and compound reactions contributed to the development of experimental psychology (q.v.). He formulated the law of eye movement, which is named after him.
Bibliography: Boring, E. G. 1950. *A history of experimental psychology.*

DONIZETTI, GAETANO (1797-1848). An Italian composer of operas. In his later years he suffered from general paralysis of the insane (q.v.) and was confined to a sanatorium at Ivry. Giuseppe Verdi (1813-1901) described his condition:

You ask me about Donizetti, and I shall tell you frankly, although it is not a pleasant story. I have not seen him yet, as it was thought ill-advised, but I assure you I very much want to, and if the opportunity presents itself for me to see him without anyone knowing of it, I certainly shall. His physical appearance is good, except that his head is constantly bowed over his chest and his eyes kept shut. He eats and sleeps well, but says hardly a word, and when he does it's very indistinct. If someone goes up to him, he opens his eyes for a moment. If they say, "Give me your hand," he extends it, and so on. Apparently this is a sign that his mind has not completely gone, although a dear friend of mine who is a doctor tells me that he does these things simply out of habit, and that it would be more encouraging if he were animated or even violently mad. There may perhaps be hope, but in his present condition it would take a miracle to improve him. Still, he is no worse now than he was six months ago, or a year ago.
[Letter to Giuseppina Appiani (*Letters of Giuseppe Verdi.* Edited by Charles Osborn.
London: Victor Gollancz Ltd., 1971.)]

Bibliography: Ashbrook, W. 1965. *Donizetti.*

DON JUAN. A legendary figure in many literary and musical works, which may be based upon the character of Don Juan Tenorio, a fourteenth-century Spaniard born in Seville. The name is used to describe insecure individuals who hide behind a façade of gallantry and boast of their amorous conquests, which constitute a never-ending search for the unattainable. Wolfgang Amadeus Mozart's *Don Giovanni* and Lord Byron's (q.v.) *Don Juan* are among the many works dealing with this theme.

DONNE, JOHN (1572-1631). English poet and dean of St. Paul's Cathedral in London. After the death of his father when he was a child, his mother married the president of the College of Physicians from whom Donne learnt medical terminology. He enjoyed an ideal marriage. In 1611, while he was in Paris, he experienced a vision of his wife carrying a dead child. A messenger from London later informed him that his wife had given birth to a dead child on the very day of his vision. When Ann died, Donne promised his children that they would never have a stepmother. From personal experience and observation, he knew that anxiety could cause sickness. He, himself, was prone to psychosomatic conditions and depression. He was forty-seven years old when he wrote a defense of suicide (q.v.) entitled *Biathanatos* (q.v.), in which he said "methinks I have the keys of my prison in mine own sword." He used poetry as a form of therapy. His preoccupation with death is reflected in the sermon "Death duel," which he preached when he was already very ill; it was his funeral oration. During the last days of his life, he asked to have his body measured in readiness for his coffin and had himself shrouded. On the day he died, he composed his hands and feet as they are usually arranged after death.
Bibliography: Bald, R. C. 1971. *John Donne: a life*.

DON QUIXOTE. A novel by Miguel de Cervantes (q.v.) in 1605. It is a parody of Spanish society of the sixteenth century. Its hero, sane in all else, is deluded in seeing wrongs where there are none and believes that it is his mission in life to put them right. Escape into fantasy relieves the pain of living in the present. Cervantes displayed a sensitive grasp of the psychology of mental illness and underlined the fact that even in psychosis (q.v.) there is an element of normal thinking.
Bibliography: Cervantes, M. 1970. *Don Quixote*, trans. J.H. Cohen.

DOORS OF PERCEPTION, THE. A book written by Aldous Huxley (q.v.) in 1954. It recounted his experiences when he was under the influence of mescaline (q.v.). He swallowed four-tenths of a gram of the drug, which changed the quality of his perception.
Bibliography: Huxley, A. 1954. *The doors of perception*.

DORA. A patient of Sigmund Freud (q.v.), the subject of a paper published in 1905. She was eighteen years old when he undertook her analysis. From the age of eight she had suffered from psychosomatic disorders culminating in periods of amnesia (q.v.) and aphonia with suicidal (*see* SUICIDE) tendencies. After three months she terminated her sessions with Freud but her neurotic (*see* NEUROSIS) symptoms never left her. Freud used her case history to demonstrate his interpretation of dreams (q.v.) and the part played by repression in emotional life.

Bibliography: Freud, S. 1905. *Fragment of an Analysis of a Case of Hysteria. The complete psychological works.* 1976. Ed. J. Stratchey.

DOREN, G.A. An American physician. He became the first superintendent of the Institution of Feebleminded Youth (q.v.) in Columbus, Ohio, which was founded in 1857. He was a founding member of the Association of Medical Officers of American Institutions for Idiots and Feeble-minded Persons (q.v.).

Bibliography: Kanner, L. 1964. *A history of the care and study of the mentally retarded.*

DORIAN LOVE. A term for male homosexuality (q.v.). The Dorians, one of the principal Hellenic races, introduced love for boys into ancient Greece. There it became fashionable and was regarded as a higher form of sexuality with no stigma attached to it.

Bibliography: Hammond, N. G. L. 1959. *A history of Greece.*

DORRIDGE GROVE. A private asylum (q.v.) in Warwickshire, England, founded in 1866 by a physician, Bell Fletcher, and a surgeon, J. Kimbell. It originally provided care for twenty idiot (q.v.) girls. It rapidly expanded, changed its name to Midland Counties Idiot Asylum, and was then supported by public subscriptions. In 1921 all female patients were moved elsewhere, but one old woman, by the name of Ada, refused to leave and remained there until her death in 1938 at the age of seventy-three; she had been in the institution a total of thirty-three years. In 1948 it was taken over by the state and it is now known as Middlefield Hospital. It offers care and rehabilitation for the mentally subnormal.

DOSTOEVSKY, FYODOR MIKHAILOVICH (1821-1881). A Russian novelist, born in Moscow. He was an extremely solitary man, who had been brought up in isolation. His father was a drunken, autocratic army surgeon, who admonished him to build a wall around himself to avoid being contaminated by others, and taught him that women should not be mentioned except in poetry. He lived in a dream world. He was in school when he was told that his father had been murdered by his serfs, and the news precipitated his first epileptic fit. He was a tortured individual searching for freedom of expression in protest against the Russian culture of his time. He was condemned to death for conspiring against the government, but he was

reprieved while facing the firing squad and sent to Siberia for four years. He married an hysterical (*see* HYSTERIA) invalid who brought more gloom to his already sad life. After her death and after a disastrous love affair, he married again, this time more successfully. He died in Saint Petersburg, and his funeral gave rise to widespread public mourning inspired by the respect and love that he had earned. Among his best known novels those of particular psychological interest are *The Idiot* (1868), *Crime and Punishment*, and *The Brothers Karamazov* (q.v.), a powerful work reflecting a deep psychological understanding. Sigmund Freud (q.v.) wrote a paper "Dostoevsky and Parricide" in which he expressed doubts about Dostoevsky's epilepsy, which he thought to be part of Dostoevsky's neuroticism. His compulsive gambling is also discussed by Freud, as well as other psychopathological traits of his personality.
Bibliography: Magarshak, D. 1962. *Dostoevsky: a life*.

DOUBLE. A duplicate of oneself. The idea of a double, as an apparition, or a hallucination of self is common to many countries and many legends. Examples can be found in Egyptian and Greek literature and in the Talmud (q.v.). In Germany it is termed the *Doppelganger*, meaning literally the "double walker." In Scotland there is the belief that a person who is about to die will see his own image, called a *fetch* or a *wraith*. Among the many writers who have used this idea in their novels, are Fyodor Dostoevsky (q.v.) and Oscar Wilde (q.v.). Painters also have employed it. Dante Gabriel Rossetti (q.v.) painted a picture of two lovers meeting their own images in a dark wood. The first reference in pathology is that of Carolus Linnaeus (q.v.), who often experienced visual hallucinations of himself. The phenomenon is clinically termed *heautoscopy*.
Bibliography: Critchley, M. 1971. Corporeal awareness. In *Modern Perspectives in World Psychiatry*, ed. J. G. Howells.

DOUCHE. A form of treatment in which water was poured on the head of a patient from a height. It was known in antiquity and continued to be used well into the nineteenth century. Jean Esquirol (q.v.) advocated it but advised great care in its administration. It was said to act morally in reducing difficult patients to obedience, but it often caused cardialgia and vomiting. (See Plate 3.)
Bibliography: Esquirol, J. E. D. 1865. Reprint 1965. *Mental Maladies*.

DOVER, THOMAS (1660-1742). English buccaneer physician, inventor of Dover's powder. He sacked Guayaquil, in Peru, cured his sailors of the plague, and rescued Alexander Selkirk (Robinson Crusoe) from a desert island. Writing in 1733 on *Hypocondriacal and Hysterical Diseases*, he asserted that the two terms referred to the same disease, "what we call hypocondriacal in men, we term hysterical in women." He added, "there is

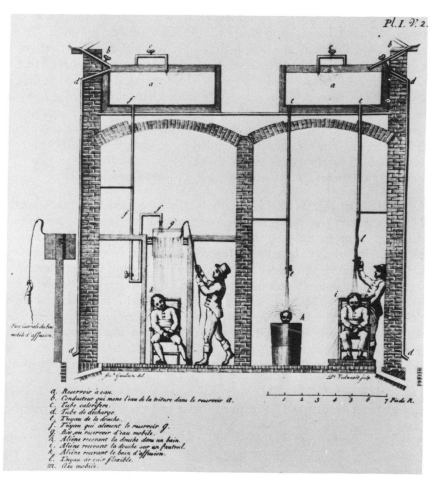

3. A DOUCHING MACHINE. Such a contraption was used for pouring water on the head of patients. The direction of the jet could be regulated. From J. Guislain, *Traité sur l'aliénation mentale et sur les hospices des aliénés*, 1826. By courtesy of the Department of Medical Illustration, Ipswich Hospital.

no disease incident to human bodies but these hystericisms will counterfeit so exactly, that without the greatest caution, the physician must be deceived." See also HYPOCHONDRIA and HYSTERIA.
Bibliography: Strong, L. A. 1955. *Dr. Quicksilver.*

DOWN, JOHN LANGDON HAYDON (1828-1896). An English psychiatrist and medical superintendent of Earlswood Asylum for Idiots. In his paper "Ethnic Classification of Idiots" he described mongolism (q.v.), now termed Down's syndrome. He believed that certain mental defectives exhibited the physical characteristics of certain races. Down believed that the Caucasian race had reached the pinnacle of evolution and argued that if a mental defective in a white race could show characteristics of a nonwhite race, then racial differences were not specific. Through this argument he tried to counter racial prejudice especially as it was related to slavery in the United States. His views were extended by Francis G. Crookshank (q.v.) in his book *The Mongol in our Midst* (1924).
Bibliography: Penrose, L. S., and Smith, G. F. 1966. *Down's anomaly.*

DOWNAME, JOHN (?-1652). An English Puritan clergyman, born in London. Among his duties was the spiritual treatment of those parishioners suffering from mental disorders that were not considered of physical aetiology. He wrote *A Treatise of Anger* (q.v.) which was published in 1609. He demonstrated his understanding of psychology in his observations and treatment of patients suffering from anger, which he termed "a short madness." In therapy he used silence and was careful not to antagonize the "chollericke man," but rather to sympathize with mild and discrete words that included wise counselling. He was aware of the futility of offering advice to an angry man.
Bibliography: Hunter, R. and Macalpine, I. 1963. *Three hundred years of psychiatry.*

DOWNSHIRE HOSPITAL. A mental hospital in Downpatrick, Northern Ireland, inaugurated in 1869 with the name of Down County Lunatic Asylum. Before that date, mental patients were cared for in private asylums (q.v.) or in the Belfast District Asylum. On the day of opening, fifty patients, twenty-five of each sex, left Belfast dressed in their best clothes. They marched in procession to the station, headed by the hospital brass band (q.v.), which, except for the leader, was also composed of patients and, on this auspicious occasion, traveled free. On their arrival at Downpatrick, they reformed ranks and joined by many spectators, proceeded to the new hospital to the lively tune of the "Donegal March." At the end of the journey, they were received by the superintendent, Dr. Tyner. The band struck up "For he's a jolly good fellow," and Tyner returned the compliment by entertaining the musicians and officials until the time of departure of the last train to Belfast.
Bibliography: Parkinson, R. E. 1969. *Historical Sketch of Downshire Hospital.*

DOYLE, ARTHUR CONAN (1859-1930). British physician and writer, born in Edinburgh, Scotland. The strong-man image that he presented to the world was only half of his personality, the other half was that of a hurt and perplexed individual. As an adult, Doyle abandoned the Catholic faith and tried to replace it with oriental religion and telepathy (q.v.). He was gullible in occult matters and even accepted the claim of two young children that they were in touch with fairy folks. After the death of his eldest son and his younger brother in World War I, he became interested in spiritualism (q.v.) and in 1926 wrote a *History of Spiritualism*. He is better known as the creator of Sherlock Holmes, the amateur detective who solves mysteries by using his powers of deduction. The character was based on Dr. Joseph Bell, whom Doyle had met in his student days at the Hospital for Sick Children in Edinburgh. Bell's uncanny knack of diagnosis had made a deep impression on Doyle. The fictional Holmes was endowed with the same foibles as Dr. Bell, including introspection and the abuse of cocaine (q.v.) as an antidepressant.
Bibliography: Symons, J. 1979. *Portrait of an artist: Conan Doyle.*

DRAGE, WILLIAM (1637-1669). An English physician and medical writer. As a believer in witchcraft (q.v.) and astrology (q.v.), he was convinced that the devil could cause all kinds of diseases and aberrations of behavior. He thought that witchcraft could afflict people "with strange and unaccustomed symptoms," that did not respond to "ordinary and natural remedies." In 1664, he published a volume entitled *A Physical Nosonomy: Or a New and True Description of the Law of God (called Nature) in the Body of Man. To Which is Added a Treatise of Diseases from Witchcraft.* In this work he described the symptomatology of demonic possession (q.v.) and suggested some forms of therapy that included punishment, imprisonment, or even execution.
Bibliography: Tourney, G. 1972. The Physician and Witchcraft in Restoration England. *Med. Hist.* 16: 143-55.

DRAMA. In the nineteenth century it was believed that theatrical presentations were damaging to people possessing nervous dispositions. Jean Esquirol (q.v.) banned all plays from his mental hospital. He wrote, "a mind at all accustomed to reflection, is astonished that theatrical representations should formerly have been permitted at Charenton; and a German author regards the multiplication of theatres as one of the causes of the great number of insane people in Germany." Psychodrama (q.v.) is now used for therapeutic purposes.
Bibliography: Esquirol, J. E. D. 1845. Reprint. 1965. *Mental Maladies: a treatise on insanity.*

DREAMS. Most primitive people and ancient civilizations have believed dreams to have a prophetic or directive value or to act as a warning. Hippocrates (q.v.) considered dreams to be produced by the mind, which during sleep was free to give expression to the individual's desires. Galen (q.v.) thought that dreams were helpful in formulating a diagnosis of a disease, as well as in arriving at a prognosis. His own personal decisions were often guided by what he had dreamed. Sigmund Freud (q.v.) gave new impetus to the study of dreams in 1900 when he published his *Interpretation of Dreams*, an accumulation of observations collected over several years.
Bibliography: Hadfield, J. A. 1954. *Dreams and nightmares*.

DREIKURS, RUDOLPH (1897-). An Austrian psychiatrist who emigrated to the United States in 1937. He was a follower of Alfred Adler (q.v.) and an early pioneer in group psychotherapy (q.v.). He thought that group psychotherapy was a natural consequence of the principles enunciated by Adler, who had "always considered man as a social being and socially motivated."
Bibliography: Dreikurs, R. 1959. Early Experiments with Group Psychotherapy. *Am. J. Psychother.* 13: 884.

DRESSER, HEINRICH (1860-1924). German discoverer of the ester of morphine (q.v.) known as heroin (q.v.) in 1898.
Bibliography: Garrison, F. H. 1929. *An introduction to the history of medicine.*

DREVER, JAMES (1873-1950). The first professor of psychology at Edinburgh University in Scotland. He was particularly interested in the problems of teaching psychology in terms that could be understood by all. *The Psychology of Everyday Life, The Psychology of Practical Life*, and *A Dictionary of Psychology* are among his works.
Bibliography: Flugel, J. C. 1945. *A hundred years of psychology.*

DRIESCH, HANS ADOLF EDUARD (1867-1941). German biologist and philosopher. He developed the theory of vitalism (q.v.), which assumes the existence of a vital force that is independent of the laws of physics and chemistry and gives direction and form to all living organisms. He was also interested in parapsychology.
Bibliography: Alexander, F. G., and Selesnick, S. T. 1966. *The history of psychiatry.*

DROPSY. The accumulation of fluid in the tissues of the body. Hippocrates (q.v.) thought that physical diseases often ameliorated mental symptoms. He believed that dropsy, when it occurred in the insane, was good.
Bibliography: Zilboorg, G. 1941. *A history of medical psychology.*

DRUGS. In medicine, substances used for healing. The use of animal, vegetable, and mineral matter as medications in the treatment of mental

disorders has been practiced from antiquity. Some of the substances used were harmful, some innocuous, and a few beneficial in as much as they relieved some symptoms. In some cultures drugs were used to achieve trance-like states, during which the intoxicated person was believed to be capable of prophesies or to be capable of committing acts alien to his nature (*see* ASSASSINS). Johann Weyer (q.v.) thought that witches (*see* WITCHCRAFT) could be people experiencing hallucinations (q.v.) after the ingestion of some intoxicating herb. In more modern times Georg E. Stahl (q.v.) and Philippe Pinel (q.v.) objected to the indiscriminate use of drugs in psychiatry. Addiction to drugs was a powerful factor in the lives of such individuals as Charles Baudelaire, Samuel Coleridge, and Thomas De Quincey (qq.v.)
Bibliography: Zilboorg, G. 1941. *A history of medical psychology.*

DRUNKEN HELOT. An expression exemplifying the idea that an example of bad behavior teaches its avoidance. The Spartans would make a helot (slave) drunk to offer their sons an example of the dangers of excessive drinking.
Bibliography: 1975. *Brewer's dictionary of phrase and fable.*

DRYDEN, JOHN (1631-1700). English poet, dramatist, critic, and translator. Born into a Puritan family, he preferred the gay life of London to the prudent ways of his native Northamptonshire. He began writing verses as a young boy and later lived by his poetry. His marriage to Lady Elizabeth Howard was unhappy, and his unsettled emotional life was reflected in his biting satire, which at times sank to indecency and lewdness. His philosophy is shown in his *Religio Leici* (1682) in which he rejected reason in the search for truth but at the same time distrusted personal interpretation of the Scriptures as well as the Roman Catholic belief in the pope's infallibility. Notwithstanding his doubts, in later life he became a Catholic. He used to be purged (*see* PURGING) and bled (*see* BLEEDING) before writing because he believed that men of genius and the insane stood near together.
Bibliography: Johnson, S. *The lives of the poets.* (1779). The World Classics 1969.

DUBINI, ANGELO (1813-1902). An Italian physician. In 1846 he described a variety of chorea characterized by sudden and violent movements. The disease was termed electric chorea and later became known as Dubini's disease.
Bibliography: Schmidt, J. E. 1959. *Medical discoveries, who and when.*

DUBOIS, JACQUES (1478-1555). A French anatomist, also called Sylvius. He was Andreas Vesalius' (q.v.) teacher in Paris. He was so devoted to Galen's (q.v.) theories that he could not bear to see his errors corrected by Vesalius. When Vesalius published his great work on anatomy, Dubois declared him insane. Although a popular teacher, he was a bigot who was harsh and miserly.

Bibliography: Zilboorg, G. 1941. *A history of medical psychology.*

DUBOIS, PAUL CHARLES (1848-1918). A Swiss neuropathologist. He believed that most mental disorders had a psychological aetiology and that psychological functions depended on the brain but could be modified by psychotherapy (q.v.). He applied psychological principles to the treatment of neurosis (q.v.) by attempting to convince the patient that his behavior and feelings were not rational. He also regarded persuasion as distinct from suggestion and hypnosis (*see* HYPNOTISM). The term "psychoneurosis" (q.v.) was introduced by him.

Bibliography: Dubois, P. C. 1905. *The psychic treatment of nervous disorders,* trans. W. A. White and S. E. Jeliffe.

DUBOIS D'AMIENS, FREDERIC (1799-1873). A French physician who wrote on hysteria (q.v.) and hypochondria (q.v.). He supported the fashionable theory of animal magnetism (q.v.). In 1833 he published a treatise entitled *Histoire Philosophique de l'Hypochondrie et de l'Histérie,* which was a comprehensive review of the literature on the subject.

DUBOIS-REYMOND, EMIL (1818-1896). German physiologist and pioneer in experimental physiology. His work included research on animal electricity (q.v.) and the physiology of nerves. He was aware that it is impossible to understand the deeper functions of the mind by biological techniques alone.

Bibliography: Haymaker, W. and Schiller, F. 1970. *The founders of neurology.* 2d ed.

DUCASSE, ISIDORE LUCIEN. *See* LAUTRÉAMONT, COMTE DE.

DUCHENNE DE BOULOGNE, GUILLAUME BENJAMIN AMAND (1806-1875). A French neurologist. In 1858 he described tabes dorsalis, a disease of the nervous system caused by syphilis (q.v.). It was later termed Duchenne's disease. In 1862, he published a collection of photographs that revealed the changes in facial expression during intense emotional states.

Bibliography: Haymaker, W., and Schiller, F. 1970. *The founders of neurology.* 2d ed.

DUCKING. A form of treatment for melancholia (q.v.) and mania (q.v.). Hermann Boerhaave (q.v.) suggested that patients should be thrown into the sea without warning and kept under the water just short of the point of drowning. Benjamin Rush (q.v.) also believed in this form of therapy, but Philippe Pinel (q.v.) was unequivocally opposed to it.

See also IMMERSION.
Bibliography: Zilboorg, G. 1941. *A history of medical psychology.*

DUENDE. An incubus (q.v.) in the folklore of Latin America. Mental illness is often attributed to his activities. His appearance, dress, habits, and behavior are defined by popular beliefs. According to these beliefs, his main activity is chasing girls for sexual purposes, although he also rides stallions by moonlight, swings from trees, and loves good music. Because he is believed to be upset by out-of-tune instruments, they are often used to drive him away. Exorcism (q.v.) is of no avail against this particular devil and those who believe in him are caused to present at psychiatric clinics with severe emotional disorders.
Bibliography: Leon, C. A. 1975. El Duende and other incubi. Suggestive interactions between culture, the devil and the brain. *Arch. Gen. Psychiat.* 32: 155-62.

DUFFIUS (?-967). A king of Scotland. He was said to be a victim of witchcraft (q.v.), which caused him to fall into a strange sickness and waste away. According to legend, a girl, who was heard uttering mysterious words, was followed to her home where her mother and other women were found slowly melting a wax image of the king. The moment the image was broken, and the old women condemned to death, the king recovered.
Bibliography: Donaldson, G. 1965. *Scottish kings.*

DUGDALE, RICHARD (fl. 1697). A self-styled prophet, born in Surrey, England. He was believed to be possessed (*see* POSSESSION) by the devil. During his hysterical (*see* HYSTERIA) fits, he would purport to be a prophet and predict all sorts of dramatic events.
Bibliography: Stephen, L. and Lee, S. 1969. *Dictionary of national biography.*

DUGDALE, RICHARD L. (1841-1883). American merchant and penologist. The Prison Association of New York appointed him to report on county jails. During the course of his visits, he found one family with no less than six members in jail, which led him to a genealogical investigation of five generations of that family. He called them the Jukes (q.v.) and concluded that crime, disease, and poverty were social conditions genetically transmitted from generation to generation and influenced by adverse environment. Of the 709 individuals he observed, only one was mentally retarded. Unfortunately this fact was overlooked by his readers, who also ignored his findings on environmental influences and concluded that social ills were always tied to retardation and genetically transmitted.
Bibliography: Dugdale, R. L. 1877. *The Jukes: a study in crime, pauperism, disease, and heredity.*

DUMAS, ALEXANDRE (DUMAS PÈRE) (1802-1870). French dramatist and novelist. His father was the illegitimate son of the marquis Antoine-

Alexandre Davy de La Pailleterie and a negress, Marie Dumas. Dumas' own liaison in Paris with Marie Catherine Labay (1794-1868) resulted in the birth of his son, Alexandre Dumas (fils) (q.v.). He later married an actress, but the marriage ended in separation, and he returned to Marie Labay. His last few years were marred by scandals and debts, until his daughter took charge of his household. Dumas' powerful imagination created suspenseful plots, although he paid little attention to psychological motivations, character analysis, or historical accuracy. During his colorful life he had many interests, from magnetism (q.v.), which he practiced, to revolution, which he experienced when he joined Garibaldi in Italy. His twenty-two volume autobiography *Mes Memoirs* (1852-1855) provides a lively record of his adventurous life and an interesting account of his odd relationship with his son with whom he shared mistresses. The phrase "cherchez la femme" was coined by him.
Bibliography: Hemming, F. W. J. 1979. *The king of romance: a portrait of Alexandre Dumas.*

DUMAS, ALEXANDRE (DUMAS FILS) (1824-1895). French novelist and dramatist, the illegitimate son of Alexandre Dumas (q.v.). His early years were marred by poverty and taunts about his illegitimacy. He never recovered from these experiences and remained a moralist all his life. His writings contain autobiographical material. *La Dame aux Camélias* (1848), which gave Giuseppi Verdi (1813-1901) the libretto for his opera *La Traviata* (1853), was largely based on his own affair with Marie Duplessis; *L'affaire Clémenceau* (1866) contains an account of his unhappy childhood and *Un Père Prodigue* (1859) is a portrait of his own flamboyant father. Most of his novels reflect nineteenth-century morality and its preoccupation with "fallen women" and dire warnings against pleasure and free love. They owe their success to their emotional appeal and Dumas' masterly handling of dramatic events.
Bibliography: Seillière, E. 1921. *La morale de Dumas fils.*

DUMMER, MRS. WILLIAM F. An American philanthropist. She was interested in juvenile delinquency and commissioned Dr. William Healy (q.v.) to do research into its causes and to devise a program of prevention. Her efforts led to the foundation of the Juvenile Psychopathic Institute of Chicago (q.v.) in 1909, which she supported financially. The institute was a forerunner of child guidance clinics (q.v.).
Bibliography: Levy, D. M. 1968. Beginnings of the child guidance movement. *Am. J. Orthopsych.* 38:799-804.

DUMPS. In the sixteenth century this term was used for slow and mournful dances or plaintive tunes, hence the expression "to be in the dumps," to be in low spirits.
Bibliography: 1978. *Brewer's dictionary of phrase and fable.*

DUNBAR, HELEN FLANDERS (1902-1959). An American psychiatrist who greatly contributed to advances in psychosomatic medicine (q.v.). She devised personality profiles, postulating that most sufferers of certain organic diseases display psychological similarities peculiar to each disorder, for example, the arthritic personality, the coronary personality, and so on. Among her works are *Emotions and Bodily Changes* (1935, revised 1954), *Psychosomatic Diagnosis* (1943), and *Psychiatry in the Medical Specialties* (1959).

DUNCAN, ANDREW (1744-1824). British physician, medical writer, and professor at Edinburgh University. He was a popular and much beloved man. He founded the Royal Public Dispensary in Edinburgh. After campaigning for a public lunatic asylum (q.v.) for many years, in 1807 he obtained a royal charter that provided for the erection of a public lunatic asylum at Morningside. It was called the Edinburgh Lunatic Asylum (q.v.) and opened in 1813. The inspiration for such an institution came to him following the death of his patient, Robert Fergusson (q.v.) in a workhouse. Duncan was a pioneer in mental welfare in Scotland and a founder of medical clubs and societies. The oldest medical dining club in Great Britain, the Aesculapian Club, was founded by him in 1773. In the same year, he founded the quarterly journal *Medical and Philosophical Commentaries*. His main work, *Elements of Therapeutics*, was published in 1770.
Bibliography: Henderson, D. K. 1964. *The evolution of psychiatry in Scotland.*

DUNCAN, ISADORA (1878-1927). An American dancer who evolved a natural style of dancing that was based on classical Greek art. She was outspoken, unconventional, and excitable. Her first two children, both illegitimate, were accidentally drowned when the car in which they were traveling fell into the Seine. The car was a covered limousine, and the accident left her with a phobia, (*see* PHOBIAS) of covered cars, and she felt suffocated every time she was compelled to enter one. In 1922, she married the Russian poet Sergei Esenin (q.v.), but they soon separated. Her life was marred to the end by accidents. She died by strangulation when her long scarf became caught in the rear wheel of the open car in which she was riding.
Bibliography: Seroff, V. 1972. *The real Isadora.*

DUNCAN, P. M. An English medical practitioner. He was physician to the Eastern Counties Asylum for Idiots and Imbeciles, at Colchester, England. In his report for 1860, congenital mental defectives were classified in three grades: simpletons, imbeciles (q.v.), and idiots (q.v.).
Bibliography: Duncan, P. M. and Millard, W. 1866. *A manual for the classification, training, and education of the feebleminded, imbecile and idiotic.*

DUNCE. A term first used in the sixteenth century, derived from John Duns Scotus (q. v.). It indicates a stupid person.
Bibliography: 1978. *Brewer's dictionary of phrase and fable.*

DUNDEE LUNATIC ASYLUM. A mental hospital in Scotland. It was developed in 1820 as a part of the General Hospital, founded in 1788. It later was called Dundee Royal Hospital and subsequently known as Gowrie House. Its foundation was sponsored by public subscription.
See also ROYAL ASYLUMS.
Bibliography: Henderson, D. K. 1964. *The evolution of psychiatry in Scotland.*

DUNGLISON, ROBLEY (1798-1869). An American physiologist. He gave the first known description of chronic hereditary chorea in 1842, which later became known as Huntington's chorea because of the more detailed description given by George Huntington (q.v.).
Bibliography: Schmidt, J. E. 1959. *Medical discoveries, who and when.*

DUNS SCOTUS, JOHN (1265?-1308). A Scholastic (*see* SCHOLASTICISM) theologian, born in Scotland. His precision and dialectical skills earned him the title of "Doctor Subtilis." He was the founder of a scholastic system termed Scotism. It tended to follow Aristotelian principles in opposition to the teaching of Saint Thomas Aquinas (q.v.) and argued that faith rests upon will. His numerous works on philosophy, religion, and logic were textbooks in the universities until the sixteenth century when they became ridiculed because they were in opposition to the new learning. The term "duns" or "dunce" (q.v.), which already indicated a hair-splitter or a caviller, became synonymous with blockhead, or an obstinate person, impervious to and incapable of learning.
Bibliography: Kanner, L. 1964. *A history of the care and study of the mentally retarded.*

DUPOTET DE SENNEVOY, J. (1796-?). A French magnetiser, descendant of an impoverished noble family. As a young man he practiced magnetism (q.v.) on two young women and became terror stricken when he could not wake them for several hours. In spite of this early experience, he believed that his mission in life was the promotion of magnetism and that he was the incarnation of it. He experimented in producing physiological changes under hypnosis.. He would draw a white circle on a black floor and make his subject stare at it until hallucinations (q.v.) were produced. His delusion (q.v.) of grandeur was evident in many of his statements.
Bibliography: Thornton, E. M. 1976. *Hypnotism, hysteria and epilepsy: an historical synthesis.*

DUPRÉ, ERNEST PIERRE (1862-1921). French physician and pyschiatrist, who taught legal psychiatry at St. Anne's Hospital (q.v.). He coined

the term "coenestopathic states" to describe certain disorders of subjective experience such as psychogenic pain.
Bibliography: Hirsch, S. R., and Shepherd, M., eds. 1974. *Themes and variations in European psychiatry.*

DUQUESNOY, FRANCESCO (1594-1643). A Flemish sculptor who worked mostly in Rome. In spite of his success, he was deeply depressed, paranoid (*see* PARANOIA), and obsessional (*see* OBSESSION). His biographer, Giovanni Passeri (1610-1679), wrote that he was:

so hesitant and careful in every particular that he wore out his life in irresolution. Nor did he ever come to a decision on anything without long and tiresome consideration which went into minutiae of no importance. This incapacity of his caused him to obtain little work and money, because his dilatoriness exasperated those who wanted his works.

Passeri also recorded that Duquesnoy suffered from continuous vertigo and that "this complaint of his progressed so much that he began to go out of his mind and to show signs of real madness, not of the impetuous and raging kind, but just wandering."
Bibliography: Wittkower, R., and Wittkower, M. 1963. *Born under Saturn.*

DURAND DE GROS, JOSEPH PIERRE (1826-1901). A French physiologist. He also wrote under the name of J. P. Philips. He became an exponent of magnetism (q.v.) and wrote about the relationship between spirit and matter. He also wrote about braidism (q.v.). To describe his own theories he coined a number of new terms; polypsychism (q.v.) was one of these. The school of Salpêtrière (q.v.) and the Nancy school (q.v.) were connected with his work.
Bibliography: Philips, J. P. 1855. *Electrodynamism vital.*

DÜRER, ALBRECHT (1471-1528). German painter and engraver. His work reflects the religious preoccupation of the time and his own personal troubled feelings about religion. He seems to have been torn between humanism and the doctrines of the Reformation as preached by Martin Luther (q.v.), whom he greatly admired. Death, pestilence, the devil, temptation, and divine punishment are much in evidence in his works. His own emotional turmoil caused unhappiness in his marriage and made personal relationships difficult. He painted his first self-portrait when he was thirteen years old and painted many more through the years. In one of them he identifies himself with Christ; in others he has a strange feminine quality. His brooding engraving of *Melencolia I* shows a dejected, enigmatic female figure surrounded by what Giorgio Vasari called "all the instruments that lead man to melancholy", stressing the belief of the time that excessive intellectual work would produce mental instability.
Bibliography: Panofsky, E. 1955. *The life and art of Albrecht Dürer.*

DURET, LOUIS (1527-1586). French physician, first physician to Henry III. In his writings he emphasized the importance of clinical observation. When Martha Brossier (q.v.) was accused of witchcraft (q.v.), he was called upon to examine her. He reported that her symptoms were due to disease and not to supernatural causes.

DURHAM DECISION, DURHAM TEST. The 1954 ruling by the United States Court of Appeals. It states that a psychiatrist may testify about the relevant details of a mental illness affecting an accused individual. Before this ruling, a psychiatrist's opinion was sought only to determine whether the accused could distinguish right from wrong or could not resist the impulse that led to his offense.

DURKHEIM, ÉMILE (1858-1917). A French sociologist, often called the father of modern sociology. Even in his youth, he was involved in politics and social questions. He believed in a collective social thought and opposed individualism. *Suicide*, one of his most important works, was published in 1897. It was the result of his investigation into the variation in the suicide (q.v.) rate among different groups, for he considered suicide a social phenomenon. In *The Division of Labour* (1893) he introduced the term *anomie* to indicate a pathological state where social norms are conflicting or nonexistent. He thought that totemism was the origin of all religions. He believed that what men called God was really society, as it had all the attributes of God.
Bibliography: Lukes, S. 1973. *Émile Durkheim: his life and work.*

DUSK OF MANKIND (MENSCHHEI TSDÄMMERUNG). Title of a German booklet written in 1929 by C. von Behr-Pinnow. It was one of the many publications of the period that expressed the international concern that mental defectives would produce more mental defectives, thus endangering civilization and mankind.
See also EUGENICS.
Bibliography: Kanner, L. 1964. *A history of the care and study of the mentally retarded.*

DUSSER DE BARENNE, JOANNES GREGORIUS (1885-1940). Dutch physiologist and psychiatrist. He demonstrated the major functional subdivisions of the sensory cortex. In 1930 he emigrated to the United States because of the intolerable religious restrictions imposed upon Dutch universities. The technique of laminar thermocoagulation came to him in a dream during a period of intense depression following the death of his wife. He had been concerned about the lack of a method for determining which

layers of the cortex were involved in sensation. He dreamed of an egg cooking slowly, which gave him the idea of applying a brass rod previously heated in boiling water to the cortex.
Bibliography: Haymaker, W., and Schiller, F. 1970. *The founders of neurology.* 2d. ed.

DVOINIK (THE DOUBLE). A novel by Fyodor Dostoevsky (q.v.) first published in 1846. It is a story of a rather insignificant office worker, Golyatkin, who slowly becomes insane. He meets a man who looks and dresses like him, and he befriends and protects this stranger. His new friend, at first humble and timid, becomes increasingly demanding and arrogant and eventually deprives him of his job, his friends, and his money. Golyatkin's confusion increases, and in the end he is sent to an asylum (q.v.). The story is an allegory of the sick self taking control of the healthy part of the individual.
See also DOUBLE.
Bibliography: Dostoevsky, F. 1945. *The Double.* In *The short novels of Dostoevsky.*

DYMPHNA, SAINT. A seventh-century Irish princess, convert to Christianity. She took refuge in Gheel, Belgium, to escape the rage and incestuous advances of her pagan father. He pursued her to her hiding place and beheaded her. She became the patron saint of Gheel. Three different versions of the legend offer reasons why Saint Dymphna became associated with mental disease: she was driven insane by her father's behavior and cruelty; her father was insane, and she forgave him; and some lunatics (q.v.) who witnessed her beheading were so affected that they recovered their reason. Gradually, a system of community care for the insane who came in pilgrimage to her shrine developed, and to this day mental patients are cared for in local households. (See Plate 4.)
See also BOARDING OUT OF MENTAL PATIENTS and GHEEL COLONY.
Bibliography: Pierloot, R. 1975. Belgium. In *World History of Psychiatry*, ed. J. G. Howells.

DYSENTERY. An intestinal disorder characterized by severe diarrhea. Hippocrates (q.v.) believed that dysentery and other physical disorders occurring in a person suffering from insanity would ameliorate his condition.
Bibliography: Hippocrates *Aphorisms* 7. 5.

DYSLEXIA. The impaired ability to understand what is read. It is due to constitutional or acquired brain dysfunction. The term was first employed in Germany by Rudolf Berlin (q.v.) in 1887.
Bibliography: Coltheart, M.; Patterson, K; and Marshall, J. C., eds. 1980. *Deep dyslexia.*
Tizard, J. 1972. *Children with specific reading difficulties.*

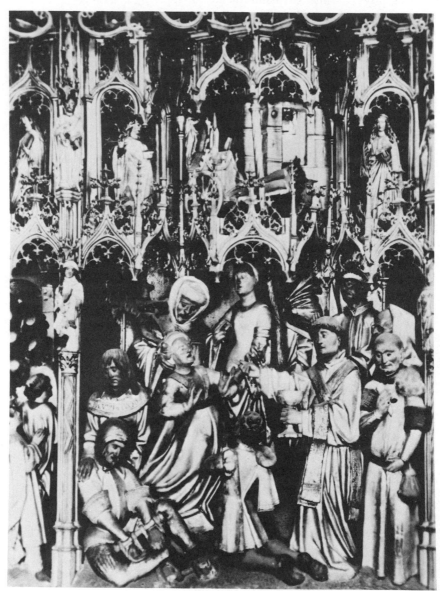

4. PILGRIMS TO ST. DYMPHNA CHURCH. A carving in the Church of St. Dymphna, Gheel, executed by Jan Wave in the sixteenth century, depicts mentally ill pilgrims, one of them with bound hands, seeking a cure at the shrine of the Saint. By courtesy of the Department of Medical Illustration, Ipswich Hospital.

DYSMNESIA. A term, derived from the Greek, indicating poor memory (q.v.). It was first introduced into medical psychology by De Valenzi (1728-1813).
Bibliography: Zilboorg, G. 1941. *A history of medical psychology.*

E

EARLE, PLINY (1809-1892). An American psychiatrist. In 1844 he became superintendent of the Bloomingdale Asylum (q.v.) in New York. He instituted manual work as a form of therapy, which may have been inspired by the work of his father, a manufacturer and improver of wool-carding machines. In 1863 he became professor of psychological medicine at Berkshire Medical Institution in Pittsfield, Massachusetts, thus inaugurating the teaching of psychiatry in medical schools in the United States. In 1864 he became superintendent of the State Lunatic Hospital at Northampton, Massachusetts, and remained for twenty-one years. Having visited many European institutions, he was well acquainted with psychiatric practice in Europe and made American psychiatrists aware of the new ideas and methods of treatment developed by European medical men. He recognized the fallacy of the curability statistics that were then fashionable and published in 1877 a critical analysis of hospital statistics under the title of *The Curability of Insanity* (q.v.). He was a pioneer in occupational therapy (q.v.) and family care and was one of the thirteen founding fathers of the American Psychiatric Association (q.v.).
Bibliography: Deutsch, A. 1949. *The mentally ill in America.*

EARTHQUAKES OF LONDON (8 February and 8 March 1750). These earth tremors were regarded by the people of London, encouraged by the preachers, as warnings from God against their way of life. A Lifeguardsman increased the general panic by running through the streets predicting a third and more disastrous earthquake in a month's time. His prediction so excited him that the day before the expected earthquake he became delirious and was admitted to Bethlem Royal Hospital (q.v.). His wife, when asked whether he had previously shown signs of madness, replied that he had not and that he was in his right mind now. The *Whitehall Evening Post*, however, reported that the man had long been affected with religious mania (q.v.) and

wild delusions. The episode was the subject of satirical drawings and comments.
Bibliography: O'Donoghue, E. G. 1914. *The story of Bethlehem Hospital.*

EASTERN STATE HOSPITAL. *See* WILLIAMSBURG EASTERN LUNATIC ASYLUM.

EAST SUSSEX ASYLUM. A mental hospital in Hailsham, England. In the nineteenth century, it pioneered a self-contained unit for short-stay cases. In 1900, the hospital changed its name to Hellingly Hospital.

EBBINGHAUS, HERMANN (1850-1909). A German psychologist. After studying philosophy, he turned to scientific psychology and applied experimental methods to higher mental processes. In this he was self-taught, but he possessed a great facility for mastering facts, extracting the essential elements from them, and expressing his findings in a lucid and precise manner. Although his scientific approach was rigid, he was a tolerant man, who never abused his intellectual gifts and overcame difficulties with his sense of humor. His greatest contribution to psychology was his experimental work on the measurement of memory (q.v.). He invented the nonsense syllables for testing memory and devised a test, known as the Ebbinghaus Completion Test, for measuring the intelligence of schoolchildren. He also postulated a theory of color vision. In 1890 he and Arthur König (q.v.) founded a new journal *Zeitschrift für Psychologie und Physiologie der Sinnesorgane* (q.v.). In 1909 he was to have spoken at Clarke University in the United States to an audience that included Sigmund Freud, Adolf Meyer and Carl Jung (qq.v.), as well as other celebrities, but he died of pneumonia shortly before the event.
Bibliography: Boring, E. G. 1950. *A history of experimental psychology.*

EBERS PAPYRUS. A sixteenth-century B.C. Egyptian papyrus on medical matters. It was named after the Egyptologist Georg Moritz Ebers (1837-1898), who acquired it in 1873. In it mental disease is attributed to possession (q.v.) by gods or to the action of evil spirits.
Bibliography: Ebbell, B., trans. 1937. *The papyrus Ebers.*

ECCLES (or EAGLES), SOLOMON (1618-1683). An English musician. In 1660 he became a fanatical Quaker (q.v.); he renounced music, burned his instruments and his books, and earned a living as a shoemaker. During the Great Plague of London he ran naked through the streets, preaching repentance and prophesying catastrophes. He added to the strangeness of his appearance by bearing a dish of burning sulphur upon his head.
Bibliography: Jeffreys, J. 1951. *The Eccles Family.*

ECKER, ALEXANDER (1816-1887). A German anatomist. In connection with his work on the anatomy of the brain, in 1869 he described the posterior occipital convolution, which is now known as Ecker's convolution. He also contributed to the understanding of cerebral development in the fetus.

ECKHART, JOHANNES (1260?-?1328). A German Dominican theologian and preacher. He was the founder of German mysticism. In 1327 he was accused of heresy because his philosophy was based on a kind of pantheistic system influenced by Arabic and Jewish conceptions. The pope accepted his declaration of orthodoxy, but after Eckhart's death twenty-eight of his propositions were condemned as heretical. Eckhart's belief that if man did not exist, God would not exist either asserted the unique importance of the individual.
Bibliography: Copleston, F. C. 1953. *A history of philosophy*, 3.

ECLECTICISM. The selection of the best philosophical doctrines handed down from classical times but diluted and altered by teachings from the East. In the period between Hippocrates (q.v.) and Galen (q.v.), philosophers and medical men gathered the best principles from each doctrine and systematized the amalgamation of them. Galen can be considered the best example of eclecticism in the field of medicine.
Bibliography: Zilboorg, G. 1941. *A history of medical psychology*.

ECLIPSES. Obscurations of the sun or the moon. Throughout history eclipses have been considered as portents and as powerful influences on the affairs, behavior, and feelings of man. William Shakespeare (q.v.), possibly awed by an eclipse of the sun in 1598, mentioned them in *King Lear*:

These late eclipses in the sun and moon portend no good to us . . . love cools, friendship falls off, brothers divide; in cities, mutinies; in countries, discord; in palaces, treason.

[*King Lear*, 1. 2.]

ECONOMO, CONSTANTIN VON (1876-1931). A neuropathologist, born into a patrician Trieste family of Greek origin. He described encephalitis lethargica (Economo disease) in detail shortly after Jean Cruchet (q.v.) in 1917. He was an assistant to Julius Wagner von Jauregg (q.v.) at the Vienna Neuropsychiatric Clinic. His major study of the cerebral cortex *Cytoarchitectonics of the Cerebral Cortex in the Adult Man*, which he began in 1912, was published and well received in 1925. Economo was particularly interested in the brain structure of very talented people and believed that

there was a special anatomy for genius (q.v.). His numerous works included research into the function of sleep and into psychiatric genetics.
Bibliography: Bogaert, L. van, and Théodoridès, J. 1979. *Constantin von Economo: the man and the scientist.*

ECPHORIA. A term meaning a lasting trace. Eugen Bleuler (q.v.), maintaining that past psychical experiences leave a permanent trace, or engram, used the expression "ecphoria of the engrams" to designate "the recurrence of a function resembling a previous experience" involved in memory (q.v.).
Bibliography: Bleuler, E. 1930. *Textbook of psychiatry,* trans. A. A. Brill.

ECPHRONIA. A term used by John Mason Good (q.v.) in his classification of mental disorders. It indicated mania (q.v.) and melancholia (q.v.), which he considered subdivisions of the class neurotica.

ECSTASY. A term derived from the Greek, originally indicating insanity or loss of consciousness. In the seventeenth century it meant a pathological state that included swooning and loss of consciousness. Later it indicated a trance, during which the soul, while separated from the body, experienced visions that often led to prophetic utterances. In this sense, ecstasy could be induced by certain rituals. In mystical language, ecstasy means a rapturous state, during which the soul is engaged in divine contemplation. It is now often used to describe the feeling of extreme delight.
Bibliography: 1978. *Brewer's dictionary of phrase and fable.*

ECSTATICI. In ancient Greece, diviners who would lie in a state of trance, during which their souls were assumed to have left their bodies. When they came out of the trance, they would recount their visions.
Bibliography: 1978. *Brewer's dictionary of phrase and fable.*

ECSTATIC VISION. A term used by James C. Prichard (q.v.) in his *Treatise on Insanity* (1835) to describe a vivid experience that lay between dream (q.v.) and hallucination (q.v.). According to Prichard, the "impressions retained after a paroxysm of ecstasy [q.v.] are so connected with external events or objects and so blended with reality," that it is difficult for the person undergoing the experience to distinguish the real from the imagined.

EDDY, MARY BAKER (1821-1910). American schoolteacher and founder of Christian Science (q.v.). As a child she had frequent temper tantrums, which would culminate in hysterical (*see* HYSTERIA) outbursts that reduced her to a semicomatose state. Her father had to persuade the local authorities to cover the surface of the road in front of their home with a material that would deaden noise because she had convulsions at the mere sound of horses'

hooves. She was also subject to auditory hallucinations (q.v.) during which she thought God spoke to her. In 1862, when she was forty years old, she met Phineas P. Quimby (q.v.), who dramatically cured her of hysterical paralysis and other incapacitating neurotic (*see* NEUROSIS) symptoms with the use of faith healing. This caused her to found a church for the propagation of the principles of Quimby's mind cure, which she expounded in a book *Science and Health*, published in 1875.
Bibliography: Dakin, E. F. 1929. *Mrs. Eddy.*

EDDY, THOMAS (1758-1827). American physician and social reformer. In 1815 he prepared a plan for the construction of an asylum (q.v.) on the lines of the Retreat (q.v.) in England. Entitled "Hints for Introducing an Improved Mode of Treating the Insane in the Asylum," the plan listed eleven points, including the abolition of physical restraint (q.v.), the introduction of moral treatment, and the keeping of case histories. Two years later, following his recommendations, construction was begun on the Bloomingdale Asylum (q.v.). The hospital was opened in 1821 with Eddy as resident physician.
Bibliography: Knapp, S. L. 1834. *Life of Thomas Eddy.*

EDGAR. A character in William Shakespeare's (q.v.) play *King Lear*. He disguises himself as a madman and models his behavior on that of a Tom o'Bedlam (q.v.). The character provides an interesting example of the way in which the Elizabethans expected a madman to behave.

EDINBURGH LUNATIC ASYLUM. A mental hospital in Scotland. It was opened in 1813 by the efforts of Dr. Andrew Duncan (q.v.) following the death of the young poet Robert Fergusson (q.v.). Bonnie Prince Charlie was also linked with the hospital, as the money for its construction was allocated to it by Parliament from the funds of Scottish estates forfeited after the rebellion of 1745. The foundation stone, with the inscription "An asylum for the cure or relief of mental derangement," was laid in 1809. In 1840 Queen Victoria became its patron and granted it the title "Royal"; it is now the Royal Edinburgh Hospital for Nervous and Mental Disorders.
See also ROYAL ASYLUMS.
Bibliography: Henderson, D. K. 1964. *The evolution of psychiatry in Scotland.*

EDINGER, LUDWIG (1855-1918). A German neurologist. In 1885, he described the ventral and dorsal spinocerebellar tracts and the grey nucleus (now known as Edinger's nucleus) under the aqueduct of Sylvius. He also was the first to distinguish the paleocerebrum and the neocerebrum. He believed that the investigation of brain anatomy should be closely linked to the study of brain function. The terms *gnosis* and *praxis* were first introduced by him and were later adopted in the description of agnosia and apraxia.

He was a superb teacher, who was much admired by his students for his lectures, as well as for his ability to draw complicated illustrations of the brain with his right hand while writing captions under the drawings with his left hand. It is reported that when the painter Louis Corinth was working on Edinger's portrait, which depicts him with a dissected brain, the brain was painted by the sitter himself. He was also well known for successfully employing hypnosis (*see* HYPNOTISM) in his practice. Like Sigmund Freud (q.v.), he collected Greek antique statuettes.
Bibliography: Haymaker, W., and Schiller, F. 1970. *The founders of neurology.* 2d. ed.

EDUCATIONAL PSYCHOLOGY. Although John Comenius (q.v.) could be considered an earlier pioneer, the value of psychology in education was first demonstrated in Germany by Johann F. Herbart (q.v.). He is regarded as the originator of educational psychology, and his doctrines provided the first example of applied psychology (q.v.).
Bibliography: Flugel, J. C. 1965. *A hundred years of psychology.*

EDWARD THE CONFESSOR (c.1002-1066). A king of England. He was called Edward the Confessor because of his saintly reputation. He was interested in religion, promoted monasticism, and took vows of chastity. He was credited with the power of experiencing visions, and on one occasion claimed he had seen the devil dancing with glee over money collected from taxes. This may have been a hallucination (q.v.) caused by guilt. He built Westminster Abbey as a penance imposed by the pope when he failed to undertake a pilgrimage to Rome. He was unable to attend the consecration of the abbey in 1065, because the humiliation of having to expel from court his unpopular favorite Tostig, earl of Northumbria, had made him ill. He was the first English king to employ the "king's touch" (q.v.), or laying of hands on the sick, to treat the scrofula (q.v.).
Bibliography: Feiling, K. 1950. *A history of England.*

EEDEN, FREDERIK VAN (1860-1932). Dutch poet and writer. Love of literature made him abandon his formal training in medicine, but he remained interested in psychiatric disorders, in the analysis of dreams (q.v.), and in hypnotism (q.v.), which he believed was a form of therapy suitable only for the lower classes because it entailed an authoritarian attitude on the part of the physician. He observed the work of Auguste H. Forel (q.v.) and in 1887 opened a "clinic of suggestive psychotherapy" in Amsterdam.
Bibliography: Eeden, F. van. 1912. *Happy humanity.*

EFFECT, LAW OF. The theory that learning is facilitated if the situation in which it occurs gives pleasure. Alexander Bain (q.v.) and Edward L. Thorndike (q.v.) both formulated this principle.
Bibliography: Watson, R. I. 1963. *The great psychologists.*

EGGER, ÉMILE (1813-1885). A French philologist. He undertook detailed research on the development of language and intelligence in children.
Bibliography: Egger, E. 1870. *Observations et reflexions sur le developpement d'intelligence et de langage chez les enfants.*

EGYPT. In ancient Egypt, life and death were believed to be part of a continuous cycle, and the importance given to the soul promoted interest in psychology, in the understanding of personality characteristics, and in the significance of dreams (q.v.). As early as 2650 B.C. Prince Ptahhotep had described senile dementia, but the first physician that can be identified as such is Imhotep (q.v.), the chief minister, magician (*see* MAGIC), architect, and physician of the pharaoh Zoser (2980-2900 B.C.). Temples of healing were established in his honor at Memphis and on the Island of Philae. Incubation (q.v.) was a form of therapy; mental disorders were not distinguished from other diseases and, therefore, were treated by physical and psychical methods. The Ebers papyrus (q.v.) mentions mental disease and attributes it to possession (q.v.) and evil spirits. The temples not only were centers for worship and teaching but also for the care of the sick. The high priests were also called physicians-in-chief. In later periods, the Egyptian temples dedicated to Saturn (q.v.) were the best asylums (q.v.). Patients spent their time in pleasant occupations, and their senses were stimulated by beautiful objects and harmonious sounds. These early examples of diversional and music therapy (q.v.) were highly organized. As Egyptian civilization declined, Greek medicine became more important, and Egyptian physicians were trained in Greece. In the Middle Ages (q.v.), Egyptian medicine was greatly influenced by Moses Maimonides (q.v.) after he settled in Cairo. Al-Mansur Hospital (q.v.) provided separate wards for the insane as early as 1283. In the fourteenth century, Kalawoun Hospital (q.v.) also had wards for mental patients. In subsequent centuries changes in Islamic society and European influence introduced new concepts that determined the development of both physical and psychological medicine. In 1876 the first European-style medical school was founded in Cairo, and the Abbasia Mental Hospital, still the largest mental hospital in the Arab (*see* ARABS) countries, was established in 1880.
Bibliography: Baasher, T. 1975. The Arab countries. In *World history of psychiatry*, ed. J. G. Howells.

EHRENBERG, CHRISTIAN GOTTFRIED (1795-1876). A German naturalist. He discovered that the brain's white matter consists of conduction fibers.
Bibliography: Flugel, J. C. 1945. *A hundred years of psychology.*

EHRENFELS, CHRISTIAN VON (1859-1932). German philosopher. In 1890 he formulated the form-quality doctrine. It asserts that form in space

or time is a new element or quality that does not depend on the sensory fundaments on which it rests. He introduced the term *gestalt* (q.v.) into psychology. His cultural interests spanned many fields; he wrote on sexual ethics, drama, Wagner, cosmology, and the theory of values. His major work was *System der Werttheorie*, which was published in two volumes between 1897 and 1898.
Bibliography: Boring, E. G. 1950. *A history of experimental psychology.*

EHRLICH, PAUL (1845-1915). German bacteriologist and pioneer in intracellular chemistry and chemotherapy. He developed salvarsan (q.v.), or arsphenamine, for the specific treatment of syphilis (q.v.) of the nervous system. Salvarsan is known also as 606, which was the number of arsenic compounds tested by Ehrlich before he arrived at the final formula.
Bibliography: Sigerist, H. E. 1933. *Great Doctors.*

EINSTEIN, ALBERT (1879-1955). A German physicist. He became a naturalized Swiss citizen when he was fifteen years old and later acquired American citizenship. He was one of the greatest thinkers of all time. Yet as a child he was late in learning to talk, and an early school report described him as "mentally slow," unsociable, and "adrift forever in his foolish dreams." He is best remembered for his theory of relativity, which gave a new direction to the study of light and allied subjects. In 1922 he was awarded the Nobel Prize for physics. He hoped to see a united world in which mankind would live in peace. As Europe prepared for war, he deplored the nationalistic thinking of scientists, and yet ironically his work contributed to the development of the atomic bomb.
Bibliography: Michelmore, P. 1963. *Einstein.*

EITINGON, MAX (1881-1943). A psychiatrist, born in Russia to a wealthy Jewish family. He moved to Germany in 1909 and studied under Eugen Bleuler (q.v.) at the Burghölzli Hospital (q.v.). Sigmund Freud (q.v.) made a great impression on him; the two men used to stroll through the streets of Vienna in the evenings. The strolls were used by Freud for analysis, and thus Eitingon became the first psychiatrist to undergo a training analysis with Freud. He was a member of the private committee of the psychoanalytic movement, which he helped financially by providing funds for the establishment of the first psychoanalytic education center. It opened in Berlin in 1920. He later lost his fortune and as a Jew following Hitler's rise had to leave Germany. He settled in Palestine and founded the Palestinian Psychoanalytic Society and the Hebrew Institute of Psychoanalysis.
Bibliography: Wulff, M. 1950. *Max Eitingon, in memoriam.*

EKADASAMUKHA. The Japanese goddess of mercy with eleven faces, worshipped in a temple at Iwakura, near Kyoto. In the eleventh century

the emperor Gosanjo sent his daughter, Daiunji (q.v.), who was sick with melancholy (*see* MELANCHOLIA), to pray to her image and drink the water of the holy fountain. She was cured and the temple became famous. A great number of mentally ill flocked to Iwakura, and soon the whole village was involved in their care, thus giving rise to a tradition of family care for the insane and the eventual establishment of Iwakura Hospital (q.v.).
Bibliography: Greenland, C. 1963. Family Care of Mental Patients. *Am. J. Psychiat.* 119: 1000.

ELAGABALUS (*or* HELIOGABALUS) (c.203-222). Roman emperor born in Syria, possibly the illegitimate son of Caracalla (q.v.). He was given to religious excesses that included perverted rites. He was irresponsible, extravagant, depraved, and possibly insane. To ward off attacks of epilepsy (q.v.), Elagabalus used remedies made from the heels of camels, the combs of live cocks, and the tongues of peacocks and nightingales. Realizing that one day his power would end, he prepared himself to commit suicide by having ready silver ropes with which to strangle himself, golden swords, poison flavored with spices, and a richly furnished high tower from which he could throw himself. But, he was murdered with his mother, and his reign ended.
Bibliography: Hyslop, T.B. 1925. *The great abnormals.*

ELAINE. The lily maid of Astolat. A character in Arthurian legend: her death was due to her unrequited love (q.v.) for Sir Lancelot (q.v.).
Bibliography: *Malory's le morte d'Arthur.* 18. 9-20.

ELAN VITAL. A term introduced by Henri Bergson (q.v.) at the beginning of the twentieth century. It indicates a kind of primordial drive.
Bibliography: Zilboorg, G. 1941. *A history of medical psychology.*

ELATION. Some physicians considered excessive elation a cause of insanity. Benjamin Rush (q.v.), who was among those who held this belief, quoted cases of insanity due to prosperity, happy marriage, and winning first prize in a lottery. In the eighteenth century, some individuals, who were admitted to Bethlem Royal Hospital (q.v.), were said to have become insane following successful speculations with the South Sea Company.
Bibliography: Kraepelin, E. 1962. *One hundred years of psychiatry.*

ELBERFELD HORSES. Trained horses named after the German town of Elberfeld. The first horse was trained in 1901 by Von Osten to carry out complex arithmetical calculations. Later Krall trained others. The animals were conditioned to tap their feet when the trainer nodded his head, the number of taps corresponding to the number of nods.
See also CLEVER HANS.
Bibliography: Katz, D. 1937. *Animals and men.*

ELBING. A town, in the domain of the Teutonic knights. In 1326 an extension was built on to the existing Georgshospital (q.v.) to house mentally ill patients.

See also DOLLHAUS.

Bibliography: Rosen, G. 1968. *Madness in society.*

EL DORADO. "The golden"; a Spanish term for a mythical city believed to exist on the shore of an inland lake in South America. The reports of such a city originated from a sixteenth-century Spanish soldier, Martinez, who claimed to have seen it. Despite futile expeditions to find it, it was marked on official maps for a long time. Stories of fantastic riches to be found in the city stimulated greed among the conquistadores, who succumbed to a collective compulsion to search for gold. Traditional beliefs could no longer restrain behavior, and they became callous psychopaths, committing deplorable acts of cruelty.

Bibliography: Leon, C. A., and Rosselli, H. 1975. Latin America. In *World history of psychiatry*, ed. J. G. Howells.

ELDER (SAMBUCUS). A deciduous shrub. The bark, the leaves the berries, and the flowers have been used in medicine since antiquity. Pliny the Elder (q.v.) mentioned elderberries in connection with Roman medicine. Martin Blockwich's *The Anatomie of the Elder* (1644) listed at least seventy diseases for which the elder was beneficial. The flowers of the elder were used to relieve asthma and epilepsy (q.v.) as well as a number of nervous disorders and psychosomatic complaints. Nicholas Culpeper (q.v.) also remarked on the elder's power to cure many ills, including hysteria (q.v.).

Bibliography: Le Strange, R. 1977. *A history of herbal plants.*

ELECTRA. In Greek drama, a figure of revenge and murder. She is obsessed (*see* OBSESSION) with her love for her father, Agamemnon, and with her hatred for her mother, Clytemnestra (q.v.). She is the driving force behind her brother Orestes' (q.v.), murder of their parents. She is driven to death by her guilt and remorse. The Greek dramatists Aeschylus, Sophocles (q.v.), and Euripides (q.v.) wrote plays around her. The German composer Richard Strauss (1864-1949) composed an opera entitled *Elektra* (1909). In psychiatry (q.v.), the Electra complex in women corresponds to the Oedipus (q.v.) complex in men and refers to a relationship between father and daughter that includes antagonism toward the mother.

Bibliography: Ellenberger, H.F. 1970. *The discovery of the unconscious.*

ELECTRICITY. Although electricity was observed and included among natural phenomena at the beginning of the seventeenth century, and the

shock produced by natural electricity had been used therapeutically even in antiquity, its scientific study did not progress greatly until the eighteenth century. John Birch (q.v.) was the first physician to treat depression by electricity at St. Thomas's Hospital. In 1767 an electric shock machine was installed in the Middlesex Hospital in England, and within a few years many hospitals possessed one. John Wesley (q.v.) advised that lunatic (q.v.) patients should be "electrified." Jean Esquirol (q.v.) recorded the use of shock machines in French mental hospitals and wrote that in the summers of 1823 and 1824 he had "submitted to the influence of electricity a large number of insane women." The results were not satisfactory as "the delirium [q.v.] persisted" in most of the patients and only one was cured. Pierre Janet (q.v.), when he was in his eighties, also became keenly interested in electroconvulsive therapy. Electroconvulsive therapy as known today was initiated by Ugo Cerletti (q.v.) in 1938.
See also ELECTROICHTHYOLOGY, BENJAMIN FRANKLIN, and MAGNETISM.
Bibliography: Adams, George. 1799. *An essay on electricity explaining the principles of that useful science; and describing its instruments.* 5th ed.

ELECTROENCEPHALOGRAM. The graphic record of the brain's electrical activity produced by means of electrodes applied to the scalp. The first such instrument was invented by Hans Berger (q.v.) in 1924.
Bibliography: Haymaker, W., and Schiller, F. 1970. *The founders of neurology.* 2d. ed.

ELECTROICHTHYOLOGY. The earliest known application of electricity (q.v.) for therapeutic purposes. Its first recorded use was by a Roman physician, Scribonius Largus (q.v.), in A.D. 46. He recommended the application of torpedo (electric fish) for the treatment of intractable headache and gout. Dioscorides (q.v.) recommended its use for complaints now associated with depression. Pliny the Elder (q.v.) also mentioned it. The Greeks, too, were aware of this form of treatment, and the Abyssinians were reported to have used the electric shock of the torpedo to cast out devils from the possessed (see POSSESSION) and to decrease fevers. Medical references to the use of the electric fish as a shock machine are found as late as 1850.
Bibliography: Kellaway, P. 1946. The part played by electric fish in the early history of bioelectricity and electrotherapy. *Bull. Hist. Med.* 20: 112-37.

ELEMENTARISM. A system of psychology that reduces everything to its basic elements in order to grasp the essential meaning of phenomena. It was championed by Edward B. Titchener (q.v.) in the early twentieth century.
Bibliography: Flugel, J. C. 1945. *A hundred years of psychology.*

ELENA, F. (1900-1927). An Italian music teacher, patient of Enrico Morselli (q.v.). She was a remarkable example of dual personality. She oscillated between a French personality and an Italian personality, each possessing the

appropriate language. Morselli used hypnotism (q.v.) in her treatment and brought to the surface the painful memories of her life, including incestuous (*see* INCEST) attacks by her father. She was gradually improving, but she died of a kidney infection before Morselli could conclude her treatment.
Bibliography: Morselli, G. E. 1930. "Sulla dissociazione mentale." *Rivista Sperimentale di Freniatria* 54: 209-322.

ELGAR, SIR EDWARD (1857-1934). A noted English composer. From 1879 to 1884 he was bandmaster of the Worcester County Lunatic Asylum (q.v.). He composed special music for this band in order to make use of whatever instruments were available. He later gave up conducting and dedicated himself solely to composing works that brought him worldwide fame.
See also BRASS BANDS.
Bibliography: McVeagh, D. M. 1955. *Edward Elgar.*

ELIOT, GEORGE. Pseudonym of **MARY ANN EVANS** (1819-1880). An English novelist. Her early life was austere and ruled by strict religious observances. Her friendship with the freethinkers Charles Bray (1811-1884) and his wife changed her outlook on life and distressed her father. Bray was a great believer in phrenology (q.v.) and to please him she had her head shaved to allow her "bumps" to be studied. She became acquainted with the writer George Henry Lewes (q.v.), and in 1854 Eliot and Lewes, who was separated from his wife, decided to live together. Encouraged by him, she wrote several classic novels, *The Mill on the Floss* (1860), *Silas Marner* (1861), and *Middlemarch* (1872), that contain a great deal of biographical material. She became extremely depressed following his death in 1878 and isolated herself from all her friends. Nevertheless, less than two years later, at the age of sixty-one, she married J. W. Cross. She died a few months after this second marriage.
Bibliography: Bennett, J. 1948. *George Eliot: her mind and art.*

ELIOT, THOMAS STEARNS (1888-1965). American-born poet and critic. Most of his life was spent in England, and he became a British subject in 1927. His mother was forty-three years old at the time of his birth and his father was an old man and completely deaf; his siblings were much older than he. He was cared for by an Irish nursemaid. He grew up in isolation, painfully shy and inhibited. In Europe he fell under the influence of Ezra Pound (q.v.), who supported and encouraged him. In 1915, he made a disastrous marriage to Vivienne, a severely disturbed young woman, who later became psychotic. She became the mistress of Bertrand Russell and for a time the three of them lived together. Eliot suffered from a number of psychosomatic complaints, was often depressed, and feared insanity. Roger Vittoz, a psychiatrist, treated him in Lausanne, Switzerland, apparently successfully, for during this period Eliot produced most of his famous poem *The Waste Land* (1922) which reflects his own psychological state.
Bibliography: Bergonzi, B. 1972. *T. S. Eliot.*

ELIZABETH, QUEEN OF BOHEMIA (1596-1662). The daughter of James I of England and VI of Scotland (q.v.). Her "hypochondriac melancholy" (*see* MELANCHOLIA) was described by John Hawkins (q.v.), who recorded the anxiety and fears that beset her. He stated that she was "troubled with various anxious and painful thoughts, almost to the point of madness . . . without manifest cause." In fact, she had much cause for depression. Her husband, Frederick V, was deposed by the Catholic league in 1620. The royal family took refuge in Holland and endured great hardship. Her eldest son died in 1629, and her brother, Charles I, was beheaded. She had thirteen children. The last year of her life was spent in England.
Bibliography: Oman, C. 1938. *Elizabeth of Bohemia*.

ELIZABETH VON R. A patient of Sigmund Freud (q.v.) whom he saw in 1892. Following her suggestion, he published her case history to illustrate his method of "free association" in 1895.
Bibliography: Breuer, J., and Freud, S. 1955. *Studies in hysteria*.

ELK. The largest existing deer, sometimes known in North America as the moose. The hoof of the elk was believed to be efficacious against epilepsy (q.v.). In the Renaissance pieces of its hoof were mounted in rings worn for this purpose.
See also DIGITUS MEDICINALIS.
Bibliography: Evans, J. 1922. *Magical jewels*.

ELLIOTSON, JOHN (1791-1868). An English physician and first professor of the practice of medicine at the University of London. He was instrumental in founding University College Hospital in London. He was a scientist, a philanthropist, and a rebel, who was willing to jeopardize his career and reputation in defense of his convictions. In the face of ridicule and objection, he was the first physician in England to use a stethoscope. He became interested in mesmerism (q.v.) after witnessing a demonstration by J. Dupotet de Sennevoy (q.v.) and did not hesitate to promote the use of magnetic sleep to alleviate pain during surgical operations and as a form of therapy for epilepsy (q.v.). Following a bitter attack by *The Lancet* and the council of the University, he was forced to resign from his post but continued to hold magnetizing sessions in his own home. In 1843 he founded the *Zoist*, subtitled *A Journal of Cerebral Physiology and Mesmerism and Their Applications to Human Welfare*. Despite strong and vicious opposition, Elliotson delivered the Harveian Oration of the Royal College of Physicians in 1843 and took the opportunity to remind his audience of the importance of mesmerism.
Bibliography: Bramwell, J. M. 1930. *Hypnotism: its history, practice and theory*.

ELLIS, HAVELOCK (1859-1939). English physician and psychologist. His mother named him after Sir Henry Havelock, hero of the Indian Mutiny. At the age of four he saw his nurse and his mother urinating, which aroused him sexually, an event that in later life made him deduce that he was somewhat "perverse." His marriage to Edith Lees (?-1916), a woman with lesbian propensities, was happy in spite of, or because of, their frequent separations. His wife had a succession of affairs with women; he, too, found comfort outside marriage, but she tried to commit suicide (q.v.) twice because of his infidelity. Sigmund Freud (q.v.) corresponded with him for thirty-five years, yet in his autobiography Ellis does not mention his name, possibly because they had a misunderstanding which broke off their connection. Following the fashionable interest in human instincts and sexuality, he undertook monumental sexological studies framed by anthropological comments. He classified varieties of human sexual expression and pleaded with society for more tolerance toward sexual deviations. His work made the discussion of sexual matters more socially acceptable. He wrote several books of which the most important is *Studies in the Psychology of Sex*, published in seven volumes between 1897 and 1928.
Bibliography: Grosskurth, P. 1980. *Havelock Ellis.*

ELLIS, SIR WILLIAM CHARLES (1780-1839). A British psychiatrist. He began his medical career as a general practitioner and gradually developed an interest in mental illness. His views were unusually enlightened for his time and led to his appointment as the first medical superintendent to two new asylums (q.v.): Wakefield Asylum (q.v.), the West Riding of Yorkshire county hospital, in 1818 to 1830, and Hanwell Asylum (q.v.), the Middlesex county hospital, where he remained until 1839. His wife helped him to run both establishments in her capacity of matron. They introduced many new and beneficial concepts. The patients were not physically restrained (*see* RESTRAINT) and were encouraged to work and earn by their efforts; nursing care, as well as the status and training of mental nurses, was greatly improved; a system of after-care was initiated; and the patients were treated with exceptional consideration and understanding. Ellis also owned a private mental hospital, Southall Park Asylum. In 1835 Ellis became the first psychiatrist to be knighted exclusively for his services to psychiatry.
Bibliography: Hunter, R. and Macalpine, I. 1963. *Three hundred years of psychiatry.*

ELSBERG, CHARLES (1871-1948). An American neurosurgeon who pioneered surgery of the spinal cord. He also carried out studies on vision and on the sense of smell.
Bibliography: Haymaker, W., and Schiller, F. 1970. *The founders of neurology.* 2d. ed.

ELSHEIMER, ADAM (1578-1610). A German painter, a founder of modern landscape painting and a forerunner of Rembrandt. At the age of twenty he went to Rome, where he spent the rest of his life. Depression so affected him that he was unable to work for long periods of time. Although he made bad friends and an unsuitable marriage and was quite incapable of facing reality and managing his domestic affairs, his landscapes were delightfully poetic. His last years were filled with depression, introspection, and lack of work. He was imprisoned for debt and became so dejected following his release that he fell ill and died.
Bibliography: Wittkower, R., and Wittkower, M. 1963. *Born under Saturn.*

ELYOT, SIR THOMAS (1490-1546). English medical writer. He was a student of medicine under Thomas Linacre (1460?-1524) but never became a physician. In 1534, he published *The Castel of Helth*, a domestic guide to simple remedies, written in English for the use of the general public. It greatly angered the physicians. He followed the humoral theory (q.v.) in explaining mental disorder, recognizing four elements and four personalities—sanguine, fleumatic, choleric, and melancholic. Melancholy (*see* MELANCHOLIA) was of two kinds, natural and unnatural. Unnatural melancholy was due to the adustion of choleric mixture and was the worse kind. He also recognized the psychological causes of depression, which he called "dolour or hevyness of mynde." For its treatment he recommended good advice from a man "well learned in morall philosophye," as well as physical remedies.
Bibliography: Hunter, R., and Macalpine, I. 1963. *Three hundred years of psychiatry.*

EL-ZAR CULT. A secret Egyptian therapeutic cult to which only women are admitted. The drinking of blood from sacrificed animals and frenzied dancing often cause such excitement that some of the participants collapse. Individuals with emotional disorders are encouraged under excitement to regress to a state of childhood and reenact painful memories.
Bibliography: Okasha, A. 1966. A Cultural Psychiatric Study of El-Zar Cult in U.A.R. *Brit. J. Psychiat.* 112: 1217-21.

EMERALD. A jewel whose green color traditionally has been associated with healing. The Romans believed it was an antidote against the evil eye (q.v.). In the seventh century, Saint Isidore (q.v.), archbishop of Seville, wrote that emeralds helped men with divination, made them eloquent and persuasive, and cured epilepsy (q.v.). A book attributed to Saint Hildegard of Bingen (q.v.) also recommended it for epilepsy: the gem should be placed in the mouth of those falling to the ground in a fit; they will soon recover and will remain well if they will say special prayers to the Holy Spirit and

carry the stone with them for nine consecutive days. The emerald was also believed to strengthen memory (q.v.) and enhance all mental powers.
See also PRECIOUS STONES.
Bibliography: Hodges, D. M. 1972. *Healing gems.*

ÉMILE, OU TRAITÉ DE L'ÉDUCATION. A book written by Jean Jacques Rousseau (q.v.) in 1762 as a treatise on education. The views expressed in it were revolutionary, and the French authorities condemned them. Rousseau advocated a return to nature, whereby children should grow up unhampered by petty restrictions and should learn by the observation of natural phenomena rather than by formal teaching. According to Rousseau, religion should not be taught until the child's reasoning powers have matured. In contrast to this enlightened program for the education of a boy (Émile), Rousseau believed that women should be taught to be submissive, docile, and mentally inferior. Although it has many obvious misconceptions, *Émile* inspired educational reforms in many countries.
Bibliography: Rousseau, J. J. 1955. *Émile,* trans. B. Foxley.

EMMANUEL MOVEMENT. A religio-psychotherapeutic movement begun in 1906 at the Emmanuel Episcopal Church in Boston, Massachusetts. Functional nervous disorders usually were treated by hypnotic (*see* HYPNOTISM) therapy administered by a team of clergymen, physicians, and social workers. Religious and medical authorities opposed the movement. After three years of popularity and wide coverage in the less sophisticated press, the movement declined.
Bibliography: Andrick, J. M. 1978. Hypnosis and the Emmanuel Movement: a medical and religious repudiation. *Am. J. Clin. Hypn.,* 20: 224-34.

EMMELOT OF CHAUMONT. A French woman who lived in the thirteenth century. She suddenly became paralyzed and recovered equally as suddenly when she was taken to the tomb of Saint Louis in Saint-Denis, France. Her miraculous cure is one of the earliest recorded cases of the cure of hysterical (*see* HYSTERIA) paralysis.
Bibliography: Zilboorg, G. 1941. *A history of medical psychology.*

EMMERICH, ANNA KATHARINA (1774-1824). A German nun. She bore the stigmata (q.v.) and became famous for her visions. Clemens Brentano (q.v.), her companion and emanuensis, spent six years recording her revelations.
Bibliography: Brentano, C. 1833. *The life of Anna K. Emmerich.*

EMMINGHAUS, HERMANN (1845-1904). A German psychiatrist who conceived a system of psychology based on natural science and emphasizing brain physiology. He was also interested in child psychiatry (q.v.) and in

1887 wrote a book entitled *Psychic Disturb...* ... presented an epidemiological study of psychiatric disor... commented on the adverse influence of poor enviro... family conditions

Bibliography: Harms, F. 1960. At the cradle of child psy...
psychiat 30: 187.

EMMY VON N. A patient of Sigmund Freud (q.v.), In his first case of cathartic (see CATHARSIS) treatment, ... history but altered dates, names, and places so heavily that ... can be drawn from the data he present...

Bibliography: Breuer, J., and Freud, S. 1955. *Studies in Hysteria*

EMOTION, THEORY OF A theory that purports to ex... by their physical accompaniments. It is also termed the James ... of emotion, as it was first developed by William James (q.v.) ... by Carl George Lange (q.v.), quite independently, in 1885.

Bibliography: Flugel, J. C. 1945. *A hundred years of psychology.*

EMPATHEMA. A nineteenth-century term meaning "ungovern... sion." It was used by John Mason Good (q.v.) in his classification of ... disorders. He used it as a subdivision in the class Neurotica.

EMPEDOCLES (c.490-430 B.C.). A Greek philosopher, physician, poet, born in Agrigentum, Sicily. He introduced the belief that earth, fire, and water were the basic elements of all things. According to ... health resulted from their balance caused by love (q.v.), and ill health fro... their imbalance caused by strife. His theory of elements was adopted b... Hippocrates (q.v.) and remained the basis of medicine until the sixteen... century. Empedocles asserted that love and hate were the basis of individual and social behaviour. He located the soul in the heart. He was held in great esteem as a physician, and he fostered a belief in his own divinity. To prove that he was a god he threw himself into the crater of Mount Etna and was seen no more. Matthew Arnold wrote a poem about his death, "Empedocles on Etna".

Bibliography: Burnet, J. 1948. *Early Greek philosophy*

ENANTIODROMIA. A term originating with Heraclitus (q.v.) and meaning "return to the opposite." Carl G. Jung (q.v.) adopted it to describe the turning of certain mental processes during unconscious thinking.

Bibliography: Ellenberger, H. F. 1970. *The discovery of the unconscious.*

ENDOCRINOLOGY. The belief that certain psychiatric illnesses can result from endocrine disorders originated in antiquity. Hippocrates (q.v.), for example, thought that insanity could be caused by body secretions.

Bibliography: Zilboorg, G. 1941. *A history of medical psychology.*

ENGELS, FRIEDRICH (1820-1895). German social philosopher and economic theorist. Until 1843 he wrote under the pseudonym of Friedrich Oswald. He and Karl Marx (q.v.) wrote the *Communist Manifesto* in 1848. His literary style helped to popularize Marx's works and to make communism known. His interest in psychology evolved from his belief that to understand people and their motivations one must analyze their thoughts and behavior.
Bibliography: Ryazanoff, D. 1927. *Friedrich Engels and Karl Marx.*

ENGLISH MALADY. In the eighteenth century there was a widespread belief that melancholy (see MELANCHOLIA) was prevalent among the English. Its cause was linked to the English climate. Charles Montesquieu (q.v.), for one, blamed the climate (q.v.) for the high rate of suicide (q.v.) among the English. The condition was well described by George Cheyne (q.v.) in his *The English Malady: or a Treatise of Spleen, Vapours, Lowness of Spirits, Hypochondriacal and Hysterical Disorders* (1733). He believed that these nervous disorders could be "computed to make almost one third of the complaints of the people of condition in England"—an estimate close to that made for neurosis (q.v.) in the twentieth century.
See also MELANCHOLIA ANGLICA.
Bibliography: Doughty, Oswald 1926. The English malady of the eighteenth century. *Review of English Studies*, 2: 257.

ENNEMOSER, JOSEPH (1787-1854). An Austrian physician. He believed in Franz Mesmer's (q.v.) theory of animal magnetism (q.v.) as a therapeutic force and used hypnotism (q.v.) in the treatment of his patients. As a Roman Catholic he tried to amalgamate the teachings of his church with those of Mesmer.
Bibliography: Galdston, I., ed. 1967. *Historic derivations of modern psychiatry.*

ENSOR, BARON JAMES (1860-1949). A Belgian painter, and a precursor of expressionism. He spent most of his life in Ostend, Belgium, his hometown. His fantastic imagination produced masks, skeletons, and gruesome satirical views of life reminiscent of the work of Hieronymous Bosch (q.v.). He satirized social and religious institutions. His paintings were rejected by his contemporaries because they presented stark and ugly realities without compromise. His macabre outlook, however, appealed to the expressionist school and to the surrealists.
Bibliography: Tannenbaum, L. 1951. *James Ensor.*

ENT, SIR GEORGE (1604-1689). An English medical writer. In 1667 he suggested to members of the Royal Society (q.v.) that experiments in blood

transfusion (q.v.) should be undertaken and that a subject should be provided from Bethlem Royal Hospital (q.v.). It was thought that the transfusion, using blood from a sheep, might even do some good to "a frantic man by cooling his blood."
Bibliography: Hunter, R., and Macalpine, I. 1963. *Three hundred years of psychiatry*.

ENTEROID PROCESSES. The convolutions of the brain that resemble the intestine. Erasistratus (q.v.) in the third century B.C. suggested the similarity between the intestine and the convolutions of the brain, but the term was first used in the nineteenth century by M. Vincenzo Malacarne (q.v.) and his pupil Luigi Rolando (q.v.).
Bibliography: Clarke, E., and Dewhurst, K. 1970. *Illustrated history of brain functions*.

ENURESIS. The involuntary voiding of the bladder. Enuresis often has a psychological cause. William Shakespeare (q.v.) mentions the sound of bagpipes as a cause of enuresis in some people:

And others, when the bagpipe sings i' th' nose,
Cannot contain their urine.

The Merchant of Venice, 4. 1.

Prescriptions for its treatment, especially in children, have exercised the minds of physicians for centuries and have included strange and repelling materials. Thomas Phaire (q.v.), for example, suggested the dried and powdered windpipe of a cock, or the "stones" of a hedgehog, likewise powdered, or the hoofs of a goat.

ÉON DE BEAUMONT, CHARLES GENEVIÈVE LOUIS AUGUSTE ANDRÉ TIMOTHÉE D' (CHEVALIER D'EON) (1728-1810). A French diplomat. He was sent as a secret agent to the court of Elizabeth of Russia, who liked her guests to dress in the clothing of the opposite sex at balls. Knowing this, he wore female clothes for his appointment with her. On his return to France he continued to dress as a woman. In 1777 a royal decree was passed that forced him to wear women's clothes for the rest of his life. His true sex was the subject of society wagers, and the chevalier did nothing to dispel the gossip. The term *eonism*, a synonym of transvestism, is derived from his name.
Bibliography: Cox, C. 1966. *The enigma of the age*.

EPICTETUS (A.D. c.55-135). A Stoic (*see* STOICISM) philosopher from Phrygia. He had been a slave but was freed and allowed to teach in Rome. He became much sought after until he was expelled by Titus Flavius Domitian (q.v.) in A.D. 94. He believed that true happiness was to be found only in complete indifference, inactivity, and withdrawal into oneself.
Bibliography: Oldfather, W. A. trans. 1925-1928. *Epictetus*.

EPICURUS (341?-270 B.C.). Greek philosopher, founder of a system of philosophy that believed man's destiny was in his own hands and that the gods would neither help nor hinder him. Introspection and contemplation were encouraged. Pleasure, which was defined as *ataraxia* (serenity), was the only good and the end of all moral considerations. It could be achieved only by leading a good life and by overcoming irrational fears. The Epicureans did not believe that the soul would survive after death or that it had any particular seat in the body. To them the soul was only a vehicle for perception. Epicurus' school at Mitylene offered guidance for mental problems through a tranquil way of life. Women and slaves were accepted by the school. Robert Burton (q.v.), quoting from Epicurus' writings, described how a depressed patient was nursed in a beautiful room, crowned with flowers, served with wine, and lulled by music and song produced by a fair maiden. Epicurus wrote on how to be happy and on fortitude against discontent of mind.
Bibliography: Strodach, G. K., trans. 1962. *The philosophy of Epicurus.*

EPIDAURUS. A town of ancient Greece. A famous temple of Aesculapius (q.v.) was established there in the sixth century B.C. Because the sanctuary had a great reputation for cures, patients went to it with confidence, which was in itself therapeutic. Dicting and bathing were preliminaries to the final sleep in the temple, during which patients were healed by divine visions. Priests, dressed as gods and accompanied by sacred serpents, walked among the sleeping patients, heightening susceptibility to miraculous cures. The sanctuary flourished for over 800 years.
See also INCUBATION.
Bibliography: Phillips, E.D. 1973. *Greek medicine.*

EPIDEMICS. Outbreaks of mass mental disorders have occurred since antiquity. They then were attributed to the intervention of gods, for example, Dionysus (q.v.). Occasional epidemics of mass suicide were known in ancient Greece. The Middle Ages (q.v.) saw epidemics of dancing mania (q.v.), visions, self-torturing, and of other forms of aberrant behavior. In the sixteenth century Johann Weyer (q.v.) recognized that epidemics of demoniacal possession (q.v.) were best treated by isolating those affected. Mass hysteria (q.v.), produced by what nineteenth-century psychiatrists called moral contagion, remains a recurring phenomenon. In the twentieth century a spectacular example of mass hysteria that ended in the death of a whole religious community occurred in 1978 at Jonestown, Guyana, when the followers of James Jones (?-1978) poisoned their children with cyanide before committing suicide.
Bibliography: Zilboorg, G. 1941. *A history of medical psychology.*

EPILEPSY. A seizure promoted by the sudden discharge of brain cells. In antiquity epilepsy was often equated with madness. The earliest recorded

mention of epilepsy is found in the 2080 B.C. code of Hammurabi, king of Babylonia. The Bible (q.v.) also contains several references to it. The ancient Greeks regarded it as a sacred disease, but Hippocrates (q.v.) asserted that there was nothing sacred about it and that it had natural causes. The Romans thought epilepsy was an omen of disaster and dismissed the meetings of the Senate whenever anyone present had an epileptic fit. Throughout the Middle Ages (q.v.) the disorder was associated with possession (q.v.) by spirits, and epileptics were regarded with fear or listened to as divinely inspired prophets. Later, physicians believed in a humoral (see HUMORS) causation of epilepsy, which remained shrouded in superstition and fear and linked to the phases of the moon (q.v.). The nineteenth century saw a multiplication of conflicting opinions. Almost all bodily organs were blamed in turn for producing the seizures; masturbation (q.v.) and sexual excesses were regarded as the commonest causes, and castration was a form of treatment often employed. Even the twentieth century has retained some misconceptions about epilepsy. In some American states epileptics are still barred from marriage. The list of remedies for epilepsy is endless. It has included peony (q.v.) root, silver (q.v.) rings, precious stones, cramp rings (q.v.), camel brain, coffin nails, heart of the hare, blood from tortoises, powder of human skull, testicles of old rams or of hippopotamuses, and berries of mistletoe (q.v.). Among famous epileptics are Hercules, Julius Caesar, Saint Paul, Dante, Martin Luther, Paracelsus, Lord Byron, and Fyodor Dostoevsky (qq.v.). Dostoevsky wrote about it with great perception in his novels, *The Idiot, The Possessed*, and the *Brothers Karamazov* (q.v.). The terms for the disease are nearly as numerous as the remedies for it. The following are only a few: sacred disease (q.v.), mal d'Hercules (q.v.), St. Valentine's disease, falling sickness, morbus demoniacus, morbus puerilis, morbus mensalis, and Saint John's evil (q.v.).
See also AURA IN EPILEPSY.
Bibliography: Temkin, O. 1971. *The falling sickness.*

EPISTAXIS. Profuse bleeding from the nose was considered beneficial in the treatment of insanity. Jean Esquirol (q.v.) reported that he had successfully treated a young man by causing epistaxis.
Bibliography: Esquirol, J. E. D. 1845. Reprint. 1965. *Mental maladies: a treatise on insanity.*

EPISTEMOPHILIC. Sigmund Freud (q.v.) used this term in one of his lectures on psychoanalysis (q.v.) to indicate an instinct that governs the need to gain knowledge.
Bibliography: Freud, S. 1955. *Introductory lectures on psychoanalysis.*

EQUINOXES. The time of the year when day and night are of equal duration. The equinoxes were believed to influence mental disorders. Jean

Esquirol (q.v.) thought that "a house for the insane is most disturbed, and requires the most careful supervision, at the period of the equinoxes."
Bibliography: Esquirol, J. E. D. 1845. Reprint. 1965. *Mental maladies: a treatise on insanity.*

ERASISTRATUS (c.310-250 B.C.). A Greek physician. He is famous for his discovery of the differences between motor and sensory cranial nerves. His work gained for him the appellation of "father of physiology," but unfortunately only fragments of it remain. Unlike his contemporaries, he gave functional significance to the substance of the brain and even expressed the view that the complexity of the human brain convolutions displayed the superiority of man over lower animals. Erasistratus thought that the seat of the soul lay in the cerebellum. He opposed the humoral theory (q.v.) of disease. Erasistratus was physician to King Seleucus of Syria and cured Antiochus (q.v.), his son, of "amorous melancholy" by persuading Seleucus to renounce his wife Stratonice and allow Antiochus to marry her.
Bibliography: Sigerist, H. E. 1933. *Great doctors.*

ERASMUS, DESIDERIUS (c.1466-1536). An early humanist, born in Rotterdam, Holland. He was one of the greatest figures of the Renaissance in northern Europe, but his brilliant intellectual gifts were at times obscured by peevishness, oversensitivity, and self-importance. In 1492 he was ordained as a priest, but the constraint of monastic life went against his passion for personal freedom. His health suffered, and he returned to secular life to dedicate himself to study. He was a wandering scholar and a prolific writer. His satiric book, *Praise of Folly* (q.v.) was written in England while visiting his friend Thomas More (q.v.) in 1509. It became one of the most read works of the time. In it he regarded madness, paradoxically, as the essence of truth and reason. The medical profession was harshly criticized by him with the comment that it was an "incorporated compound of craft and imposture." He also advocated suicide (q.v.) in intolerable conditions, feeling it was more praiseworthy to die than to continue to live in unhappiness.
Bibliography: Sowards, J. K. 1976. *Desiderius Erasmus.*

ERASTUS, THOMAS (1524-1583). German-Swiss philosopher, theologian, and physician. He was professor of medicine and ethics at the University of Basle. His real surname was Liber, Liebler, or Lüber. He denied the church's power of excommunication and did not believe that the devil was connected with mental disease.
Bibliography: Wesel-Roth, R. 1954. *Thomas Erastus.*

ERB, WILHELM HEINRICH (1840-1921). A German neurologist remembered for his work on neuropathology connected with muscular dystrophy. He was an authority on electrotherapy. Sigmund Freud (q.v.) read

his textbook, but concluded that any success attributed to electrotherapy was actually the effect of suggestion on the part of the therapist.
Bibliography: Haymaker, W., and Schiller, R. 1970. *The founders of neurology*, 2d ed.

ERFURT. A German town. In 1385, during the rebuilding of the Grosse Hospital, a special hut was erected to house the insane. It was referred to as the *Tollkoben* (q.v.) or mad hut.
Bibliography: Rosen, G. 1968. *Madness in society*.

ERGOT POISONING. A form of intoxication due to a fungus found on infected rye. It was common in the Middle Ages (q.v.) and a number of epidemics of St. Anthony's fire (q.v.) were caused by it. Those affected had symptoms of gangrene, hallucinations (q.v.), delirium (q.v.), and convulsions. An outbreak of the disease occurred in 1951 at Pont St. Esprit in the south of France, when, to avoid tax, some grain was sold illegally without having been inspected. Investigations on the chemistry of ergot led to the discovery of LSD, lysergic acid diethylamide (q.v.).
Bibliography: Bové, F. J. 1970. *The story of ergot*.

ERHARD, JOHN BENJAMIN (1776-1827). German physician and philosopher. He devised a classification of mental disorders based on symptomatology. Erhard thought that there were three types of melancholia (q.v.): hypochondriaca, thanatophobia (q.v.), and demonomania (q.v.).
Bibliography: Zilboorg, G. 1941. *A history of medical psychology*.

ERICHSEN, SIR JONATHAN ERIC (1818-1896). An English surgeon, surgeon extraordinary to Queen Victoria. He described and named Railway spine, a disorder associated with the then current theories of meningeal irritation and ascribed to concussion of the spine. Railway spine was a mythopathology couched in scientific language and covering a multitude of hysterical (*see* HYSTERIA) symptoms. His theories were opposed and destroyed by Furneaux Jordan and Herbert Page.
Bibliography: Erichsen, J. 1875. *On concussion of the spine*.

ERIKSON, ERIK HOMBURGER (1902-   ). A neo-Freudian psychologist born in Germany of Danish parents. After wandering through Europe, he settled in Vienna and, with Peter Blos, ran a progressive school sponsored by Anna Freud (q.v.), who later analyzed him. He studied clinical

psychoanalysis (q.v.) with a number of brilliant teachers and was influenced by Maria Montessori's (q.v.) system of education. In 1933 he emigrated to America. For a time he worked in Boston at Massachusett General Hospital and at the pioneering Judge Baker Child Guidance Center. Most of his work has been in the field of developmental psychology (q.v.), for example, *Childhood and Society* (1950), but his numerous books also include historical research, *Young Man Luther* (1959), and a biography of Gandhi, *Gandhi's Truth* (1969).
Bibliography: Coles, R. 1970. *Erik H. Erikson: the growth of his work.*

ERINYES *or* **FURIES.** Hideous avenging goddesses of Greek mythology. They were considered to be the daughters of night, or of darkness. Their numbers varied, but it was usually agreed that there were three: Alecto, Tisiphone, and Megaera. They personified curses or the spirits of murdered people. They tortured those who had committed a crime, never letting them forget their guilt and eventually driving them to madness. The Erinyes were represented with serpents in their hair and blood pouring from their eyes.
See also ALCMAEON and ORESTES.
Bibliography: Guthrie, W.K.C. 1968. *The Greeks and their gods.*

ERLANGER, JOSEPH (1874-1965). American physiologist, renowned for his contributions to neurology (q.v.) and his research on the transmission of impulses through single nerve fibers. He was awarded the Nobel Prize for discoveries in the field of neurophysiology.
Bibliography: Haymaker, W., and Schiller, F. 1970. *The founders of neurology.* 2d. ed.

EROS. A god in Greek mythology. He represented the passion of love, and his images were worshipped by males and females alike. He was also a god of fertility. He was considered cunning and cruel, a peril to those he affected in mind and body, and a punisher of those who resisted him. Hesiod, in the eighth century B.C., described him as the god who "loosens the limbs and damages the mind." His role as an emotion was recognized by Plato (q.v.) as a force in the life of the individual and of society. In his classification of madness, he attributed the madness of lovers to Eros and Aphrodite. Sigmund Freud (q.v.) regarded Eros as synonymous with libido (q.v.) and as a primary instinct that tries "to establish ever greater unities and to preserve them thus, in short, to bind them together."
Bibliography: Freud, S. 1974. *The complete psychological works.*
Guthrie, W.K.C. 1968. *The Greeks and their gods.*

EROTOGRAPHOMANIA. The morbid compulsive impulse to write love letters. A famous example is the correspondence between Abelard (q.v.) and Heloise. In more recent times, the wife of Tchaikovsky (q.v.) could be said to have suffered from it; she addressed her love letters indiscriminately to a number of men.

EROTOMANIA. Love insanity. The term was used in the English title of a volume by Jacques Ferrand (q.v.). The English translation was subtitled *A Treatise Discoursing of the Essence, Causes, Symptoms, Prognosticks, and Cure of Love or Erotique Melancholy.* The original was published in Paris, in 1623, and the translation appeared in London in 1640.
Bibliography: Hunter, R., and Macalpine, I. 1963. *Three hundred years of psychiatry.*

ERSKINE OF RESTORMEL, THOMAS (1750-1823). A British criminal lawyer, famous for his brilliant oratory. His eloquence and skill contributed to changes in the criminal law relating to insanity. He defended James Hadfield (q.v.), who was accused of shooting at George III (q.v.). Erskine asserted that total insanity was not the essential excuse from responsibility as it rarely occurred, whereas "in other cases, reason is not driven from her seat, but distraction sits down upon it along with her, holds her, trembling upon it, and frightens her from her property." He also thought that if the accused suffered from delusion (q.v.), his judgment was not under his own control. The conclusions of such a person, he argued, would be logical, but the premises from which he reasoned would be uniformly false. Lord Erskine's arguments convinced the courts to accept delusions as a component of legal insanity. He also worked towards the emancipation of the Negro. His last speech in the House of Lords (1820) was in defense of Queen Caroline, wife of George IV.
Bibliography: Walker, N. 1968. *Crime and insanity in England.*

ERWARTUNG (EXPECTATION). An opera by Arnold Schönberg (1874-1951). The work depicts the gradual disintegration of a woman's mind, culminating in her intense terror and final mental collapse when she finds her lover's dead body in a dark forest.
Bibliography: Rosenthal, H., and Warrack, J. 1964. *Concise Oxford dictionary of opera.*

ESCHENMAYER, ADAM KARL AUGUST VON (1768-1852). A German metaphysician and one of the first physicians to teach psychiatry. His beliefs were a mixture of the occult and scientific ideas. He practiced hypnosis (*see* HYPNOTISM) and wrote a book entitled *Animal Magnetism* (1806) in which he described the effects of magnetism (q.v.) on the feelings and behavior of a person. The relationship between the body and the mind was one of the fields he investigated. He thought that mental illness occurred when the ego was repressed. His works reflect his conviction that faith is above philosophical speculations.
Bibliography: Eschenmayer, A. K. A. von. 1830. *Fundamentals of psychiatry.*

ESDAILE, JAMES (1808-1859). An English surgeon who practiced in India. Risking his professional reputation, he reported that he had performed more than 250 operations on Hindu convicts using mesmerism (q.v.) to anesthetize them. His report was met with hostility and scepticism, and the government closed the small mesmeric hospital in Calcutta, even though they had received a petition signed by over three hundred people. A new mesmeric hospital was founded by private funds and placed under the direction of Esdaile. In 1851 he left India and moved to Scotland, where he continued to pursue his interest in mesmerism. He was a firm supporter of John Elliotson (q.v.) and corresponded with him for many years.
Bibliography: Esdaile, J. 1846. *Mesmerism in India, and its practical application in surgery and medicine.*

ESENIN, SERGEI (1895-1925). A Russian poet, known as "the poet laureate of the Revolution" until he rejected the Bolshevik regime. Esenin's way of life was disorderly and rowdy. In 1922, he married Isadora Duncan (q.v.), seventeen years his senior; their union was not harmonious and they soon separated. He then married Leo Tolstoy's (q.v.) granddaughter, but this marriage also was unsuccessful and possibly illegal as it is not certain that he was divorced. One woman, Galina Benislavskaya (?-1926) loved him devotedly and unselfishly all her life; she shot herself on his grave in 1926. Toward the end of his life, Esenin's mental health deteriorated; he found that alcohol was no longer an antidote to depression and insecurity. He hanged himself in a Leningrad hotel after writing a last poem in his own blood. His poetry reflects a tragic outlook on life; his sensitive verses contain striking and daring imagery and deep emotional statements, often disguised by blasphemy and cynical overtones.
Bibliography: Poggioli, R. 1960. *The poets of Russia: 1890-1930.*

ESMARCH, JOHANNES FRIEDRICH AUGUST VON (1823-1908). German surgeon and medical writer. In 1863, with Peter Willers Jessen (q.v.), he suggested that syphilis (q.v.) was the essential cause of general paralysis of the insane (q.v.).
Bibliography: Zilboorg, G. 1941. *A history of medical psychology.*

ESPINAS DE LA CABEZA. A disease recognised by Mayan Indians. It is said to be the consequence of fright, which causes loss of soul. The prognosis is poor.
Bibliography: Gillin, J. 1948. Magic fright. *Psychiatry*, 2: 387.

ESQUIROL, JEAN ÉTIENNE DOMINIQUE (1772-1840). A French psychiatrist, born in Toulouse. He was a pupil of Philippe Pinel (q.v.). Esquirol, like others before him, tried to classify mental disorders in the same way that Carolus Linnaeus (q.v.) had classified animals and plants, according to families, types, species, and varieties. Thus he fell into the error of ascribing fixed and unchanging characteristics to illnesses, but his acute sense of observation often allowed him to disregard tradition and arrive at his own conclusions. He greatly influenced his students, who learned from him to observe and describe accurately symptoms of mental illness. He revolutionized the traditional ideas of asylums (q.v.), believing that they should offer not only custody but also effective treatment. Magnetism (q.v.) was fashionable during his lifetime, and he tried to use it but was unable to put his patients into trances. His efforts to directly influence patients through personal contact with them laid the basis for individual psychotherapy (q.v.). Due to his efforts the reforms recommended by Pinel were implemented in many French asylums. He was the first to differentiate between illusions and hallucinations (q.v.). Esquirol is regarded as one of the founders of modern psychiatry.

Bibliography: Esquirol, J.E.D. 1845. Reprint. 1965. *Mental maladies: a treatise on insanity.*

ESSAY CONCERNING SELF-MURTHER, AN. A work condemning suicide (q.v.). It was written by a clergyman named Adams and published in England in 1700. It was meant as a reply to the *Biathanatos* (q.v.) of John Donne (q.v.).

Bibliography: Fedden, H. R. 1938. *Suicide.*

ESSAY ON CLASSIFICATION OF THE INSANE. A short work by Matthew Allen (q.v.) written in 1837. It contained a plea for voluntary treatment, a revolutionary idea at a time when strict certification was regarded as an essential safeguard to the public.

Bibliography: Hunter, R., and Macalpine, I. 1963. *Three hundred years of psychiatry.*

ESSAY ON THE ART OF INGENIOUSLY TORMENTING. A publication first issued in 1753 in England. Its author Jane Collier seems to have enjoyed creating emotionally damaging situations. The subtitle informs the reader that the essay contains *Proper Rules for the Exercise of that Pleasant Art . . . with some General Instructions for Plaguing all your Acquaintances.* The front of the volume shows an engraving of a cat tormenting a mouse.

Bibliography: Collier, Jane 1753. *Essay on the art of ingeniously tormenting.*

ESTATE OF THE IDIOTS AND INSANE. During the reign of Edward II (1284-1327), a law was passed in England that allowed the estates of "idiots" or "natural fools" to be vested in the king, after provision was made for the welfare of the patient. This was a considerable source of revenue for the crown. The estate of a lunatic (q.v.), one who had lost his reason, was administered by the crown on his behalf, and an account of it was given to his heirs after his death. The British legal system still provides a guardianship for the property of insane patients.

See also CHANCERY LUNATICS.

Bibliography: Barr, M. W. 1904. *Mental defectives.*

ESTELLE (1825-?). The daughter of a Swiss merchant, born in Paris. As a child she became a patient of the magnetizer Antoine Despine (q.v.), following a fall that caused her to become paralyzed and to experience excruciating pain. The journey from Neuchatel to Aix, where Despine lived, took five days, and the patient traveled by coach in a padded basket. Despine treated her with magnetism (q.v.), and eventually he thought that her healthy personality, which appeared during hypnotic (*see* HYPNOTISM) sleep, fused with the sick personality that she exhibited when awake. Despine wrote a remarkable book about her in 1840 and described in detail for the first time a case of multiple personality.

Bibliography: Despine, A. 1840. *De l'emploi du magnétisme animal et des eux minérales dans le traîtment des maladies nerveuses.*

ETHER. In the first half of the nineteenth century an American dentist, William Morton (1819-1868) discovered the anesthetic properties of ether. Mesmerism (q.v.) ceased to be used in surgery. Sniffing ether became a kind of parlor game and ether parties became an accepted form of social entertainment.

Bibliography: MacQuitty, B. 1969. *The battle for oblivion.*

ETTLINGER, MAX EMIL (1877-1929). A German psychologist. He tried to reconcile Platonic-Aristotelian theories with modern science. He is also remembered for his work on animal psychology and science of education.

ETTMÜLLER, MICHAEL (1644-1683). A German physician and medical writer. He distinguished delirium (q.v.) from melancholy (*see* MELANCHOLIA), stating that the former succeeded the latter. Because he was a member of the iatrochemical school, he recommended blood transfusions (q.v.) in the treatment of insanity in his book *Chirurgia Transfusoria* (1682).

Bibliography: Zilboorg, G. 1941. *A history of medical psychology.*

EUGENICS. The term was introduced in 1883 by Sir Francis Galton (q.v.). He defined it as "the science which deals with all influences that improve the inborn qualities of the race." A number of works, for example the investigations on the Jukes (q.v.) and the Nams (q.v.), caused widespread alarm, and the feebleminded, who might produce more defectives, were regarded as a menace to society. Segregation and sterilization (q.v.) were advocated. Sterilization was made legal for the whole of the United States in 1927, and some European countries, among them Denmark, Switzerland,

and Finland, introduced similar legislation. Countries that were predominantly Catholic resisted this trend because of the church's theological teachings.

See also HILL FOLK, KALLIKAK FAMILY, MARKUS FAMILY, PINEYS, SAM SIXTY, and ZERO FAMILY.

Bibliography: Kanner, L. 1964. *A history of the care and study of the mentally retarded.*

EURIPIDES (c.480-406 B.C.). A Greek dramatist. His tragedies reflect his deep understanding of human nature evident in the discussions on everyday problems that he presented through his characters. He was particularly interested in feminine psychology, which he portrayed in superb detail in the characters of Phaedra (q.v.) and Medea (q.v.) among others. Insanity was a recurring theme in his ninety-two plays of which only eighteen survive, including *Electra* (q.v.) and *Bacchanals* (q.v.).

Bibliography: Way, A. S., trans. 1912. *Euripides.* 4 vols.

EVACUANTS. Substances causing the expulsion of the contents of the digestive system. From antiquity and until the nineteenth century purging (q.v.) was considered an appropriate form of treatment for insanity. Emetics, causing vomiting, were equally popular, as both, according to the aetiological ideas of the time, either cast out the devils or evacuated the humors (q.v.). Jean Esquirol (q.v.) was perhaps one of the first to question their usefulness; he thought that "far from being adapted to all cases, they may augment the evil."

EVELYN, JOHN (1620-1706). An English author. He is remembered principally for his diary. On April 21, 1657, he recorded his visit to Bethlem Royal Hospital (q.v.) and stated he had seen "several poor miserable creatures in chains; one of them was mad with making verses." On April 18, 1678, he repeated his visit, and by this time the hospital had been rebuilt: "I went to see new Bedlam hospital, magnificently built, and most sweetly placed in Moorfields since the dreadful fire in London."

Bibliography: Evelyn, J. 1955. *Diary (1620-1706),* ed. E. S. De Beer.

EVIL EYE. The belief that some people have the power to harm others by their glance. This superstition, which is widespread in many primitive cultures, is associated with witchcraft (q.v.). Archeological excavations of the Sumerian civilization have produced the earliest written references to it. Special charms against the evil eye are still worn today by less educated Europeans, for instance, a little horn made of coral is the charm of choice in Italy. In the Islamic world many amulets (q.v.), beads, shells, charms, and the color blue-green are believed to keep the evil eye at bay. Any expression of admiration of a child or an animal is permissible only if prefaced by saying, "Not my eye but the eye of the Prophet."

Bibliography: Gifford, E. S. 1958. *The evil eye.*

EWALD, JULIUS RICHARD (1855-1921). German physiologist and professor of physiology at Strasburg. His interest in the physiology of the end-organs and of sensation led him to the pressure-pattern theory of hearing that bears his name.
Bibliography: Boring, E. G. 1950. *A history of experimental psychology.*

EWLIYA, EFFENDI (1611-1679). A Turkish traveler and chronicler. He left a description of the mental hospital built in 1500 by the Sultan Bayezid II (q.v.) in Adrianopolis. Acording to him, the hospital offered a relaxed atmosphere in pleasant surroundings; music, perfumes, special diets, and baths were among the methods of therapy used.
Bibliography: Galdston, I., ed. 1967. *Historic derivations of modern psychiatry.*

EXCELSIOR. One of the earliest asylum magazines. It was begun by the patients at Murray Royal Hospital (q.v.) in 1857 and continued to appear until 1917.
See also JOURNALS BY PATIENTS.

EXCITABILITY. The eighteenth-century theory of excitability of the tissues, propounded chiefly by Albrecht von Haller (q.v.) in 1757 was acceptable to psychiatrists because many mental disorders were characterized by states of excitement and depression. These states of excitement and depression were linked by John Brown (q.v.) to irritability (q.v.) and exhaustion of the nervous system.
Bibliography: Zilboorg, G. 1941. *A history of medical psychology.*

EXE VALE HOSPITAL. A mental hospital in Exeter, England, first planned in 1795 and finally opened in 1801. The first section was rebuilt at Wanford in 1869 for paying patients, and it still stands. The second section, at Exminster, was opened in 1846 for paupers. The first patient for this section was admitted from sixty miles away, arriving at the hospital naked and strapped in the back of a cart. John Bucknill (q.v.) was the first superintendent. The third section, at Digby, was opened in 1886 and was also dedicated to the care of pauper lunatics (q.v.).

EXHIBITIONISM. An anomalous form of sexual behavior. It was clinically described for the first time in 1877 in a paper by Ernest Lasègue (q.v.), who coined the term. One of the earliest accounts of it can be found in the 1550 Court Reports of the Republic of Venice. It is recorded that a certain Domenego, "with temerity and impudence," went about exposing his pudendal member in the churches of the city where pious ladies were hearing masses; he was imprisoned and banned from the republic for ten years. Another famous exhibitionist was Sir Charles Sedley (q.v.).

EXISTENTIALISM. A system of philosophy, essentially European in origin, developed by Søren Kierkegaard, Martin Heidegger, and Jean-Paul Sartre (qq.v.) among others. Developed at the end of World War I, it rejects the view that what cannot be thought cannot be real and regards existence as a reality, rather than a subject for speculation. In psychiatry existential analysis attempts an approach to the patient that takes into account his modes of existence in the world.
Bibliography: Condrau, G., and Boss, M. 1968. Existential analysis. In *Modern perspectives in world psychiatry*, ed. J. G. Howells.

EXNER, SIGMUND (1846-1926). Austrian physiologist and professor of physiology at Vienna University. He worked on the physiology of the senses, the relationship between processes in the central nervous system and psychic phenomena, and the psychology of motivation. His reaction experiment demonstrated that reaction is mostly automatic and depends upon predisposition. He founded the first archive in Vienna to preserve examples of dying dialects and the voices of famous people.
Bibliography: Boring, E. G. 1950. *A history of experimental psychology.*

EXORCISM. Although demoniac possession (q.v.) had been acknowledged since antiquity, European consciousness of Satan reached its zenith in the twelfth and thirteenth centuries. Exorcism, which is supposed to drive the devils from the body of the possessed, consisted of singing ancient incantations that had been handed down from the time of Solomon (q.v.), who was himself a composer of them. The odor of certain roots was believed to draw the devils out through the nostrils. Holy relics were used sometimes, and the patient, who often was subjected to preliminary fasting and long prayers, was touched with the relics and covered by the stole of the officiant. Exorcists had considerable showmanship ability and their activities included many elements of entertainment for the onlookers. Music was another medium often used in exorcism. William Shakespeare (q.v.) gave examples of exorcism in *The Comedy of Errors* (4.4) and in *Twelfth Night* (4.2). The Elizabethans frequently used a book entitled *The Treasury of Exorcism*, which offered numerous incantations and epithets against the devil. The Viennese were more scientific and kept statistics. We are told that in 1583 no less than 12,652 devils had been exorcised by the effort of their holy men. As late as the nineteenth century, Emil Kraepelin (q.v.) reported first-hand knowledge of cases of mental patients who were treated with holy water and exorcised on admission to asylums (q.v.).
Bibliography: Woolley, R. 1932. *Exorcism and the healing of the sick.*

EXPERIMENTAL PSYCHOLOGY. The work of Ernst Weber (q.v.) usually is regarded as the foundation stone of experimental psychology, although the official date of its birth often is taken to coincide with that of

the publication of *Elemente der Psychophysick* (1860) by Gustav Fechner (q.v.).
See also PSYCHOLOGY.
Bibliography: Boring, E. G. 1950. *A history of experimental psychology.*

EXPRESSIONISM. An art movement founded by Wassily Kandinsky (1866-1944) and represented by Vincent Van Gogh (q.v.), Paul Gauguin (q.v.), Henri Matisse (1869-1954), Toulouse-Lautrec (q.v.), and Edward Munch (q.v.) among others. In music and painting, it is represented by Schönberg (1874-1951) and in literature by Franz Kafka (q.v.) and James Joyce (q.v.). It sought to give expression to personal, intimate emotions. To make a greater impact on feelings, it used a style based on simple line and unsubtle colors. The term *expressionism* was first used by German critics in 1911 to describe those painters who were opposed to impressionism.
Bibliography: Myers, B. S. 1958. *Expressionism.*

EXPRESSION OF THE EMOTIONS IN MAN AND ANIMALS. A book written by Charles Darwin (q.v.) in 1872. Among other things, he describes the muscular hyperactivity that is the first response to grief; this is then followed by a period of inaction with sorrow and despair. He also described the typical facial features that accompany various emotions.
Bibliography: Darwin, C. 1872. *Expression of the emotions in man and animals.*

EXTRA SENSORY PERCEPTION (ESP). Perception supposedly occurring outside the known sensory channels. The term, coined by Joseph B. Rhine (q.v.), covers telepathy (q.v.), clairvoyance (q.v.), precognition and psychokinesis (the ability to control the movement of physical objects by power of concentration). Scientific interest in the subject dates from the early part of the twentieth century. Sigmund Freud (q.v.) considered the implications of telepathy and its relevance to psychoanalysis (q.v.) and especially the interpretation of dreams (q.v.). Carl Jung (q.v.) accepted the reality of telepathy and developed a system to explain it. Alfred Adler (q.v.) rejected ESP and regarded any claim of telepathy as a manifestation of compensatory neurosis (q.v.). The work of J. Eisenbud and J. Ehrenwald in America in the 1940s gave new impetus to interest in ESP and its psychiatric implications. New studies on the subject have attempted to arrive at scientific explanations of phenomena that do not yet fit in with the known working of the psyche (q.v.).
Bibliography: Hansel, C. E. M. 1966. *Extra sensory perception.*

EXTROVERT TYPE. A term used by Carl G. Jung (q.v.) to describe one of the types in his classification of personality.
See also INTROVERT TYPE.
Bibliography: Jung, C. G. 1923. *Psychological types,* trans. H. G. Baynes.

F

FABRE, JEAN HENRI (1823-1915). A French naturalist. He studied the behavior, habits, and social life of insects, emphasizing the differences between their behavior and that of men. His work *Souvenirs Entomologiques* was published in ten volumes between 1879 and 1904.
Bibliography: Legros, G. V. 1921. *Fabre, poet of science.*

FACTOR SCHOOL. A school of psychology founded in London by Charles E. Spearman (q.v.). It was based on his views of the "abilities of man" and attracted many students from all over the world. Spearman postulated a general factor of mental ability or energy that varied in individuals. In addition there were a number of specific abilities.
Bibliography: Burt, C. 1940. *The factors of the mind.*

FADEYEV, ALEXANDER ALEXANDROVICH (1901-1956). A Russian novelist. His youth was spent in Siberia. He was influenced by Leo Tolstoy (q.v.), and his novels show a particular understanding of psychological situations. He was not always politically acceptable in Russia, and he committed suicide (q.v.) in Moscow when accused of political crimes.
Bibliography: Bodorykin, V. G. 1968. *Alexander Fadeyev.*

FAIRBAIRN, W. RONALD (1889-1964). A British psychoanalyst. He suggested a new approach to ego psychology, maintaining that the theory of impulses needed reformulating on the basis of structural theory. He thought that the theory of internalized objects had followed Sigmund Freud's (q.v.) psychology of impulses without adding anything new to it.
Bibliography: Fairbairn, W. R. 1954. *An object relation theory of personality.*

FAITHFUL BRETHREN OF BASRA. A secret fraternity in Iraq active in the middle of the tenth century. The members of the fraternity were based

mostly in Basra and Baghdad. They wrote about fifty-one anonymous epistles that described their ideas and tried to reconcile a rational philosophy
with Islamic doctrine. Their writings, which were divided into four groups,
superficially covered practically all contemporary science. The first group
concerned figures, letters, music, and mathematics; the second, man's progress from material elements to spirituality; the third psychology and reason;
and the fourth divinity, the order of the universe, magic (q.v.), and super-
human beings in which they believed.
Bibliography: Mcdonald, D. B. 1903. *Muslim theology.*

FAITH HEALING. The seeking of divine intervention to remedy physical
or mental illness. In primitive people it is associated with exorcism (q.v.),
charms, and the intervention of medicine men, or shamans (q.v.). All great
religions in the East and in the West have employed faith healing. Mind
cure movements often are centered in a sect (Christian Science [q.v.]) or in
a shrine (Lourdes [q.v.]). Psychological and medical theories to explain the
phenomenon vary and have evolved from studies in hypnosis (*see* HYP-
NOTISM), suggestion, and psychosomatics.
Bibliography: Weatherhead, L. D. 1952. *Psychology, religion and healing.*

FAKIR. Hindu or Moslem holy man. Fakirs are believed to possess miraculous powers that allow them, for example, to be insensitive to pain, walk
on fire, or rest on beds of nails. They are able to produce mass suggestion
in the credulous uneducated masses, and they have been known to use this
ability to intervene in political issues.
See also ASCETICS.
Bibliography: Akhilananda, S. 1946. *Hindu psychology.*

FALCONER, WILLIAM (1744-1824). A British physician who practiced
in Chester and Bath. In 1788 he wrote an essay entitled "Dissertation on
the influence of passions upon disorders of the body," which received the
first psychiatric prize ever given and won for him the Fotheringillian Medal
of the Medical Society of London. The theme set to the competitors was,
"What diseases may be mitigated or cured, by exciting particular affections
or passions of the mind?". Falconer wrote that there were two types of
emotions; those that excite the "vital system" and those that depress it. He
discussed their effects on various pathological states, including gout, toothache, typhus, and scurvy, as well as depression and mania (q.v.). He was
well aware of the influence of suggestion and devised experiments to demonstrate it.
Bibliography: Leigh, D. 1961. *The historical development of British psychiatry.*

FALCONRY. The hunting of wild quarry with trained birds of prey. In
1250, Frederick II (q.v.) wrote a book on falconry entitled *De Arte Venandi*

cum Avibus, in which he listed various practices based on a system of technology of animal behavior. He advised systematic desensitization of the falcon to certain stimuli, followed by conditioning and positive reinforcement. The falcons were never punished, and the emperor warned that a bad-tempered falconer would not succeed in training such a sensitive bird. The work is possibly the earliest example of a systematic plan of conditioning and imprinting (q.v.).

Bibliography: Frederick II. c.1250. *De arte venandi cum avibus*, trans. C. A. Wood and F. M. Fyfe. 1943. *The art of falconry.*

FALLOWES, THOMAS (fl.1705). A self-styled M.D. who established a private madhouse in Lambeth Marsh in London. He treated lunacy with an ointment he had invented. It was called Oleum Cephalicum (q.v.), and it was rubbed into the shaven scalp until pustules were formed, which he claimed released the "black vapors" responsible for madness. The use of the ointment was standard procedure in his establishment, and his patients were treated with kindness. According to his advertisement, they were not kept short of food. The Oleum Cephalicum was also sold to users outside his madhouse and was widely used. Fallowes even wrote a book on his "incomparable oleum cephalicum," describing its advantages.

Bibliography: Hunter, R., and Macalpine, I. 1963. *Three hundred years of psychiatry.*

FALRET, JEAN PIERRE (1794-1870). French physician, pupil of Jean Esquirol (q.v.) and chief physician at the Salpêtrière (q.v.). He presented an early clinical exposition of *folie circulaire* (q.v.) (manic depressive psychosis) and established definite diagnostic criteria for general paralysis of the insane (q.v.). He believed that mental illness was an alienation from the social environment and therefore used the term "mental alienation" from which the term "alienist" (q.v.) is derived. He was the first to publish statistical data on suicide (q.v.), which he believed to be a disease of the brain.

Bibliography: Falret, J. 1822. *De l'hypochondrie et du suicide.*

FALRET, JULES PH. J. (1824-1902). A French psychiatrist. In addition to his studies on manic-depressive psychoses (q.v.) and on general paralysis of the insane (q.v.), he contributed to psychiatry by a description of a mutually induced neurosis (q.v.), a phenomenon implying psychological contagion. He and Ernest Lasègue (q.v.) termed it *folie à deux* [q.v.] *ou folie communiquée.*

Bibliography: Lasègue, C., and Falret, J. 1877. La folie à deux (ou folie communiquée). *Annls. med.-psychol.* 18:321.

FAMILY CARE. Boarding of mental patients in private families has a long tradition and some examples of this practice are several centuries old. One

of the oldest centers is at Iwakura near Kyoto, in Japan. According to tradition, it originated in 1070, following the cure of Daiunji (q.v.), the emperor's daughter, who had been sent there to drink the water of a holy fountain. The Gheel colony (q.v.), in Belgium, also originated in the eleventh century; the miraculous cures there were attributed to Saint Dymphna (q.v.), who lived in the seventh or eighth century. In the nineteenth century the tradition was revived and other family-care villages were developed in Scotland, Holland, and Norway, as well as other places. The first program in the United States was begun in Massachusetts in 1885.
See also BOARDING-OUT OF MENTAL PATIENTS and COTTAGE SYSTEM.
Bibliography: Crutcher, H.B. 1944. *Foster home care for mental patients.*

FARADAY, MICHAEL (1791-1867). An English scientist, renowned for his many discoveries in chemistry and physics. In 1839 he suffered an undefined illness which affected his mental faculties and prevented him working for about three years. He complained of giddiness, headaches, and most of all, of loss of memory. This state so concerned him that he withdrew almost completely from society. Even after recovery he was never fully free from these symptoms. Two years before his death he became demented.
Bibliography: Williams, L. P. 1965. *Michael Faraday: a biography.*

FARIA, JOSÉ CUSTODIO DE (1754-1819). An Indian priest born in the village of Candolim in Bardez, Goa. He went to Rome, where he obtained a degree in theology, and thence to Paris, where he became interested in the hypnotic practices of Franz Mesmer (q.v.) and Amand-Marie-Jacques Puysegur (q.v.). His experiments with mesmerism (q.v.) led to his appointment as professor of philosophy at Marseilles. He was the first to prove that hypnotic states had nothing to do with magnetic fluid but rather were the result of direct suggestion on impressionable subjects. He also discussed the link between somnambulism (q.v.) and anaemic conditions and the psychological mechanism of somnambulism. His work "De la cause du somneil lucide" was published in 1819. He died that year of apoplexy.
Bibliography: Sharma, S. 1973. Abbé de Faria: the true founder of the doctrine of suggestion from the East. *Proceedings of the Fifth World Congress of Psychiatry, Mexico City.*

FARINELLI, CARLO (*original surname* **BROSCHI**) (1705-1782). An Italian male soprano, castrated at the age of seven. It was said that his singing could relieve the chronic melancholy of Philip V of Spain (q.v.). He was offered 50,000 francs a year if he would remain in Spain. He accepted and stayed for twenty-five years, singing the same four songs every night to the king. He achieved power approaching that of a prime minister. Ferdi-

nand VI (q.v.) also found relief in his songs. In 1761 he retired to a castle in Bologna, Italy, where he died.
Bibliography: Osborn, M. L. 1975. Pseudohermaphrodites with the golden voices. *World Medicine*. 11: 55.

FARMING. In his *Mental Maladies: A Treatise on Insanity*, Jean Esquirol (q.v.) quoted the cures obtained by a Scottish farmer who forced mental patients to work in his fields. The occupation of patients on farms has been a feature of the management of mental patients until recent times. With more concentrated therapy, especially occupational therapy (q.v.), there has been a tendency to abandon it.
Bibliography: Henderson, D. K. 1964. *The evolution of psychiatry in Scotland.*

FARNHAM, RICHARD (?-1642). A weaver from Colchester, in Essex, England. He suffered from delusions (q.v.) and believed himself to be inspired by God and by Him commanded, like the biblical Hosea, to marry an unfaithful woman. Unfortunately, he picked the wife of a sailor who did not share his religious aspirations. In 1637 he was accused of bigamy and sent first to Newgate prison and then to Bethlem Royal Hospital (q.v.). He was discharged after a year and continued to preach, gathering a number of followers. After his death, his followers continued to believe that he was alive. They justified his absence by saying that he had gone to Israel to preach and regularly drank to his health. Some hysterical women even testified to his resurrection a year after his death.
Bibliography: O'Donoghue, E. G. 1914. *The story of Bethlehem Hospital.*

FAROUK I (1920-1965). A king of Egypt. As a child he was spoiled by his mother, who fostered his interest in superstition by taking him to seances. His father, too, was superstitious; having been told that the letter "F" would bring him luck, he chose names beginning with "F" for all his children. Farouk suffered from insomnia and violent dreams. He became king when he was sixteen years old and at seventeen married a fifteen-year-old girl, who had to change her name to Farida to conform to the "F" rule. She also had to comfort him whenever he was rejected by one of his many mistresses. His poor education made him feel inferior, and he compensated by being flamboyant, dressing in gaudy uniforms, womanizing, gambling, and drinking excessively. His obesity has been linked to his anxiety. From an attractive adolescent, he rapidly degenerated into a gross and repulsively fat adult. In 1952 he was forced to abdicate in favor of his baby son Fuad. Farouk died in Rome, in the arms of a mistress, in comparative poverty.

FASCIOLA HEPATICA. The sheep liver fluke. It is discharged in the mucus of a snail, which then is eaten by an ant. The fluke attacks the ant's nervous system and causes an aberration of behavior whereby the ant climbs

blades of grass and remains at the top of them until eaten by cattle or sheep, which in turn become infected.
Bibliography: Carr, D. E. 1971. *The deadly feast of life.*

FASTING. Abstinence from food and drink. Fasting is practiced at stated periods in most religions. During the sixteenth and seventeenth century when so-called miraculous happenings were a common phenomenon, many people were said to survive prolonged periods of fasting. Barbara Kremers (q.v.) was one such famous case. Johann Weyer (q.v.) investigated her claims and was prompted to write an essay '*De Commentitiis Jejuniis*, on alleged fasting, which was published in 1577. He reviewed the various instances of fasting in the Bible (q.v.) and presented the Barbara Kremers case, concluding that these phenomena were not supernatural but were due to malingering. In 1869, a similar case was provided by a Welsh girl, Sarah Jacob (q.v.).
Bibliography: Zilboorg, G. 1941. *A history of medical psychology.*

FATHER DIVINE (c. 1880-1965). The assumed name of George Baker, an American Negro. After being given the title of "God in the Sonship Degree" by Samuel Morris in the Baptist Church Colored of Baltimore, he moved to New York and proclaimed himself God, Father Divine. His followers, mainly Negroes, were called "angels"; they were obliged to renounce all family ties and sexual relationships. Their meeting places were called "heavens."
Bibliography: Harris, S. 1954. *The incredible Father Divine.*

FATUA. According to Saint Isidore of Seville (q.v.), she was a seeress in Roman religion whose prophesies caused a state of stupefaction in those listening. Listeners were called "fatui," a term that was later used for mental defectives. The word "infatuation" has the same origin.
Bibliography: Kanner, L. 1964. *A history of the care and study of the mentally retarded.*

FATUITATE ALPINA. A term derived from Fatua (q.v.) and used to designate a type of cretinism (q.v.) allied with endemic goiter. It was commonly found in alpine valleys.
Bibliography: Abercrombie, J. 1803. *De fatuitate Alpina.*

FAULKNER, BENJAMIN (?-1799). English owner of a private madhouse at Little Chelsea in London. Following an arrangement common to his time, he provided only nursing care for mental patients and left treatment to their own doctors. He believed that psychic treatment should be tried before putting the patient in an asylum, where the sudden change of environment

and the absence of family and friends could worsen his condition. Visitors, relations, and friends were freely admitted in his establishment.
Bibliography: Hunter, R., and Macalpine, I. 1963. *Three hundred years of psychiatry*.

FAULKNER, WILLIAM (1897-1962). Major American poet and novelist, recipient of the 1949 Nobel Prize for literature and the Pulitzer prizes in 1955 and 1963, posthumously. He changed his name from Falkner when he published his first book of poems in 1924 and said, "I myself really don't know the true reason." Before he settled down to writing, he had many different occupations including three years as postmaster at the University of Mississippi, from which he was discharged because, as he put it, he had been accused of "throwing all in coming mail into (the) garbage can." His style of writing was influenced at first by T. S. Eliot (q.v.) and James Joyce (q.v.). He gradually evolved his own style which was often obscure and was often referred to as "stream-of-consciousness" writing. His writing was very immediate and involved the reader in participating in the thoughts of his characters; these often tended to be brutal and depraved. One of the characters in his main work *The Sound and the Fury* (1929) was an idiot (q.v.).
Bibliography: Millgate, M. 1966. *The achievement of William Faulkner*.

FAUNI. In ancient Roman folklore, spirits of the woods. They were believed to cause mental illness. Pliny the Elder (q.v.) used the term *ludibria faunorum*, or "mockeries of the fauni" for certain mental disorders.
Bibliography: Zilboorg, G. 1941. *A history of medical psychology*.

FAUST. A legendary figure who sold his soul to the devil in exchange for supernatural power. The legend reflects the ambivalent feeling toward power, desired yet feared. The most likely source of the legend is Johann F, or Faustus (c. 1488-1541) a magician born in Swabia. He was a student of necromancy (q.v.) and assumed the roles of diviner, astrologer, alchemist, or medium to swindle gullible people. Over the years, the story of Faust has inspired many writers and musicians, for example, Christopher Marlow (1564-1593) in the sixteenth century and Johann von Goethe (q.v.) in the seventeenth century, as well as Louis Berlioz, Franz Liszt, and Richard Wagner (qq.v.).
Bibliography: Palmer, P., and Moore, R. 1936. *The sources of the Faust tradition*.

FAUSTINA AUGUSTA (c. 125-c.175 A.D.). A Roman empress, wife of Marcus Aurelius Antoninus (q.v.). Her passionate desire for a gladiator (q.v.) so overwhelmed her that she became dangerously ill. She confessed her lust to her husband. Following the advice of a physician, he had the

gladiator killed and Faustina's body anointed with his warm blood. Her passion abated and she was cured.
Bibliography: Boccaccio, G. 1962. *Concerning famous women*, trans. G. Guarino.

FAWCETT, BENJAMIN (1715-1780). An English clergyman. Despite being a man of the Church, he realized that excessive preoccupation with religion is pathological and wrote a book entitled *Observations on the Nature, Causes and Cure of Melancholy, Especially of That Which is commonly Known as Religious Melancholy* in 1780.

FAXENSYNDROM. A German term used by Eugen Bleuler (q.v.) to describe a form of psychosis (q.v.) occurring in prisoners whose behavior becomes clownish because of dissociation.

FAYETTE HOSPITAL. A mental hospital founded in the United States in the early 1800s. It was a group venture in public service, but it did not prosper and was never completed. In 1824 the unfinished and unoccupied building was taken over by the Kentucky Lunatic Asylum (q.v.).
Bibliography: Deutsch, A. 1949. *The mentally ill in America*.

FEAR WATER. Water contained in a bottle hidden in a cemetery. In ancient Russia, patients suffering from nervous disorders or epilepsy (q.v.) were sent by folk healers to search for it at the dead of night. The more scared and superstitious the patients, the more likely it was that a cure would ensue. Yakut and Buriat shamans (q.v.) used this method to treat nervous disorders in general.
Bibliography: Kourennoff, P. M., and St. George, G. 1970. *Russian folk medicine*.

FECHNER, GUSTAV THEODOR (1801-1887). German physician, psychologist, physicist, and philosopher. His father, a progressive man, was a village pastor, who shocked his parishioners by preaching without a wig and by installing a lightning rod on the church tower. After qualifying in medicine, Fechner became interested in physics and mathematics and went on to become professor of physics in Leipzig in 1834. He resigned five years later, exhausted by overwork. His condition was diagnosed by William James (q.v.) as "habit neurosis." After this crisis, Fechner recovered and turned his attention to spiritual problems: he affirmed that mind and matter are identical. He studied sensations, introduced experimental methods into the study of psychological phenomena, and has been regarded as the father of experimental psychology (q.v.) because of his book *Elemente der Psychophysik*, published in 1860. From time to time he wrote under the pseudonym of "Dr. Mises".
Bibliography: Boring, E. G. 1950. *A history of experimental psychology*.

FEDERN, PAUL (1871-1950). Austrian physician and one of the first pioneers of psychoanalysis (q.v.) as well as a founding member of the Vienna

Psychoanalytic Society. He was a gentle, sensitive, romantic, and melancholy man whose dark beard made him appear somewhat fierce. He married Wilma Bauer, who had loved him since her childhood. She was a poet and playwright of merit, but Federn would not consent to the publication of her work. He was a great admirer of Sigmund Freud (q.v.) and regarded him as his teacher. Freud, after being struck with cancer, appointed Federn as his representative in the Vienna society. Federn was an ardent patriot; when the First World War was declared, he invested heavily and disastrously in Austrian War Bonds. He had a casual attitude toward money and often did not bother to charge fees for treatment, thus incurring Freud's disapproval. In 1938 he left Vienna for New York, where he obtained a licence to practice medicine in 1946. In the same year he was reunited with his son Ernst, recently freed from a concentration camp, but his life now entered a sad last phase: his chronically ill wife died in 1949, and he himself had to limit his professional activities because of advanced cancer of the bladder. On the day he should have undergone an operation he shot himself in his office. His concern for others prevailed even in his last hour, as he warned in the note he left that the gun contained another bullet. His studies are mainly concerned with analysis of the ego and descriptions of inner experiences and how these could be applied to the treatment of psychosis (q.v.). His book, *Ego Psychology and the Psychoses* is an important contribution to the psychological analysis of the ego.

Bibliography: Alexander, F.; Eisenstein, S.; and Grotjahn, M., eds. 1966. *Psychoanalytic pioneers.*

FEIGNED INSANITY. There are many examples of feigned insanity in history. King David (q.v.) pretended insanity to escape Achish; Lucius Junius Brutus, the Roman consul, feigned insanity to expel the Tarquins; Ulysses (q.v.) pretended to be mad to avoid going to war; Solon of Athens feigned insanity to raise his fellow citizens to war. In William Shakespeare's (q.v.) plays, Edgar (q.v.) in *King Lear*, and Hamlet (q.v.) in *Hamlet* feign madness. A rapid pulse and an inability to reword a sentence were considered proof of genuine insanity by the Elizabethans, hence Hamlet's offer to be put to the test:

My pulse as yours, doth temperately keep time.
. . . bring me to the test
And I the matter will reword: which madness would gambol from.

Hamlet, 3. 4.

In the nineteenth century, the spinning chair (q.v.) was sometimes used as a test. Its effects were so unpleasant that no one had the strength to act insane after two minutes in it.

FÉLIDA, X. (1843-?). A patient of Etienne Azam (q.v.). At thirteen, after a difficult childhood, she developed a case of double personality—each unaware of the other and quite different. She suffered from pulmonary and gastric hemorrhages, but no lesions could be discovered. Blood flowed constantly from her mouth during her sleep. After a crisis culminating in a lethargic sleep, she would awaken elated, free from her usual physical symptoms and unaware of her recent condition. Despite her disabilities she married, had eleven children, and worked extremely hard. Azam observed her from 1858 to 1893 and published her case history with an introduction by Jean-Martin Charcot (q.v.).
Bibliography: Azam, E. E. 1887. *Hypnotisme, double conscience et altération de la personnalité.*

FELO DE SE. An Anglo-Latin expression meaning suicide (q.v.). It reflects the view that self-destruction is a crime, or a felony against oneself.

FELTRINI, ANDREA (1477-1548). An Italian painter. He was pathologically insecure and depressed. Feltrini was highly regarded by Giorgio Vasari (1511-1574), who praised him in his *Lives of the Artists* (1550). Vasari, however, also wrote:

he was of such a timid nature that he would never undertake any work of his own account, because he was afraid of exacting money for his labours. Tortured by a melancholic humour, he was often on the point of taking his life, but he was so closely watched and so well guarded by his companion Mariotto that he lived to be an old man.

Bibliography: Wittkower, R., and Wittkower, M. 1963. *Born under Saturn.*

FENICHEL, OTTO (1898-1946). An Austrian pioneer in psychoanalysis (q.v.) and the author of the first textbook on psychoanalysis, *The Outline of Clinical Psychoanalysis*, which was published in 1934. His book *The Psychoanalytic Theory of Neuroses*, written in 1945, has become a classic. He was a forceful, critical, and direct man; a brilliant teacher, who could convey his ideas concisely and clearly; and a humanitarian clinician, who felt deep concern for his patients. He did not believe in the therapeutic value of insight but rather thought that patients could be better helped by emotional experiences. At the age of forty-seven, when he was already a famous psychoanalyst and teacher, he decided to obtain an American medical degree and began the prescribed year of internship at the Cedars of Lebanon Hospital in Los Angeles, California. He felt that he would be better able to further the cause of psychoanalysis in America with an American degree, but his self-imposed task remained uncompleted because he died before finishing his internship.

Bibliography: Alexander, F.; Eisenstein, S.; and Grotjahn, M., eds. 1966. *Psychoanalytic pioneers*.

FERAL CHILD. A child brought up by a species other than his own. Examples of feral children are found mostly in legend, for example, Romulus (q.v.) and Remus, who were said to have been fostered by a she-wolf. Between 1344 and 1961 some fifty-three feral children have been described. The term was first used by Carolus Linnaeus (q.v.) in 1758. The wolf child of Hesse, the wild boy of Aveyron and the wild boy of Salvador (qq.v.) are some of the most famous examples.

See also BOVINUS BAMBERGENSIS, MARIE LEBLANC, OVINUS HIBERNUS, URSINUS LITHUANUS, WOLF CHILDREN OF MIDNAPORE.

Bibliography: Malson, L. 1972. *Wolf children*.

FERDINAND VI (1713-1759). A king of Spain. In the later years of his life he became increasingly melancholy (*see* MELANCHOLIA) and was considered insane. Like his father, Philip V (q.v.), he benefited from the singing of the Italian castrato Carlo Farinelli (q.v.).

FERENCZI, SANDOR (1873-1933). A Hungarian psychoanalyst, born in Miskolc, Hungary. There were eleven children in the family. He spent most of his childhood among books, as his father ran a bookstore, which may explain the wide range of his interest in literature and art. Early in his medical career he became interested in mental disorders and neurotic difficulties. He became a prominent pioneer in psychoanalysis (q.v.) and was considered by many second only to Sigmund Freud (q.v.) whom he met in 1908. He was called by Freud "my dear son" and underwent a personal analysis with him. He was a prolific writer. Some of his works expanding Freud's theories and developing many new aspects of them are considered masterpieces in the field of psychoanalysis. His ideas, which were expressed in a dramatic and arresting style, were based on his clinical practice. The boldness of his ideas attracted great attention and generated much controversy. He investigated the development of a sense of reality, sexual habits, and therapeutic methods. He was a charming, colorful, and warm person who many people admired; his lectures were always well attended. However, when he lectured in the United States, he encounterd some strong professional opposition because he supported analysis by lay people such as educators. During the last few years of his life, Ferenczi's relationship with Freud became strained after Freud seriously criticized some of his experiments in technique. He

also wrote some poetry, which so far remains unpublished. He died of pernicious anaemia, and the neurological complications resulting from it.
Bibliography: Alexander, F.; Eisenstein, S.; and Grotjahn, M., eds. 1966. *Psychoanalytic pioneers.*

FERGUSSON, ROBERT (1750-1774). A Scottish poet. He was a popular man, whose health was damaged by excess of conviviality. Paradoxically, he was given to religious melancholy (*see* MELANCHOLIA). He was said to have become deranged following a head injury. Dr. Andrew Duncan (q.v.) found him suffering from "furious insanity" and in need of hospitalization. He was admitted to the workhouse of Edinburgh where a few stone-floored cells were reserved for the mentally ill. He died there on a bed of straw at twenty-four years of age. The lack of suitable accommodation and his lonely death inspired Duncan to found the Edinburgh Lunatic Asylum (q.v.) in order that the mentally ill could be properly treated. A locket with a lock of Fergusson's hair and his portrait by Henry Raeburn still sits on the mantelpiece of the hospital's drawing room.
Bibliography: Henderson, D. K. 1964. *The evolution of psychiatry in Scotland.*

FERNEL, JEAN (FERNELIUS) (1497-1558). French physician, mathematician, and astronomer. He believed that disease was caused by disordered humors (q.v.) and that symptoms were to be found by the observation of bodily functions. He opposed bleeding (q.v.) and made the best classification of diseases between Galen's (q.v.) and Felix Plater's (q.v.). He classified mental disorders according to the sites where they originated, hence: lesions of the meninges of the brain, aphalalgia, hemicrania, cephaleia; lesions of the substance of the brain, phrenitis, delirium, lycanthropy, mania, stultitia (qq.v.), amentia, oblivio; and lesions of the ventricles, epilepsy (q.v.), incubus (q.v.), apoplexy. Although he made a fortune with his clinical practice, Fernel wasted most of his money indulging his passion for astronomy. His patients included Catherine de Medici, whom he cured of sterility, and Diane de Poitiers, mistress of Henry II. Although frequently melancholy, he would always come out of his depression for the sake of a patient, and patients would always be treated, no matter how poor they might be. His main work is *Universa Medicina* (1554).
Bibliography: Sherrington, Charles. 1946. *The endeavour of Jean Fernel.*

FERRAND, JACQUES (fl. 1604-1630). A French physician. He seems to have appreciated the importance of giving insight to his patients. He cured two young women of the delusion that the devil lay with them every night by reasoning with them. After recovery, they admitted that "it was all a depravity of their imagination" - the first recorded case of patients gaining insight through medical treatment. He wrote a treatise *De la Maladie d'Amour, ou Mélancholie Érotique* in 1623, to offer specific advice on the treat-

ment of love melancholy and to confound those physicians "who prescribe for the cure of this disease, Lust, and Fornication." He realized that love melancholy was different in aetiology and pathology from the disorders of "other melancholics and madmen." His book was translated into English in 1640 with the title of *Erotomania*.
Bibliography: Stafford-Clark, D. 1952. *Psychiatry to-day*.

FERRI, ENRICO (1856-1929). Italian criminal lawyer and psychiatrist, pupil of Cesare Lombroso (q.v.). He represented a school of criminology that paid attention to the biological and anthropological aspect of the individual offender. He considered prevention, education, and rehabilitation a greater deterrent to criminal behavior than punishment.
Bibliography: Ferri, E. 1917. *Criminal sociology*.

FERRIAR, JOHN (1761-1815). Scottish physician and medical writer. He was particularly interested in psychology and was physician to the Manchester Lunatic Asylum (q.v.). He tried to explain in physiopathological terms phenomena that were then believed to have supernatural causes. He advised psychiatrists to rely on direct observation rather than on accepted theories. Having assessed many traditional remedies for insanity he expressed the opinion that they were useless as were emetics and bleeding (q.v.). He introduced the term "hysterical conversion" (q.v.) and was one of the first physicians to advocate isolation of violent patients rather than restraint (q.v.). He also advocated the provision of separate accommodations for convalescing patients. His observations were based on experience and were published in 1795 with the title *Medical Histories and Reflections*.
Bibliography: Hunter, R., and Macalpine, I. 1963. *Three hundred years of psychiatry*.

FERRIER, SIR DAVID (1843-1928). A Scottish neurologist who worked in England. His studies of localization of cerebral functions laid the basis for future knowledge in this field and demonstrated the importance of the central nervous system. His book *Functions of the Brain* was published in 1876.
Bibliography: Haymaker, W., and Schiller, F. 1970. *The founders of neurology*, 2d. ed.

FERRUS, GUILLAUME MARIE ANDRÉ (1784-1861). A French physician. He gained his doctorate in medicine at the age of twenty. Like his father, he was involved in politics and followed the fortunes of Napoleon (q.v.) as a surgeon in his army. In 1818 he joined Philippe Pinel (q.v.), and eight years later he became physician-in-chief at Bicêtre (q.v.). He visited asylums (q.v.) in France and in England and was shocked to find that criminals and the insane were often kept together. He separated them at Bicêtre and solved the problem of overcrowding by setting the less severely ill patients to work in farms and workshops, thus instituting an early system of occupational therapy (q.v.). He was a devoted and insightful physician. Ferrus never hesitated to express his opinion even when it was against the current trend, as in the case of complete nonrestraint, which he considered detrimental to the patient. He believed mental disorders had an exclusively organic aetiology. In 1835, he was appointed inspector general of all mental institutions in France, and in 1847 he became the first president of the Société Medico-psychologique (q.v.). Forensic psychiatry (q.v.) was advanced by him and especially by his insistence that the criminally insane should receive treatment.

Bibliography: Semelaigne, R. 1930. *Les pionniers de la psychiatrie française.*

FETCH. The ghost of a living person. According to superstition, it appears to distant relations or friends at the moment when the person it represents dies.

Bibliography: 1978. *Brewer's dictionary of phrase and fable.*

FETISH. A term derived from the Portuguese *fetico*, meaning a "charm." In psychiatry it refers to an object that has become emotionally charged and, in some cases, is the source of perverted sexual gratification. Alfred Binet (q.v.) first used the term in this sense in 1888.

Bibliography: 1978. *Brewer's dictionary of phrase and fable.*

FEUCHTERSLEBEN, ERNST VON (1806-1849). An Austrian psychiatrist. His first book of psychological interest was *On the Dietics of the Soul* (1838), which was translated into several languages. He approached the study and treatment of mental disorders from a psychosomatic point of view, believing that body and mind were "a single phenomenon, invariably one and indivisible" and therefore mental illness and personality disturbances were linked. He coined many terms: psychiatrics, psychosis (q.v.), psychopathy (q.v.), psychopathology, and psychological physician, as well as others. By psychopathy or psychosis he meant disorders that are not characterized by pathological changes in the nerves. He divided these disorders into: folly, fixed delusions (q.v.), mania (q.v.), and idiocy (*see* IDIOT). His therapeutic methods employed colors and sounds and accepted smoking as a measure useful in "dissipating thoughts." He favored asylums (q.v.) situated in the country so that the patients would not be upset by the bustle of the town, and the town would not be disturbed by the presence of lunatic patients. His book *Lehrbuch der ärztlichen Seelenkunde* was published in Vienna in 1845. It covered the whole field of psychological medicine, history, physiology and pathology of the mind, and treatment, including psychotherapy (q.v.). Two years later the book was translated into English and published by the Sydenham Society of London, an honor usually reserved

to works proved successful by time. He was a poet, a philosopher, and an educational reformer as well as a medical writer.
Bibliography: Feuchtersleben, E. von. 1847. *The principles of medical psychology.*

FEUERBACH, PAUL JOHANN ANSELM, VON (1775-1833). A Bavarian jurist and philosopher. He specialized in criminology and legal reform and advocated the abolition of torture, which he wished to replace with psychological coercion, an approach he pioneered. In 1832, he reported the case of Kaspar Hauser (q.v.).
Bibliography: Goldenson, R. M. 1970. *The encyclopedia of human behavior.*

FEVER THERAPY. From Hippocrates (q.v.) onward it has been noted that an acute infection accompanied by a high temperature may produce an improvement in the condition of a mentally ill patient. Galen (q.v.), Hermann Boerhaave (q.v.) and later workers cited cures brought about by so-called quartan agues. As a result of these observations, infections were deliberately introduced in a patient's system by means of injections producing typhus, tuberculosis (q.v.), or malaria. Malaria therapy (q.v.) was particularly popular as a form of treatment for general paralysis of the insane (q.v.).
Bibliography: Rudolf, G. de. 1927. *Therapeutic malaria.*

FICHTE, JOHANN GOTTLIEB (1762-1814). A German philosopher, disciple of Immanuel Kant (q.v.). His ideas contain the rudiments of existentialism (q.v.). According to him, the ego is the only reality, and it affirms itself through consciousness; the non-ego is the world of experience. He later developed his philosophy to a point where the ego became a symbol of the German nation. In 1810 he became the first rector of the newly founded University of Berlin. His main work, *Uber den Begriff der Wissenschaftslehere*, was published in 1794.
Bibliography: Engelbrecht, H. C. 1933. *Johann Gottlieb Fichte.*

FICINO, MARSILIO (1433-1499). Italian humanist and head of the Neo-Platonic academy of Florence. He is remembered for his translations of Plato (q.v.) and other Greek philosophers, as well as for his own philosophical writings in which he asserted that man could find eternal truth through his own efforts. This statement caused him to be accused of heresy. He was also a physician and in 1482 wrote *De Studiosorum Sanitate Tuenda* in which he offered advice to all those engaged in intellectual occupations and subjected to a particular type of stress of a nonphysical nature. He

attempted to find a rational explanation for supernatural phenomena and opposed witchcraft (q.v.).
Bibliography: Jayne, S. R. 1963. *John Colet and Marsilio Ficino.*

FIGS. The Brahmans and Buddhists regard the fig tree as sacred. In the sixteenth century, figs were recommended in the treatment of epilepsy (q.v.), but the melancholy man was advised to avoid them in his diet.
Bibliography: O'Hara-May, J. 1977. *Elizabethan dyetary of health.*

FILICIDE. The killing of a child by his own parents as an offering to the gods or as an act of vengeance. It has many examples in antiquity. In Greek mythology, Medea (q.v.) is the prototype of the murdering mother. In the Bible (q.v.) Abraham nearly killed Isaac to prove his complete devotion to God. In the first century B.C., Diodorus of Sicily wrote about the practices of the Carthaginians, who periodically sacrificed first-born sons to the god Baal Hammon. His account was given credulity in 1963 when a burial ground containing the remains of about 3,000 children was unearthed. The inscriptions on the urns stated that they had been strangled and their bodies burned in religious ceremonies. In other cultures, children have been enclosed in the foundations of buildings as a propitiatory measure. The Romans gave the father the legal right of killing his children. In China (q.v.), as in some other countries, female children were often destroyed at birth—a practice still in existence at the end of the nineteenth century. In many cultures deformed children were destroyed and so were twins who were considered monstrous births. In psychiatry and in legal practice infanticide has special implications of deep conflict between parents and their children.
Bibliography: Piers, M. W. 1978. *Infanticide: past and present.*

FILIGER, CHARLES (1863-1928). A French symbolist painter, follower of Paul Gauguin (q.v.). His art reflects his psychopathology: he suffered from paranoia (q.v.). After a disordered life, he completely isolated himself and finally committed suicide (q.v.).
Bibliography: Bader, A. 1971. Decouverte Psychopathologique de Charles Filiger. *Confin. Psychiat. (Basel)* 14:18-35.

FINAN, SAINT (?-661). Irish bishop of Lindisfarne, Ireland, famous for his zeal, learning, and prudence. A lunatic asylum in Killarney, Saint Finan Hospital, was dedicated to him when it opened in 1847, shortly after the Great Famine.
Bibliography: Anon. 1971. *Saint Finan's Hospital, Killarney.*

FINCH FAMILY. An English family whose members kept several madhouses since the later part of the eighteenth century. Both Fisherton House

(q.v.) and Laverstock House in Wiltshire were operated by them as was a house in Kensington and another in Chelsea.
Bibliography: Parry-Jones, W. Ll. 1972. *The trade in lunacy.*

FINDLATTER, LORD. An Elizabethan nobleman. After trying to seduce his stepmother, he schemed to drive his father mad by keeping him awake and walking in a dark house until he became insane. The plot was discovered, and his father disinherited him.
Bibliography: Sitwell, E. 1962. *The queens and the hive.*

FIRE. As late as the last century, fire was applied to the head and neck of the insane as a form of therapy. Jean Esquirol (q.v.) reports applying red hot irons to the neck of some of his manic patients "with success."
See also CAUTERIZATION.
Bibliography: Esquirol, J. E. D. 1845. *Mental maladies.* Reprint, 1965.

FIRST LINES ON THE PRACTICE OF PHYSICS. A treatise by William Cullen (q.v.), first published in 1777. It presented a new system of classification of diseases based on symptoms, methods of diagnosis, and treatment and covered practically all the disorders then known. Mental diseases were classified under the term neuroses (see NEUROSIS), which was subdivided into four orders: comata (q.v.), adynamias (q.v.), spasms, and vesanias (q.v.). Cullen's work exercised great influence on the theory and practice of psychiatry both in England and abroad. Philippe Pinel (q.v.) was much impressed by this book and based many of his own ideas on it.
Bibliography: Leigh, D. 1961. *The historical development of British psychiatry.*

FISHER, JOHN ARBUTHNOT, LORD FISHER OF KILVERSTONE (1841–?1920). A British admiral. He became first sea lord. He was responsible for building a new British fleet on modern lines and was an advocate of the submarine. He was a restless, imaginative, and impatient man whose unconventional behavior in the later part of his life made many people think that he was going mad even before his mind became unhinged. The phrase "sack the lot" was coined by him.
Bibliography: Mackay, R. F. 1973. *Fisher of Kilverstone.*

FISHER HOUSE. A private madhouse in Islington, England, licensed to Ann Holmes. Mary Lamb (q.v.) was a patient there, and her brother Charles Lamb (q.v.) wrote to Samuel Coleridge (q.v.) that "the good lady of the madhouse and her daughter love her and are taken with her amazingly, and I know she loves them."
Bibliography: Lucas, E. V., ed. 1935. *The letters of Charles and Mary Lamb.*

FISHERTON HOUSE. A private asylum (q.v.) in Wiltshire, England, established by the Finch family (q.v.) in the early part of the nineteenth

century and used by the government. It had special wards for criminal lunatics (q.v.) who had been transferred there from Bethlem Royal Hospital (q.v.) and other asylums because of overcrowding.
Bibliography: Parry-Jones, W. Ll. 1972. *The trade in lunacy.*

FISHPONDS PRIVATE LUNATIC ASYLUM. *See* MASON'S MADHOUSE.

FITZGERALD, FRANCIS SCOTT KEY (1896-1940). An American novelist. He was only twenty-four years old when he became a celebrity, following the publication of his first novel, *This Side of Paradise* (1920). *The Great Gatsby*, which he wrote in 1925, is now considered a classic. In 1920 he married Zelda Sayre, who later became a patient of Oscar Forel and Adolph Meyer (q.v.). She spent much of her life in mental hospitals. He became an alcoholic (*see* ALCOHOLISM), and many of the characters in his book are drunkards. He seems to have regarded drunkenness as an achievement and used to pretend to be more inebriated than he was, introducing himself as "F. Scott Fitzgerald, the well-known alcoholic." He and his wife were notorious for their unconventional behaviour, their histrionics and their public fights. His fame declined with his fortune. In his thirties he became hypochondriacal and suffered from insomnia. He died of a heart attack when he was forty-four.
Bibliography: Turnbull, A. 1962. *Scott Fitzgerald.*

FITZ-JAMES COLONY. A famous institution for the insane based on the cottage system (q.v.). It was founded privately in 1847 and situated near Clermont, France. The patients were engaged mainly in agricultural work, but other trades were also encouraged, according to the physical and mental conditions of the patients.
Bibliography: Tuke, D. H. 1892. *A dictionary of psychological medicine.*

FITZ-MARY, SIMON (fl.1240). A wealthy, influential, and devout Englishman. In 1247 he heard the encyclical of Pope Innocent IV (q.v.) read in the churches of London. The pope asked that the brothers of St. Mary of Bethlehem should be given hospitality wherever they went. Fitz-Mary was inspired to give land for a priory to be founded in London for their use. The priory later became Bethlem Royal Hospital (q.v.).
Bibliography: O'Donoghue, E. G. 1914. *The story of Bethlehem Hospital.*

FIVE WITS, THE. The five senses, or the five faculties of the mind—common sense, imagination, fantasy, estimation and memory (q.v.). Stephen Hawes included them in his *Passetyme of Pleasure*, a long allegorical poem dedicated to Henry VII, written in 1507.
Bibliography: 1978. *Brewer's dictionary of phrase and fable.*

FIXING. "Fixing, or setting the patients by the eye". Catching and holding a patient's attention by a piercing look. William Pargeter (q.v.) favored this

method and claimed he could calm maniac patients in this fashion. He described his method in a book entitled *Observations on Maniacal Disorders* published in 1792. Fixing gained favor with those who preferred to manage patients by humane methods rather than by force.
Bibliography: Tuke, S. 1813. Reprint. 1964. *Description of the retreat.*

FLAGELLANTS. A masochistic (*see* MASOCHISM) and hysterical (*see* HYSTERIA) sect that came into existence in the thirteenth century following the Black Death. It spread throughout Europe from Italy. Its members flagellated themselves until blood spurted from their bodies in the belief that the Lord would accept their sufferings and stop the plague. They wore dark cloaks with a red cross on their breast. For a time they gained many followers, but in 1349, because of their extreme behavior and the looting, vandalism, and rape that they perpetrated, the sect was declared heretical and collapsed. Some medieval hospitals were founded by them.
Bibliography: Cooper, W. M. 1908. *Flagellation and the flagellants.*

FLAGELLATION. Erotic flagellation as an aid to sexual excitement was part of many rites in antiquity. The Greek and Roman rituals in honor of Dionysus (q.v.) included flagellation. Epidemics of self-torture leading to ecstasy (q.v.) occurred both in antiquity and in medieval times.
See also FLAGELLANTS.
Bibliography: Robinson, V., ed. 1936. *Encyclopaedia sexualis.*

FLANNAGAN, JOHN BERNARD (1895-1942). An American sculptor. He regarded his sculptures as a species of occult fossil. He relied on the subconscious for inspiration and thought that the act of becoming is a traumatic experience. Rebirth motifs recur in his work, and his technique strives to let the spirit emerge from inert matter. He committed suicide (q.v.).
Bibliography: Miller, D. C. 1942. *The sculpture of John B. Flannagan.*

FLAUBERT, GUSTAVE (1821-1880). A French novelist born in Rouen, the son of a doctor. As a child he had a morbid interest in sickness, insanity and corpses. At the age of fifteen he conceived an unrequited passion for Elisa Schlesinger, and this passion greatly influenced the formation of his character. He suffered from epilepsy (q.v.) and experienced his first seizure on hearing that he had failed an examination. Flaubert abandoned his study of law in order to dedicate himself to writing. His great novel *Madame Bovary* (1856) reflected insight and knowledge of the manners of the time, as well as his intense hatred of the bourgeoisie. Because the novel was considered immoral, its publication caused a scandal, and both author and publisher were prosecuted. The book was a realistic and sordid tale of bourgeois life that related the fall into vice of the heroine and her final, vividly described, suicide (q.v.). Flaubert was said to be a shy, and morose man, ready to satirize the world and never satisfied with his own work, which cost him much effort. He died of apoplexy.

See also BOVARISM.

Bibliography: Steegmuller, F. 1939. *Flaubert and Madame Bovary.*

FLECHSIG, PAUL EMIL (1847-1929). A German neuroanatomist. He is remembered for his contribution to the localization of motor, sensory, and inexcitable areas of the brain and for his numerous autopsies of patients who had died from organic disorders of the brain. Emil Kraepelin (q.v.) worked under him in Leipzig. Daniel Paul Schreber (q.v.) was a patient of Flechsig and in his memoirs described the period spent in the Leipzig psychiatric clinic. Flechsig was a large man, who tended to be abrupt and dogmatic especially about his aversion to socialism. During the autopsy of a well-known socialist, he remarked that his brain had "dysharmonic convulutions". When Flechsig retired from the University of Leipzig, he refused to leave the cottage he occupied on the grounds of the university and had to be evicted.

Bibliography: Haymaker, W., and Schiller, F. 1970. *The founders of neurology.* 2d. ed.

FLEISCHL-MARXOW, ERNST VON (1846-1891). Austrian physiologist and physicist. At the age of twenty-five he had to undergo repeated amputations on his right hand because of an infection contracted during research at the physiological institute in Vienna. He was a charming, handsome, and brilliant man, as well as colleague and close friend of Sigmund Freud (q.v.). He became addicted to morphine (q.v.), and Freud tried to cure him by substituting cocaine (q.v.), which he thought was nonaddictive. As a result, Fleischl became deeply addicted to cocaine.

Bibliography: Jones, E. 1956. *Sigmund Freud: life and work.*

FLEMING, SIR ALEXANDER (1881-1955). Scottish surgeon and bacteriologist. His discovery of penicillin contributed to psychiatry by providing a form of treatment for syphilis (q.v.) and the organic psychosis (q.v.) related to it.

Bibliography: Maurois, A. 1959. *The life of Sir Alexander Fleming.*

FLEMMING, KARL FRIEDRICH (1799-1880). A German physician. After working for some time in mental hospitals, he became director of a new asylum (q.v.) near Schwerin. He was a pioneer in the direct observation of mental patients and promoted a scientific approach in psychiatry. He also was interested in forensic medicine and legislation concerning the insane.

His writings contain an early description of the manifestations of anxiety; he introduced the term "precordial anxiety" (q.v.).
Bibliography: Flemming, K. F. 1859. *Pathologie und therapie der psychosen.*

FLEMYNG, MALCOLM (?-1764). An English physician. He observed that "intermittent fevers strengthen the nerves," thus providing a historical precedent for the observations of other physicians a century or more later when malaria therapy (q.v.) was introduced in the treatment of general paralysis of the insane (q.v.). He was also the author of a medical poem in Latin entitled *Neuropathia.* In it he discussed hypochondriasis (q.v.) and hysteria (q.v.), which he regarded as functional disorders of nerves. The nerves, according to the theories of his time, could be hollow and contain a nervous fluid, or the nervous impulses could flow on their surface by vibration; whatever the structure, for him nervous disorders were literally related to tense nerves.
Bibliography: Hunter, R., and Macalpine, I. 1963. *Three hundred years of psychiatry.*

FLEURY (*or* ROBERT-FLEURY), JOSEPH NICHOLAS ROBERT (1797-1890). A German-French painter. His works include one famous painting of psychiatric interest: Philippe Pinel (q.v.) striking off the chains of the insane at Bicêtre (q.v.).
Bibliography: Roback, A. A., and Kiernan, T. 1969. *Pictorial history of psychology and psychiatry.*

FLEXIBILITAS CEREA. A waxlike flexibility of the limbs. Felix Plater (q.v.) gave an early description of this phenomenon occurring in catalepsy.

FLIBBERTIGIBBET. One of the several fiends that were believed to possess the insane. It was mentioned by William Shakespeare (q.v.) (*King Lear,* 4.1) as one of the five fiends that had taken possession (q.v.) of "poor Tom."

FLIESS, WILHELM (1858-1928). A German ear and nose specialist. He was consulted by Sigmund Freud (q.v.) about his own condition and the conditions of some of his patients. Fliess was said to have a fascinating personality, and he soon became a close friend of Freud. Freud's letters to him contain biographical material and references to his self-analysis and interpretation of dreams (q.v.). Fliess, whose interests covered a wide field, believed in a kind of sexual mysticism and developed a theory of human bisexuality based on periodicity and the computation of certain numbers (twenty-eight for females and twenty-three for males), which allowed him to calculate biological occurrences. He introduced the term "nasal reflex neurosis" for a syndrome he described in 1893. He had a dogmatic attitude

toward his own theories and was unable to accept any criticism, which eventually led to his break with Freud.
Bibliography: Jones, E. 1956. *Sigmund Freud: life and work.*

FLOGGING. Much has been written about the cruel treatment of the insane in the past, and flogging has been cited as an example of what they often endured. Certainly flogging was cruel, yet in the Middle Ages (q.v.) it was not intended as a punishment but rather as an effort to expel the devil. Later, it became a misguided but well-meant form of shock therapy. Whipping posts, to which individuals who were to be flogged were tied, were used in the treatment of lunatics in England until the seventeenth century.
Bibliography: Rosen, G. 1968. *Madness in society.*

FLOURENS, MARIE JEAN PIERRE (1794-1867). A French physiologist. He is regarded as the founder of the theory of brain function, as accepted today. By excising a part of the brain in animals, he demonstrated the importance of the cerebellum and the equipotentiality of the hemispheres.Most of his experiments were conducted on pigeons. He was a concise and lucid writer, a popular lecturer, and a formidable opponent. His theories were accepted, and they superseded those of Franz Gall (q.v.). In 1840 he was elected to the Académie de France. His main works include *Recherches expérimentales sur les propriétés et les fonctions du système nerveux* (1824); *Expériences sur le système nerveux* (1825) and *De la vie et de l'intelligence* (1849).
Bibliography: Boring, E. G. 1950. *A history of experimental psychology.*
Haymaker, W., and Schiller, F. 1970. *The founders of neurology.* 2d ed.

FLOURNOY, THÉODORE (1854-1920). Physician, philosopher, and professor of psychology at the University of Geneva in Switzerland. He was particularly interested in phenomena related to multiple personality and parapsychology and tried to apply to them the techniques of experimental psychology (q.v.) that he had learnt from Wilhelm Wundt (q.v.). He investigated the medium Catherine Muller (q.v.) for five years and published his conclusions in a book entitled *From India to the Planet Mars*—a reference to her so-called previous lives. His studies of the unconscious contributed to a better understanding of psychic phenomena and inspired other workers in the same field. His cousin Édouard Claparède (q.v.) was one of his pupils. Jean Piaget (q.v.) was guided by him.
Bibliography: Claparède, E. 1923. Théodore Flournoy: sa vie et son oeuvre. *Archive de psychologie* 18:1-125.

FLUDD (FLUD *or* FLOID), ROBERT (1574-1637). An English physician, mystic philosopher, and author of many books. He based his theories on the Scriptures, which he considered superior to the evidence of the senses.

He rejected the humoral theory (q.v.) of Aristotle (q.v.) and Galen (q.v.) and thought that the basic elements of nature were darkness, light, and water; God, world, and man were the three cosmic elements. He was influenced by Paracelsus (q.v.) and supported sympathetic medicine. Fludd was the first to agree in print with William Harvey's (q.v.) discovery of the circulation of the blood. He related it to his own theory that all life depends on a circular motion. He was also interested in occult sciences, and at one point in his studies he was accused of witchcraft (q.v.). Fludd was an early theorist in the field of animal magnetism (q.v.).
Bibliography: Craven, J. B. 1902. *Doctor Robert Fludd: the English rosicrucian.*

FLÜE, NICHOLAS VON DER (1417-1487). Swiss farmer, mystic, and hermit. Although he could neither read nor write, his reputation for wisdom and goodness led the authorities of the Swiss cantons to consult him in 1481, when civil war was threatened. His advice preserved the peace and unity of the country. In 1467 he left his wife and ten children to dedicate himself to a religious life in a lonely cottage, following a frightening vision in the shape of a mandala (q.v.) with God at the center. After this experience his facial expression remained that of a terrified man for the rest of his days.
Bibliography: Fordham, F. 1953. *Introduction to Jung's psychology.*

FLUTE. A musical instrument. In symbolism it is equated with anguish and extreme emotions. In Greco-Roman mythology the Sirens were said to use flutes, because the sound appealed to the emotions and seduced the senses.
Bibliography: Cooper, J. C. 1978. *An illustrated encyclopedia of traditional symbols.*

FLY AGARIC. *Amanita muscaria.* A poisonous mushroom, containing muscarine and having hallucinogenic (*see* HALLUCINATION) properties. It has been suggested that the fighting fury of the Vikings was induced by ingestion of fly agaric.
Bibliography: Retterstøl, N. 1975. Scandinavia. In *World History of Psychiatry*, ed. J. G. Howells.

FLYING SAUCERS. In the 1950s and in later years many people claimed to have seen saucer-shaped objects traveling through the air. These reports usually are the results of hallucinations (q.v.) and suggestion. Only occasionally have people actually witnessed unusual atmospheric phenomena that are "as real as rainbows are real" according to Dr. Menzel of Harvard University.
Bibliography: Michel, A. 1957. *The truth about flying saucers.*

FODÉRÉ, FRANÇOIS EMMANUEL (1764-1835). A Savoyan physician and professor of forensic medicine. He was particularly interested in mental

disorders. He wrote a book on mental deficiency, *Traité du goître et du crétinism*, based on his observations and autopsies of cretins (*see* CRETINISM) in the Alpine valleys. This work so impressed King Vittorio Amedeo III of Savoy that he granted Fodéré funds for research and travel. Fodéré regarded mental disease as a state in which "the internal senses were asleep whilst the external senses were awake"—a statement remarkable for its similarity to the later theory of loss of appreciation of reality and retreat into a world of fantasy. Despite the fact that his wife was cousin to the wives of the King of Spain and the King of Sweden, Fodéré never used this tie with royalty to gain advancement.
Bibliography: Fodéré, F. E. 1817. *Traité du delire applique à la medicine, à la morale et à la legislation.*

FOERSTER, OTFRID (1873-1941). A German neurosurgeon. He was physician to Nikolai Lenin (q.v.) and closely supervised his treatment during the last year of his life, practically living in a room next to that occupied by Lenin, at times watching him through a keyhole to avoid interrupting him. He was particularly interested in therapy and often succeeded where others had failed. Rhyzotomy treatment for spastic paralysis was pioneered by him and was one of many innovations he introduced and financed. He was a very sick man, who often was in pain, but he was able to disregard his physical condition and dedicate himself completely to his work.
Bibliography: Haymaker, W., and Schiller, F. 1970. *The founders of neurology.* 2d. ed.

FÖHN (*or* FOEHN). A strong, hot, dry wind, that blows down Alpine valleys. It brings physical discomfort and depression to the inhabitants of the valley.

FOIX, CHARLES (1882-1927). A French physician. His research on brain lesions, which he approached from the point of view of arterial occlusion, was an important contribution to the field of neurology (q.v.). He collected many case histories of patients who had died of focal brain lesions and compared the findings during their illness with those discovered at the time of autopsy. Foix was a lively individual, well liked by patients and students for his kindness and his sympathetic understanding. He was also an accomplished writer of verses.
Bibliography: Haymaker, W., and Schiller, F. 1970. *The founders of neurology.* 2d ed.

FOLIE À DEUX. Psychological contagion. The term *folie à deux* was first used in 1877 by Ernest Lasègue (q.v.) and Jules Falret (q.v.) in a paper entitled "La Folie à deux ou folie communiquée." Mutually induced neurotic (*see* NEUROSIS) symptoms have been recognized since at least the seventeenth cen-

tury when Sir Kenelm Digby (q.v.) gave a good account of what he called "contagion of the imagination" (q.v.). Prosper Despine (q.v.) referred to it as "contagion morale" in 1870. Folie à deux also plays a role in suicide (q.v.) pacts.
Bibliography: Lasègue, C., and Falret, J. 1877. La folie à deux (ou folie communiquée). *Ann. med.-psychol.* 18: 321. English trans. R. Michaud. 1964. *Suppl. Am. J. Psychiat.* 121, No. 4.

FOLIE À DOUBLE FORME. A type of mental disorder characterized by alternating changes of mood from elation to depression. The term was first used by Jules Baillarger (q.v.) in 1851 and was later superseded by manic-depressive psychoses (q.v.).
Bibliography: Zilboorg, G. 1941. *A history of medical psychology.*

FOLIE CIRCULAIRE. Term used by Jean Falret (q.v.) to describe a mental disease characterized by the alternation of elation and depression. His observations were published in 1854 in a paper entitled "De la folie circulaire." *See also* MANIC-DEPRESSIVE PSYCHOSES.
Bibliography: Zilboorg, G. 1941. *A history of medical psychology.*

FOLIE LUCIDE. Ulysses Trélat (q.v.) used this term in the nineteenth century to describe a condition in which emotional turmoil, rather than lack of reasoning power, produced antisocial behavior. He argued that individuals so affected were not legally responsible for their actions.
Bibliography: Zilboorg, G. 1941. *A history of medical psychology.*

FOLKLORE. Folk wisdom and learning. The study of folklore is important to psychiatry as a branch of ethnological psychology that records and interprets myths, beliefs, medical remedies, and patterns of behavior handed down from generation to generation by various races.
Bibliography: Sumner, W. G. 1906. *Folkways.*

FØLLING, IVOR ASBJØRN (1888-   ). A Norwegian biochemist. In 1934 he discovered a reversible metabolic disturbance, phenylpyruvic acid oligophrenia (*see* PHENYLKETONICS), that causes mental retardation. His work gave great impetus to further research in the field of mental deficiency.
Bibliography: Kanner, L. 1964. *A history of the care and study of the mentally retarded.*

FONTANA, FELICE (1730-1805). An Italian naturalist and physiologist. He was the first to give an accurate description of nerve fibers and nerve sheaths and to recognize the degeneration and loss of function of nerves separated from their centers. His views on the theory of irritability (q.v.) appeared in 1767 in a treatise entitled *De Irritabilitatis Legibus.*
Bibliography: Haymaker, W., and Schiller, F. 1970. *The founders of neurology.* 2d ed.

FONTHILL GIFFORD. An early private asylum (q.v.) in England. It was founded in Wiltshire in 1718. The patients were subjected to severe restraint (q.v.). They frequently were kept in chains in unsanitary conditions and allowed out only occasionally. By 1828 standards had improved, and the county records of private asylums for that year state that more consideration was shown for the welfare of the inmates and that "a canary and other singing birds" were kept to amuse the patients.

Bibliography: Parry-Jones, W. Ll. 1972. *The trade in lunacy.*

FOOL OF QUALITY, THE. The title of a novel written by Henry Brooke (1703?-1783) in 1766. The hero is Henry, son of an earl of Moreland. He is rejected by his family, because they consider him unintelligent, and he is brought up by a foster mother. Under her care, he becomes a kind and generous man, a champion of the oppressed, the sick, and the poor. The novel offers a good example of the success obtained by loving foster-parents, where the natural unloving parents had failed, and describes what today we would call "psychogenic retardation".

Bibliography: Harvey, P. 1967. *The Oxford companion to English literature.* 4th ed.

FOOLS. Individuals, often with misshapen bodies, kept by kings and important people as sources of amusement. If the fools were not genuine mental defectives, they might assume the cloak of folly in order to behave and speak with greater license. In ancient cultures, the fool was often a scapegoat (q.v.) who was killed in ritual sacrifices. Ancient Sanskrit, Greek, Latin, and Mexican literature mention fools. Marcus Valerius Martialis (c.A.D. 40-c.104), a Roman poet, makes several references to mental defectives and describes their appearances. In one of his epigrams he complained that the fool he bought in the market was not a genuine fool, thus reflecting the custom of keeping defectives as household objects of amusement. Fools also were known in Islamic culture. In the ninth century, Buhlul gained fame as a fool at the court of Harun al-Rashid (q.v.), while in India during the same period the character of the dwarf Viduska appeared as a fool in many dramas. Medieval manuscripts often contain illustrations representing defectives, usually in the illuminated ornamentation of the letter "D"—a reference to the beginning of Psalm 53: "Dixit inspiens in corde suo non est Deus" [the foolish has said in his heart that there is no God].

Rigoletto (q.v.) in Giuseppe Verdi's (1813-1901) opera, *Rigoletto*, is an example of a deformed jester. Other fools and jesters were very astute and accumulated large fortunes. Rahere (q.v.), the court jester of Henry I of England, founded Royal Hospital of St. Bartholomew's (q.v.) in London in 1123. John Heywood, one of the fools of Henry VIII, had considerable literary talent, and Richard Tarlton became a well-known actor. At Glamis Castle, Scotland, is preserved a dress which had belonged to the resident jester; it is of fine material and tiny bells are stitched onto it. The last private

fool on record in England was a Dick Pierce who belonged to the household of Lord Suffolk and died in 1728.
Bibliography: Welsford, E. 1935. *The fool.*

FOOL'S CAP. A conical cap adorned with bells, ribbons, and feathers worn by court jesters, or fools (q.v.). In 1795 the fool's cap was used as a watermark in paper, and the term has remained to indicate a certain size of paper sheet.

FORCELLINI, EGIDIO (1688-1768). An Italian philologist. In 1771 he published a Latin glossary, *Totius Latinitatis Lexicon*, in which he distinguished between *fatuous* and *stultus*, defining *fatuous* as "an individual with no intellect" and *stultus* as "an individual with an obtuse intellect".
Bibliography: Kanner, L. 1964. *A history of the care and study of the mentally retarded.*

FORDYCE, GEORGE (1736-1802). A British physician. He was educated in Edinburgh and later studied under William Hunter (1718-1783) in London. He was a somewhat eccentric man, but was liked despite his untidy way of dressing and strange habits. For instance, he ate only one very large meal a day, at Dolly's Chop-house, and with it he consumed a tankard of ale, a bottle of port, and a quarter of a pint of brandy. His lectures on the practice of physic, materia medica, and chemistry occupied more of his time than his clinical practice. He wrote an early work on the symptomatology of febrile deliria, discussing hallucination (q.v.) and delusion (q.v.) in clinical terms; it was published in 1798 with the title *A Third Dissertation on Fever.* John Haslam (q.v.) was one of his pupils.
Bibliography: Hunter, R., and Macalpine, I. 1963. *Three hundred years of psychiatry.*

FOREEST, PIETER VAN (FORESTUS) (1522-1597). Dutch physician and medical writer. He believed insanity to be a mixture of depressive thoughts, fear, and delirium (q.v.). He discussed hysterical (*see* HYSTERIA) fits and reported cases that had been precipitated by anger and other strong emotions. He also wrote on lycanthropy (q.v.) from personal observations and studied mental deficiency and its characteristics. His *Observationum et curationum medicinalium* was published in 1587.
Bibliography: Beek, H. H. 1969. *Waanzin in de middeleeuwen.*

FOREL, AUGUSTE HENRI (1848-1931). A Swiss psychiatrist. As a child he suffered from an inferiority complex (q.v.) and tried to compensate for it with an interest in insects. He studied ants, and later became the greatest authority on their behaviour. After qualifying in medicine, he became well known for his studies of cerebral anatomy. He was appointed professor of psychiatry at the University of Zurich and director of the Burghölzli Hos-

pital (q.v.) to which he introduced many reforms that gained world fame for this hospital. He went to Nancy to observe the work of Hippolyte-Marie Bernheim (q.v.) and to learn about hypnotism (q.v.) , which he later introduced as treatment for a wider field of ailments. He described three stages of hypnosis, drowsiness, hypotaxy, and somnambulism (q.v.), and maintained that the study of hypnosis would lead to a better understanding of the physiology of the brain and human psychology (q.v.). He studied memory (q.v.), instinct, alcoholism (q.v.), crime, and sexual problems and promoted occupational therapy (q.v.), community mental health, and social reforms.
Bibliography: Ellenberger, H. F. 1970. *The discovery of the unconscious.*

FORMAN, SIMON (1552-1611). An English astrologer (*see* ASTROLOGY) and unqualified practitioner of medicine. His father died when he was young, and he was brought up by an unsympathetic mother. He hungered for learning but had to rely on self education. Although he managed to get to Oxford University, he did so only as a servant. He wrote an autobiography (unusual in Elizabethan times) that shows his compulsive need to reveal himself and dwell on his frustration and paranoia (q.v.). He was small of stature and felt so insecure toward women that he avoided sexual experiences until he was thirty years old. He did, however, more than make up for this late start and became an irresistible seducer. From poverty, persecution, and occasional imprisonment, he rose to riches and respectability. He had a large medical practice from all strata of society. His diagnoses were mostly based on astrology, urology, and intuition and his treatment relied on herbs more than on bleeding (q.v.). His case books are an interesting psychological and social record of Elizabethan life.
Bibliography: Rowse, A. L. 1974. *The case books of Simon Forman.*

FORMICARIUS (THE ANTHILL). A book by Johannes Nider (q.v.). It was published in 1435 and had been reprinted six times by 1692. It described the superstitious practices of his time and dealt with witchcraft (q.v.), witches' trials, and the problems that faced the church in distinguishing between heretics and deluded people. It was often appended to the *Malleus Malefi-carum* (q.v.) and became a kind of handbook of antisatanism.
Bibliography: Robbins, R. H. 1959. *Encyclopedia of witchcraft and demonology.*

FORMICATION (*also known as* **COCAINE BUG**). The sensation of insects crawling and biting experienced by cocaine (q.v.) addicts during withdrawal from the drug.

FORRESTAL, JAMES VINCENT (1892-1949). An American investment banker. In 1947 he became the first American secretary of defense, a position that placed him under considerable strain. He is said to have become paranoid (*see* PARANOIA) and believed that he was being spied upon constantly. His behavior became strange, mannerisms and feelings of guilt hampered his work, and he became increasingly unable to concentrate or to remember important events. Even after resigning, his depression continued to grow, and he committed suicide (q.v.).

FORSTER, THOMAS IGNATIUS MARIA (1789-1860). English astronomer and naturalist. He was a many-sided man and an eccentric. He studied with Johann Spurzheim (q.v.) in Edinburgh and wrote on the anatomy and physiology of the brain. He was interested in phrenology (q.v.) and is credited with coining the term. He thought phrenology had great social value and could be used to advise people about appropriate careers, assist in criminology and explain the psychology of dreams. He believed that periodic insanity and atmospheric changes were linked and wrote a book on this belief. He left his mark in the field of astronomy by discovering a comet in 1819.
Bibliography: Forster, T. 1817. *Observation on the causal and periodical influence of particular states of the atmosphere in human health and diseases, particularly insanity.*

FOTHERGILL, JOHN (1712-1780). English physician and Quaker (q.v.). In 1778 he gave the first accurate descriptions of migraine (q.v.), which he called "sick headache," and facial neuralgia. His London practice benefited from his famous botanical garden, as it provided herbal remedies for his patients. He was also the first in England to recognize diptheria. He published an account of it in 1748. The use of coffee was popularized by him.
Bibliography: Foa, R. H. 1919. *Dr. John Fothergill and his friends.*

FOUNTAIN HOSPITAL. A hospital established in Tooting, England, in 1911 by the Metropolitan Asylums Board. At first patients were housed in huts that previously had been used for isolating infectious patients. It was dedicated exclusively to children and was an important center for study and research in mental deficiency until it closed in 1963.
Bibliography: Ayers, G. M. 1971. *England's first state hospitals and the Metropolitan Asylums Board, 1867-1930.*

FOUNTAIN OF YOUTH. A mythical magic fountain whose water had the power of restoring youth to those who bathed in it. In the Middle Ages (q.v.) it was believed to be a side stream of the Euphrates in which Alexander the Great (q.v.) and his army were rejuvenated. After the discovery of America, it was believed to be located in the Bahamas and expeditions were organized for its discovery.
Bibliography: Harvey, P. 1967. *The Oxford companion to English literature.* 4th ed.

FOURNIER, JEAN ALFRED (1832-1914). A French syphilologist. He was a professor in Paris. His lessons were said to penetrate even the dullest

minds because of his clarity and his harmonious and precise voice. In 1894 he demonstrated statistically that syphilis (q.v.) is related to tabes dorsalis and to general paralysis of the insane (q.v.). His studies of syphilis contributed to the clinical and social understanding of this disease.
Bibliography: Fournier, J. A., and Raymond, F. 1905. *Paralysis générale et syphilis.*

FOUR TANTRA (ROOTS). The Tibetan translation of a Sanskrit work by an unknown author in the eighth century A.D. It is used in the teaching of medicine in Hindu temples. According to the *Four Tantra*, all diseases are caused by three psychic factors, sensuality or desire, excitement or anger, stupidity or ignorance, which, in turn, are related to three bodily humors: wind, bile, and phlegm.
Bibliography: *The history and philosophy of the brain and its functions.* 1959. Symposium.

FOVILLE, ACHILLE L. (1799-1878). A French neurologist. He described a syndrome, which later was named after him, that is a variant of hemiplegia with paralysis of the abducens and facial nerves.
Bibliography: Haymaker, W., and Schiller, F. 1970. *The founders of neurology.* 2d. ed.

FOWLER, ORSON SQUIRE (1809-1887). An American phrenologist. He and his younger brother, Lorenzo, popularized phrenology (q.v.) in the United States, wrote extensively about it, and founded the *American Phrenological Journal*, which was published from 1838 to 1911.
Bibliography: Boring, E. G. 1950. *A history of experimental psychology.*

FOWLER, RICHARD (1765-1863). An English physician. He was interested in Luigi Galvani's (q.v.) experiments with animal electricity (q.v.) and in many aspects of psychological phenomena. He wrote on the mental state of the blind and the deaf and dumb and on the physiological processes of thinking in people with defective sensory organs. He was a Fellow of the Royal Society (q.v.) and a member of the celebrated Speculative Society.
Bibliography: 1900. *Dictionary of national biography.*

FOWLER, THOMAS (?-1801). A British physician. He qualified in medicine in Edinburgh and for a time was an apothecary in York. When the Quakers (q.v.) opened the York Retreat (q.v.) in 1796, Fowler was appointed first physician because of his personal qualities as well as his medical skill. He was a benevolent and open-minded man, prepared to work hard and to try new methods. He was disappointed by the rate of cures brought about by the usual contemporary prescriptions for insanity and came to the conclusion that bleeding (q.v.), blistering, and purging (q.v.) were of little use. He introduced a better and more plentiful diet, which promoted sleep with-

out the administration of opium (q.v.), abolished chains and corporal punishment, successfully employed moral medicine (q.v.), and classified the patients, separating them into groups according to their symptoms. Solution of arsenic was introduced into the British pharmacopoeia by him in 1786.
Bibliography: Hunter, R., and Macalpine, I. 1963. *Three hundred years of psychiatry.*

FOX, EDWARD LONG (1760-1835). A British Quaker (q.v.) and physician to the Bristol Royal Infirmary. He was a colorful and energetic man. In 1804 he opened the first purpose-built private asylum, Brislington House (q.v.), in which he invested a large sum of money. His progressive ideas were embodied in the way in which he ran the establishment: patients were classified and separated according to diagnosis; a scale of charges was devised (the most expensive rooms were those at the top of his own house); no coercion was imposed; and patients suitable for manual work were encouraged to occupy themselves in gardening, farming, and other jobs. According to Fox, it was difficult to find suitable employment for "gentlemen" patients. In 1811, Fox was asked to supervise the treatment of George III (q.v.) but declined.
Bibliography: Hunter, R., and Macalpine, I. 1963. *Three hundred years of psychiatry.*

FOX, GEORGE (1624-1691). The founder of Quakerism. He was the son of an English weaver. He wandered about the country searching for religious enlightenment. As an adolescent he had suffered from hallucinations (q.v.), and these continued into adulthood. In 1651, he fell into a trance and ran barefooted through the frozen streets of Litchfield crying, "Woe to the bloody city," as the town seemed to him to be covered in blood. He was imprisoned several times for blasphemy and disturbing the peace. His emotional experiences are related in his *Journal*, which was published in 1694, after it was edited by a committee of Friends headed by William Penn (1644-1718), the famous Quaker who founded the proprietary colony of Pennsylvania.
Bibliography: Van Etten, H. 1959. *George Fox and the Quakers.*

FOX, MARGARET (1833-1893). An American spiritualist medium (q.v.). In 1848, while living with her sisters Leah and Kate in a house in Hydesville, New York, she reported mysterious rappings, which she claimed were supernatural messages from the world of the dead. Shortly afterward the theory that the dead could communicate through a medium (q.v.), became widely accepted and aroused much interest. Spiritualistic phenomena were investigated in many parts of the United States and Europe. The Fox sisters undertook many tours to demonstrate their powers, but in 1888 they con-

fessed that they had operated a clever imposture. They later retracted this admission.
Bibliography: Podmore, F. 1963. *Mediums of the 19th century.*

FRACASTORO, GIROLAMO (1483?-1553). Italian physician and humanist, professor of logic, astronomer, poet, and theologian. He studied contagious diseases and, in advance of his time, talked of germs. In 1530 he gave the disease syphilis (q.v.) its name in a poem entitled *Syphilis sive morbus gallicus.* Syphilus, a shepherd, was punished with the disease for worshipping a mortal king rather than Apollo (q.v.). The poem summarized the knowledge about syphilis available in the sixteenth century. In another work *Sympathy and Antipathy of Things* (1546) he discussed many psychological aspects of human behavior.
Bibliography: Wynne-Finch, H. trans. 1935. *Fracastoro: Syphilis or the French disease.*

FRANCIA, FRANCESCO RAIBOLINI (1450-1517). An Italian painter, particularly well known for his madonnas. Francia was killed by his own capacity to feel deeply. He was said to have been so overwhelmed by the sight of a painting by Raphael (1483-1520) that he died of joy.
Bibliography: Wittkower, R., and Wittkower, M. 1963. *Born under Saturn.*

FRANÇOIS-FRANK, CHARLES ÉMILE (1849-1921). A French physician. He contributed to the field of neurology (q.v.) with his original work on vasomotor nerves and the functioning of the sympathetic system. In 1887 he published a book entitled *Leçons sur les fonctions motrices du cerveau* in which he discussed the motor functions of the brain and the localization of cerebral functions; Jean-Martin Charcot (q.v.) wrote the preface to the volume.
Bibliography: Haymaker, W., and Schiller, F. 1970. *The founders of neurology.* 2d ed.

FRANK, JOHANN PETER (1745-1821). A German physician. He is regarded as the founder of pathology of the spinal cord. He was critical of the care that mental patients received and believed that physicians should study mental disorders as much as they studied other diseases. He was the first to put forward the theory that some skin diseases have a psychological aetiology. He wrote a *Complete System of Medical Policy* in which he proposed a community health service and a review of public health hazards.
Bibliography: Zilboorg, G. 1941. *A history of medical psychology.*

FRANKENSTEIN OR, THE MODERN PROMETHEUS. A novel by Mary W. Shelley, wife of Percy Bysshe Shelley (q.v.). It was written during a rainy holiday in Switzerland, when the Shelleys and Byron (q.v.) were amusing themselves by composing ghost stories. In the novel, Frankenstein is a Swiss student of natural philosophy. He creates a creature in the image of a man from bones collected in a charnel house and, knowing the necessary secret, gives it life. The creature is so ugly that it is loathed by all and in its loneliness reacts with hatred and wishes for revenge. It murders Franken-stein's brother, his young bride, and finally, before disappearing, destroys its creator, who has pursued it to the Arctic. The novel was published in 1818.

Bibliography: Shelley, M. W. 1818. *Frankenstein, or the modern Prometheus.*

FRANKLIN, BENJAMIN (1706-1790). American journalist, statesman, and scientist. He was one of seventeen children and started his working life as an apprentice printer and from printing moved on to journalism and to politics. He was a complex individual, and his life was marked by many contradictions. His studies of electrical phenomena gained him a F.R.S. At one point during his experiments with electricity (q.v.), he was knocked unconscious and suffered retrograde amnesia (q.v.), which led him to suggest that electric shock should be tried on the insane as a form of therapy. While ambassador to France, he was invited by Louis XVI to head a commission investigating animal magnetism (q.v.) and the practices of Franz Mesmer (q.v.). Franklin asserted that magnetism (q.v.) had no curative qualities and credited any therapeutic results to suggestion. He proposed the establish-ment of the Pennsylvania Hospital (q.v.) on the lines of hospitals he had observed in England.

Bibliography: Van Doren, C. 1948. *Benjamin Franklin.*

FRANZ, SHEPHERD IVORY (1874-1933). An American neurologist who devised new techniques for testing, learning, and discrimination. He studied and became an authority on the functions of the cerebrum and the frontal lobes in relation to the production and retention of simple sensory habits. He found that lobectomy of both frontal lobes in animals made them forget recent habits but not old ones and that the recent habits so lost could be relearned. Lobectomy carried out on one lobe only diminished efficiency but did not cancel the memory.

Bibliography: Franz, S. I. 1912. *The handbook of mental examination methods.*

FRAZER, SIR JAMES GEORGE (1854-1941). A Scottish social anthro-pologist renowned for the wealth of material he studied in the field of comparative folklore (q.v.), religion, and magic (q.v.). Sigmund Freud (q.v.) found support for his social theory in Frazer's anthropological findings. Frazer's most famous work, *The Golden Bough*, was published in 1890. The title is derived from the golden bough in the sacred grove at Nemi;

the work presents an extensive study of early religions, superstitions, and social groups.
Bibliography: Downie, R. A. 1940. *James George Frazer: the portrait of a scholar.*

FRAZIER, CHARLES HARRISON (1870-1936). American surgeon and pioneer of neurosurgery. During World War I, he became interested in peripheral nerve injuries and gunshot wounds of the head. With William G. Spiller (q.v.), he introduced a surgical technique for the relief of trigeminal neuralgia and cordotomy.
Bibliography: Haymaker, W., and Schiller, F. 1970. *The founders of neurology.* 2d ed.

FREDERICK II (1194-1250). A Holy Roman emperor, born in Ancona, Italy. He was an enlightened but cruel individual. The regulations he introduced for medical education have lasted to this day (five years training, one year internship). He was also the founder of the University of Naples. He was said to have regarded Moses, Christ, and Mohammed as impostors who damaged men. Although he was a freethinker, he persecuted heretics. Wanting to know what behavior was learned, what innate, and what language children brought up in silence spoke, he had a group of children cared for by nurses who were not allowed to speak to them. His experiment was a failure, as all the children are said to have died for lack of petting and loving words.
See also FALCONRY.
Bibliography: Masson, G. 1957. *Frederick II of Hohenstaufen: a life.*

FREDERICK THE GREAT (1712-1786). A King of Prussia. He was the fourth of fourteen children, only ten of whom survived infancy. He was delicate, small for his age, nervous, and shy and a complete contrast to his brutal father, whom he detested. Despite his physical weakness he managed to survive his childhood, probably because of his nurse's devotion and care. In his adolescence he was often depressed and ill and found comfort in homosexual relationships. He was made so unhappy by his father that he planned to escape to England. When his plan was discovered, his accomplice and friend Hans Herman von Katte (1704-1730) was beheaded in his presence. This action so affected Frederick that he submitted to his father's wishes in a state of dazed indifference. A bride was chosen for him, but he never loved her, nor did he consummate the marriage. He remained a misogynist in an almost totally masculine household. He was a great admirer and friend of Voltaire (q.v.). Fredrick worried so much about illness that his court physician was ordered to have remedies for every possible disorder

ready at all times. As he grew older, his dissatisfaction with life did not lessen, notwithstanding his success as an intellectual and as a king.
Bibliography: Ritter, G. 1968. *Frederick the Great: a historical profile*, trans. P. Paret.

FREE HOUSE. A term applied to those nineteenth-century private nursing homes in England that provided mental patients with board, lodging, and nursing care but left clinical responsibility with the patient's own physician, who would visit the premises when required.
See also ASYLUMS.
Bibliography: Hunter, R., and Macalpine, I. 1963. *Three hundred years of psychiatry.*

FREEMAN, JOHN (fl. 1600). A resident of Sittingbourne, in Kent, England. He had been engaged successfully in the practice of medicine for some time, when he was granted a special license in 1600 by the archbishop of Canterbury to "practice and exercise" the art of medicine among "the melancholy and mad," because he had shown particular skill in their treatment. Thus, he may have been the first licensed English psychiatrist.
Bibliography: Hunter, R., and Macalpine, I. 1963. *Three hundred years of psychiatry.*

FREEMAN, WALTER (1895-1972). An American neurologist and psychiatrist, well known for his research in psychosurgery (q.v.). From observations of lobotomized patients, he worked out a hierarchy of functions dependent on the frontal lobe and how these are related to social adjustment.
Bibliography: Freeman, W. 1952. *Plane of section in leucotomy in relation to social adjustment—a follow-up study of 1,000 cases.*

FRENCH PROTESTANT HOSPITAL. A foundation for poor French Protestants in Great Britain. It was established in London in 1716 by a bequest of M. de Gastigny (?-1708). In 1736 it was considerably enlarged to include poor French Protestants with minds disordered as a consequence of the privations and tortures suffered in France for their religious beliefs.
Bibliography: Poynter, F.N.L., ed. 1964. *The evolution of hospitals in Britain.*

FRENCH REVOLUTION. According to Jean Esquirol and Philippe Pinel (qq.v.) the turbulent events in the years 1789 to 1795 caused many French people to become insane and led to a remarkable number of suicides (q.v.). Marc-Antoin Petit of Montpellier wrote about the effects of the revolution on mental health in a book entitled *Discours sur l'influence de la Revolution française sur la Santé publique* (in *Essai sur la Médicine due Coeur* . . . Lyon, 1806).
Bibliography: Rosen, G. 1968. *Madness in society.*

FREUD, ANNA (1895-1982). An Austrian psychoanalyst, daughter of Sigmund Freud (q.v.). In 1939, she emigrated with her father to London.

During World War II, she organized residential nurseries for homeless children. Her clinical work with children led to the foundation of the Hampstead Child Therapy Clinic, which provides facilities for treatment and research on normal and abnormal child development, as well as training courses for child psychoanalysts. Her works include: *The Ego and the Mechanisms of Defence* (1936), *The Psycho-Analytical Treatment of Children* (1946), and *Normality and Pathology in Childhood* (1965).

FREUD, SIGMUND (1856-1939). Austrian Jewish physician, neurologist, psychiatrist, and founder of psychoanalysis (q.v.). Inspired by Johann Wolfgang von Goethe's (q.v.) essay on nature, Freud decided to study medicine. He began his studies with an interest in physiology and discovered the analgesic qualities of cocaine (q.v.). Soon neurology (q.v.) attracted his attention, and he went to Paris to study under Jean-Martin Charcot (q.v.). From Paris, he went to Nancy to learn the hypnotic (*see* HYPNOTISM) techniques of Ambroise-August Liebeault and Hippolyte-Marie Bernheim (qq.v.). Having become disappointed in the results obtained from hypnosis, he de-veloped a new method of treatment for neuroses called free association (*see* ASSOCIATIONISM), which he used in connection with an explanation of dreams (q.v.). At first his work was rejected and condemned especially for what seemed to be an excessive emphasis given to sexual impulses, but by 1909 it had gained an international reputation, and Freud was invited to lecture in the United States. The next twenty years saw not only the development and maturation of his ideas, but also the first disagreements with his associates. Freud managed to retain his leadership in the field of psychoanalysis (q.v.) by organizing what amounted to a secret inner circle. This circle consisted of seven individuals: Freud himself, Otto Rank, Hans Sachs, Karl Abraham, Max Eitingon, Sandor Ferenczi and Ernest Jones (qq.v.). To each of these men Freud gave a copy of his own antique ring, which enclosed an Egyptian stone carved with the features of an old man. Yet, eventually even this inner circle collapsed because of disagreements. The last twenty years of Freud's life were marred by his ill health; cancer of the mouth caused him intense pain and he underwent a series of operations. Despite this, he continued to work intensively until 1939 when the Nazi horror finally became unbearable, and he fled to London for a final peaceful year. His views released a flood of writing both by himself and others.

Bibliography: Freud, S. 1966. *Complete psychological works. Standard Edition*, ed. J. Strachey.

Clark, R. W. 1979. *Freud: The man and the cause.*

FREY, MAXIMILIAN VON (1852-1932). An Austrian physiologist who was an authority on touch. He wrote on cutaneous sensitivity and tried to correlate sensations to particular types of sense organs. He developed a

technique for measuring the threshold of skin sensitivity to cold, heat, pressure, and pain.
Bibliography: Boring, E. G. 1950. *A history of experimental psychology.*

FREYJA. A Scandinavian divinity, goddess of sexual love, more or less equivalent to Eros (q.v.).
Bibliography: Sykes, E. 1968. *Everyman's dictionary of nonclassical mythology.*

FRIEDLÄNDER, KATE (1903-1949). An Austrian physician, the daughter of Jewish parents. After qualifying in medicine she went to Germany and worked at the psychiatric university clinic of Berlin with Karl Bonhoeffer (q.v.). In the early 1930s she emigrated to Britain where she continued her psychoanalytic work and was instrumental in establishing a clinic for Hampstead Child Therapy Course trainees under the guidance of Anna Freud (q.v.). She was a talented woman, interested in many practical and intellectual pursuits, and full of enthusiasm for whatever she did. She was an authority on the various aspects of juvenile delinquency, which she discussed in her book *The Psychoanalytical Approach to Juvenile Delinquency* (1947). She died of a brain tumor.
Bibliography: Alexander, F.; Eisenstein, S., and Grothjan, M., eds. 1966. *Psychoanalytic pioneers.*

FRIEDMANN, MAX (1858-1925). A German neurologist. He described the clinical manifestations of traumatic encephalopathy, which include headache, fatigue, insomnia, vertigo, impaired memory (q.v.) and intellect, and emotional instability. The condition is known as Friedmann's complex and is commonly seen in boxers.

FRIEDREICH, JOHANNES BAPTISTA (1796-1862). German physician and medical historian. In his book *Exposition of the Theories upon the Nature and the Seat of Mental Disease* (1836), he opposed the psychical theories of Johannes Heinroth (q.v.), declaring them to be immoral and diabolical. He believed that all mental disorders were caused by somatic conditions and were the end product of a chain of events; if physical abnormalities were not found at the time of autopsy, then the observer had missed them. He considered the assumption that mental illness might have a psychological cause sacrilegious because he believed psychic matters appertained to the soul, which could not become sick as it was immortal. According to him, half insanity was possible because the brain is divided into two halves. He stressed the importance of taking the family history of the patient and devised one of the earliest systematic methods of exploring and examining psychiatric patients. He was also the author of a history of psychiatry.
Bibliography: Zilboorg, G. 1941. *A history of medical psychology.*

FRIEDREICH, NIKOLAUS (1825-1882). A German physician. He was influenced by the work of Rudolf Virchow (q.v.) and contributed valuable

observations on neuropathological conditions. He wrote on intracranial tumors, muscular dystrophy, and hereditary spinal ataxia. Paramyoclonus multiplex, a condition first described by him in 1881, is now known as Friedreich's disease.
Bibliography: Haymaker, W., and Schiller, F. 1970. *The founders of neurology.* 2d. ed.

FRIENDS' ASYLUM. The second oldest American institution for the mentally ill established in Frankford, Pennsylvania, in 1817. Thomas Scattergood, a Quaker (q.v.) minister, is said to have proposed the project to the Philadelphia Society of Friends after a visit to the Retreat (q.v.) in York, England. An appeal for funds, furniture, and domestic items was launched, and each prospective contributor was given an abridged edition of *Description of the Retreat* by Samuel Tuke (q.v.). The hospital was a three-story building with ample grounds and accommodations for forty paying patients. The first patients were all Quakers, but later patients were drawn from a wider circle. In addition to medical care, the hospital provided "tender and sympathetic attention and religious oversight." Chains were not used, but leather straps were employed to restrain (*see* RESTRAINT) patients. A crude classification system was used—mild cases housed at the top of the building, violent and noisy cases at the bottom.
Bibliography: Dain, N. 1964. *Concepts of insanity in the United States, 1789-1865.*

FRIERS, JAKOB FRIEDRICH (1773-1843). German philosopher and psychologist. He was a follower of Immanuel Kant (q.v.). His philosophy was based on the belief that reality could be understood only through self-observation, a concept later embraced by experimental psychology (q.v.). His writings on psychology were mainly in the form of papers that were published in *Schmids Psychologisches Magazin.*

FRITSCH, GUSTAV THEODOR (1838-1897). German anatomist and anthropologist. With Eduard Hitzig (q.v.), he applied electrical stimulation to the brains of dogs and in 1870 published his findings, which described the "electrical excitability" of the brain and the connection of different areas with certain movements. It can be said that he was the father of experimental neurophysiology.
Bibliography: Haymaker, W., and Schiller, F. 1970. *The founders of neurology.* 2d. ed.

FROBENIUS, LEO VIKTOR (1873-1938). A German ethnologist. Carl Jung (q.v.) was influenced by his book *Epoch of the Sun God* (1904). In it Frobenius developed the theory that mankind had gone through three basic stages of worship: during the first stage, men worshipped animals; in the second stage, the dead, and in the third the Sun-God, who was followed

by the souls of the dead to a dark domain from which they reemerged to a new life.
Bibliography: Frobenius, L. 1904. *Das zeitalter des sonnegottes.*

FRÖBES, JOSEPH (1866-1947). An Austrian psychologist. He was brought up in an intensely religious atmosphere. He was educated by the Jesuits and became a Jesuit priest and a teacher of mathematics, physics, and chemistry. He later taught philosophy, which also included psychology (q.v.), and this led to his lifelong interest in experimental psychology (q.v.). He regarded it as a science concerned with all mental and emotional expressions. He contributed to the literature on psychophysiology and wrote on the psychology of sensation and of reason.
Bibliography: Murchison, C., ed. 1936. *A history of psychology in autobiography.*

FROEBEL, FRIEDRICH WILHELM AUGUST (1782-1852). A German educational psychologist. He lost his mother in infancy and his stepmother neglected him. This experience made him protective toward young children whose happiness he was anxious to promote. He became a teacher and organized an educational community. His system of teaching, which was based on free play and direct experience, rather than on the mechanical imparting of information, was influenced by the ideas of Jean Jacques Rousseau (q.v.) and Johann Pestalozzi (q.v.) . Froebel thought that children like flowers would prosper when looked after by interested people who encouraged them to grow naturally. He called his system *Kindergarten* (q.v.) (garden of children), a term reflecting his adolescent apprenticeship to a forester. The first kindergarten was opened in Blankenburg in 1837. The Prussian police closed all Froebel's schools in 1851, accusing them of atheism and socialism, but the public opinion against such ridiculous accusations prevailed, and they were reopened in 1860. The Froebel system became accepted throughout the world. The kindergarten opened in London in 1851 was visited and admired by Charles Dickens (q.v.), who described it in "Household Words."
Bibliography: Lilley, I. M. 1967. *Friedrich Froebel.*

FROG. In Chinese symbolism, a frog in a wall represents a person of poor understanding and limited vision.
Bibliography: Cooper, J. C. 1978. *An illustrated encyclopaedia of traditional symbols.*

FRÖHLICH, ALFRED (1871-1953). An Austrian neurologist associated with adiposogenital dystrophy, later known as Frohlich's syndrome. He first described it in 1901 in a work entitled "Tumor of the Hypophysis without Acromegaly."
Bibliography: Schmidt, J. E. 1959. *Medical discoveries: who and when.*

FROMM, ERICH (1900-1980). A German-born psychoanalyst who immigrated to the United States in 1934. He was a neo-Freudian and applied psychoanalytic theory to ethics, sociology, and philosophic anthropology. Fromm was interested in social reform related to psychodynamics, in problems of motivation, in Zen Buddhism, and in the concept of a "sane society." His first book, *Escape from Freedom*, was published in 1941 and has been widely read; it was followed by numerous volumes including *The Sane Society* (1955), *Zen Buddhism and Psychoanalysis* (1960), and *You Shall Be as Gods* (1966). Fromm became director of the Mexican Psychoanalytic Institute in 1962.

FROMM-REICHMANN, FRIEDA (1890-1957). A German psychoanalyst who immigrated to the United States in 1934. Her work was mainly concerned with schizophrenia (q.v.), which she believed could be treated by psychotherapy (q.v.). She advocated a close relationship between patient and therapist.
Bibliography: Fromm-Reichmann, F. 1953. *Principles of intense psychotherapy.*

FRUGARDI, ROGERIUS. *See* ROGER OF SALERNO.

FRY, ELIZABETH (1780-1845). An English Quaker (q.v.), daughter of John Gurney, a rich banker, and wife of a successful London merchant. After a visit to Newgate Prision in 1813 she was so moved by the conditions under which the women and children were imprisoned that she dedicated the rest of her life to improving prisons. She also founded hostels for vagrants and an order of nursing sisters.
Bibliography: Rose, J. 1980. *Elizabeth Fry.*

FULLER, THOMAS (1608-1661). An English divine and antiquary, writer of many books and chaplain to Charles II. He believed in witches (*see* WITCHCRAFT) but distinguished between "black," or bad witches, and "white," or good witches. He attributed to the latter the power to "heal those that are hurt". He expatiated these ideas in a book entitled *The Holy State and the Profane State* (1642).
Bibliography: Lyman, D. B. 1935. *The Great Tom Fuller.*

FUMIGATION. The application of fumes or smoke. This was a worldwide and ancient practice against many diseases, but it was especially employed in demoniacal possessions (q.v.). In Arab countries the fumes of mastic, alum, and benzion were believed to drive away evil spirits; the inhalation of the smoke from a piece of burning paper on which verses from the Koran (q.v.) had been written was an even stronger remedy for mental disorders. In Saxon times, after certain herbs were gathered, scattered on hot stones, and then had cold water poured on them, the patient was made to sit in the hot steam. From the Middle Ages (q.v.) into the seventeenth century, fumigation was considered efficacious treatment for the insane, who were

believed to be possessed by the devil or affected by black bile (q.v.). The patient was held over a cauldron of smoking brimstone until he vomited and expelled the devil, or the black bile.
Bibliography: Rohde, E. S. 1974. *The old English herbals*.

FUROR. A Latin term indicating a condition in which the individual has lost his intellectual capacity and is not responsible for his actions. Cicero (q.v.) preferred this term to the Greek one, *mania* (q.v.). Roman law divided the insane into two groups: the *mente capti*, feebleminded, and the *furiosi*, maniacal and violent. Both were considered legally irresponsible.
Bibliography: Zilboorg, G. 1941. *A history of medical psychology*.

FUSELI, JOHN HENRY (1741-1825). A Swiss painter, whose original name was Johann Heinrich Füssli. In 1763 he immigrated to England where he became famous. His work often represents such dramatic subjects as madness, hallucination (q.v.), and nightmare (q.v.). He illustrated William Shakespeare's (q.v.) plays and John Milton's (q.v.) *Paradise Lost*.
Bibliography: Tomory, P. 1972. *The life and art of Henry Fuseli*.

FUTURISM. An art movement initiated by the Italian writer Emilio Filippo Tommaso Marinetti (1876-1944), a friend of Benito Mussolini. It glorified aggression, violence, war, and the age of the machine. It favored fascism and came to an end with the beginning of World War II.
Bibliography: Clough, R. T. 1942. *Looking back at futurism*.

G

GAGATES LITHOS. Bitumen from Gagas, Cilicia, first used around A.D. 200 by Dioscorides (q.v.) of Cilicia as a test for epilepsy (q.v.). He recommended a "suffumigation" of the stone, which involved passing it through fire to be smelted and then holding under the nostrils; if the patient suffered from epilepsy, he would fall to the ground. Alexander of Tralles (q.v.) also advised its use.
Bibliography: Whitwell, J. R. 1936. *Historical notes on psychiatry.*

GAGE, PHINEAS P. (?-1861). An American citizen who was injured while blasting rock in 1848. The explosion caused a crowbar to transfix his skull and left frontal lobe. The iron bar, weighing 13¼ pounds and measuring 3 feet 7 inches in length, was picked up some distance away from him, smeared with blood and particles of brain. Gage recovered consciousness within a few minutes and made a dramatic recovery. His behavior, however, changed after this event and from an "active, steady, alert workman" he became "restless, adventurous, and unreliable," and "he was very profane." He spent some years traveling from place to place and charging a fee to the curious who wanted to see his perforated head and the crowbar. He later settled down to farmwork. His case was cited as clinical proof that frontal lesions of the brain cause changes in behavior but do not damage simple functions. His skull and the crowbar are preserved at the Warren Anatomical Museum of the Harvard Medical School.
Bibliography: Jackson, J. B. S. 1870. *Descriptive catalogue of the Warren Anatomical Museum.*

GAIT. Manner of walking. Moses Maimonides (q.v.) remarked that the gait of a person could indicate whether he was sane or was of unsound mind.

He quoted the words of Solomon (q.v.) in the Old Testament, "Even when he walks along the road, the fool shows no sense. . ." (Eccles. 10:3).
Bibliography: Maimonides, M. 1904. *The guide for the perplexed*, trans. M. Friedlander. 2d. ed.

GALACTITE. A gem that in antiquity was believed to induce those who carried it to forget their sorrows.
See also PRECIOUS STONES.
Bibliography: Evans, J. 1922. *Magical jewels.*

GALE, THOMAS (1507-1586). An English surgeon. He introduced Girolamo Fracastoro's (q.v.) term "syphilis" (q.v.) into the English language in his book, *Certaine Works of Chirurgerie*, published in 1563.
Bibliography: Schmidt, J. E. 1959. *Medical discoveries: who and when.*

GALEN (GALENUS CLAUDIUS) (A.D. c. 129-199). A Greek physician, born at Pergamum in Asia Minor, the son of a calm, considerate father whom he loved, and a passionate, quarrelsome mother whom he disliked. He was educated in philosophy but encouraged to study medicine by his father, who had dreamed that this was his son's destiny. He studied in Alexandria for five years and then became surgeon to the gladiators at Pergamum. He devised for them the first recorded football rules. In 162 he went to Rome where he acquired a fashionable clientele and was appointed court physician to Marcus Aurelius (q.v.). He lectured and wrote on philosophy and medicine. Although he was influenced by Hippocrates (q.v.), Plato (q.v.), and, to a lesser extent, Aristotle (q.v.), he contributed many original observations that he had made during systematic investigations and dissections of animals. He collected, codified, synthesized, and coordinated practically all the medical knowledge of his time in some 400 works. They remained the unchallenged textbooks in medicine for about fifteen hundred years, thus discouraging further research. His physiological schema involved three kinds of spirit: natural spirit from the liver; vital spirit from the lung; and animal spirit from the brain. He emphasized the link between soul, mind, and body and believed that the seat of the soul lay in the substance of the brain and not in the ventricles. He regarded disorders of the soul as consequences of bodily dysfunction and therefore accepted the humoral theory (q.v.) of mental disorder. According to him, black bile (q.v.) collected in the cavities of the brain and affected its substance because of an imbalance. He classified mental disorders as follows: 1) Anoia (diverse forms in which reasoning is affected); 2) Moria (retardation is a feature); 3) Phrenitis (q.v.); 4) Melancholia (q.v.), often associated with mania [q.v.]; 5) Mania; 6) Lethargus (stupor); 7) Hysterical (*see* HYSTERIA) conditions, male as well as female; and 8) Epilepsy (q.v.). The treatment he advised included bleeding, drugs, and diet (qq.v.). Many anecdotes attributed to Galen show his awareness of psychological matters, but his contribution to the understanding of mental disorders was minimal, and his approach to this field was more philosophical than medical.

Bibliography: Temkin, O. 1973. *Galenism: rise and decline of a medical philosophy.*

GALILEI, GALILEO (1564-1642). Italian astronomer, experimental philosopher and mathematician. He studied medicine at the University of Pisa before turning to other sciences. As a child he daydreamed and was given to hearing strange sounds and to having visions. He was a self-assured man, who proudly presented his inventions and revolutionary discoveries to an incredulous and superstitious world that regarded him with enmity and was intolerant of his biting satire. The Inquisition (q.v.) persecuted him for asserting truths that contradicted the Scripture, and he was compelled to abjure his discovery of the movement of the earth as heretical. The study of human behavior was influenced through his ideas of subjectivity of perception, the essential reflexive character of all behavior, and contiguity as the basic principle in association of ideas.

Bibliography: Seeger, R. J. 1966. *Galileo Galilei: his life and works.*

GALL. A term for bile (q.v.). In antiquity it was associated with grief and bitterness. In the Bible (q.v.) gall is used to denote a state produced by sin: "For I perceive that thou art in the gall of bitterness, and in the bond of iniquity" (Acts 8:23).

Bibliography: 1978. *Brewer's dictionary of phrase and fable.*

GALL, FRANZ JOSEPH (1758-1828). A German physiologist. He was primarily concerned with the study of the head and the brain. As a boy he had believed that there were some correlations between the shape of his schoolmates' heads and their mental characteristics. He continued to investigate this theory, as an adult. After observing the inmates of prisons and asylums (q.v.), he tried to relate personality to the shape of the skull and psychological functions to parts of the brain. He stated, for example, that suicide (q.v.) was more frequent in people with thick craniums. He taught brain physiology in Vienna from 1796 until 1801 when the government stopped his lectures because the church regarded his ideas as too materialistic. With Johann Kaspar Spurzheim (q.v.) he laid the foundations for phrenology (q.v.). After settling in Paris in 1807, Gall acquired a fashionable practice and published his most important book, *Anatomie et Physiologie du Systeme Nerveux en Général* (1810-1819). Although his conclusions were inaccurate, his work on pathology and comparative anatomy gave a new importance to the brain and initiated a series of studies on cerebral localization. It is said

that Napoleon I (q.v.), who was notorious for not recognizing the achievements of foreigners, prevented the Institut de France from honoring him.
Bibliography: Watson, R. I. 1963. *The great psychologists.*

GALT, JOHN MINSON (1819-1862). An American physician. In 1841 he became superintendent of the Williamsburg Eastern Lunatic Asylum(q.v.) in Williamsburg, Virginia, and continued a family tradition that was to give a total of eighty-nine years of medical service to the same hospital. He greatly improved conditions in the hospital. He believed that "if you wish to benefit the insane, you must love him and devote yourself to him." His commentaries on insanity were embodied in his principal treatise entitled *Treatise of Insanity*, published in 1848. However, due to his reserve, anxiety and introspection, he was not a good administrator, and during his time funds fell so low that the patients' diets, as well as other material aspects, deteriorated dangerously. He was one of the original thirteen founders of the American Psychiatric Association (q.v.).
Bibliography: Dain, N. 1971. *Disordered minds.*

GALTON, SIR FRANCIS (1822-1911). An English biologist, a cousin of Charles Darwin (q.v.), and a member of a family famed for its illustrious members. He was a hypochondriac (*see* HYPOCHONDRIA) with a tendency toward recurrent nervous breakdowns, which usually were precipitated by overwork and remedied by trips abroad. His childless marriage was not happy because his wife's beliefs were in opposition to his own. She liked children, music, and religion; he did not. Influenced by the theory of evolution, he tried to establish a relationship between heredity and intelligence by measuring certain faculties in children and their parents. In 1869 he published his findings in a book entitled *Heredity of Genius*. He also studied human facial characteristics and tried to group people accordingly. He established in London the first anthropometric laboratory (q.v.) which is now known as the Galton Laboratory at University College. He also devised a way of classifying fingerprints and pointed out their importance as a means of identification. He strongly advocated the concept of eugenics (q.v.), a term coined by him for his book *Human Faculty and its Development* (1883).
Bibliography: Forrest, D. W. 1974. *Francis Galton: the life and work of a Victorian genius.*

GALTON BAR. An apparatus devised by Francis Galton (q.v.) for determining the thresholds of estimation of linear distances.
Bibliography: Boring, E. G. 1950. *A history of experimental psychology.*

GALTON WHISTLE. A device designed by Francis Galton (q.v.) for determining sensitivity to very high-pitched notes.
Bibliography: Boring, E. G. 1950. *A history of experimental psychology.*

GALVANI, LUIGI (1737-1798). An Italian physiologist and professor of anatomy at the University of Bologna. He is known for his experiments on

"animal electricity," which were the results of his experiments on preparations of the muscles and nerves of frogs. His work stimulated many scientists to search for an explanation of his findings and led to the detection of electricity (q.v.) in nerves.
Bibliography: Galvani, L. 1953. *Commentaries on the effect of electricity on muscular motion*, trans. R. M. Green.

GAMBLERS ANONYMOUS. An association organized on the lines of Alcoholics Anonymous (q.v.). Using group therapy, discussions, and support, it tries to help chronic compulsive gamblers and their families. The association was formed in 1957 in southern California, spread across the United States, and opened a branch in London in 1964.
Bibliography: Bergler, E. 1970. *The psychology of gambling*.

GAMLE BAKKEHUS. The first institution in Denmark for the feeble-minded. Due to the efforts of Dr. Jeans R. Hübertz (q.v.), it was opened at a farm in 1855.
Bibliography: Barr, M. W. 1904. *Mental defectives*.

GANNEAU, JEAN SIMON (?-?). A pretender to the French throne in the 1840s. He believed that he was the reincarnation of Louis XVII and that his wife was Marie Antoinette, the mother of the same king. He called himself Mapah, using the first letters of Maman and Papa.
Bibliography: Hall, A. 1976. *Strange cults*.

GANSER, SIGBERT JOSEPH MARIA (1853-1931). A German psychiatrist. He described a form of hysterical (*see* HYSTERIA) reaction that is often observed among prisoners and characterized by deviously relevant answers. It is now known as the Ganser syndrome, or the nonsense syndrome.
Bibliography: Enoch, M. D., and Trethowan, W. H. 1967. *Uncommon psychiatric syndromes*.

GAP (GROUP FOR THE ADVANCEMENT OF PSYCHIATRY). An organization founded in 1946 by fifteen psychiatrists under the chairmanship of Dr. William G. Menninger. It hoped to provide professional leadership and to advance psychiatry through study and report.
Bibliography: Deutsch, A. 1959. *The story of GAP*.

GARGOYLISM. Coarse facial characteristics that are associated with some forms of mental deficiency, for example, Hurler's disease (q.v.). The term derives from the gargoyle waterspouts projecting from church and cathedral roofs. In Gothic architecture the churches were ornamented with grotesque

figures of goblins, monsters, and legendary animals that symbolized evil spirits flying from the church.
Bibliography: MacGillivray, R. C. 1952. "Gargoylism." *J. Ment. Sci. 98*, 687-696.

GARIOPONTUS (?-c.1050). An Italian physician and medical writer. He gathered together Galenic (*see* GALEN) and Byzantine writings on medicine in a treatise entitled *Ad Totius Corporis Aegritudines Remediorum*. He claimed that epilepsy (q.v.), which he attributed to the viscidity of the blood, was caused by black bile (q.v.) reaching the brain and disturbing the soul residing therein. He recognized three kinds of epilepsy: *analepsia*, when the patient is deprived of perception; *catalepsia*, when fever and frothing at the mouth are present; *epilepsia*, when all the mental faculties are affected. Herbal concoctions, vomiting and sneezing, diet (q.v.), purging (q.v.), and bleeding (q.v.) were the recommended treatments. He also described melancholia (q.v.), which he believed was more frequent in males than in females. He believed it was caused by black bile, occurred mainly in autumn and winter, and was cured by bleeding. Lethargy (q.v.) was the term he used for a condition characterized by acute fever, slow pulse, and prostration. In these cases the recommended treatment consisted of keeping the patient in a well lit room and rousing him frequently by shaking and calling him. Mania (q.v.), in his treatise, was an alienation of mind without fever but accompanied by fear, rage, or hilarity, and it was caused by poor digestion or too much drink. It was also common in those who took drugs such as opium (q.v.) and mandrake, and those who engaged in intellectual pursuits.
Bibliography: Whitwell, J. R. 1936. *Historical notes on psychiatry.*

GARLAND, AGNES. A Londoner. In the law court records of 1612 she is mentioned as the keeper of Stone House (q.v.).
Bibliography: O'Donoghue, E. G. 1914. *The story of Bethlehem Hospital.*

GARLIC. A perennial plant known since antiquity. An old folk remedy used in Russia consisted of crushed garlic bulb boiled in milk; it was used to stop nervous spasms and seizures.
Bibliography: Kourenoff, P., and St. George, G. 1970. *Russian folk medicine.*

GARNET. A gem listed in the lapidaries of the seventeenth century as an efficient remedy against melancholia (q.v.) when worn round the neck.
See also PRECIOUS STONES.
Bibliography: Evans, J. 1922. *Magical jewels.*

GARRICK, DAVID (1717-1779). English actor and playwright. He attributed his successful performance of Lear in *King Lear* to his study of a distracted friend. The friend had lost his reason when his only daughter was

killed by falling out of his arms and through a window onto the paving below.
Bibliography: Barton, M. 1948. *Garrick*.

GARZONI, TOMASO (1549-1589). An Italian monk, author of *L'Hospidale de Pazzi Incurabili (The Hospital of Incurable Fools)* first published in 1586 and subsequently translated into English and French. In it, the author described several types of mental disorders: idiocy (*see* IDIOT), dementia, delusional (*see* DELUSIONS) states, manic-depressive psychoses (q.v.), melancholia (q.v.), and psychopathic (*see* PSYCHOPATHY) personalities among others. He established a kind of classification of mental disorders and gave a vivid clinical picture for each group. He also distinguished between demoniacal possessions (q.v.) and natural causes.
Bibliography: Garzoni, T. 1601. Reprint 1967. *L'Hospidale de Pazzi incurabili*.

GASKELL, SAMUEL (1807-1886). A British physician and superintendent of the Lancaster Moor Hospital. He introduced in England special care and training for feebleminded children. He also advocated voluntary admission to public hospitals for nonpauper patients suffering from mild or incipient mental disorders. He was the first medical superintendent to be appointed a commissioner in lunacy and held the position from 1849 to 1866. The Royal College of Psychiatrists commemorates his work with the Gaskell Medal and prize, which was established in 1886 by members of his family. It is presented annually to the most successful candidate in a specially designed examination on psychiatry.
Bibliography: Hunter, R., and Macalpine, I. 1963. *Three hundred years of psychiatry*.

GASKELL, WALTER HOLBROOK (1847-1914). An English physiologist. His studies of the autonomic nervous system were a notable contribution to the field of neurology (q.v.). He was a pioneer of the theory of functional nerve components. His best-known textbook is *The Involuntary Nervous System*.
Bibliography: Haymaker, W., and Schiller, F. 1970. *The founders of neurology*. 2d. ed.

GASSER, HERBERT SPENCER (1888-1963). An American physiologist. He studied under Joseph Erlanger (q.v.) and in 1944 shared a Nobel Prize in physiology with him. With Erlanger, he developed the cathode ray oscillograph, which was capable of recording the exact pattern of nerve impulses. This instrument made possible the understanding of nerve conduction.

He is famous also for his laboratory work on nerve fibers and their relation to specific sensory and motor functions.
Bibliography: Haymaker, W., and Schiller, F. 1970. *The founders of neurology.* 2d. ed.

GASSNER, JOHANN JOSEPH (1727-1779). A German country priest. He believed that some illnesses had supernatural causes and employed exorcism (q.v.) in their treatment. He ascertained that the patient was possessed (*see* POSSESSION) by asking the demon to make the symptoms of the disease appear. If the symptoms appeared, he considered it proof of the presence of evil spirits and would proceed with exorcism. If they did not, the patient's disease was considered natural, and the patient was sent to a physician. For a time Gassner was famous; he had a fashionable clientele and many honors. Franz Mesmer (q.v.), however, asserted that Gassner was using animal magnetism (q.v.) in an unscientific way, and the Bavarian court and even the pope investigated his activities. He was eventually discredited and sent to a small community with orders to desist from his exorcising practices. However, fame remained at his side after death and his tombstone describes him as the most celebrated exorcist who ever lived.
Bibliography: Ellenberger, H. F. 1970. *The discovery of the unconscious.*

GATES, ELMER (1859-1923). An American psychologist. He thought that the structural elements of the brain cells could be developed by systematic means, which would improve skill and mental capacity. His experiments were aimed at making a more efficient use of the mind.
Bibliography: Gates, E. *The art of mind building.*

GAUB, HIERONYMUS DAVID (GAUBIUS) (1705-1780). A German physician and medical writer, greatly influenced by Hermann Boerhaave (q.v.). He believed that irritability (q.v.), or muscular contraction, was a pathological increase of vital power. He extended this principle to all diseases. According to him, vital power, or psychological factors, influenced all physiological functions. His book *On the Duty and Office of Physicians of the Mind* (c. 1750) stated that "the care of the human mind is the most noble branch of medicine."
Bibliography: Garrison, F. H. 1929. *An introduction to the history of medicine.*

GAUDÍ Y CORNET, ANTONIO (1852-1926). A Spanish architect. His childhood was difficult and unhappy. His mother, a brother, and a sister died when he was young. His family was too poor to pay for his training, so he worked and studied at the same time. His ability and originality led him to collaborate with noted Spanish architects, and he became involved in the brilliant and worldly social life of Barcelona's intellectuals. In contrast, in his last years he was completely isolated, infatuated with religion, alienated

from society. The most extreme elements of his designs anticipate surrealism (q.v.) and were explained by him in terms of mysticism and symbolism. The best-known example of his work is the Expiatory Temple of the Sagrada Familia in Barcelona. Like many of his buildings, it can have a disorientating and disturbing effect on the onlooker, because of its persevering motifs reminiscent of schizophrenic (see SCHIZOPHRENIA) drawings. Gaudí died in Barcelona Hospital for the Poor, after he had been knocked down by a tram; his shabby clothing and neglected appearance had hidden his identity.
Bibliography: Masini, L. V. 1970. *Gaudí*.

GAUGUIN, EUGÈNE HENRI PAUL (1848-1903). A French painter. His grandmother was a revolutionary; his grandfather was imprisoned for shooting her in a fit of jealousy; his mother was nearly seduced by her father; and the rest of the family was hardly more conventional. He was three years old when his parents sailed for Peru, and his father died during the journey. A few years later mother and son returned to France. Despite some fluctuations in their circumstances, he became a conventional and successful stockbroker and a typical middle-class husband and father. His hobby was painting and buying works by the impressionists. Eventually painting became his full-time occupation, and the family suffered financially. They went to live with his wife's parents in Denmark, but his pictures shocked the Danes. Taking one of his children with him, he returned to Paris and lived in extreme poverty. His behavior became odd, he suffered from insomnia, and restlessness eventually drove him to leave France for Panama and then Martinique where he painted his first exotic pictures. Back in France he renewed his friendship with Vincent Van Gogh (q.v.) and for a time lived with him, passionately arguing most the time and leaving when Van Gogh was taken to an asylum (q.v.). Tahiti was his next refuge, a native hut his abode, and a local girl his companion. He fathered several half-caste children and became syphilitic (see SYPHILIS). His return to France was painful, for his paintings were not appreciated, and his bizarre behavior caused comment and rejection. For the second time he went to Tahiti, and eventually received the news of his favorite daughter's death. In despair he attempted suicide, but he took too much arsenic and merely vomited. He lived on to take sides with the natives in their struggle against the authorities. His activities on their behalf caused his imprisonment and a serious deterioration in health. He died of a heart attack in Dominica. His life has been the subject of many novels, including *The Moon and Sixpence* by William Somerset Maugham (q.v.).
Bibliography: Boudailles, G. 1966. *Gauguin: his life and work*.

GAUPP, ROBERT EUGEN (1870-1953). A German psychiatrist, pupil of Emil Kraepelin (q.v.). In his research he always considered man in his totality, investigating his past, his culture, and his personality. He is re-

membered for his work on progressive paralysis, paranoia (q.v.), depressive disorders, and homosexuality.
Bibliography: Zilboorg, G. 1941. *A history of medical psychology.*

GAUSTAD ASYLUM. A public institution for the care of the mentally ill established near Christiania (now Oslo), Norway in 1855. It was the first Norwegian psychiatric hospital, and its planners sited it outside the town among pleasant green hills.
Bibliography: Letchworth, W. P. 1889. *The insane in foreign countries.*

GAUTIER, THÉOPHILE (1811-1872). French poet, novelist, critic, and journalist. As a young man he was garish and eccentric. He studied painting and was attracted to romanticism (q.v.), especially to the more lurid branch, which emphasized vampirism, satanism, and other horrific expressions. He was a fanatical admirer of Victor Hugo (q.v.). By 1830 he had turned to writing. For a time, he remained interested in the macabre, and his novels were often aimed at shocking the middle class whom he despised. At one time he was addicted to cannabis indica (q.v.) and wrote vivid descriptions of the sensations he experienced while intoxicated. He was a member of the Club des Haschichins (q.v.).
Bibliography: Richardson, J. 1958. *Théophile Gautier: his life and times.*

GAY, JOHN (1685-1732). An English poet. He was feckless and lazy and loved food and wine overmuch. His first published poem *Wine* was in praise of alcohol consumption and affirmed the belief that those who drank water would never be successful writers. In his *Trivia* (1716), subtitled *The Art of Walking the Streets of London*, he satirically wrote of Bedlam (q.v.):

> Through famed Moorfields, extends a spacious seat
> Where mortals of exalted wit retreat;
> Where wrapped in contemplation, and in straw,
> The wiser few from the mad world withdraw.

His financial speculations in the South Sea Bubble (q.v.) ended in disaster, but he recovered his fortunes by writing *The Beggar's Opera* (1728) and a sequel *Polly* (1729), which received a great deal of publicity when it was prohibited.
Bibliography: Irving, W. H. 1940. *John Gay.*

GAZETTE DE SANTÉ. A French medical journal. Philippe Pinel (q.v.) was the editor of it from 1784 to 1789 and contributed several articles to it. Parts of his unpublished book "Hygiène" also appeared in the journal.
Bibliography: Zilboorg, G. 1941. *A history of medical psychology.*

GAZING CRYSTAL. A mirror or a crystal (q.v.) used in hypnoanalysis with subjects who are in a deep trance. The patient is instructed to open his

eyes and gaze into the crystal, where he will see past events of his life which he will describe to the therapist.
See also HYPNOTISM.
Bibliography: Wolberg, L. R. 1945. *Hypnoanalysis*.

GEHUCHTEN, ARTHUR VAN (1861-1914). A Belgian physician who dedicated himself to neurology (q.v.) . One of his most important contributions was his work on the structure of nerve cells. In 1900 he founded the journal *Le Névraxe* in which many of his papers were published. He was professor of descriptive anatomy at Louvain, where many scientists came to his laboratory, and maintained an active clinical practice. His life was simple, almost ascetic, yet he was happy in his work; he would sing all the time while preparing his experiments. At the beginning of World War I, after he had lost his laboratory and most of his notes, he emigrated to England and worked at Cambridge until his untimely death by heart failure.
Bibliography: Haymaker, W., and Schiller, F. 1970. *The founders of neurology*. 2d. ed.

GELB, ADHÉMAR MAXIMILIAN MAURICE (1887-1936). A Russian psychologist. He was educated in Germany and worked there for most of his life. His research was in the field of sense perception. He described space perception dependent on time experience, which is now known as the Gelb phenomenon.

GÉLINEAU, JEAN BAPTISTE ÉDOUARD (1859-192?). A French neurologist. Idiopathic narcolepsy was first described by him in 1880.
Bibliography: Schmidt, J. E. 1959. *Medical discoveries: who and when*.

GELLO. A female demon who steals children. She appeared in the folklore (q.v.) of ancient and medieval Greece from the time of Sappho (q.v.) onward. She was believed to have been a woman who suffered an untimely death.
Bibliography: Hammond, N.G.L. and Scullard, H. H., eds. 1973. *The Oxford classical dictionary*.

GENERAL PARALYSIS OF THE INSANE. A form of paralysis associated with syphilis (q.v.). Although John Haslam (q.v.) is credited with the first clinical description of paresis in his *Observations on Insanity with Particular Remarks on the Disease and an Account of the Morbid Appearance on Dissections*, published in London in 1798, Louis Florentin Calmeil (q.v.) also studied paralysis in the insane and gave the disease the name of general paralysis of the insane. Antoine Bayle (q.v.) was the first to affirm that the paralysis and the mental disorder were one disease entity. He published his findings in 1822 under the title *Recherche sur l'arachnite chronique*. Through a series of experiments, Richard von Krafft-Ebing (q.v.) established the

definite relationship between syphilis and general paralysis in 1897. At first the treatment of choice was mercury (q.v.), because mercury was used in the therapy of other mental disorders irrespective of their aetiology. Later, malaria therapy (q.v.) was used because the high fever it produced was considered therapeutic. In 1910, Paul Ehrlich (q.v.) revolutionized the treatment of GPI by discovering salvarsan (q.v.), which was based on arsenic. *See also* INSANITY, PARALYTIC.
Bibliography: Zilboorg, G. 1941. *A history of medical psychology.*

GENIUS. 1) In classical times, the guardian spirit assigned to each person at birth to determine his character and the events in his life. It was also the spirit connected with a place, a house, or an event. In ancient Rome, every household worshipped its own familial genius, which was personified in the capacity to reproduce the family. 2) Extraordinary intellectual power limited to heredity. One of the first scientific studies on the genetics of intelligence was conducted by Sir Francis Galton (q.v.), who published his findings in 1869 in a volume entitled *Heredity of Genius.*
Bibliography: Galton, F. 1869. *Heredity of genius.*

GEORGE II (1683-1760). A king of Great Britain and Ireland, elector of Hanover. He was disliked by his father and in turn hated his own son, wishing him dead and not regretting his early demise. He was tactless, short-tempered, and arrogant. His propensity for mistresses did not prevent frequent fits of depression, which were relieved by music (*see* MUSIC THERAPY).
Bibliography: Fraser, A., ed. 1975. *The lives of the kings and queens of England.*

GEORGE III (1738-1820). A king of Great Britain and Ireland and elector of Hanover. He ascended the throne in 1760. It is believed that in his youth he married Hanna Lightfoot, a Quaker (q.v.), by whom he had a daughter. In 1761, he married Charlotte Sophia of Mecklenburg-Strelitz, who gave him fifteen children. When he was twenty-seven he had his first of five attacks of a mental disorder. Each attack lasted several months and finally culminated in a chronic state in 1811. In 1788 he came under the care of the Rev. Francis Willis (q.v.), who ran a private madhouse. The treatment used by Willis included drugs (q.v.), exercise, bleeding (q.v.), a straitjacket, and a special chair of coercion. To celebrate the king's temporary recovery in 1789, special medals were issued. Dr. Willis provided one with his own portrait and the inscription, "Britons Rejoice, Your King's Restored." At the time, the illness was called manic-depression (*see* MANIC-DEPRESSIVE PSYCHOSES). It puzzled the attending physicians, distressed his family, and grieved the nation, but the controversy over the royal malady benefited psychiatry, as it focused attention on mental disorders and stimulated interest in them. The illness now is believed to have been caused by a metabolic disorder known as porphyria (q.v.). The attempted assassination of George III

by James Hadfield (q.v.) in 1800 unwittingly offered another opportunity for progress in the approach to mental disorders. The trial of Hadfield, who was defended by Lord Thomas Erskine (q.v.), resulted in the amendment of the laws relating to criminal responsibility and insanity. In old age, the king had to bear the burden of blindness in addition to many other calamities, but despite his illness and the treatment he received, he lived to be eighty-two years old.
Bibliography: Macalpine, I., and Hunter, R. 1969. *George III and the mad-business.*

GEORGET, ÉTIENNE (1795-1828). A French physician, a pupil of Philippe Pinel (q.v.) and Jean Esquirol (q.v.). As a young man he defended magnetism (q.v.). His essay on autopsies conducted on insane patients made him the first to win a prize established by Esquirol. Georget described mental disorders very accurately and asserted that all mental diseases were different stages of the same process. In 1820 his main work *Traité de la Folie* was published in Paris and attracted international interest. It was illustrated by Jean Gericault (q.v.).
Bibliography: Zilboorg, G. 1941. *A history of medical psychology.*

GEORGIA LUNATIC ASYLUM. An American mental hospital established in Milledgeville, Georgia, in 1837 and opened in 1842.
Bibliography: Deutsch, A. 1949. *The mentally ill in America.*

GEORGSHOSPITAL. A dollhaus (q.v.), or madhouse, was erected in 1326 as part of this hospital at Elbing.
Bibliography: Rosen, G. 1968. *Madness in society.*

GERARD, JOHN (1545-1612). English barber-surgeon and herbalist. His famous *Herball*, based on that of Rembert Dodoens (q.v.), was first published in 1597 and went through many reprints because of its popularity. In the enlarged version of 1633, he described 2,850 plants. Gerard wrote that "a purgation of Hellebore is good for mad and furious men, for melancholy, dull and heavie persons, and briefly for all those that are troubled with the falling sickness, and molested with melancholy."
Bibliography: Woodward, M. 1971. *Gerard's Herball: the essence thereof distilled by Marcus Woodward.*

GERARD, MARGARET (1894-1954). An American pioneer in child psychiatry (q.v.). She contributed to the field of psychosomatic medicine (q.v.) in children with her study of enuresis (q.v.). She believed that free play was not synonymous with overpermissiveness; the latter would cause a child to feel insecure and lead to character disintegration.
Bibliography: Alexander, F. G., and Selesnick, S. T. 1966. *The history of psychiatry.*

GÉRICAULT, JEAN LOUIS ANDRÉ THEÓDORE (1791-1824). A French painter. He was a depressive, who courted death and attempted

suicide (q.v.). His style was sombre and realistic. It reflected his close observation of details and his preoccupation with death. His work often met with hostility because of the macabre subjects he chose to depict, such as the cadavers in the *Raft of the Medusa*. In his last years he painted vivid portraits of the insane, five of which are in the Lyons Museum. Among them there is a particularly striking portrait of a woman who had murdered her child. He also illustrated *Traité de la Folie* written by Étienne Georget (q.v.).
Bibliography: Berger, K. 1956. *Théodore Géricault*, trans. W. Ames.

GERSHWIN, GEORGE (1898-1937). An American composer. When he developed symptoms of abnormal behavior he underwent psychoanalysis (q.v.) for two years and refused to undergo any diagnostic tests and any form of treatment. His friends eventually persuaded him to see a surgeon, who diagnosed a malignant frontal lobe tumor, but by then it was too late to save his life.
Bibliography: Behrman, S. N. 1972. *The Gershwin years*.

GERSON, JEAN LE CHARLIER DE (1363-1429). A French philosopher, mystic, and medical writer. He wrote three tracts on self-abuse which were printed in Cologne, Germany, possibly in 1467, thus claiming to be some of the oldest printed medical books and anticipating the nineteenth-century preoccupation with masturbation as a cause of mental illness.
Bibliography: Connolly, J. L. 1928. *John Gerson, mystic and reformer*.

GESELL, ARNOLD LUCIUS (1880-1961). An American psychologist and pediatrician. In 1911 he founded and directed the Yale Clinic of Child Development, where, in 1920, he conducted a survey on normal behavior in children from birth to six years. The importance of his work rests on his assertion that normality must be understood before studying deviations.
Bibliography: Gesell, A. L. 1934. *An atlas of infant behavior*.
Gesell, A. L. 1940. *The first five years*.

GESNER, CONRAD (1516-1565). A Swiss naturalist of great erudition. Although he is known as a botanist, he graduated in medicine in 1541. He reported using antimony (q.v.) "with happiest results" for the treatment of melancholia (q.v.) and for the treatment of those patients contemplating suicide (q.v.).
Bibliography: Whitwell, J. R. 1936. *Historical notes on psychiatry*.

GESTALT. A term introduced into psychology in 1890 by the German philosopher Christian von Ehrenfels (q.v.). He used it to denote an integrated whole that is more than a sum of parts.
Bibliography: Boring, E. G. 1950. *A history of experimental psychology*.

GESTALT PSYCHOLOGY. A school of psychology developed in 1912 by Max Wertheimer, Wolfgang Köhler, and Kurt Koffka (qq.v.). The idea

for this new system, which was based heavily on perception, came to Wertheimer in 1910, during a train journey when he conceived of a new approach to the problem of seen movement.
Bibliography: Boring, E. G. 1950. *A history of experimental psychology*.

GESTATION. Aulus Cornelius Celsus (q.v.) recommended "gestation," or gentle oscillation of the patient in a suspended bed, in cases of mental disorder. Similar methods were popular in the nineteenth century.
Bibliography: Spenser, W. G., trans. 1971. *Celsus—de medicina*.

GESUALDO, CARLO, PRINCE OF VENOSA (1560-1613). An Italian composer and musician. He was pathologically sensitive, and his neurotic personality found an outlet in the dramatic madrigals he composed. He ordered the murder of his young wife and her lover, Fabrizio Carafa, and then married Eleonora d'Este. He was brilliant in music but unbalanced in everyday life and considered himself above the judgment of others. The tortured complexity of his compositions had no precedents and no imitators.
Bibliography: Watkins, G. E. 1973. *Gesualdo*.

GEYA (GHEYN), JACOB DE (1565-1629). Flemish engraver and painter. Among his works are four engravings representing the temperaments and their corresponding elements. He depicted melancholy (*see* MELANCHOLIA) as a dejected man, sitting on a terrestrial globe (earth is the element of melancholy), surrounded by a gloomy landscape that is made still more oppressive by a dark sky. Underneath the engraving there is a Latin inscription that reads, "Melancholy, the most unfortunate affliction of the soul and of the mind often oppresses men of talent and of genius."
Bibliography: Wittkower, R., and Wittkower, M. 1963. *Born under Saturn*.

G FACTOR. A term used by Charles Spearman (q.v.) to indicate general intelligence in his two-factor theory of intelligence. The term "S Factor" indicated specific abilities.
See also O FACTOR, P FACTOR, and W FACTOR.
Bibliography: Flugel, J. C. 1945. *A hundred years of psychology*.

GHEEL COLONY. A system of foster family care (q.v.) for the mentally ill that developed around the cult of Saint Dymphna (q.v.) in Gheel, Belgium. The shrine of Saint Dymphna has been known for its miraculous cures since the eleventh century. In the thirteenth century a hospital was built next to the chapel for the care of the pilgrims. In less than a century the numbers of pilgrims seeking cures, especially for mental disorders, had overwhelmed the hospital, making it necessary to lodge them with local families and thus originating a system of family care. At first the pilgrims received no medical care: they merely passed under the tomb of the saint daily and often spent

the rest of the time chained in dark rooms. Eventually proper psychiatric care was organized, although in 1821 Jean Esquirol (q.v.) visited the hospital and found its facilities inadequate. By 1937 the number of patients in fostercare was over 4,000. This number has declined since the 1950s due to increased industrialization and changed cultural patterns, but mental patients are still fostered in the town under the supervision of the Belgium Ministry of Health, which insures that they are given up-to-date psychiatric treatment.
Bibliography: Meeus, F. 1921. *L'histoire de la colonie de Gheel.*

GHOST-DANCE RELIGION. A term applied to epidemics of mental disorders that occurred among American Indians in the latter part of the nineteenth century. Those affected made objects representing dancing figures and other things seen in visions or dreams (q.v.).
Bibliography: Mooney, J. 1965. *The ghost-dance religion and the Sioux outbreak of 1890*, ed. A.F.C. Wallace.

GIDDINGS, FRANKLIN HENRY (1855-1931). American sociologist who worked in the field of political sociology and developed the concept of "consciousness of kind."
Bibliography: Giddings, F. H. 1924. *The scientific study of human society.*

GIDE, ANDRÉ PAUL GUILLAUME (1869-1951). A French author. He rebelled against the puritanical and orthodox atmosphere in which he was raised. When he was in his twenties, he visited North Africa, where he met Oscar Wilde (q.v.) and Lord Alfred Douglas. Under their influence he was able to acknowledge his latent homosexuality (q.v.), which had been a cause of inner guilt and torment. His writings were often attacked as shamelessly immoral. Gide was a creature of conflict, half puritan, half hedonist (*see* HEDONISM), and in perpetual oscillation between the Bible (q.v.) and Johann Wolfgang von Goethe (q.v.), sensuality and austerity. He was equally attracted by God and the devil. He was awarded the Nobel Prize for literature in 1947. His biography and diaries are of outstanding frankness.
Bibliography: Cordle, T. 1976. *André Gide.*

GIFT EXCHANGE. Bronislaw Malinowski (q.v.), M. Mauss, and G. Homans, as well as other students of behavior, have been impressed by the possibility of considering gift exchange as the basis for social organization, because it represents a basic form of transaction met in every society.
Bibliography: Mauss, M. 1954. *The gift*, trans. I. Cunnison.

GILBERT, MARIE DOLORES ELIZA ROSANNA (1818?-1861). A British dancer, born in Ireland. She assumed the name of Lola Montez. She was a tumultuous woman of incredible vitality. Her beauty, wit, charm, and ambition led her into several adventures. She was the mistress of Franz

Liszt (q.v.), Alexandre Dumas père (q.v.) and Ludwig I (1786-1868) of Bavaria, who was so bewitched by her that he allowed her to rule his kingdom until the revolution of 1848, which forced her to leave Bavaria. She went to California, joined the gold rush, and opened a frontier saloon. Her behavior began to show signs of mental stress: she plotted to become queen of California and turned to mysticism and astrology (q.v.). After an Australian tour, she settled in New York and devoted herself to the rescue of prostitutes. At forty-one she is said to have become schizophrenic (*see* SCHIZOPHRENIA) and could be seen shuffling along the sidewalks of New York imploring divine forgiveness for her sins. She died of a stroke when she was forty-three years old.

Bibliography: Ross, I. 1972. *The uncrowned queen.*

GILBERT, WILLIAM (1544-1603). An English physician to Queen Elizabeth I and a scientist. He studied electricity (q.v.) and was the first to distinguish electricity from magnetism (q.v.). He ruled that matter is not animated by a soul and that electricity is a natural phenomenon. His book *De Magnete, Magneticisque Corporibus* (1600) was the first major scientific work to be published in England. He advocated experimental methods in science and provided information that served as a stimulus for new investigations.

Bibliography: 1959. *The History and philosophy of the brain and its functions.*

GILBERTUS ANGLICUS (fl.1250). An English author of several works on medicine. The oldest manuscript of his most famous work, *Compendium Medicinae*, is dated 1271. Among other things it contains discussions of mental illness. He considered mania (q.v.) a disorder of the imagination and melancholia (q.v.) a disorder of reason, both due to affections of the brain. Gibertus Anglicus identified many kinds of mental disorders and gave vivid examples of their symptomatology. He also suggested suitable forms of treatment, including special diet (q.v.), wine, music (*see* MUSIC THERAPY), reassurance for the anxious, and rational arguments for the paranoid (*see* PARANOIA). His theories were derived primarily from Galen (q.v.) and Constantine the African (q.v.), but unlike others of his time he did not recognize diabolic possession as a cause of insanity. Geoffrey Chaucer (q.v.) mentioned Gilbertus among the famous writers studied by his "doctor of Physik".

Bibliography: Talbot, C. H. 1967. *Medicine in mediaeval England.*

GILLES DE LA TOURETTE, GEORGES (1857-1904). A French physician, disciple of Jean Martin Charcot (q.v.). He synthetized and defended Charcot's work in a treatise on hysteria (q.v.) entitled *Traité Clinique et Thérapeutique de l'Hysterie*, published in Paris in 1891. In 1885, he had published a study of eight patients suffering from a syndrome that usually began in childhood and was characterized by involuntary jerking, and noises, coprolalia and echolalia; the disorder is now known as Gilles de la Tourette syndrome. With Dr. Gabriel Legues he wrote *Soeur Jeanne des Agnes*, an account of the epidemic hysteria among the Loudun nuns in the 1630s. In 1893 a young woman patient, who was reminiscent of Soeur Jeanne, believing that she was under Dr. Gilles de la Tourette's hypnotic (*see* HYPNOTISM) influence and frustrated in her paranoid (*see* PARANOIA) love for him, shot him three times. He never recovered from the brain injury she inflicted.

Bibliography: Enoch, M. D. and Trethowan, W. H. 1979. *Uncommon psychiatric syndromes*.

GILLESPIE, ROBERT DICK (1897-1945). An English practitioner of psychiatry (q.v.). He was trained by Adolf Meyer (q.v.) at the Henry Phipps Psychiatric Clinic (q.v.) in the United States. In 1927 with David Kennedy Henderson (q.v.) he wrote *A Textbook of Psychiatry*, which had one section devoted to child psychiatry (q.v.) and influenced the establishment of this branch of psychiatry. He also wrote on depression in adults and children.

Bibliography: Gillespie, R. D. 1939. *A survey of child psychiatry*.

GILLRAY, JAMES (1757-1815). An English caricaturist. His talents often were employed in castigating the social follies of his time. His caricatures sometimes exceeded the boundaries of satire and were cruel and brutal. George III (q.v.) was one of the individuals he ridiculed. Gillray's career ended in 1811 when he became insane.

Bibliography: Hill, D. 1965. *Mr. Gillray, the caricaturist*.

GIN. An alcoholic beverage that was invented originally as a diuretic by Franciscus de la Boë (q.v.). It is a distillation of grain flavored with juniper. In the eighteenth century gin intoxication was common especially among the poorer classes of London. Some people were said to live exclusively on it. William Hogarth's (q.v.) famous drawing *Gin Lane*, one of a series entitled *The Four Stages of Cruelty*, vividly depicted the degradation and child neglect brought about by cheap gin. Gin was given even to small children as a sedative and hypnotic. In 1751 the British Gin Laws raised the price and restricted the sale of spirits, thus reducing the incidences of drunkenness and the number of deaths directly and indirectly caused by alcoholic intoxication.

GIOCONDA, LA. An opera by the Italian composer Amilcare Ponchielli (1834-1886). Gioconda is torn between love and jealousy; in her despair and anguish she sings a dramatic soliloquy invoking suicide (q.v.), "Suicido . . . in questi fieri momenti to sol mi resti" (Act 2). Faced with no escape from the psychopathic (*see* PSYCHOPATHY) Barnaba, she stabs herself. Fear of

witchcraft (q.v.), suspicion, superstition, and the use of a powerful narcotic are other items of psychopathological interest.
Bibliography: Harewood, ed. 1969. *Kobbé's complete opera book.*

GIOTTO (GIOTTO DI BONDONE) (1267-1337). Italian painter and architect. He developed the trend begun by his master Cimabue that replaced symbolism with expression. The expressions shown on the faces of his subjects depict anguish, suffering, joy, and other emotions. By discarding superfluous details and intensifying the essential elements, he was able to produce dramatic works of art.
Bibliography: Battisti, E. 1966. *Giotto.*

GIRALDUS CAMBRENSIS, *or* GERALD DE BARRI (c.1146-c.1220). A Norman-Welsh ecclesiastic and writer. In his *Topographia Hibernica,* an account of the people and natural history of Ireland, he referred to lunatics (q.v.) "Those are called lunatics where attacks are exacerbated every month when the moon is full."
Bibliography: Tuke, D. H. 1882. *History of the insane in the British Isles.*

GISSING, GEORGE (1857-1903). An English writer. His promising scholastic career was curtailed when he was found stealing to assist a prostitute and was expelled from Owens College in Manchester. He went to America where he quickly became destitute and nearly starved. He then returned to London, married the prostitute he had helped, and experienced the squalor and ugliness of life in slums. His alcoholic (*see* ALCOHOLISM) wife died miserably and he again married unhappily. His novels are full of social criticism derived from the psychological evils he saw. His themes are developed with great insight into human nature and display a pathological gloom and pessimism.
Bibliography: Tindall, G. 1974. *The born exile.*

GJESSING, LIEV ROLVSSÖN (1889-1959). A Norwegian physician. His work advanced the understanding of those metabolic diseases that cause mental symptoms. In 1932 he described Gjessing's syndrome, a catatonic (*see* CATATONIA) stupor or excitement in schizophrenics (*see* SCHIZOPHRENIA). He attributed it to disorders of nitrogen metabolism. He continued to publish papers on this subject until his death.
Bibliography: Gjessing, R. 1938. Disturbances of Somatic Function in Catatonia with Periodic Course and their compensation. *J. ment. Sci.*, 84: 608-21.

GLADIATOR. The warm blood of a gladiator killed in the arena was one of the remedies used by the Romans for insanity.
See also FAUSTINA AUGUSTA.

GLANVILL, JOSEPH (1636-1680). English divine, philosopher, and Fellow of the Royal Society (q.v.). Like many of his contemporaries, he thought that science should not deny supernatural phenomena and held that a belief in witches (*see* WITCHCRAFT) and apparitions should be defended, as it rested on the same principles as the theory of the soul's immortality. He stated his arguments in an essay entitled *Philosophical Considerations Touching Witches and Witchcraft*, which was first published in 1666.
Bibliography: (1900). *Dictionary of national biography.*

GLANVILLE FRITILLARY. A pale brown and yellow butterfly. It was named after Lady Glanville, an enthusiastic collector of butterflies in the eighteenth century. Her absorption in this pursuit added to her relatives' conviction that she was insane, and after her death they contested her will.

GLASGOW ASYLUM FOR LUNATICS. An institution in Scotland begun in 1810 by private enterprise. The funds for it were collected from the community by a prominent Glasgow citizen, Robert M'Nair, in order to provide a better place for the insane who were kept in the cellars of the town's hospital. Unfortunately when the tide of the nearby river was abnormally high those cells were flooded. The Glasgow Asylum was designed by William Stark (q.v.) and opened in 1814. The various wings were arranged so that they radiated from an observation center placed in the middle. In 1843 the hospital was replaced by a new building at Kelvinside and given a royal charter. In 1960 the institution was renamed the Gartnavel Royal Hospital and became one of the Scottish Royal Hospitals.
See also ROYAL ASYLUMS.
Bibliography: Henderson, D. K. 1964. *The evolution of psychiatry in Scotland.*

GLEN-NA-GALT. The Irish "Valley of the Lunatics," beautifully situated in County Kerry, near Tralee. It was believed that every lunatic (q.v.), if left to himself, would eventually come to this valley. It acquired its curative reputation when Gall, the son of the king of Ulster, became deranged after a battle, plunged into the valley, and there recovered his sanity. Those entering the valley had to ford a stream at the Ahagaltaum (Madman's Ford) and pass by the Gloghnagalt (Standing Stone of the Lunatics) to reach Tobarna-galt (Wells of the Lunatics), where they would drink their curative waters and eat the watercress that grew beside them.
Bibliography: Tuke, D. H. 1882. *History of the insane in the British Isles.*

GLINKA, MIKHAIL IVANOVICH (1804-1857). A Russian composer. He is considered the father of Russian operatic music. He was employed in government administration but poor health forced him to travel to Italy where he met Vincenzo Bellini (1801-1835) and Gaetano Donizetti (q.v.). His musical genius was in contrast to his character. His life was trivial, and

he was continuously preoccupied with hypochondriacal (*see* HYPOCHON-DRIA) disorders.
Bibliography: Brown, D. 1973. *Glinka.*

GLISSON, FRANCIS (1597-1677). An English physician, one of the founders of the Royal Society (q.v.), and a president of the Royal College of Physicians. He greatly contributed to anatomy, physiology, and pathology. His notion of irritability (q.v.), which he thought was a quality of all the tissues, was a variant of the vital spirits theory of his time.
Bibliography: 1900. *Dictionary of national biography.*

GLOSSOLALIA. A term meaning "speaking in tongues," a widespread ecstatic (*see* ECSTASY) phenomenon observed in those who speak while in a state of trance. In antiquity it was believed that prophets, possessed (*see* POSSESSION) by a god, produced divine revelations in these unintelligible sounds. The Bible (q.v.) gives instances of glossolalia in Isaiah. Similar phenomena occurred in the seventeenth century when French Huguenot children were said to utter prophesies in foreign languages while in a religious trance. The belief persisted in such other religious sects as the Shakers (q.v.), the Quakers (q.v.), the Methodists (*see* METHODISM) and the Mormons.
See also CAMISARDS.
Bibliography: Cutten, G. B. 1927. *Speaking with tongues: historically and psychologically considered.*

GLOUCESTER LUNATIC ASYLUM (*now* HORTON ROAD HOSPITAL). One of the oldest county asylums (q.v.) in England still in use. Plans for it were approved in 1793 but were not executed until enough funds had been collected through voluntary subscriptions in 1823. At the end of 1824 the hospital report stated that accommodations had been provided for three classes of patients: "24 Opulent Patients, 36 Charity Patients and 60 Pauper Patients." Each class had its own accommodations: the stucco-fronted section was for private patients, the back-to-back cells were for paupers, and some cells under the forecourt were reserved for refractory patients. In 1849 cholera struck the city of Gloucester, but not a single case arose in the asylum. In the report for the same year, it is proudly noted that no form of restraint (q.v.) was used even in cases of violence, "not even a glove being fastened to the hand of any patient."
Bibliography: 1963. *Horton Road and Coney Hill Hospital reports 1823-1963.*

GLOVER, MARY (fl. 1602). A young London girl. In 1602 she claimed she had been bewitched by an old woman named Elizabeth Jackson. Edward Jorden (q.v.) gave evidence at the trial that Mary Glover's symptoms were

not due to supernatural intervention but rather to "hysterical passion" (*see* HYSTERIA). Even with this evidence, Elizabeth Jackson was found guilty.
Bibliography: Thornton, E. M. 1976. *Hypnotism, hysteria and epilepsy: an historical synthesis.*

GLOVER, MARY (?-1688). An American laundress, born in Boston. She was tried for witchcraft (q.v.) and executed in 1688. She was accused of having bewitched the Goodwin children, who had exhibited various hysterical (*see* HYSTERIA) symptoms. Her confession was so wild and incoherent that it should have proved her derangement rather than her guilt. Cotton Mather reported her trial and execution in his *Memorable Providences relating to Witchcraft and Possessions* in 1689.
Bibliography: Deutsch, A. 1949. *The mentally ill in America.*

GOAT'S MILK. Andrew Boorde (q.v.) recommended goat's milk with sugar for "frantic" patients.
Bibliography: Poole, H. E. 1936. *The wisdom of Andrew Boorde.*

GODDARD, HENRY HERBERT (1866-1957). An American psychologist and director of the psychological laboratory (q.v.) at the Training School for the Feebleminded at Vineland, New Jersey, where he introduced the Simon-Binet mental age test. He devised a classification of mental defectives that included three grades: 1) idiot (q.v.) with a mental age of up to two years; 2) imbecile (q.v.) with a mental age of three to seven years; and 3) moron (q.v., a term introduced by him) with a mental age of eight to twelve years. He believed that mental deficiency was hereditary and expounded this theory in a genetic investigation on a feebleminded family that he named the Kallikak family (q.v.). He derived the name from two Greek terms *kalos* (beautiful) and *kakos* (bad).
See also EUGENICS, JUKES, and NAM.
Bibliography: Goddard, H. H. 1912. *The Kallikak family: a study in the heredity of feeblemindedness.*

GOES, HUGO VAN DER (1435?-1482). A Flemish painter and monk. While on a journey, his mind became deranged, and he became convinced that his sins would lead to the damnation of his soul. The prior of his religious order recognized that he was sick, compared his disorder to that of King Saul (q.v.), and tried to cure it by the same method, music (*see* MUSIC THERAPY), to which he added other forms of entertainment. The monk in charge of the sick, Gaspar Ofhuys (q.v.), treated him according to the guidelines of Bartholomaeus Anglicus (q.v.) but thought that the disorder in this case was sent by God to chasten brother Hugo, who re-

covered as soon as he ceased to think too much of himself. His last painting, *Death of the Virgin*, is a tense work expressing violent grief.
Bibliography: Rosenberg, C. E., ed. 1978. *Healing and history.*

GOETHE, JOHANN WOLFGANG VON (1749-1832). German poet, dramatist, scientist, and philosopher. There was some abnormality in his family: his father was eccentric and his sister died insane. Goethe suffered from depression from an early age and maintained that sometimes he could see himself approaching in hallucinatory experiences. A series of unsatisfactory love affairs was the stimulus for some of his works. The *Sorrows of Young Werther*, written in 1774, reflects his hopeless love for Charlotte Buff, the fiancee of a friend. Werther (q.v.) solved his problems by committing suicide (q.v.), but Goethe merely left the area. *Werther* was widely read and it sparked off a number of suicides, especially among the young, who killed themselves with a copy of the book in their pockets. In 1776 Goethe accepted a position at the court of the duke of Weimar. There, under the influence of Charlotte von Stein (1742-1827), he became more tranquil but less creative. His scientific approach to the study of nature gained respect for his theory of the metamorphosis of parts, according to which the skull is essentially a developed vertebra. Sigmund Freud (q.v.), who interpreted Goethe's life and identified with him during his own self-analysis, was so influenced by him that he imitated his literary style and often quoted him. Goethe also was one of Alfred Adler's (q.v.) favorite authors and Carl Jung (q.v.) encouraged the rumor that his grandfather was an illegitimate son of Goethe. He too quoted and imitated him. Goethe's masterpiece is *Faust*, a drama rich in symbolism, often obscure.
Bibliography: Hatfield, H. 1963. *Goethe.*

GOGOL, NIKOLAI VASILYEVICH (1809-1852). A Russian novelist and playwright. He was brought up in fear of the devil and hell-fire by an overreligious mother. He started to write poetry when he was five. To avoid punishment at school, he pretended to be insane and was kept in a school sanatorium for two months. In adolescence he experienced sexual difficulties and was often moody and depressed. Later in life the religious and moral scruples that are reflected in his tormented writings assailed him. His doubts, his fears, hallucinations (q.v.) and obsessions (q.v.) are mirrored in *Selected Passages from Correspondence with Friends* (1847) and *The Diary of a Madman* (1835). He was so afraid of attacks from behind that he would walk sideways and try to keep his back to a wall at all times. He burned many of his manuscripts in fits of depression and guilt over his own sinfulness.
Bibliography: Troyat, H. 1974. *Divided soul: the life of Gogol.*

GOHL, JOHANN DANIEL (1674-1731). German physician and medical writer, also known as Ursinus Wahrmund. He was interested in mental

disorders which he regarded within the scope of medicine and encouraged a scientific approach to their assessment and therapy.
Bibliography: Gohl, J. D. 1735. *Medicina practica, clinica et forensis.*

GOLDEN BOUGH, THE. A monumental work by Sir James Frazer (q.v.) originally published in two volumes in 1890. It was revised and expanded into twelve volumes in 1915. It is a study of primitive customs, superstitions, and institutions of mankind. The title is taken from the golden bough that symbolized the link between this world and the next in ancient mythologies.
Bibliography: Frazer, J. G. 1915. *The golden bough.* 12 vols.

GOLDEN GATE BRIDGE. A famous bridge in San Francisco, California, begun in 1933 and completed in 1937. Many individuals have committed suicide (q.v.) by leaping to death from its 240 foot height. By 1973, 500 people had died in this way, and seven had survived the experience. Suicide prevention patrols and closed circuit television scanning the bridge footpaths are among the precautions employed to prevent would-be suicides.

GÖLDI, ANNA (?-1782). A Swiss servant girl who was accused of witchcraft (q.v.) and beheaded. She was probably the last woman in Europe to be executed after a legal trial for witchcraft.
Bibliography: Werlinder, H. 1978. *Psychopathy: a history of the concepts.*

GOLDSMITH, OLIVER (1728-1774). Irish novelist, playwright, and poet. From an early age he was an academic failure, rejected by the church, the law, and medicine, which he studied for two years in Edinburgh. He tried to earn a living by practicing medicine, by ushering, and by occasionally contributing articles to the press, but what he earned he quickly lost by gambling. He was always in debt and sometimes so poor that he had to pawn his clothes. He toured Europe roaming on foot, with a flute. In 1759 his writings and plays began to attract attention, and his luck turned. Because he was never able to write to order and remained an erratic character, unreliable and irritable yet compassionate and warmhearted, Horace Walpole referred to him as "the inspired idiot." The family depicted in his novel *The Vicar of Wakefield* (1766) is partially modeled on his own family.
Bibliography: Rousseau, G. S. 1974. *Oliver Goldsmith.*

GOLDSTEIN, KURT (1878-1965). A German psychiatrist. His work has been particularly important to the fields of brain lesions, schizophrenia (q.v.), and speech disorders. He thought that the effects of leucotomy are due to an impairment of abstract thought. He affirmed the importance of the psychological assessment of patients with brain lesions.
Bibliography: Galdston, I., ed. 1979. *Historic derivations of modern psychiatry.*

GOLEM. According to Jewish legends from the Middle Ages (q.v.), an enormous man-shaped brutish creature. Its creation was based on super-

natural power. Traditionally it was said that the first golem was made from clay by Elijah of Chelm in the sixteenth century. Another famous golem legend also belongs to the sixteenth century. This golem was said to have been made by Rabbi Judah Löw ben Bezalel in Prague, Czechoslovakia.
Bibliography: Baynes, H. G. 1940. *Mythology of the soul.*

GOLGI, CAMILLO (1844-1926). An Italian cytologist. His description of nerve cells and their functions contributed to a better understanding of the nervous system. For a brief period he worked with Cesare Lombroso (q.v.). Golgi made valuable observations on mental disorders and their manifestations in patients suffering from pellagra (q.v.). He also developed a new method of staining nerve tissue with silver nitrate, and developed the theory that the neurons formed a reticular network.
Bibliography: Haymaker, W., and Schiller, F. 1970. *The founders of neurology.* 2d. ed.

GOLL, FRIEDRICH (1829-1903). Swiss physician and neurohistologist. He prepared over 2,000 tissue samples of the spinal cord and described the structure of nerve fibers. The median portion of dorsal funiculus of spinal cord is named after him.

GOLTZ, FRIEDRICH LEOPOLD (1834-1902). A Polish physiologist. His studies on decorticated dogs, which he kept alive for up to three years, demonstrated the importance of the central nervous system.
Bibliography: Haymaker, W., and Schiller, F. 1970. *The founders of neurology.* 2d. ed.

GONCHAROV, IVAN ALEKSANDROVICH (1812-1891). A Russian novelist, famous for his profound psychological study of a lazy and idle man, *Oblomov* (1855). The hero, Oblomov, subsequently became the Russian symbol of pathological laziness.
See also OBLOMOVSHTCHINA.
Bibliography: Goncharov, I. A. 1954. *Oblomov*, trans. D. Magarshack.

GONCOURT, JULES ALFRED HUOT DE (1830-1870). A French novelist whose work was based on a detailed study of neurotic characters and contemporary life. He wrote in collaboration with his elder brother Edmond (1822-1896). After Jules' death, Edmond published their diary, which contains a vivid description of his brother's illness. Jules died of general paralysis of the insane (q.v.) and the last period of his illness was marked by a rapid deterioration in mental faculties and a change in personality that included moodiness and brutish behavior; these symptoms so affected Edmond that he contemplated suicide (q.v.) and the destruction of his sick brother. In

the end, Jules' speech disintegrated and his features changed beyond recognition. He died in a coma.
Bibliography: Critchley, M. 1979. *The divine banquet of the brain and other essays.*

GONZALES HENRIQUES, RAUL (1906-1952). A Mexican psychiatrist, a director of psychiatric services for the Mexican Social Security Institute, and one of the founders of the Association Psiquiatrica de America Latina. He was interested in research and teaching and was a brilliant organizer. Psychoanalysis (q.v.) was introduced into Mexico by him.
Bibliography: Leon, C. A. and Rosselli, H. 1975. Latin America. In *World history of psychiatry*, ed. J. G. Howells.

GOOCH, ROBERT (1784-1830). An English physician who practiced in London as a male midwife and lectured in midwifery at the Royal Hospital of Saint Bartholomew (q.v.). He was particularly interested in the psychiatric problems arising in obstetric practice and wrote on puerperal insanity (q.v.), giving it a poor prognosis. He described its onset and course with illustrations drawn from his own clinical experience. He first presented his findings in a paper *Observations on Puerperal Insanity* that was read to the College of Physicians in 1819. He later expanded his findings into a book entitled *An Account of Some of the Most Important Diseases Peculiar to Women* (1829).
Bibliography: 1900. *The dictionary of national biography.*

GOOD, JOHN MASON (1764-1827). English physician and medical writer who devised a classification of mental disorders, which he arranged into classes and orders, according to the symptoms presented.
Bibliography: 1900. *The dictionary of national biography.*

GORDON, ADAM LINDSAY (1833-1870). An Australian poet. He tried a number of occupations, and was in succession a police-trooper, a horse-breaker and a stablekeeper. Eventually he became the best steeplechase rider in Australia. Following a fall and some financial difficulties, he developed acute anxiety about his poetry and in a fit of depression shot himself. His poetry is permeated with a deep pessimism.
Bibliography: Sladen, D. 1934. *A. L. Gordon: a study.*

GORDON, ALFRED (1874-1953). An American neurologist. He described the reflex seen in pyramidal-tract disease (Gordon reflex) whereby there is dorsal extension of the great toe, if the calf muscle is compressed.

GORDON, BERNARD DE (?-c.1320). A physician possibly born in Scotland. He practiced in France and taught at Montpellier. He was a medical reformer and his book *Lilium medicinae* was circulated in manuscript form,

and in 1480 was printed for the first time in Naples. He recognized the following mental disorders: lethargia vera (eyes closed), lethargia nonvera (eyes open), stupor, mania (q.v.) and melancholia (q.v.) (corruptions of the mind), phrenesis, incubus (q.v.), and epilepsy (q.v.) . His novel treatment for lethargia consisted of rubbing the extremities with salt and vinegar "without pity" and tormenting the patient with the squealing of little pigs; trumpets and drums also could be employed to keep the patient awake. He suggested treating patients with mania and melancholy with every consideration, unless they were disobedient. Under those circumstances he advised binding and thrashing them.
Bibliography: Whitwell, J. R. 1936. *Historical notes on psychiatry.*

GORDON, LORD GEORGE (1751-1793). A British nobleman who was an ardent agitator on political and religious matters. In 1780 he led the No-Popery Riots (the Gordon Riots [q.v.]), championing the Protestant cause. Later he became a Jew. He was tried for treason and acquitted because of the efforts of Thomas Erskine (q.v.), but in 1788 he was imprisoned for libeling Marie Antoinette and the British government. He spent the remainder of his life languishing in Newgate Prison as a pauper lunatic (q.v.). He died there of typhus.
Bibliography: Colson, P. 1948. *Private portraits.*

GORDON RIOTS. Instigated by Lord George Gordon (q.v.) in London in 1780 to demand the repeal of the act that had returned political rights to Roman Catholics. The rioters threatened to burn down Bethlem Royal Hospital (q.v.) and to release the insane. Their threat was not put into action, but it produced great anxiety in the citizens of London, who were terrified at the thought of mad people set free.
Bibliography: O'Donoghue, E. G. 1914. *The story of Bethlehem Hospital.*

GORKY, MAXIM (1868-1936). A Russian writer. His real name was Alexei Maximovich Peshkov; he adopted the pseudonym Maxim Gorky (Maxim the Bitter) when he published his first story in 1892. His father died when he was five, and his mother took him to live with her parents. In his autobiography *Childhood* he wrote that his grandfather's house was "filled with hot vapors of hostility," and the fighting and wrestling of his relatives were so upsetting that even as an adult he could not bear to think about them. He spent his adolescence in a number of menial trades. A drunken cook on a steamer taught him to read. At one point he was so miserable that he tried to commit suicide (q.v.) by shooting himself; he survived despite a pierced lung. With other manual workers, he founded a study circle and unsuccessfully approached Leo Tolstoy (q.v.) naively expecting him to give a small piece of land for the project. By 1900 his political sympathies aroused the suspicion of the police and he was kept under close observation. After

the 1905 revolution failed, Gorky escaped abroad but met open hostility in the United States when it was revealed that he was not married to his companion. He moved to Capri, Italy, where he lived undisturbed for seven years before returning to Russia. After the death of Nikolai Lenin (q.v.), he became a personal friend of Joseph Stalin (1879-1953) whom he glorified, even approving of the forced labor camps. His writings are at times violent, depicting man crushed by his environment, nature equated with beauty, humanity with frailty and ugliness, and life endowed with "the burden of great and inexorable sorrow."
Bibliography: Levin, D. 1967. *Stormy petrel: the life and works of Maxim Gorky.*

GOSSE, SIR EDMUND WILLIAM (1849-1928). English poet, author, and critic. His parents were Plymouth Brethren, who lived by their interpretation of the Scripture and made his childhood lonely and miserable with their restrictions and their ban on all amusements. He said that his childhood was "long, long with interminable hours." His father would cane him and then quote from the Book of Proverbs, "spare the rod and spoil the child." He felt murderous hatred for his father and described this and other negative emotions from his childhood in his book *Father and Son*, which he published anonymously in 1907. He had a distinguished career as an author and a lecturer; among his best known works are his lives of John Donne, Thomas Gray, and Sir Thomas Browne (qq.v.). His collected poems were published in 1911.
Bibliography: Charteris, E. 1931. *Life and letters of Sir Edmund Gosse.*

GOTHAM. A village in Nottinghamshire, England, proverbial for the stupidity of its inhabitants. According to tradition, the inhabitants feigned folly to dissuade King John from establishing a hunting lodge there. Many tales of their foolish doings were circulated, and in 1550 they were collected (possibly by Dr. Andrew Boorde [q.v.]) in a book entitled *Merie Tales of the Mad Men of Gotam*. New York is sometimes nicknamed Gotham, following Washington Irving calling it so in *Salmagundi* (1807-8).
See also COGGESHALL.
Bibliography: 1978. *Brewer's dictionary of phrase and fable.*

GOWERS, SIR WILLIAM RICHARD (1845-1915). An English neurologist. In 1880 he was the first to describe the bundle of nerve fibers in the spinal cord, now known as Gowers' tract. In 1881 he described the tetanic nature of convulsions in epilepsy (q.v.). He was obsessed by shorthand, which he used to take notes on his patients. He would stop complete strangers in the street to ask them if they were proficient in it. His opinion of the startled individuals then depended on whether they did or did not write shorthand. His numerous contributions to medicine include *Diagnosis of*

Diseases of the Brain, which was published in 1885, and a *Manual of the Diseases of the Nervous System*, published in 1886.
Bibliography: Critchley, M. 1949. *Sir William Gowers, 1845-1915: a biographical appreciation.*

GOYA Y LUCIENTES, FRANCISCO JOSÉ DE (1746-1828). A Spanish painter. Lustiness, pride, and swings of mood have been regarded as the main characteristics of his long life. As court painter he portrayed the royal family and the nobility but despite the social rank of his subjects he did not hesitate to represent them with cruel truthfulness. In middle age he became deaf; it has been suggested that the breakdown in health that he suffered at this time was due to syphilis (q.v.). His children, perhaps as many as twenty, all died young with the exception of one. Although personal tragedy and political unrest left him isolated, they also seem to have sharpened his awareness. He reacted with violent bitterness to the injustices and the atrocities of the Spanish War of Independence. Goya's work during this period is full of violence and psychopathology (q.v.); his hideous themes include madness, torture, rape, and satanism (q.v.). They represent not only an almost journalistic reportage of contemporary events but also sensual excitement. He fought superstition, yet he could not reject it. He was old when he fell disastrously in love with the dazzling and inconstant Duchess of Alba; the series of etchings *Los Caprichos*, which he had intended to call *The Sleep of Reason produces Monsters*, are a comment on a society that produced the woman he had to share with bullfighters and others. When the civil war broke out in Madrid, he went into exile in Bordeaux. When his daughter-in-law and his grandchildren reluctantly came to see him he was so overjoyed at the long-delayed visit that he had a seizure and died.
Bibliography: Harris, E. 1969. *Goya.*

GRACIÁN, BALTASAR (1601-1658). Spanish writer, philosopher, and Jesuit theologian. His work is didactic and shows a strong Jesuit ideology aimed at adapting means to ends. He deliberately used a writing style that had to be read slowly, because he believed the consequent mental effort helped to fix his meaning in the mind. In his book *The Manual Oracle and Art of Prudence* (1647), he gave advice on how to forget the painful episodes in life:

The things which are better forgotten are those we remember best; memory [q.v.] is not merely a rogue in failing us when it is most needed, but a fool in turning up at inconvenient times; in matters which will prove troublesome, it is long, and in those which ought to be a source of pleasure it is heedless. Sometimes the cure for misfortune consists in forgetting it, and the remedy is forgotten; it is advisable,

therefore, to train the memory to good habits, for it can turn life into a heaven or a hell.
Bibliography: Hafter, M. Z. 1967. *Gracián and perfection: Spanish moralist of the 17th century.*

GRADIVA. The title of a novel by the German writer Wilhelm Jensen (1837-1911). It was published in 1903. The hero falls in love with a Roman sculpture of a young woman whom he calls Gradiva. Following his fantasy, he goes searching for her in Pompeii and finds among the ruins his forgotten childhood sweetheart, Zoe. He believes that she is Gradiva, and at first she enters into his delusion (q.v.), but she soon brings him back to reality, and they are married. Sigmund Freud (q.v.) greatly admired this novel and wrote a psychoanalytic interpretation of the dreams (q.v.) and delusions of the protagonist.
Bibliography: Freud, S. 1907. *Delusions and Dreams in Jensen's Gradiva.* In 1959 *Complete Psychological Works*, ed. Strachey, J. vol. 9.

GRAF, HERBERT. *See* LITTLE HANS.

GRAHAM, JAMES (1745-1794). A professional charlatan, born in Edinburgh, Scotland. He pretended to be a doctor of medicine and practiced in London. He gathered a fashionable clientele who were attracted by his claims of cures through the use of electricity (q.v.). His establishment, The Temple of Health, boasted an "electrical bath," a "magnetic throne," and a "celestial bed with magnetic properties." The latter was in an elaborately decorated room, which was rented for enormous sums to those seeking a cure for infertility. Further stimuli were provided by erotic lectures, in which Graham was assisted by a so-called goddess of health, who danced thinly veiled. She was Emma Lyon, later Emma Hamilton (c.1765-1815). In 1792, Graham was granted an audience with George III (q.v.) and presented to him one of his works. He had previously produced a prayer and a pamphlet that purported to explain the causes of the king's insanity and how it could be cured. He also offered his services for the treatment of the mad queen of Portugal, Maria I (q.v.), but they were not accepted. In the last period of his life he became morbidly religious and followed a diet of vegetables, milk, and honey.
Bibliography: Eden, M., and Carrington, R. 1961. *The philosophy of the bed.*

GRAHAMSTOWN, SOUTH AFRICA. The site of the first mental hospital in South Africa. It was established in 1875 on the English model.
Bibliography: Hurst, L. A., and Lucas, M. B. 1975. South Africa. In *World history of psychiatry,* ed. J. G. Howells.

GRAINGER, PERCY ALDRIDGE (1882-1961). An Australian musician and composer. His mother so wanted her child to be artistic that when she was pregnant with him she gazed on a statue of a Greek god every night before going to sleep. His father was an alcoholic (*see* ALCOHOLISM); his mother horsewhipped her husband and, occasionally, her son also. This may have given him a taste for flagellation (q.v.) to which he was so addicted that even on tour he took whips with him. Mother and son were very dependent on each other; she would lie on the floor feigning illness to test his reactions. She finally committed suicide (q.v.), and her son set up a museum in Melbourne in memory of her. He was fanatically interested in athletics, walking miles between concerts and running to recitals in shorts.

Bibliography: Bird, J. 1976. *Percy Grainger.*

GRANADA. Mohammed V, an Arab caliph, built a mental hospital in Granada, Spain, in 1365. It was modeled on the lines of the Cairo lunatic asylums (q.v.) and was called "the house of the insane and the innocents." It was two stories high and included porticos and galleries where convalescent patients could walk. Water was piped from the mouths of two stone lions that are still in existence, although they have been moved in front of the Ladies' Tower in the Alhambra.

Bibliography: Lopez Ibor, J. J. 1975. Spain and Portugal. In *World history of psychiatry*, ed. J. G. Howells.

GRANDE HYSTÉRIE. Term used by Jean Charcot (q.v.). He gave the first full description of hysterical-crisis (*see* HYSTERIA) and distinguished it from a true epileptic (*see* EPILEPSY) crisis but oversimplified his observations because they were based on a small number of cases. Patients used for clinical demonstrations often produced symptoms for payment or to please the physicians.

Bibliography: Ellenberger, H. F. 1970. *The discovery of the unconscious.*

GRAND HYPNOTISME. The name given to the school created by Jean Charcot (q.v.) and his followers. Patients were treated by hypnosis (*see* HYPNOTISM) and obediently went through the three stages of lethargy (q.v.), catalepsy, and somnambulism (q.v.) because they were expected to produce the appropriate phenomena during clinical demonstrations.

Bibliography: Tinterow, M. M. 1970. *Foundations of hypnosis: from Mesmer to Freud.*

GRANVILLE, JOSEPH MORTIMER (1833-1900). English physician. He introduced nerve vibration as a method of treatment for functional and organic nervous disorders and invented a hammer for giving vibratory massage. With the help of Andrew Wynter (q.v.), he wrote *The Borderlands*

of Insanity, and Other Papers. As a member of the Lancet Commission he helped to investigate asylums in 1877.
Bibliography: Schmidt, J. E. 1959. *Medical discoveries: who and when.*

GRAPHOLOGY. The study of handwriting in relation to personality traits. It has existed for at least nine centuries. It was practiced in China (q.v.) as early as the eleventh century, and it became fashionable in Europe during the seventeenth century. The term "graphology" was coined by the French physician Pierre Michon (q.v.). A German graphological society was founded in 1897 by Ludwig Klages (q.v.).
Bibliography: Rand, H. A. 1962. *Graphology.*

GRASHEY, HUBERT VON (1839-1914). A German psychiatrist, a professor of the department of psychiatry at Munich University, and a pioneer in psychological testing. He was the son-in-law of Bernhard von Gudden (q.v.). He investigated aphasic and agnostic conditions following post-traumatic brain conditions with a testing procedure that he had devised. His test of perceptual integration consisted of a slotted sheet of paper through which letters, words, or parts of a picture were shown to the patient. The patient was then asked to integrate the single elements into meaningful vowels.
Bibliography: Bondy, M. 1974. Psychiatric antecedents of psychological testing (before Binet). *J. Hist. Behav. Sci.* 10:187-94.

GRASSET, JOSEPH (1849-1918). A French physician. Although he was an authority on neural diseases, his investigations covered a wide field that included hypnotism (q.v.), spiritualism (q.v.), and occultism. He wrote *Des localisation dans les maladies cérébrales* in 1878 and *Anatomie clinique des centres nerveux* in 1900, as well as works on physiopathology and biology.

GRATIOLET, PIERRE (1815-1865). A French neuroanatomist. His life was spent mostly in poverty and neglect, even though he made significant contributions to neurology (q.v.), especially in the field of comparative anatomy of the nervous system. He described the cerebral folds in man and primates and pointed out their differences and their similarities. He also tried to justify the belief that some races are superior to others by describing the developmental features of the skull and the brain, but his assertion contained obvious weaknesses.
Bibliography: Haymaker, W., and Schiller, F. 1970. *The founders of neurology.* 2d ed.

GRAY, JOHN PERDUE (1825-1886). An American psychiatrist. He was superintendent of the New York State Lunatic Asylum in Utica, and he introduced new ideas in asylum construction, such as better ventilation and

steam heat. He abolished as far as possible physical restraint (q.v.) of violent patients but was irremittently against moral medicine (q.v.). He was a strong-supporter of the organic approach in mental disorders and believed that psychosis (q.v.) was due to specific brain lesions. From 1854 to 1886 he was editor of the *American Journal of Insanity* (q.v.), which he used to propagate his ideas.
Bibliography: Dain, N. 1964. *Concepts of insanity in the United States, 1789-1865.*

GRAY, THOMAS (1716-1771). An English poet, born in London. He was the only survivor of twelve children. It was said that the others had died of suffocation due to too much blood and that his mother had saved his life by opening one of his veins when he had a fit. His father, a scrivener, had a violent temper and was so cruel that his wife was forced to leave him. Thomas Gray had a colourless life, the greatest event of it being a tour of Europe with his friend Horace Walpole. He was a solitary man who lived and worked in Cambridge, where, it is said, he kept a rope ladder by his window as a precaution against fire of which he had a morbid fear. A lifelong sufferer of poor health and depression, his melancholy (*see* MELANCHOLIA) is reflected in his verses, which he wrote with exhausting effort. The best remembered of his poems is *Elegy in a Country Churchyard* (1751), which ends with the author's supposed death, burial, and epitaph.
Bibliography: Golden, M. 1964. *Thomas Gray.*

GREATFORD. A village near Stamford, Lincolnshire, England. The Reverend Francis Willis (q.v.) instituted a system of boarding-out of mental patients (q.v.) there. Each patient was housed in a cottage with a keeper and was encouraged to take long walks. If a patient escaped, his keeper lost his wages and was responsible for the expenses of his recapture. Violent patients were handled with violence because fear of beating was considered beneficial to their condition.
Bibliography: Parry-Jones, W. Ll. 1972. *The trade in lunacy.*

GREATRAKES, VALENTINE (1629-1683). An Irish empiric physician. He achieved great fame for the cures he brought about by his touch and by stroking. His power of suggestion was enhanced by the fact that he firmly believed God had endowed him with the power to cure illness. In 1666 he was summoned to the presence of Charles II to give a demonstration of his methods, but he failed to produce a cure. He answered his critics in a short volume entitled *Brief Account* (1666).
Bibliography: Laver, A. B. 1978. Miracles no wonder! The mesmeric phenomena and organic cures of Valentine Greatrakes. *J. Hist. Med. & All. Sci.* 33:35-46.

GRECO, EL (1541-1614). "The Greek," the Spanish name for the painter Domenicos Theotocopoulos. It was given to him because of his Cretan

origin. El Greco, after leaving his native Crete, went to Venice and from there settled in Toledo, Spain, a walled and insular city. He ended his life there in mystical solitude. His style of painting accentuated certain features and gave maximum emphasis to the emotional content of his subject. It is believed that he painted the inmates of Saint James Asylum in Toledo, where many of his canvases remained until that institution was dissolved in 1840. The mentally ill appear in a considerable number of his works.
Bibliography: Wethey, H. 1973. *El Greco and His School.*

GREDING, JOHANN ERNST (1718-1775). A German physician, author of *Medical Aphorism on Melancholy* (1781), in which he described the appearance of the brain in over 200 cases of insanity. Sir Alexander Crichton (q.v.) added an English translation of this work to his own book on mental disease.
Bibliography: Hunter, R., and Macalpine, I. 1963. *Three hundred years of psychiatry.*

GREENFIELD, GODWIN (1884-1958). A British neuropathologist. He had little enthusiasm for experimental work and preferred to relate his pathological findings to clinical work. He classified spinocerebellar degenerations and was particularly interested in encephalitis and a wide range of other topics on the pathology of the nervous system. His laboratory at the National Hospital in Queen Square, London, became a center of interest for many international workers. With E. A. Carmichael, he wrote *Pathology of the Nervous System* in 1921.
Bibliography: Haymaker, W., and Schiller, F. 1970. *The founders of neurology.* 2d. ed.

GREGORY I *or* **GREGORY THE GREAT, SAINT** (c.540-604). A pope born in Rome. He enforced papal supremacy and established the pope's temporal position. He gave his wealth away and retired to a monastery. He wanted to convert England to Christianity and on being prevented from leaving Rome, entrusted Augustine with the mission. Among other works, Gregory wrote a treatise on *Pastoral Care* in which he covered many aspects of support and counseling so thoroughly that it amounted to psychotherapy (q.v.).
Bibliography: Richards, J. 1980. *Consul of God: the life and times of Gregory the Great.*

GREGORY IX (1148-1241). The Pope excommunicated Frederick II (q.v.) for refusing to go on a crusade, ordered the refutation of Aristotle (q.v.), and instituted the Holy Office of the Inquisition (q.v.), thus interfering with

free thought. He also encouraged the formation of mendicant religious orders that contributed to the care of the sick in body and mind.
Bibliography: Ullmann, W. 1971. *A short history of the papacy in the Middle Ages.*

GREGORY, JOHN (1724-1773). A Scottish physician, professor of medicine at Aberdeen University, and later a professor of the practice of physics at the University of Edinburgh. He was a firm believer in the amalgamation of the medicine of the mind with that of the body and asserted that the physician should be versed in both. He thought that comparative psychological studies would facilitate the understanding of human behavior better than the theoretical speculations of the German school of philsophy of his time. He wrote on this subject in a book entitled *A Comparative View of the State and Faculties of Man with Those of the Animal World* in 1765. In 1770 he published another volume entitled *Observations on the Duties and Offices of a Physician and the Method of Prosecuting Inquiries in Philosophy.* In this work, he stressed the importance of a good rapport between doctor and patient and the need for sympathy in cases of nervous complaints, which he considered the most lucrative diseases in the practice of medicine.
Bibliography: 1900. *The dictionary of national biography.*

GREGORY OF NYSSA, SAINT (331?-?394). A Greek ecclesiastical writer, bishop of Nyssa in Cappadocia. He refuted the belief that the soul resided in the heart, arguing that the heart was affected by emotion only as a secondary phenomenon that was dependent on the contraction or dilation of the vessels. He believed that in grief the vessels contracted and impeded evaporation so that moisture was then transformed into tears; in joy the vessels dilated, more air was inhaled and when expelled it produced laughter. He gave similar explanations for palpitations of the heart, pallor, and other phenomena.
Bibliography: Goggin, T. A. 1947. *The life and times of St. Gregory of Nyssa.*

GREGORY OF TOURS, SAINT (GEORGIUS FLORENTIUS) (538?-594). Frankish ecclesiastic and historian. He was cured of illness by a pilgrimage to the grave of Saint Martin of Tours and, because of his cure, dedicated himself to the church. He became bishop of Tours in 573. He thought that the best treatment for physical and mental disorders was the application of relics of saints.
Bibliography: Wallace-Hadrill, J. M. 1962. *The long-haired kings.*

GRENVILLE, ANNE (?-1691). Youngest daughter of John Cosin (1594-1672), bishop of Durham, England, and wife of the Reverend Denis Grenville. When the bishop failed to pay Grenville the agreed dowry, Grenville publicized the fact that he had been burdened with a deranged wife. She was overexcitable, garrulous, violent, could not sleep, and was given to depression with morbid delusions (q.v.). A family quarrel grew around her: her father and sister insisted that she was perfectly sane. Two doctors stated that she had "suffered of old, and at varying intervals from melancholy [*see* MELANCHOLIA], hypochondria [q.v.] and hysteria [q.v.]" mostly caused by "various humours (of bile [q.v.], black bile, salt, nitre and the incinerated portion)" which "fermented and degenerated into a true melancholic juice." She was subjected to bleeding (q.v.), purges (q.v.), and emetics, but she managed to escape before trepanation (q.v.), salivation by mercury (q.v.), and excision of the temporal artery were tried on her. More doctors stated that she was insane, while her father remained unconvinced and her husband had a nervous breakdown. In 1679 she was placed in the custody of Dr. William Cole (q.v.) in his house in Worcester.

Bibliography: Dewhurst, K. A. 1962. A 17th century symposium on manic-depressive psychosis. *Brit. J. med. Psychol.*, 35:113-25.

GRIESINGER, WILHELM (1817-1868). A German psychiatrist. He is regarded as the father of German psychiatry because of his research into the aetiology and therapy of mental disorders. He was perhaps the first German physician to dedicate himself fully to psychiatry. He was a professor at the University of Berlin, where he reorganized the psychiatric department. He believed that symptoms could not be properly understood unless it was known on which organ they depended; he was a convinced supporter of the organic aetiology of psychiatric conditions but thought that suicide (q.v.) was caused by psychological disorders. His book *Pathology and Therapy of Mental Diseases* was published in 1845, when he was twenty-eight years old. He distinguished three forms of mental disorders: states of depression, states of exaltation, and states of mental weakness. He regarded all these as organic conditions, but he did not exclude moral medicine (q.v.) in their management. In 1867 Griesinger founded the *Archiv für Psychiatrie* and the Berlin Psychiatric Association.

Bibliography: Griesinger, W. 1867. Reprint. 1965. *Mental Pathology and Therapeutics*, trans. C. L. Robertson and J. Rutherford.

GRILLPARZER, FRANZ (1791-1872). Austrian dramatist and poet. His life was a series of unhappy events. His father's death forced him to abandon his studies, his mother committed suicide (q.v.), and his brother soon followed her example. He became a high official in the civil service but hated his job. He was so insecure that he could never make decisions even in his personal life, which was embittered by unsatisfactory and sordid love affairs. Although engaged to Käthe Fröhlich, he never married her and ended up as her lodger. Grillparzer was, however, a successful playwright; his works reflect sensitivity, bitterness, and renunciation. Among the English trans-

lations of his writings are *A Dream is Life, The Poor Minstrel,* and *The Jewess of Toledo.*
Bibliography: Yates, D. 1946. *Franz Grillparzer.*

GRIMALDI, JOSEPH (1779-1837). An English clown of great repute. His father combined dentistry with a theatrical career and Joseph first appeared on the stage at the age of two. Although he could make everybody laugh, offstage he was a quiet, nervous, and melancholy man. When he consulted a doctor about his depression, he was advised to go and see Grimaldi and exclaimed "I am Grimaldi!" Charles Dickens (q.v.) edited *The Memoirs of Grimaldi* in 1838.
Bibliography: Findlater, R. 1979. *Joe Grimaldi: his life and theatre.*

GRIMES, JAMES STANLEY (1807-1903). An American philosopher, called "the erratic philosopher." For a time he taught medical jurisprudence, but his main interest was in science and the discussion of speculative problems. He was a student of phrenology (q.v.), of an early theory of evolution, and of the methods of Franz Mesmer (q.v.). He approached mesmerism (q.v.) with a practical mind and ascribed phenomena to the power of suggestion. However, he could not resist introducing into its explanation a so-called occult fluid. According to him, the medulla oblongata was the seat of consciousness. He also wrote on spiritualism (q.v.). His main work was *The Mysteries of Human Nature Explained by a New System of Nervous Physiology,* which was published in 1857.
Bibliography: Tinterow, M. M. 1970. *Foundation of Hypnosis: from Mesmer to Freud.*

GRINSHTEIN, ALEKSANDR MIKAILOVICH (1881-1931). A Russian neuropathologist. His work included research on the influence of the cerebral cortex on autonomic innervation. He demonstrated that abnormally intense hunger is a symptom of hypothalamic lesions and that the same symptom appears in epileptic aura. His best known work is entitled *Routes and Centres of the Nervous System.*

GRISELDA. A long-suffering and virtuous heroine, subject of many medieval romances. She was blessed with endless patience, submissively bearing all kinds of trials and humiliations. James Putnam (q.v.) called Griselda complex the father's unconscious reluctance disguised as solicitude to give up his daughter to another man.
Bibliography: Jones, E. 1949. *Hamlet and Oedipus.*

GRODDECK, GEORG (1866-1934). A German physician. He attributed his understanding of man's bisexual nature to his close relationship with his sister Lina. His parents, his three brothers, and his sister died early, leaving

him as the only survivor of his family. He became the owner of a small sanatorium, and his fame spread throughout Europe. Groddeck was a pioneer of psychosomatic medicine (q.v.) and thought of bodily sickness as a reaction to trauma expressing inner needs. At first he attacked psychoanalysis (q.v.), but in fact his concepts were close to its principles. The term "the id" (q.v.) was originated by him and gratefully borrowed from him by Sigmund Freud (q.v.) for his work *The Ego and the Id* (1923). Freud called him "an analyst of the first order," and the two men enjoyed many years of mutual respect and friendship, although there were some disagreements. Groddeck was a man of passionate temperament, courage, and integrity. His written work, which he regarded as wild and artistic, was not particularly scientific, but it was always honest and dignified.
Bibliography: Groddeck, G. 1928. *The book of the Id.*

GROOS, FRIEDRICH (1768-1852). German physician and psychiatrist-philosopher of the romantic school. He attempted to combine philosophical principles with physiological reactions and considered psychology a biological science. According to him, mental disorders resulted from inner obstacles to the physiological forces that determined man's behavior. In 1814 he was appointed director of the asylum (q.v.) for the insane and infirm at Pforzheim. He lectured in psychiatry and wrote several books, of which the most important is *Outline of a Philosophical Foundation for the Doctrine of Mental Disease*, published in 1828.
Bibliography: Zilboorg, G. 1941. *A history of medical psychology.*

GROOS, KARL THEODOR (1861-1946). German philosopher and psychologist. He tried to combine psychology and biology with metaphysics. He was particularly interested in the significance of play, which he believed to be a form of preparation for adult activities. He expounded this theory in *Play of Animals* (1898) and *Play of Man* (1901).
Bibliography: Flugel, J. C. 1945. *A hundred years of psychology.*

GROSS, HANS (1847-1915). Austrian jurist and criminologist. He believed that frustrated sexual drives could cause crime and thought that those involved in the administration of justice should be aware of symptoms masking frustrated sexuality (q.v.). He is regarded as the founder of judicial psychology.
Bibliography: Gross, H. 1898. *Criminalpsychologie.*

GROUNDSEL. The popular name for *Senecio viscosus*. Nicholas Culpeper (q.v.) believed it to be beneficial in the treatment of hysterical (*see* HYSTERIA) disorders.
Bibliography: Le Strange, R. 1977. *A history of herbal plants.*

GROUP PSYCHOTHERAPY. In 1855 William Browne (q.v.) started discussion groups with patients at the Crichton Royal Hospital (q.v.). This approach had not been tried before, and the venture can be regarded as the first attempt at group psychotherapy.

GRUHLE, HANS WALTHER (1880-1958). A German psychiatrist. He belonged to a school of psychiatry which regarded man in his totality and took into consideration civilization, culture, and psychobiological factors in the past, as well as in the present. His field of research included psychopathology, criminology, schizophrenia (q.v.), suicide (q.v.), and the history of psychology. His collected works were published in 1953 under the title *Verstehen und Einfühlen*.
Bibliography: Zilboorg, G. 1941. *A history of medical psychology.*

GUAINERIO, ANTONIO (fl.1447). An Italian medical writer. His classification of mental disorders recognized frenesis, vera and nonvera; lethargia, vera and nonvera; incubus (q.v.); epilepsy (q.v.); melancholia (q.v.); mania (q.v.); and stupor. As a follower of Rhazes (q.v.), he believed that frequent flogging (q.v.) could be beneficial for melancholy patients. He also advocated cautery (*see* CAUTERIZATION) applied to the skull. His tests for epilepsy were the smell of fresh parsley (q.v.) or the smoke of the scorched horn of a she-goat applied to the nostril. If the patient failed to fall to the ground, he was considered cured.
Bibliography: Whitwell, J. R. 1936. *Historical notes on psychiatry.*

GUDDEN, BERNARD ALOYS VON (1824-1886). A German psychiatrist. He was among the first to teach psychiatry at the newly opened University of Zürich. Emil Kraepelin (q.v.) became his assistant in Munich. Gudden was well known for his work on the histology of the brain and mapped out the motor and sensory areas of the cerebral cortex. He was psychiatrist to Ludwig II of Bavaria (q.v.) and drowned with him in a lake near Berg.
Bibliography: Blunt, W. 1970. *The dream king.*

GUGGENBÜHL, (JOHANN) JAKOB (1816-1863). A Swiss physician. He became interested in the mentally retarded when he "saw an old cretin who was stammering a half-forgotten prayer before an image of the Virgin, at Seedor in the canton of Uri. This sight excited my feelings in favour of those unhappy creatures and fixed my vocation." In 1842, he founded the Abendberg Institution for cretins (*see* CRETINISM) in the Interlaken district. His pioneering work attracted many observers and stimulated research in the field of mental retardation. He believed that mentally retarded children could be given some education and could lead near-normal lives. His treatment consisted in strengthening the body before beginning a program of instruction and education. He wrote and lectured on cretinism and feeblemindedness. His work and enthusiasm made various governments aware of their responsibilities for the mentally retarded.

Bibliography: Kanner, L. 1964. *A history of the care and study of the mentally retarded.*

GUILD OF FRIENDS OF THE INFIRM IN MIND. A society founded in England in 1871 by the Reverend Henry Hawkins (q.v.). It offered voluntary help in asylums (q.v.). It also pioneered the after-care movement (q.v.) for discharged mental patients.

Bibliography: Deutsch, A. 1949. *The mentally ill in America.*

GUILLAIN, GEORGES (1876-1951). A French neurologist. He was an authority on the spinal column and the first to describe the polyradicular syndrome.

Bibliography: Haymaker, W., and Schiller, F. 1970. *The founders of neurology.* 2d. ed.

GUILLOTIN, JOSEPH IGNACE (1738-1814). A French physician, remembered for his support of judicial assassination, which he believed would be humanized by his invention of an instrument of decapitation, called guillotine after him. He was a member of a committee, appointed by the Paris faculty of medicine, which with the Academie des Sciences (q.v.), investigated magnetism (q.v.) as practiced by Charles Deslon (q.v.).

Bibliography: Zilboorg, G. 1941. *A history of medical psychology.*

GUISLAIN, JOSEPH (1797-1860). A Belgian psychiatrist. He believed that all mental disorders were preceded by depression, which was often dependent on such factors as family problems, the political situation, and unemployment. In his opinion, depressed patients should be confined to bed. He was greatly influenced by phrenology (q.v.). Guislain not only was instrumental in bringing about changes in the Belgian legislation relating to mental patients but also introduced more humanitarian methods of care in mental hospitals.

Bibliography: Boismont, A. B. de. 1867. *Esquisses de medecin mentale: Joseph Guislain, sa vie et ses ecrits.*

GUITEAU, CHARLES JULIUS (1840?-1882). The American lawyer who shot James Garfield, president of the United States, in 1881. Guiteau had received little love in his childhood, he lost his mother when he was seven, acquired a stepmother and was so ill-treated that he ran away from home. In his youth he joined a religious sect, the Oneida Community, which preached free love. He left the community after five years and attacked it in letters in the newspapers. His professional activities were dishonest, while his attendance to prayer meetings was meticulous. His lectures on religion

brought about the comment that he was "not so much deranged as very badly arranged." His plea of insanity was supported by the fact that several of his relations had been insane. On the evidence of a physician, his own father was said to have been deluded and to have thought himself endowed with the power to exorcise, (see EXORCISM) the devils possessing (see POSSESSION) the insane. His sister was certified insane and became a patient in the state asylum of Illinois; she wrote a confused book entitled *The Stalwarts: or, Who were to Blame?*, in which she related the events surrounding the assassination. Guiteau diagnosed himself as suffering from "Abrahamic insanity," arguing that like Abraham he had been commanded by God to kill but asserting that he was sane both before and after the deed. The jury found him guilty, and he was condemned to death.
Bibliography: Ireland, W. W. 1889. *Through the ivory gate.*

GUJER, JAKOB (1716-1785). A Swiss farmer also known as Kleinjogg, or Little John. He was an early source of Adolf Meyer's (q.v.) concepts. Guyer first gained recognition in his country for his enlightened farming methods and for introducing the cultivation of potatoes in the canton of Zürich. His commonsense approach and his success in breaking away from tradition extended to the working community that he created and inspired with his example. His advice was much sought after, and his visitors included Johann Pestalozzi (q.v.) and Johann Wolfgang Von Goethe (q.v.). Meyer became connected with Kleinjogg through his grandfather, who acquired some of the farm's land. Later the two families became related through marriage. Meyer's approach to psychiatry reflected the common sense and the unprejudiced evaluation that was the tradition of Kleinjogg. It was not until after his death, however, that he became world famous through a book that Hans Kaspar Hirzel, a Zürich doctor, wrote about him in 1792.
Bibliography: Bleuler, M. 1962. Early sources of Adolf Meyer's concepts. *Am. J. Psychiat.* 119: 193.

GULL, SIR WILLIAM WITHELY (1816-1890). An English physician. He was an admirer of John Conolly (q.v.) whose lectures he attended. Gull noted and described several disorders, among which is anorexia nervosa (q.v.), a term introduced by him in 1873. He was a gifted lecturer and a man of wit whose imposing appearance fascinated patients and pupils. His temper made him less acceptable to his colleagues. Gull's management of neurotic patients (see NEUROSIS) made him successful with psychosomatic disorders, and Queen Victoria and the Prince of Wales were among his patients. When he died he left £344,000, a record for a physician of that time.
Bibliography: Leigh, D. 1961. *The historical development of British psychiatry.*

GUNASEELAM SHRINE. A Hindu shrine on the northern banks of the Cauvery river. It is often visited by Hindus suffering from psychiatric disorders. The presiding divinity is also believed to help those with marriage difficulties. The patients are first purified by the waters of the Cauvery and then taken to the temple where they stay for several days. Their diet (q.v.) is controlled and no intoxicants are allowed. Women are forbidden to wear flowers or perfume. If no cure is achieved, the priests explain that the disease is retribution from God and hence incurable.

Bibliography: Somasundaram, O. 1973. Religious treatment of mental illness in Tamil Nadu. *Indian J. Psychiat.* 15: 38-48.

GUNTER, ANNE (fl. 1600). A young Englishwoman who was said to be possessed (*see* POSSESSION) by the devil. In 1604, the bishop of London asked the College of Physicians of London to investigate her. They reported that she was not possessed by the devil but that she was a cheat, who simulated symptoms, including insensibility to pinpricks. James I of England and VI of Scotland (q.v.) investigated Anne and wrote a report (the only psychiatric report ever written by a king of England) in which he too stated that "she was never possessed by any devil, nor bewitched" and that she had confessed her fraud to him. The king noted that the periodic "swelling of her belly" was occasioned by "the disease called the mother" (i.e., hysteria [q.v.]) and that the girl was passionately in love with a servant whom she wished to marry. Dr. Edward Jorden (q.v.) came to the same conclusions and included her case history in his book *A Discourse of Natural Bathes and Mineral Waters*. She was in the limelight again in 1616, when William Harvey (q.v.) mentioned her insensibility to pinpricks in his famous lecture on the circulation of the blood.

Bibliography: Hunter, R., and Macalpine, I. 1963. *Three hundred years of psychiatry.*

GURNEY, IVOR BERTIE (1890-1937). An English composer and poet, highly esteemed as a songwriter. During World War I he served in the British army and wrote some remarkable war poems. His output was curtailed by the onset of schizophrenia (q.v.), and the last fifteen years of his life were spent in mental hospitals.

Bibliography: Hurd, M. 1978. *The ordeal of Ivor Gurney.*

GUSTAVUS I (GUSTAVUS VASA) (1496-1560). A king of Sweden. He was particularly concerned with the care of the mentally ill. In 1551, he established the Holy Ghost House (q.v.) at Danviken, Stockholm.

Bibliography: Retterstøl, N. 1975. Scandinavia. In *World History of Psychiatry*, ed. J. G. Howells.

GUTHLAC, SAINT (c.673-714). A monk and hermit, born in the Anglo-Saxon kingdom of Mercia. His life was very austere; he even refused to

drink wine. He was reputed to be able to cure madmen by exorcising (*see* EXORCISM) the devil that possessed (*see* POSSESSION) them.
Bibliography: Congrave. E., ed. 1956. *Felix's life of St. Guthlac.*

GUTTMANN-MACLAY COLLECTION. A collection of art objects made by mental patients. It is designed to show the change in artistic production occurring with mental illness. It was begun in the 1930s by Dr. Eric Guttmann and Dr. Walter Maclay. In addition to paintings and drawings it contains pieces of embroidery, music, and other objects. The work of Louis Wain (q.v.) is well represented by a number of his pictures. Presently it is housed at the Maudsley Hospital (q.v.) in London, England.

GUY, THOMAS (1645?-1724). English bookseller, printer, and member of Parliament for Tamworth. He built Tamworth's town hall. He founded an almshouse and built and furnished three wards of St. Thomas' Hospital in London. He is best remembered as the founder of Guy's Hospital. He accumulated his large fortune by holding the right to print Bibles for Oxford University and by financial speculations with South Seas shares (*see* SOUTH SEA BUBBLE). Despite his wealth, he lived like a miser. A story circulated about his parsimony; a collector for funds for Bethlem Royal Hospital (q.v.) approached his house but hesitated when he heard Guy scolding a servant for wasting a match. To his surprise, however, Guy contributed a bag of money to the collection, saying that he kept his house in his own way so that he might spend his money in his own way. In his will he made a provision for insane and incurable patients to be kept in his hospital.
Bibliography: Cameron, H. C. 1954. *Mr. Guy's hospital.*

GYMNASIUM OF CYNOSARGES. A Greek institute near Athens where the Cynic school was founded by Antisthenes in 366 B.C. It laid the foundations for the psychological study of man as it stressed the importance of feelings, behavior, and relationships between people.
Bibliography: Zilboorg, G. 1941. *A history of medical psychology.*

GYMNOSOPHISTS. A term meaning "naked sages" that was used by the Greeks to indicate those Hindu philosophers, who regarded clothes and food as hindrances to purity of thought. Their asceticism caused them to live like hermits and at times to burn themselves to death in order to achieve a state of perfect purity.
Bibliography: Esquirol, J. E. D. 1845. Reprint. 1965. *Mental maladies: A treatise on Insanity.*

GYRATOR. An apparatus devised by Benjamin Rush (q.v.). The patient was placed on a horizontal board that revolved round a pivot at the foot end. Rapid gyration caused centrifugal force to send the blood to the head.

Thus, according to Rush, shocking the blood vessels into their normal function and curing the insanity caused by their malfunction.

Bibliography: Wittels, F. 1946. The contribution of Benjamin Rush to psychiatry. *Bull. Hist. Med.* 20:157.

H

HAAKON THE GOOD (914-961). A ruler of Norway. He serves as an early example of reactive depression mistaken for insanity. He was banished to Denmark; there, he brooded until he became deeply depressed and was believed to be insane. He recovered after a few months when his hopes rose again.
Bibliography: Retterstøl, N. 1975. Scandinavia. In *World history of psychiatry*, ed. J. G. Howells.

HABERLIN, PAUL (1878-1960). A well-known Swiss philosopher. He was interested in children with behavior problems and dedicated himself to their education, allowing two to three of these children to live in his own home. Although he met Carl Jung (q.v.) and Sigmund Freud (q.v.), he remained critical of psychoanalysis (q.v.) and accepted only some elements of it. He believed that anxiety stemmed from guilt and depression from arrogance toward life. He wrote on many subjects, including the psychology (q.v.) of marriage, characterology, and education.
Bibliography: Ellenberger, H.F. 1970. *The discovery of the unconscious*.

HACKET, WILLIAM (?-1591). An English fanatic. Believing himself to be a prophet of God and king of Europe, he persuaded two other individuals to propagate these ideas in a kind of *folie à trois*. When he was arrested and tried for treason, his behavior induced the judges to think that he was assuming madness to escape justice. Hacket was hanged, although popular opinion held that he was insane. One of his accomplices starved himself to death in Bridewell (q.v.) prison, and the other lived to repent his actions. An account of the trial was written by Richard Cosin (q.v.).
Bibliography: Hunter, R. and Macalpine, I. 1963. *Three hundred years of psychiatry*.

HADFIELD, JAMES (c. 1771-1849). An English war veteran. While serving in Flanders, he received severe head injuries, which were believed to have

caused the insanity that led to his discharge from the army. In 1800 he shot at George III (q.v.) hoping to be put to death for it. He believed that in this way he could achieve martyrdom and save the world. His trial is of great importance to British criminal law because it led to the admission of partial insanity as a plea for criminal irresponsibility. Hadfield was defended by Lord Thomas Erskine (q.v.), who so eloquently unfolded the story of his client's illness that the trial was stopped and the jury was directed to find the prisoner not guilty. Hadfield was committed to Bethlem Royal Hospital (q.v.) for the remainder of his life.
Bibliography: Macalpine, I. and Hunter, R. 1969: *George III and the mad-business.*

HAECKEL, ERNST HEINRICH (1834-1919). A German naturalist and philosopher. He was the first German to advocate a theory of organic evolution. According to him, each individual animal repeated in his development the stages through which the species has passed and thus recapitulated the developmental history of the species (Haeckel's biogenetic law). He believed that "the child is on a lower developmental level of mankind than the adult" and that all the criminal drives of humanity are latent in him.
Bibliography: Haeckel, E. H. 1879. *Evolution of man.*

HAËN, ANTON DE (1704-1776). A Dutch physician and follower of Hermann Boerhaave (q.v.). He was said to be quarrelsome, pragmatic (q.v.), and a rabid defender of the belief in witchcraft (q.v.). He was the author of a voluminous treatise on hospital treatment that was published in fifteen volumes between 1758 and 1769. Haën considered clinical experience far superior to experimentation and was an early user of the thermometer and electrotherapy.
Bibliography: Garrison, F. H. 1929. *An introduction to the history of medicine.*

HAGEN, FRIEDRICH WILHELM (1814-1889). A German psychiatrist. In 1844 he visited mental hospitals in England, France, and Germany. He later became the director of two asylums (q.v.) in Germany in which he introduced humane methods of treatment. Hagen believed in the psychic importance of the brain and in the influence of mood shifts on biological functions. According to him, psychotic delirium was a form of dreaming in a waking state.
Bibliography: Zilboorg, G. 1941. *A history of medical psychology.*

HAGGARD, SIR HENRY RIDER (1856-1925). An English writer. In one of his novels, *She*, published in 1887, he created the character of a fascinating woman, Ayesha (q.v.), who destroys men unless they overcome her spells. Ayesha was regarded by Carl Jung (q.v.) as an anima (q.v.) figure.

Haggard was said to have written the book in a kind of trance, after sudden inspiration.
Bibliography: Cohen, M. 1960. *Rider Haggard: his life and works.*

HAHNEMANN, SAMUEL (1755-1843). A German physician and founder of homeopathy. After reading that Peruvian bark (quinine, or cinchona) provoked in healthy people the symptoms that were treated by it in the sick, he experimented with other drugs and concluded that they could be used in minute quantities to treat the conditions similar to the ones they caused in healthy individuals. Apothecaries refused to dispense the small doses that he prescribed and he was prosecuted when he dispensed them himself free of charge. He expounded his theories in a volume entitled *Organon of the Rational Art of Healing,* published in 1810.
Bibliography: Alexander, F. G. and Selesnick, S. T. 1966. *A history of psychiatry.*

HAINDORF, ALEXANDER (1782-1862). A German physician and author in 1811 of the first German textbook of psychiatry *Versuch einer Pathologie und Therapie der Gemüths und Geisteskrankheiten.* He discussed the physiological origins of drives, related them to different areas of the brain, and outlined their influence on reasoning. He tried to devise a characterology and to explain how mental diseases have psychological, as well as physiological, causes. Haindorf regarded man as a psychophysical unity. He was one of the first to believe that emotional conflicts disturb the balance of the organism and cause mental disorders.
Bibliography: Zilboorg, G. 1941. *A history of medical psychology.*

HAIR-RAISING. A psychosomatic reaction. As an expression, it denotes something terrifying. An early example is found in the Bible (q.v.), "Fear came upon me and trembling . . . and the hair of my flesh stood up" (Job 4: 15). William Shakespeare (q.v.) gave many examples of this phenomenon (Henry VI, Part 2, III, ii; Hamlet, I, v and III, iv; Tempest, I, ii; Macbeth, I, iii).
Bibliography: *Brewer's dictionary of phrase and fable* 1978.

HAIZMANN, CHRISTOPH (? - 1700). A painter born in Bavaria. During a nervous breakdown, he produced nine illustrations depicting his visions of the devil. These, with the painter's account of his life and illness, and some writings by contemporary observers, were discovered in the National Library of Austria at the beginning of the twentieth century by Payer-Thurn the library's director. He sent them to Sigmund Freud (q.v.), who, after studying the manuscript, analyzed it in a paper entitled "A Neurosis of

Demoniacal Possession in the Seventeenth Century" (1923). Using it as his basis, Freud extended his theory of paranoia (q.v.).
Bibliography: Macalpine, I., and Hunter, R. A. 1956. *Schizophrenia 1677: a psychiatric study of an illustrated autobiographical record of demoniacal possession.*

HALE, SIR MATTHEW (1609-1676). An English judge and author. He was elected lord chief justice of the King's Bench is 1671. In his *History of the Pleas of the Crown* in 1678 he discussed criminal responsibility. According to him, a person was legally irresponsible only if totally deprived of memory (q.v.) and understanding. Lord Thomas Erskine (q.v.) refuted his doctrines in 1800. In Hale's opinion there were three types of mental disorder: idiocy (*see* IDIOT), madness, and lunacy (*see* LUNATIC). He defined madness as permanent, while lunacy consisted of alternate periods of mental incapacity and lucidity. He believed that the moon (q.v.) influenced all diseases of the brain and that insane individuals "commonly in the full and change of the moon, especially about the equinoxes and summer solstice, are usually at the height of their distemper." He was in charge at the Bury St. Edmunds witch trial of 1662. He avoided summing up the case but reminded the jury that two points had to be considered: whether or not the children were truly bewitched and whether or not the two accused were witches. He did not question the existence of witches, because both the Scriptures and the laws of the country recognized their existence.
Bibliography: Ray, I. 1838. Reprint 1962. *A treatise of jurisprudence of insanity*, ed. W. Overholser.

HALE, RICHARD (1670-1728). An English physician. He was the second physician to Bethlem Royal Hospital (q.v.) after the death of Edward Tyson (q.v.). He advocated visiting by friends and relations and considered "jollity and merriment and even a band of music" beneficial for depressed patients. His staff discovered that suicide attempts were more frequent on Sunday, when visitors were excluded and the patients had a duller day. Hale, however, believed that happy events also could derange the mind and said that he had many patients who had become deranged after acquiring great fortunes in the South Sea Bubble (q.v.) enterprise. He claimed that they exceeded in number those who had become deranged from the loss of money in the same venture.
Bibliography: O'Donoghue, E. G. 1914. *The story of Bethlehem Hospital.*

HALFORD, SIR HENRY (1776-1844). A British physician and president of the College of Physicians. He was one of the doctors in charge of George III (q.v.) during his periods of insanity; he reported to Parliament on the state of the king's health. Halford believed that music could help mitigate mental disorders and advocated visiting by friends and relations in order to remove the superstition and shame connected with mental disorders. The monarchs of England from George III to Queen Victoria (1819–1901) were among his patients.

Bibliography: Halford, H. 1933. *On the treatment of insanity, particularly the moral treatment.*

HALL, BASIL (1788-1844). A Scottish author and captain in the navy. In 1827 he toured North America and visited the Hartford Retreat (q.v.), which he described in a book about his travels. He commented favorably on its management and recorded its high rate of recovery for patients (over 90 percent). The book was widely read, and through it the Hartford Retreat gained the reputation of being the most successful mental institution in the world. This led to competition among asylums (q.v.). New and better ones were built and statistics were compiled in such a way that it appeared more cures had occurred than actually had taken place. In later life, Hall became insane and died in Haslar Hospital.

See also CURABILITY OF INSANITY, THE

Bibliography: Hall, B. 1829. *Travels in North America in the years 1827 and 1828.*

HALL, GRANVILLE STANLEY (1844-1924). An American psychologist. His highly educated mother supported his desire to go to college to study theology, but his first sermon was so poor that his colleagues knelt in prayer for his soul. He turned to philosophy, which he studied in Germany. On his return to the United States, he became a preacher in New York for a short time before returning to Germany to study with Wilhelm Wundt (q.v.). He eventually achieved a doctorate in philosophy and psychology at Harvard University. In 1883 he created the first American psychological laboratory (q.v.). He established the concept of child-study in psychology by using questionnaires and advocated the understanding of normal behavior as well as abnormal behavior. In 1888 Hall became the first president of Clark University in Worcester, Massachusetts. Four years later, in July 1892, he founded the American Psychological Association (q.v.). He also founded several journals: the *American Journal of Psychology*, the *Pedagogical Seminary* and the *Journal of Applied Psychology* (qq.v.).

Bibliography: Hall, G. S. 1923. *Life and confessions of a psychologist.*

HALL, JOHN (1575-1635). A British physician who practiced in Stratford-upon-Avon. He married Susanna Shakespeare (1583-?), the elder and favorite daughter of William Shakespeare (q.v.). Hall left a collection of case histories that demonstrate his awareness of emotional disorders. He recorded cases of melancholia (q.v.), hysteria (q.v.), and insomnia, as well as other disorders, and often briefly described the personality of patients in his clinical notes.

Bibliography: Howells, J. G., and Osborn, M. L. The incidence of emotional disorder in a seventeenth-century medical practice. *Med. Hist.* 14: 142-98. Joseph, H. 1964. *John Hall: man and physician.*

HALL, JOHN (1733-1793). An English physician, the son of a barber-surgeon. He was in charge of the Newcastle Lunatic Asylum (q.v.) in New-castle-upon-Tyne, and in 1766 he opened Saint Luke's House (q.v.), a private asylum. He became a friend of James Boswell (q.v.) and treated his younger brother John Boswell (q.v.), who suffered from recurring periods of mad-ness. James Boswell described Hall as a "sensible, pretty kind of man and of a humane appearance." Hall was very much involved in the activities of Newcastle-upon-Tyne. In 1781 he founded the public baths and from 1786 to 1787 he was president of the Newcastle Philosophical and Medical Society.

Bibliography: Hall, J. 1767. *A narrative of the proceedings relative to the establish-ment of St. Luke's House.*

HALL, JOSEPH (1574-1656). An English divine, bishop of Exeter and Norwich. In 1642 he was imprisoned for defending the canons of 1640; in 1643 his cathedral was desecrated, he lost his episcopal revenues, and he was expelled from his palace. These anxious events of his life are reflected in his writings. He wrote about insomnia, which he regarded as a symptom of mental disorder, and noted that it was often caused by the fear of not being able to sleep. Sleep deprivation (q.v.), according to him, often made people confess acts which they had never done.

Bibliography: Hunter, R. and Macalpine, I. 1963. *Three hundred years of psychiatry.*

HALL, MARSHALL (1790-1857). An English physician who specialized in the treatment of mental disorders. He demonstrated that reflexes are produced more readily by stimulation of the nerve endings than by stim-ulation of the nerves and established the difference between voluntary and reflex movement. He firmly opposed the claims of mesmerism (q.v.) and insisted that patients who claimed to feel no pain when mesmerized during surgical operations were imposters. He also encouraged a more rational treatment of epilepsy (q.v.).

Bibliography: Haymaker, W. and Schiller, F. 1970. *The founders of neurology.* 2d. ed.

HALL, RADCLYFFE (MARGARET RADCLYFFE HALL) (1886-1943). An English writer. As a lesbian, (*see* LESBIANISM) she preferred to be called John. Her first serious love affair was with Mabel Batten known as Ladye. When Una Troubridge took Batten's place Batten suffered a fatal stroke and

Hall and Troubridge felt so guilty about her death that they sought reassurance through the services of a medium. After hearing that Ladye was happy in the other world, they settled into a homosexual marriage. Hall enjoyed the furor created by her book *The Well of Loneliness* (1928), which was an impassioned defense of lesbianism, which she claimed resulted in contentment and the ability to improve the mental balance of the partners. Havelock Ellis (q.v.) stated that her book had great psychological and sociological significance.
Bibliography: Dickson, L. 1975. *Radclyffe Hall and the Well of Loneliness; a sapphic chronicle.*

HALL, SPENCER TIMOTHY (1812-1885). An English mesmerist and the author of various works on mesmerism (q.v.) and phrenology (q.v.). He was said to have cured the economist and novelist Harriet Martineau (1802–1876) of her continuous poor health and deafness.
Bibliography: Hall, S. T. 1845. *Mesmeric experiences.*

HALLARAN, WILLIAM SAUNDERS (1765?-1825). An Irish physician. He was the first physician of the second asylum to be established in Ireland at Cork (the first was Saint Patrick's Hospital [q.v.]). He enlarged the hospital and introduced policies of nonrestraint and occupational therapy (q.v.), including farming and other occupations for his patients. He was an enthusiastic advocate of the swing, a contraption that revolved patients at the rate of one hundred times per minute, and adapted the model made by Joseph Cox (q.v.). In 1810 Hallaran wrote a book on insanity, the first to be written by an Irish physician — *Practical Observations on the Causes and Cure of Insanity.*
Bibliography: Hunter, R., and Macalpine, I. 1963. *Three hundred years of psychiatry.*

HALLER, ALBRECHT VON (1708-1777). A Swiss physician and poet. He was a pupil of Hermann Boerhaave (q.v.), and his extensive systematic work in the field of physiology gained him the name of Father of Experimental Physiology. He developed the concept of the irritability of living tissue, especially nerves, which influenced psychiatric thought for a long time, as many mental disorders displayed states of excitement. He studied cretins (*see* CRETINISM) in the Alps and reported his findings in 1772.
See also IRRITABILITY.
Bibliography: Sigerist, H. E. 1933. *Great doctors.*

HALLER, BERTOLD (1492-1528). A Swiss clergyman. He was influential in securing the acceptance of the principles of the Reformation. He developed a pathological guilt complex and believed that God and all humanity were against him because of his sins and heretical writings. He lived in terror and could be calmed only by frequent and large doses of opium (q.v.) and reassurance from fellow priests.

Bibliography: Hyslop, T. 1925. *The great abnormals.*

HALLIDAY, SIR ANDREW (1781-1839). A British physician. He was deputy inspector general of army hospitals and was not directly connected with the treatment of mental disorders until 1838, when he was appointed consulting physician to Crichton Royal Institution (q.v.). As a student, however, he had seen asylums (q.v.), and he had not forgotten the impression they made on him. Thus he wrote on lunatic (q.v.) asylums in Britain, in Europe, and in India, advocating state control and inspection of all such institutions. His reports contributed to the establishment of the Commissioners in Lunacy (q.v.).

Bibliography: Halliday, A. 1828. *A general view of the present state of lunatics, and lunatic asylums, in Great Britain and Ireland, and in some other kingdoms.*

HALLUCINATIONS. The term "hallucination" as it is now understood, was first introduced into medicine by Jean Esquirol (q.v.). He defined it as a pseudosensory product of mental disorder and differentiated it from illusion, which he defined as false perception. Eugen Bleuler (q.v.) defined hallucinations as "perceptions without corresponding stimuli from without." Among the early medical writers who referred to hallucinations, Aesculapius (q.v.) differentiated them from delusions. Sir Thomas Browne (q.v.) defined hallucination in his *Pseudodoxia Epidemica* (1646) as follows: "If vision be abolished, it is called caecitas, or blindness, if depraved and receives its objects erroneously, hallucination." Jacques Moreau de Tours (q.v.) described the occurrence of hallucinations under a wide variety of conditions including drugs (q.v.). Alexander Brierre de Boisemont, Pierre Janet, Francis Galton, and John Hughlings Jackson (qq.v.) all contributed to theories on hallucinations.

Bibliography: West, L. J., ed. 1962. *Hallucinations.*

HALS, FRANS (1580?-1666). A Dutch painter. He was said to be a heavy drinker, constantly in debt, and unable to manage his family affairs. In addition to the children of his first marriage, he had ten children by his second wife. One of his daughters was so unruly that his wife applied to the mayor of Haarlem to have her admitted to the workhouse. One son was a mental defective who so disrupted the household that the family had to ask for help from the town authorities. Hals was often so drunk that his pupils had to take him home from the tavern and put him to bed. As he grew old, his paintings changed from merry, robust themes to bitter psychological portraits of old people and rigid, frustrated, prim women, such as those in his 'Regentesses of the Old Men's Alms House.' In spite of his

fame, which brought him many commissions, he had to be supported from public funds in his old age.
Bibliography: Slive, S. 1971. *Frans Hals*. 2 vols.

HAMILTON, SIR WILLIAM (1788-1856). A Scottish philosopher. His contributions to psychology include a theory of free association, a study of unconscious mental modifications, and the concept of the inverse relation of perception and sensation. He disapproved of phrenology (q.v.), which he regarded as "not discovered, but invented."
Bibliography: Mills, J. S. 1865. *Examination of Sir William Hamilton's philosophy*.

HAMLET. A Danish prince first mentioned in a history of Denmark written in the twelfth century by Saxo Grammaticus. The character Hamlet in William Shakespeare's (q.v.) *Hamlet* is derived from him. Shakespeare may have based his psychological portrayal on the description of depression symptoms found in *A Treatise of Melancholie* (q.v.) by Timothy Bright (q.v.). Shakespeare's Hamlet is an inadequate young man, indecisive, at times agitated, driven to suicide (q.v.) by a deep reactive depression. The observations on mental disorders in the play reflect the opinions of the period. Ophelia's madness and suicide, for example, are attributed to rejected love (q.v.). The opera *Hamlet* by Charles Louis Ambroise Thomas (1811-1896), a French composer, ends with Ophelia's mad scene. She moves among the courtiers distributing her posy of wild flowers and sadly singing a ballad about a water sprite who lures untrue lovers to their death. ('Partagez-vous mes fleurs: et maintenant écoutez ma chanson' Act IV.)

HAMMOND, WILLIAM ALEXANDER (1828-1900). An American neurologist. He was only thirty-four years old when he was nominated surgeon general by President Abraham Lincoln (q.v.) in 1862. In 1864 he was court-martialed and dismissed for alleged irregularities in the purchase of medical equipment. Fifteen years later his case was reviewed, and he was reinstated with the rank of brigadier general. He became professor of nervous and mental diseases at Bellevue Hospital in New York, and, as such, he initiated a systematic course of lectures. He was one of the founders of the American Neurological Association (q.v.). His books *Treatise on Diseases of the Nervous System* (1871) and *Insanity in its Medical Relations* were widely used as textbooks.
Bibliography: Haymaker, W., and Schiller, F. 1970. *The founders of neurology*, 2d ed.

HAMPTON COURT. An ancient manor on the River Thames acquired by Cardinal Wolsey (q.v.) in 1514. He built a sumptuous palace there and later presented it to Henry VIII, who enlarged it. The gardens include the famous maze that was used as a model for the maze test devised by William S. Small (q.v.).

HANDCUFFS. A means of physical restraint (q.v.). Metal handcuffs linked by iron rings to an abdominal belt that also was made of heavy iron were a standard part of the equipment of most asylums (q.v.) until the middle of the nineteenth century.
Bibliography: Leigh, D. 1961. *The historical development of British psychiatry.*

HANDEL, GEORGE FREDERICK (1685-1759). A German-born English composer. His unmusical parents beat him to make him give up music, but, even as an eight-year-old child, he was a clever composer and performer and was firmly determined to have a musical career. When he was fifty years old he suffered a paralytic seizure that completely changed him. He became reclusive, suffered from anxiety, and was given to stormy outbursts and irrationality.
Bibliography: Hyslop, T. 1925. *The great abnormals.*

HANNIBAL (247-182 B.C.). A Carthaginian general and implacable opponent of the Romans. Because of opposition at home and defeat of his ally, Antiochus III of Syria, he sought refuge with Prusias, King of Bithynia in 183 B.C. When an agreement was made to return him to the Romans, he committed suicide (q.v.) by poison.
Bibliography: Rosen, G. 1971. History in the Study of Suicide. *Psychol. Med.* 1:267-85.

HANSEN, CARL. A Danish stage hypnotist. In the 1880s his performances attracted the attention of several neurologists, who then began to investigate hypnosis (*see* HYPNOTISM) and experiment with it. In London, Hansen gave instruction in hypnotism to Daniel H. Tuke (q.v.). Hansen's exaggerated claims of his power to heal patients under hypnosis often caused riots and mass hysteria (q.v.).
Bibliography: Thornton, E. M. 1976. *Hypnotism, hysteria and epilepsy: an historical synthesis.*

HANSEN, C. F. (?-1861). A German physician. He was particularly interested in mentally retarded children and spent all his savings in building a small institution for them at Eckernförde. When the building was destroyed by fire before opening, he began again. Eventually the institution opened with eleven children. After his death, his widow continued the work for a year before transferring it to another physician.
Bibliography: Kanner, L. 1964. *A history of the care and study of the mentally retarded.*

HANWELL ASYLUM. An asylum founded in England in 1831 for the county of Middlesex. Restraint (q.v.) in the form of handcuffs (q.v.) and

leg-locks (q.v.) was widely employed until John Conolly (q.v.) became the superintendent in 1839. He abolished restraint and instituted a more humane regime that included music, dancing, and other entertainments (see Plate 5), as well as an improved diet (q.v.). Many of his reforms were described in his book *The Construction and Government of Lunatic Asylums and Hospitals for the Insane*, which was first published in 1847.
Bibliography: Leigh, D. 1961. *The historical development of British psychiatry.*

HAPPY PUPPET SYNDROME. A condition in children in which mental subnormality is associated with epilepsy (q.v.), jerky movement of the limbs, and developmental anomalies of the skull and facial bones. H. Angelman first drew attention to these children in 1965 and called them "puppet children." Because they were subject to paroxysms of uncontrollable laughter, they were later called "happy puppets."
Bibliography: Angelman, H. 1965. "Puppet" children. A report on three cases. *Developmental Medicine and Child Neurology.* 7:681.

HARA-KIRI. A Japanese custom of suicide (q.v.). Obligatory hara kiri was abolished in 1868. The first sword cut was self-inflicted and followed by a final blow dealt by a friend if the courage of the condemned person failed. A recent occurrence of hara-kiri was the suicide of Yukio Mishima (q.v.), who disembowelled himself with his Samurai sword.

HARALD I (HAARFAGER) (c.850-933). The founder of the kingdom of Norway. According to legend, he became so deeply depressed following the death of Snefrid, his favorite concubine, that he was believed to be insane.
Bibliography: Retterstøl, N. 1975. Scandinavia. In *World history of psychiatry*, ed. J. G. Howells.

HARDY, GATHORNE, EARL OF CRANBROOK (1814-1906). A British politician. He influenced the movement toward the founding of state hospitals and worked for the introduction of legislation that would provide special establishments for so-called poor law lunatics (q.v.) and imbeciles (q.v.).
Bibliography: Ayers, G. M. 1971. *England's first state hospitals and the Metropolitan Asylums Board.*

HARE. In the Middle Ages the hare was considered to be a melancholy animal, and it was believed that its flesh would cause depression in those who ate it because it created an excess of black bile (q.v.). Hares are said to be "mad" possibly because their behavior becomes frantic when they have no cover.
Bibliography: 1978. *Brewer's dictionary of phrase and fable.*

HARMAN, THOMAS (fl. 1567). A magistrate and country gentleman who lived in Kent. In 1566 he wrote a book on beggars in which he recounted

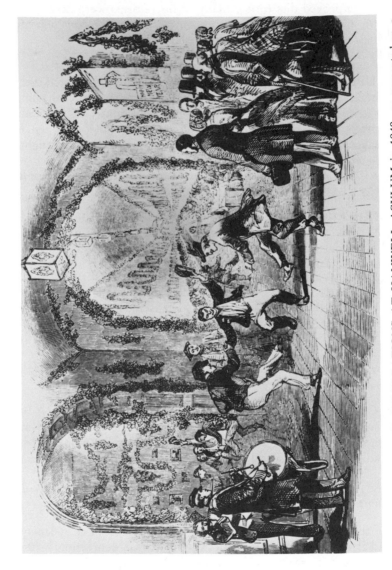

5. TWELFTH NIGHT CELEBRATIONS AT HANWELL ASYLUM in 1848, as presented in a contemporary issue of the *Illustrated London News*. By courtesy of the Department of Medical Illustration, Ipswich Hospital.

a story of Tom O'Bedlam (q.v.), who came begging at his house. Harman checked the beggar's story with the keeper of Bethlem Royal Hospital (q.v.), who stated that patients were not sent out to beg. The beggar, one Nicholas Jennings, had never been in Bethlem Royal Hospital, nor was he epileptic, as he had claimed, but, in fact, was well off. He was sent to Bridewell (q.v.) where he was set in the pillory and whipped through the streets of London.
Bibliography: O'Donoghue, E. G. 1914. *The history of Bethlehem Hospital.*

HARMSWORTH, ALFRED, VISCOUNT NORTHCLIFFE (1865-1922). An Irish publisher and owner of many newspapers, including the *Times.* Throughout his life he was an unstable and eccentric character who reacted to stress with psychosomatic illnesses. Fond of secrecy and of impressing people, he kept a dummy telephone on his desk in order to pretend that he was speaking with important people. He had several nervous breakdowns, and it is believed that he became insane and died of general paralysis of the insane (q.v.).
Bibliography: Ferris, P. 1971. *The house of Northcliffe.*

HARPER, ANDREW (?-1790). An Anglo-American physician. He believed that mental illness was a psychic disorder that should be treated at home rather than in asylums (q.v.). He was against restraint (q.v.), confinement, and isolation and advocated a plan of treatment that would attempt to discover the source of distress. The patient was advised to avoid exhausting his mind with unpleasant or irritating thoughts; physical remedies were secondary. In 1789 Harper published a book entitled *A Treatise on the Real Cause and Cure of Insanity.*
Bibliography: Hunter, R., and Macalpine, I. 1963. *Three hundred years of psychiatry.*

HARRINGTON (or HARINGTON), JAMES (1611-1677). An English political philosopher. He became convinced that diseases disguised themselves as flies and bees. To protect himself from their attacks he went about with a long broom.
Bibliography: Hyslop, T. O. 1925. *The great abnormals.*

HARRISON, CATHARINE. *See* CAPPE, CATHARINE.

HARRISON, ROSS GRANVILLE (1870-1959). An American scientist. He studied at Johns Hopkins University and in Germany, where he obtained his medical degree, although he never practiced medicine. After he had mastered the latest microsurgical methods, he was able to demonstrate the cellular origin of the components of the nervous system in vertebrates, thus advancing the study of neuroembryology. As a scientist, Harrison was unusually well read, spoke several languages, and wrote with exemplary clarity and logic. He illustrated his material with his own skilled drawings. Yet,

he was a shy and unassuming man, who said little but was interested in open air pursuits as well as literature and music.
Bibliography: Haymaker, W., and Schiller, F. 1970. *The founders of neurology.* 2d. ed.

HARSNETT, SAMUEL (1561-1631). An archbishop of York, England. He was unpopular with the Puritans because he did not believe in witchcraft (q.v.), demonaic possession (q.v.) and wrote against exorcism (q.v.). In a pamphlet written in 1599, to expose the exorcist John Darrell (q.v.), he stated: "They that have their brains baited and their fancies distempered with the imaginations and apprehensions of witches, conjurors and fairies, and all that lymphatic chimera, I find to be marshalled in one of these five ranks: children, fools, women, cowards, sick or black melancholic discomposed wits."
Bibliography: 1900. *The dictionary of national biography.*

HARTFORD RETREAT. An American asylum in Connecticut. It was opened in 1824. The name was adopted from the York Retreat (q.v.), in England, which it tried to emulate. Its first superintendent was Dr. Eli Todd (q.v.), who had vigorously worked for its creation. The American asylum became famous for its high rate of so-called cures, which promoted the theory of curability (q.v.) of mental disorders. Charles Dickens (q.v.) visited the Retreat during his visit to America and found it one of the few institutions worthy of his praise.
See also INSTITUTE OF LIVING
Bibliography: Braceland, F. J. 1972. *The Institute of Living: The Hartford Retreat 1822-1972.*

HARTLEY, DAVID (1705-1757). An English philosopher and physician. He was unable to enter the Church because, being a benevolent and tolerant man, he found it impossible to agree with eternal punishment. He became a physician and was said to dispense philosophical advice for mental disorders in the same way that others dispensed drugs (q.v.). He greatly admired the theory of the association of ideas developed by John Locke (q.v.) and adapted it into a formal doctrine, thus becoming the founder of associationism (q.v.). In 1749 he published his book *Observations on Man, his Frame, his Duty, and his Expectations* in which he discussed his belief that the mind is a mosaic of sensations that are produced by vibrations in the nervous system.
Bibliography: Rand, B. 1923. *Early development of Hartley's doctrine of association.*

HARTMANN, KARL ROBERT EDUARD VON (1842-1906). A German philosopher. By a process of abstract reasoning, he came close to the concept of the unconscious (q.v.) that Sigmund Freud (q.v.) developed. Hartmann believed that the unconscious was the origin of being. According to him there were three levels of unconscious: the absolute, which was the

substance of the universe; the physiological, which was the basis of all organic life; and the relative, or psychological, from which conscious mental processes and behavioral patterns developed. In 1869 he published *Philosophy of the Unconscious* (q.v.) in which he expounded his theories and discussed emotions, association of ideas, personality, destiny, perception, instinct, and the role of the unconscious in many spheres of life. After an initial success the book was attacked by philosophers and scientists.
Bibliography: Schnehen, W. von. 1929. *E. von Hartmann.*

HARUN AL-RASHID (c.763-809). A caliph of Bagdad. Under his rule, the Eastern caliphate attained its greatest power. He figures prominently in the *Arabian Nights*. His wife was said to have been mentally ill and to have been cured by a physician from the medical family of Bukht Yishu (q.v.).
Bibliography: Philby, H. St. J. B. 1933. *Harun-al-Rashid.*

HARVEY, GIDEON (1637?-1700). An English physician. He wrote on what he called "hypochondriack melancholy," a complaint that combined gastric disorders with depression. He thought that it was caused by "passions", including fear, anger, jealousy (q.v.), and despair. His work *Morbus Anglicus, or a Theoretick and Practical Discourse of Consumptions, and Hypochondriack Melancholy* was published in 1672.
See also HYPOCHONDRIA.
Bibliography: Hunter, R., and Macalpine, I. 1963. *Three hundred years of psychiatry.*

HARVEY, WILLIAM (1578-1657). An English physician and the discoverer of the circulation of the blood. He described his discovery in 1628 in *Exercitatio De Motu Cordis et Sanguinis*, a work that tended to make bleeding (q.v.) even more fashionable as a treatment for mental disorders. Harvey was aware of the effect of emotions on cardiac activity and thought that sexual disorders could cause mental illness. He described two cases of pseudocyesis (q.v.) and advised the parents of a hysterical (*see* HYSTERIA) girl to provide her with a husband. When his advice was followed, she recovered.
Bibliography: Keynes, G. 1949. *The personality of William Harvey.*

HASHISH. The Arab term, meaning "dried herb," for the resin of *Cannabis sativa* (q.v.). It produces mental exaltation. It was used by a ruthless band of Persians, hashashins, or assassins (q.v.), to help them commit acts of terrorism. The term was introduced to the West by Marco Polo (1254?-?1324) after his travels in Persia in 1271. Johann Weyer (q.v.) theorized that witches (*see* WITCHCRAFT) were women under the influence of hashish or suffering from its after effects. He also applied this theory to the sorcerers

mentioned in the Bible (q.v.) and claimed that the Hebrew word for sorcerer had been mistranslated.
Bibliography: Emboden, W. 1972. *Narcotic plants*.

HASLAM, JOHN (1764-1844). An English medical writer and apothecary at Bethlem Royal Hospital (q.v.). His work allowed him to study carefully many mental disorders, which he described in minute detail, and his methods of investigation were the most scientific of his period. He was among the first to describe general paralysis of the insane (q.v.), although he remained unaware of its cause. He also gave accurate descriptions of childhood schizophrenia, obsessional neurosis, and manic-depressive psychoses (qq.v.), as well as writing vivid accounts of the autopsies he performed. He wrote a case history of a psychotic (*see* PSYCHOSIS) patient, James Tilley Matthews (q.v.), in his *Observations on Insanity*, which was published in 1798. Haslam contributed to forensic psychiatry, with his work entitled *Medical Jurisprudence, As It Relates to Insanity, According to the Law of England* (1817). He seems to have been more interested in research than in day-to-day management. Although he advocated moral treatment, convalescence, and aftercare facilities, he was also the inventor of a "key" to force open the mouths of recalcitrant patients. Following the case of William Norris (q.v.), he was dismissed from Bethlem by the governors. According to Edward G. O'Donoghue, the Bethlem historian, Haslam was an innocent scapegoat. He was forced to sell his beloved books to make ends meet. His son, John, often acted as locum for him, and his daughter, Henrietta, became matron at Bethlem. She too was accused of neglecting her duties and was forced to resign.
Bibliography: Hunter, R., and Macalpine, I. 1963. *Three hundred years of psychiatry*.

HASTINGS, SIR CHARLES (1794-1866). A British physician. In 1832 he founded the Provincial Medical and Surgical Association, which became the British Medical Association in 1856. He also founded the journal of the association, the *British Medical Journal* in 1840. Hastings was physician to the Worcester Infirmary and the owner of a private asylum called Droitwich Lunatic Asylum, which had been in existence since 1791.
Bibliography: 1900. *Dictionary of national biography*.

HATSHEPSUT (1503-1482? B.C.). A Queen of Egypt. As the ruler of her country she promoted a policy of peace and economic development. She assumed male attributes and was seen in male clothes and with a beard. Nevertheless, she married and produced children.
Bibliography: Petrie, W. M. F. 1894-1925. *A history of Egypt*. 6 vols.

HATTER, JOHN (fl. 17th cent.). Also known as John Hodgson. An eccentric living in the seventeenth century. He is mentioned in the dedication of the English translation (1660) of *The Hospital of Incurable Fools* (q.v.) written by Tomaso Garzoni (q.v.) in 1586. According to William Hazlitt (q.v.) , the expression "Mad as a Hatter" may have originated with him. *See also* MAD HATTER.

HATTON ASYLUM. A mental hospital near Warwick, England, opened in 1852. It followed an enlightened policy of care for the mentally ill. The first superintendent, Dr. William Henry Parsey (1821-1884), introduced recreational activities, occupation, chapel services, reading, and weekly dances for the patients. A brass band (q.v.) was also part of the hospital enterprises; in addition to other duties, the band used to meet Dr. Parsey's carriage when he returned from leave. It would accompany him up the drive to the strains of "See the Conquering Hero Comes"—a sign of his popularity. The hospital also used to brew its own beer, as the brewer was a patient. After many changes, Hatton is now known as the Central Hospital. It offers psychiatric services to a large area.

HAUFFE, FRIEDERICKE (1801-1829). The daughter of a gamekeeper in Prevorst, a village in Würzttemberg, Germany. She experienced religious visions and premonitions that culminated in convulsions and catalepsy with fever and hemorrhages. She acquired a reputation as a seeress and offered advice and cures. She also displayed a prodigious memory (q.v.) while in a trance and spoke in pure German in contrast to the village dialect that she usually spoke. She became a patient of Andreas Justinus Kerner (q.v.) , who wrote her story and treated her with magnetism (q.v.). Theologians and physicians became interested in her, and several mediums (q.v.) imitated her activities.
Bibliography: Kerner, A.J.C. 1845. *The seeress of Prevorst*, trans. Mrs. Crowe.

HAUSER, KASPAR (1812?-1833). The name given to a young man found incarcerated in a Nuremberg dungeon in 1828. He claimed that he had been kept in complete isolation from his childhood until he was found at the age of approximately seventeen. His attendants never spoke to him, and his cell was so small that he could neither stand nor lie down in it. He was said to have been imprisoned because he was the heir to a small principality in Germany. His appearance was brutish, and he could not talk, walk properly, or understand the spoken word. He soon learned to speak German and mastered Latin, proving that his intelligence had not been affected by his long isolation. He wrote an account of his years in prison, but he was assassinated before it was published. Many plays and books have been based on the events of his life. In 1908 Jakob Wasserman (q.v.) wrote a novel about him entitled *Caspar Hauser*.
Bibliography: Goldenson, R. M. 1970. *The encyclopedia of human behaviour.*

HAVISHAM, MISS. A character in *Great Expectations* (1860-1861) by Charles Dickens (q.v.). Abandoned at the altar by her bridegroom, she

remained a withered bride for the rest of her life, permanently dressed in her wedding dress and lived among the relics of the untouched wedding banquet. She is a prime example of women who become eccentric recluses, imprisoned by self-preoccupation and unable to progress with time. They have a distorted body concept of themselves.
Bibliography: Critchley, M. 1979. *The divine banquet of the brain and other essays.*

HAWKER, ROBERT STEPHEN (1803-1875). An English clergyman and poet of great eccentricity. As a child, he ran away from several schools; at nineteen he became happily married to a woman of forty and took her to Oxford. He was ordained into the Church of England and became curate of Morwenstow, a village high on the cliffs of Cornwall. He rebuilt the church and the vicarage as well as the road leading to it, created a bridge, a school, and a house for its master, and wrote poetry. He helped the villagers fight disease, poverty, corruption, and natural disasters. Between 1824 and 1874 more than eighty ships foundered on that coast, and Hawker witnessed the recovery of many terribly mutilated corpses, which he then had to bury. The horror of wrecks preyed on his mind, and he came to dread the sound of approaching storms. He found the nursing of his beloved dying wife a great strain, and, after her death, he happily married a woman forty years his junior. To his eccentricity of dress and behavior he added addiction to opium (q.v.). Toward the end of his life he became a Roman Catholic.
Bibliography: Brendon, P. 1975. *Hawker of Morwenstow.*

HAWKES, JOHN (fl. 1850s). An English physician and assistant medical officer for the Wiltshire County Asylum. He believed that the increased pace of living brought about by the industrial revolution was responsible for the increase in mental illness and proposed a preventive program based on improved social conditions.
Bibliography: Hawkes, J. 1857. On the increase of insanity. *J. Psychol. Med. ment. Pathol.* 10: 508-21.

HAWKINS, HENRY (1826-1904). An English clergyman and chaplain to Colney Hatch Asylum (q.v.) . His pleas for convalescent homes and after-care services for mental patients led to the foundation of the Mental After-Care Association (q.v.) in 1879. Prior to this, he had founded a group known as Guild of Friends of the Infirm of Mind (q.v.), who offered voluntary help in asylums.
See also AFTER-CARE MOVEMENT.

HAWKINS, JOHN (fl. 1620). An English physician. He was forced to leave England because of his religious beliefs. He wrote a Latin treatise on melancholy (*see* MELANCHOLIA) entitled *Discursus de Melancholia Hypochondriaca Potissimum*, which was published in Germany in 1633. Basing his

observations on the illness of Elizabeth, queen of Bohemia (q.v.), daughter of James I of England and VI of Scotland (q.v.), he described the anxiety and depression accompanied by gastric disorders and insomnia that are typical symptoms of hypochondriac melancholy.
Bibliography: Hunter, R., and Macalpine, I. 1963. *Three hundred years of psychiatry.*

HAWTHORN. One of the oldest English hedge trees. It is connected with Henry VII of England (1457-1509), who retrieved his crown from a hawthorn tree after Richard III (q.v.) was killed at Bosworth Field. Herbalists have regarded this plant as useful in the treatment of nervous debility, and helpful in the relief of severe emotional stress and depression.
Bibliography: Leyel, C. F. 1949. *Hearts-ease.*

HAWTHORNE EXPERIMENTS. A series of investigations conducted in the United States by the Western Electric Company between 1924 and 1927. Among other things, the investigators measured the effect of light on a group of girl workers and found that improved lighting increased productivity, but they also discovered that reduced lighting or no change in lighting produced the same effect. Eventually it was realized that the increased productivity was due to the presence of the research workers.
Bibliography: Galdston, I., ed. 1967. *Historic derivations of modern psychiatry.*

HAYDON, BENJAMIN ROBERT (1786-1846). An English painter of historical subjects. He is famous for his *Flight into Egypt,* and the *Judgement of Solomon,* among other works. Even though he was successful and enjoyed the patronage of George IV (1762-1830) who purchased one of his works, he was so poor that he was arrested for debt. He was given to paroxysms of rage and was a bitter, disappointed, and lonely man. In 1846 he shot himself. At the inquest upon his death, the coroner's jury found that he committed suicide (q.v.) while of unsound mind.
Bibliography: Winslow, L.S.F. 1898. *Mad humanity: its forms, apparent and obscure.*

HAYGARTH, JOHN (1740-1827). An English physician. He was skeptical of the cures brought about by metallic tractors (q.v.) and constructed similar ones out of wood painted to look like metal. As they had the same effect on patients, he concluded that they acted on the patients' imaginations. He published his findings in 1800 in *Of the Imagination, as Cause and As Cure of Disorders of the Body; Exemplified by Fictitious Tractors, and Epidemical Conclusions.*
Bibliography: Hunter, R., and Macalpine, I. 1963. *Three hundred years of psychiatry.*

HAZARD, THOMAS ROBINSON (1797-1886). An American reformer. He retired as a successful businessman, at the age of forty-three and dedicated himself to a number of public causes. He supported reforms in education, the abolition of capital punishment, and women's rights. The Rhode Island legislature asked him to investigate the conditions of the poor and the insane in the state, and his *Report on the Poor and Insane in Rhode Island* was published in 1851.

Bibliography: Deutsch, A. 1949. *The mentally ill in America.*

HAZLITT, WILLIAM (1778-1830). An English essayist and literary critic. His infatuation with a tailor's daughter caused him to obtain a divorce from his wife by providing proof of adultery with a one-eyed prostitute in Edinburgh. The tailor's daughter, Sarah Walker, turned him down, however, for a richer suitor. He was so distressed by her actions that he wandered about London telling his tale to strangers. He also wrote the whole story of his woes in *Liber Amoris*, which was published in 1823. His friends believed that his behavior was due to temporary insanity. He eventually married a charming widow, who also tired of him and left him. Notwithstanding these events, he died murmuring "I have had a happy life."

Bibliography: Baker, H. 1962. *William Hazlitt.*

HEAD, HENRY (1861-1940). An English neurologist. He conducted original research on pain, peripheral nerve injuries, and sensory nerve function. As an experiment, he had the radial and external cutaneous nerves of his own forearm divided and resutured, and he kept careful notes on the process of recovery. He developed the theories of the protopathic and epicritic sensibility of nerves. He also confirmed that the thalamus is a seat of feeling and emotion. Head wrote a major work on aphasia entitled *Aphasia and Kindred Disorders of Speech*, which was published in 1926.

Bibliography: Haymaker, W., and Schiller, F. 1970. *The founders of neurology.* 2d ed.

HEADDRESS OF PAUPER LUNATICS. According to John Bucknill (q.v.) in the first issue of the English *Asylum Journal* (q.v.) in 1853, "nothing determines the character of a man's appearance more than the garment which he wears upon his head. . . ." His article described the hats provided for male pauper lunatics (q.v.) in county asylums (q.v.). Stout felt hats were found to be too expensive and "some patients were apt to use them as depositories for rubbish," therefore fustian caps were adopted. Bucknill described them as "shaped like a forage cap, but the sides are cut deep and stiffened, so that the crown is maintained at a little distance from the vertex."

HEAD SURGERY. Surgery of the head for the treatment of mental disorders has been practiced since prehistory. In early times its objective was the release of demons. Medieval miniatures illustrate a procedure in which the top of the head was incised in the shape of a cross and the cranium carefully perforated. In the fourteenth century, Rogerius Salernitanus described the operation in a manuscript of Montpellier. As there was no anesthesia (q.v.), the patient was held in chains.

See also TREPANATION.

Bibliography: MacKinney, L. 1965. *Medical illustrations in medieval manuscripts.*

HEALY, WILLIAM (1869-1963). An English physician and psychologist. He emigrated to America early in life and became a pupil of William James (q.v.). In 1909 he founded the Chicago Juvenile Psychopathic Institute (q.v.) which was to help the juvenile court investigate young first offenders and prevent them, through rehabilitation, from becoming adult criminals. The institute became a model for child guidance clinics (q.v.), and Healy is regarded as the founder of the child guidance movement in the United States. Using techniques derived from psychoanalysis (q.v.), he rejected the idea that juvenile delinquency was due to hereditary factors and believed it to have a socioeconomic aetiology. In 1917 Healy was appointed director of the Judge Baker Guidance Center in Boston, and he spent the next thirty years of his life as its director.

Bibliography: Healy, W., and Bronner, A. 1926. *Delinquents and criminals: their making and unmaking.*

HEART. Throughout history the heart has been considered the seat of the soul where moral courage as well as hope and love reside. To die of a broken heart meant to die of disappointment, or sorrow. Many sayings reflect these beliefs, for example, "take heart" (have courage), "lose one's heart" (fall in love), and "take to heart" (feel deeply). Aristotle (q.v.) regarded the heart as the *sensorium commune* (q.v.), and Galen (q.v.) sited the irrational (emotional) soul in it.

Bibliography: Zilboorg, G. 1941. *A history of medical psychology.*

HEARTSEASE. Also known as wild pansy. Herbalists have used the plant since antiquity for the treatment of many ailments, including convulsive disorders and epilepsy (q.v.). The ancient Greeks used it to moderate anger and to promote sleep. They had such regard for its powers that it became the symbol of Athens. The Anglo-Saxons regarded it as an antidote to spells and a protection against evil spirits. During the sixteenth century, a decoction was made from its flowers and leaves for treatment of venereal diseases. John Gerard (q.v.) wrote that it "assuageth the pains of the head" and "causeth sleep."

Bibliography: le Strange, R. 1977. *A history of herbal plants.*

HEAT. Since antiquity it has been believed that excessive warmth could cause insanity. Jean Esquirol (q.v.) stated that "the continuance of warmth augments excitement."

Bibliography: Esquirol, J.E.D. 1845. Reprint. 1965. *Mental maladies: a treatise on insanity.*

HEATHER. *Calluna vulgaris,* a plant found on hillsides and moorlands. Herbalists attribute medical properties to it and use it as a tonic in nervous

disorders and as a remedy for depression and migraine (q.v.). It is also used to promote sleep in those suffering from insomnia.
Bibliography: de Baïracli Levy, J. 1974. *The illustrated herbal handbook.*

HEBB, DONALD OLDING (1904-   ). A Canadian psychologist. He has conducted many experiments on sensory deprivation and has proved that it affects thought processes and produces hallucinations (q.v.), as well as abnormal emotional responses.
Bibliography: Hebb, D. O. 1949. *The organisation of behavior: a neuropsychological theory.*

HEBEPHRENIA. The term used by Ewald Hecker (q.v.) in 1871 to describe a psychosis (q.v.) appearing in puberty and resulting in rapid clinical deterioration. "Hebe" is derived from Hebe, the Greek goddess of youth.
Bibliography: Hecker, E. 1871. Die hebephrenie. *Archive für pathologische anatomie und physiologie.* 52.

HECATE. A Greek goddess of the underworld. She was regarded as the patron of witches (*see* WITCHCRAFT) and associated with ghosts and sorcery. She was represented with three heads and was worshipped at crossroads (q.v.). In Shakespeare's *Macbeth* she directs the witches.
Bibliography: Kraus, T. 1960. *Hekate.*

HECKER, EWALD (1843-1909). A German psychiatrist and an assistant to Karl Kahlbaum (q.v.) . In 1871 he described a mental disorder related to puberty and adolescence and leading to rapid deterioration. He coined the term *Hebephrenia* (q.v.) to describe the condition.
Bibliography: Hecker, E. 1871. Die hebephrenie. *Archive für pathologische anatomie und physiologie* 52 .

HECUBA. A legendary queen of the Trojans. She represented misery and disaster because her whole life was said to have been clouded by a series of tragedies that destroyed her family. Her great sorrows deranged her mind, and she wandered through the Thracian fields howling like a dog. According to Greek mythology (q.v.), she was changed into a bitch and threw herself into the sea. Several Greek tragedies feature her sorrows.
Bibliography: Hammond, N.G.L., and Scullard, H. H. 1970. *The Oxford classical dictionary.*

HEDONISM. A philosophic doctrine going back to the third century B.C. It presents pleasure or happiness as the supreme good. In the eighteenth century it was regarded as the basis of all human motivation, and it was said that men were prepared to suffer present pain in order to win pleasure in

the future. In psychiatry hedonism refers to the search for goals that will afford gratification.
Bibliography: Boring, E. G. 1950. *A history of experimental psychology.*

HEEMSKERCK, MAERTEN JACOBSZ VAN (1498-1574). A Dutch painter who was pathologically anxious. He was so afraid of soldiers and the sound of their guns that during military parades he went into hiding. Anxiety about his old age made him a miser, and he always carried gold coins hidden in his clothes.
Bibliography: Wittkower, R., and Wittkower, M. 1963. *Born under Saturn.*

HEEP, URIAH. A character in *David Copperfield* (1849-1850) by Charles Dickens (q.v.). He was a cringing, malicious hypocrite whose psychopathic (*see* PSYCHOPATHY) behavior eventually caused his own downfall. He is described as having closely cropped hair and "hardly any eyebrows, and no eyelashes, and eyes of a red brown, so unsheltered and unshaded" that one wondered how he ever managed to sleep.

HEGEL, GEORG WILHELM FRIEDRICH (1770-1831). A German philosopher. His philosophical system was based on reason and supported authoritarian institutions rather than democratic ones. According to him, a group had more reality than the individuals within it. He advanced the idea of evolution in sociology. Hegel believed that man was alienated, or estranged, from himself because he had projected his own image onto God whom he then worshiped outside himself. His main works were *Phenomenology of Spirit* (1807), *Science of Logic* (1812-16), and *Philosophy of Right* (1821), which contains his political views.
Bibliography: Taylor, C. 1975. *Hegel.*

HEIDEGGER, MARTIN (1889-1976). German philosopher and founder of the phenomenological school of philosophy. His new method of analyzing the phenomena of human existence led to the development of existential analysis in psychiatry. According to his doctrine, despair, or anxiety, was caused by the fear of not existing, as opposed to the experience of "being in the world."
See also EXISTENTIALISM.
Bibliography: Biemel, W. 1977. *Martin Heidegger.*

HEIDENHAIN, RUDOLF (1835-1897). A German physiologist. He became interested in animal magnetism (q.v.) and the practices of Franz Mesmer (q.v.). In 1880 he wrote a book *Animal Magnetism* in which he tried to explain magnetism by a complicated and farfetched system of physiology of the nervous system.

Bibliography: Thornton, E. M. 1976. *Hypnotism, hysteria and epilepsy: an historical synthesis.*

HEILPÄDAGOGIK (REMEDIAL EDUCATION). A movement by German, Austrian, and Swiss educators to study and help mentally handicapped children. It originated in Germany and received its impetus from the introduction of the Binet-Simon tests (q.v.) in 1914.

Bibliography: Kanner, L. 1964. *A history of the care and study of the mentally retarded.*

HEINE, HEINRICH (1797-1856). A German poet. As a young man he graduated in law, but, inspired by the French revolution of July 1830, he turned his attention to poetry and to politics. He converted from Judaism to Christianity in the hope of greater acceptance, but he lost the support of his own people and had to leave Germany because of his political sympathies. He experienced several unsatisfactory love affairs in which his mistresses were women who were as unlike his mother as possible. For at least the last ten years of his life, he suffered from depression and was confined to bed by a paralysis that was attributed to syphilis (q.v.) or porphyria (q.v.). His spine was subjected to frequent cauterization (q.v.) as part of the treatment, and, to overcome the pain he suffered, he took large doses of opium (q.v.). Fame came too late for him to enjoy it. The last comfort of his life was his "Lotus-flower," a beautiful young girl engaged to read to him. She had been a patient in a mental hospital and was a sensitive woman whom he passionately loved and immortalized in his poetry. Sigmund Freud (q.v.) quoted him frequently.

Bibliography: Critchley, M. 1979. *The divine banquet of the brain and other essays.*

HEINEKEN, CHRISTIAN (1721-1725). A child genius (q.v.), born at Lübeck, Germany. It was said that he could talk within a few hours of his birth and could retell poems and stories by the time he was a year old. Soon after his first birthday he had memorized the whole Bible (q.v.), and by the time he was three years old he had mastered three languages (including Latin), as well as geography, history, and anatomy. He had also memorized hundreds of songs and poems. He demonstrated his skills at the court of Denmark in Copenhagen. He was just over four years old when he died.

Bibliography: Strauch, A. 1924. Christian Heineken. *Am. J. Dis. Chil.* 27: 163.

HEINROTH, JOHANN CHRISTIAN (1773-1843). A German psychiatrist. He was against a somatological theory of mental disorders and considered the soul to be all important. He tried to establish a unity of psychological phenomena and studied the pathological mental processes of

the mentally ill. In the Lutheran tradition, Heinroth thought that mental disorders were caused by sin and consequent guilt. His classification listed forty-eight mental disorders associated with several kinds of sin. Using a religious-moralistic terminology, he pointed to inner conflict as a primary cause of mental disorders. He advised that treatment should consist of correction of judgment and inculcation of moral principles.
Bibliography: Kraepelin, E. 1962. *One hundred years of psychiatry.*

HELD, JAN THEOBALD (1770-1851). A Czech physician. He is regarded as the first Czech psychiatrist. He was in charge of the department for mentally ill priests in the hospital of the Brothers of Charity in Prague, Czechoslovakia. He advocated a program of occupational therapy (q.v.) and established a library and a music room in the hospital for the benefit of the patients. He treated Josef Dobrovsky (q.v.) during his derangement.
Bibliography: Vencovsky, E. 1975. Czechoslovakia. In *World history of psychiatry,* ed. J. G. Howells.

HELIOGABALUS. *See* ELAGABALUS.

HELL, MAXIMILIAN (fl.1750). A Jesuit priest and court astrologer (*see* ASTROLOGY) to Maria Theresa of Austria (1717-1780). He claimed to have discovered animal magnetism (q.v.) and was attacked by Franz Mesmer (q.v.), who claimed the honor for himself. Hell used steel magnets to accomplish his so-called cures.
Bibliography: Ehrenwald, J., ed. 1976. *The history of psychotherapy.*

HELLEBORE. Black hellebore, also known as the Christmas Rose, was used as a herbal remedy against madness in ancient Greece. It was found in Greece at Anticyra (q.v.) and to say to anybody "sail to Anticyra" was equivalent to saying "you are mad, go and eat hellebore." Melampus (q.v.) was said to have used it to cure the mad women of Argos. Robert Burton (q.v.) recommended its use in his *Anatomy of Melancholy*, and John Gerard (q.v.) wrote, "a purgation of Hellebore is good for mad and furious men, for melancholy, dull and heavie persons, and briefly for all those that are troubled with black choler, and molested with melancholy." Nicholas Culpeper (q.v.) also thought that it was effective against madness. The use of hellebore in psychiatry lasted even into the nineteenth century because it was considered "specifically anti-maniacal." Benjamin Rush (q.v.) was among those who prescribed it.
Bibliography: le Strange, R. 1977. *A history of herbal plants.*

HELLER'S DISEASE. Dementia infantilis (q.v.), named after Theodore Heller (fl. early twentieth century), an Austrian neuropsychiatrist, who de-

scribed the disease in a classic paper that appeared in the *Zeitschrift fuer Kinderforschung* in 1930.
Bibliography: Heller, T. 1969. About Dementia Infantilis. In *Modern perspectives in international child psychiatry*, ed. J. G. Howells.

HELLPACH, WILLY (1877-1955). A German psychologist. He was especially interested in anthropology and social psychology (q.v.). He believed that social class was an influence in the aetiology of hysteria (q.v.) and was an early supporter of the theory of sexuality (q.v.) and neurosis (q.v.) proposed by Sigmund Freud (q.v.).
Bibliography: Hellpach, W. 1953. *Kulturpsychologie.*

HELMHOLTZ, HERMANN LUDWIG FERDINAND VON (1821-1894). A German physiologist, physicist, and psychologist and professor of physics at Berlin. His physiological work was connected with the eye, the ear, and the nervous system. Helmholtz discovered that objects are perceived as they should be and not as they impress the sensory organs. His *Handbuch der physiologischen Optik* (1856-1866), is regarded as the greatest classic in the field of sense perception.
Bibliography: Haymaker, W., and Schiller, F. 1970. *The founders of neurology*, 2d. ed.

HELMONT, FRANCISCUS MERCURIUS VAN (c.1614-1699). A Flemish physician and mystic philosopher, the son of Jan Batista van Helmont (q.v.). He believed that the mind influenced the body in producing and curing diseases. Like his father, he recommended that "fools and distracted" patients should be "ducked" and kept under water until unconscious, although he admitted that this treatment was unsuitable for those who had been born foolish. He claimed that melancholics (*see* MELANCHOLIA) should be made to cry as their tears would dissipate the watery humor that caused melancholy. He investigated the physiology of speech and devised methods of instruction for the deaf and dumb.
Bibliography: Hunter, R., and Macalpine, I. 1963. *Three hundred years of psychiatry.*

HELMONT, JAN BATISTA VAN (1577-1644). A Flemish physician and chemist. After studying the works of Hippocrates, Galen, and Avicenna (qq.v.), he turned to the writings of Paracelsus (q.v.) but later rejected them also, gave away all his books, and refused to take any degree. He regarded the brain as an executive organ closely linked to the stomach, which, in turn, was the starting point of abnormal appetites in pregnancy, hysteria (q.v.), and epilepsy (q.v.). He thought that asthma was similar in principle to epilepsy and called it "the falling sickness of the lungs." He advised sudden and prolonged immersion (q.v.) in cold water for cases of mental derangement. Helmont believed that the human body radiated a magnetic

fluid, which could be focused through an act of will on the bodies or the minds of other people to cure illness. He attributed the cures produced by saints' relics to this power. Franz Mesmer's (q.v.) use of magnets (q.v.) in therapy was influenced by Helmont's theories. He is regarded as the father of biochemistry because he studied phenomena related to the human body in terms of chemistry. He introduced the word *gas*, modified from the Greek *chaos*, to describe aeriform fluids. His works *Ortus Medicinae, vel Opera et Opuscula Omnia* were published by his son in 1648.
Bibliography: Sigerist, H. E. 1933. *Great doctors.*

HELVETIUS, CLAUDE ADRIEN (1715-1771). A French philosopher. His theories were based on the senses as the sources of all intellectual activity. He thought that the differences among individuals were due to differences in education and that the mind began as a *tabula rasa* (q.v.). A perfect man would be the product of perfect education. According to him, man is motivated by the wish to be powerful and, therefore, able to gratify his passions. His work *De l'esprit*, which was published in 1758, was condemned by the Sorbonne as too materialistic and publicly burnt by the hangman. This action greatly publicized the work and assured a widespread readership.
Bibliography: Smith, D. W. 1965. *Helvetius.*

HEMINGWAY, ERNEST MILLAR (1899-1961). An American writer. Courage, violence, stamina, and independence are recurrent themes in his writings. He had a compulsion to search for dangerous situations and used hunting, fishing, fighting, brawling, and hard drinking to assert his virility. He boasted that he had slept with all the girls he wanted and some that he did not want. He was married four times and had no compunction in publicizing his erotic feats. Yet, he was insecure, depressed, and full of self-hatred. In 1960 because of depression he was admitted to the Mayo Clinic in Rochester, Minnesota. In 1961 Hemingway committed suicide (q.v.) by shooting himself. Among his works are *For Whom The Bell Tolls* (1940), *The Old Man and the Sea* (1952), which was specifically mentioned in his 1954 Nobel Prize award, and the autobiographical *A Moveable Feast*, published posthumously in 1964.
Bibliography: Baker, C. 1972. *Ernest Hemingway: a life story.*

HEMORRHOIDS. Varicose veins of the anus. They were regarded as beneficial in the treatment of insanity. Jean Esquirol (q.v.) quoted Hippocrates, Celsus, and Hermann Boerhaave (qq.v.) as followers of this theory. Hemorrhoids were even provoked by cupping to achieve a cure, and

their suppression was believed to produce melancholy (*see* MELANCHOLIA) and dementia.
Bibliography: Esquirol, J.E.D. 1845. Reprint. 1965. *Mental maladies: a treatise on insanity.*

HEMP. *See* CANNABIS SATIVA.

HENBANE. *Hyoscyamus Niger,* an annual plant. It grows to a height of five feet, is hairy and fetid, and often thought to look sinister. It is possibly the oldest narcotic known to man and has been widely used, although it can produce delirium (q.v.) and convulsions. The Romans, the Greeks, the Babylonians and ancient Egyptians knew its qualities as a painkiller. In the Middle Ages (q.v.) its juice was used in the anaesthetic sponge and in witchcraft (q.v.) to cause hallucinations (q.v.), frenzy, and convulsions. In the sixteenth century, it was often put into beer illegally to make it more intoxicating. In Eastern medicine it is still used for maniacal excitement, epilepsy (q.v.), dementia, insomnia, and hysteria (q.v.), as well as for many physical disorders.
Bibliography: le Strange, R. 1977. *A history of herbal plants.*

HENDERSON, SIR DAVID KENNEDY (1884-1965). A Scottish psychiatrist. He was trained by Adolf Meyer (q.v.) and became the senior resident physician of the Henry Phipps Psychiatric Clinic (q.v.). He was superintendent of the Glasgow Asylum for Lunatics (q.v.), later known as the Glasgow Royal Mental Hospital, and later professor of psychiatry at the University of Edinburgh. He collaborated with Robert D. Gillespie (q.v.) to write *A Textbook of Psychiatry for Students and Practitioners,* which was published in 1927. His *The Evolution of Psychiatry in Scotland* (1964) is a valuable contribution to the history of psychiatry.

HENRY I (1068-1135). A king of England and the son of William the Conqueror (1027-1087). He reformed the English legal system. The *Leges Henrici Primi,* 78. 7 state that the mentally ill are to be cared for by their parents: "insanos et ejusmodi maleficos debent parentes sui misericorditer custodire."
Bibliography: Walker, N. D. 1968. *Crime and insanity in England.*

HENRY IV (1367-1413). A king of England during a turbulent period. In 1403 he ordered two of his chaplains to inquire into the affairs of Bethlem Royal Hospital (q.v.) because of reported mismanagement involving those in charge of the patients. Although an intelligent and able ruler, toward the end of his life Henry lost his sense of judgment through an obsessive (*see*

OBSESSION) fear of losing the throne. In his last years he became senile, and it is said that he suffered from fits and trances.
Bibliography: Kirby, J. L. 1970. *Henry IV of England.*

HENRY VI (1422-1471). A king of England. He succeeded his father when he was less than twelve months old. A pious and weak-minded man, he was ruled by his uncles and by his strong-willed and power-hungry wife, Margaret of Anjou (1430?-1482). He was a protector of learning and founded Eton and King's College in Cambridge. In 1453, he became insane, lost his memory (q.v.), and was paralyzed, which led to the election of Richard of York (1411-1460) as protector. The Privy Council gave John Arundell (q.v.) and other physicians the authority to treat Henry. They used the then standard treatment of purges (q.v.), baths, and shaving of the head. Henry recovered for a brief period and resumed power but again suffered episodes of insanity with visual and auditory hallucinations (q.v.) that lasted until his death. He was imprisoned in the Tower of London by his rival, Edward (1442-1483), son of Richard of York, who had him murdered. For some time after his death he was considered a saint and a martyr.
Bibliography: Christie, M. E. 1922. *Henry VI.*

HENRY OF FORDWICH. In the chronicle edited by E. A. Abbot *Life and Miracles of Saint Thomas of Canterbury* (Thomas à Becket [1118?-1170], it is reported that a madman, Henry of Fordwich, was dragged struggling and shouting to the tomb of the saint. He spent a day and a night in the church and returned home cured. A painted window in the Trinity chapel of Canterbury Cathedral (q.v.) commemorates a similar miracle.
Bibliography: O'Donoghue, E. G. 1914. *The story of Bethlem Hospital.*

HENRY PHIPPS PSYCHIATRIC CLINIC. A psychiatric unit attached to Johns Hopkins Hospital in Baltimore, Maryland. It was planned by Adolf Meyer (q.v.), who was its medical director, and founded by Henry Phipps. When the clinic was opened in 1913, the *American Journal of Psychiatry* (q.v.) dedicated a special issue to the addresses delivered by the many distinguished figures at its inauguration.

HENRY THE NAVIGATOR (1394-1460). A Portuguese prince, son of King John of Portugal (1357-1433) and Philippa of Lancaster. He and his four brothers disliked women. His palace housed mostly young men who were trained to undertake voyages of discovery. The Madeira Islands were discovered by his sailors in 1418 and Sierra Leone in 1460, but Henry himself disliked the sea and never sailed on a voyage of discovery. It has been argued that he was a homosexual (*see* HOMOSEXUALITY).
Bibliography: Ure, J. 1977. *Prince Henry the Navigator.*

HENSCHEN, SALOMON (1847-1930). A Swedish physician, professor of medicine at the University of Uppsala in Sweden, and a pioneer in modern

neurology (q.v.). He wrote on aphasia, agraphia, and the pathways of the senses, as well as on the histology of the cerebral cortex and idiocy (*see* IDIOT). Many of his findings were not immediately accepted, and he was compelled to defend his ideas. Henschen was an indefatigable campaigner against prostitution and alcoholism (q.v.). When Nikolai Lenin (q.v.) showed signs of cerebral disorder, he was one of the specialists consulted.
Bibliography: Haymaker, W., and Schiller, F. 1970. *The founders of neurology.* 2d. ed.

HENSING, JOHANN THOMAS (1683-1726). A German physician and professor of medicine at the University of Glessen. In 1719 he published a monograph on his chemical examination of the brain. He succeeded in isolating phosphorus from the brain tissue and speculated on the purpose of this substance in brain functioning.
Bibliography: Haymaker, W., and Schiller, F. 1970. *The founders of neurology.* 2d. ed.

HEPBURN, JAMES, EARL OF BOTHWELL (1536?-1578). Third husband of Mary Queen of Scots (1542-1587). He married her in 1567 after an irregular divorce from his wife. He was involved in numerous plots and intrigues and was suspected of murdering Lord Henry Darnley (1545-1567), the Queen's previous husband. In 1570 his divorce from Mary was granted by the Pope. The last ten years of his life were spent in prison, where he gradually became insane.
Bibliography: Fraser, A. 1969. *Mary, Queen of Scots.*

HERACLES. A mythological Greek hero, said to be the son of Zeus and Alcmene. He was called Hercules by the Romans. His main characteristic was exceptional strength, which he used in many dangerous undertakings. According to various myths, he suffered from periodic insanity, and was said to have killed his friend Iphitus and his own children in fits of insane fury. Presumably this caused him to be considered epileptic (*see* EPILEPSY) and hence the term *Mal d'Hercules* for epilepsy. Heracles went to Delphi for a cure and, in the midst of a fit, smashed the sacred tripod. It was also said that he killed his teacher Linus by throwing a musical instrument at his head. After his fits he was said to fall asleep and awake unaware of his acts, which is symptomatic of postepileptic confusional states. Euripides (q.v.) described a number of his attacks, and Seneca (q.v.) based his tragedy *Hercules Furens* on these descriptions. His jealous wife Deianira sent him a shirt steeped in the blood of a centaur in the hope of regaining his affection, but the garment was poisoned and caused Heracles so much agony that he elected to die. Deianira hanged herself in guilt and remorse.
Bibliography: Euripides. *Madness of Hercules*, trans A. S. Way.

HERACLITUS (c.536-470 B.C.). A Greek philosopher and scientist born in Ephesus. Because of his gloomy view of life, he is known as the "weeping

philosopher." His pronouncements were always cryptic. He attacked religious practices, the belief in prophetic dreams (q.v.), and the cult of images. He based his theories on the rhythm of nature: life and death, health and disease, sleeping and waking. According to him fire (q.v.) was the fundamental element, and mental health depended on the fire within man. A dry soul was healthy, while a humid one would produce insanity or idiocy (*see* IDIOT). He was probably the first Greek philosopher to assert that each individual is different. He originated the term *enantiodromia* (q.v.), which Carl G. Jung (q.v.) used to denote a return to the opposite after a journey through the unconscious (q.v.).
Bibliography: Kirk, G. S., ed., 1954. *Heraclitus: the cosmic fragments.*

HERBART, JOHANN FRIEDRICH (1776-1841). A German philosopher-psychologist. He was educated by his mother and did not go to school until he was twelve years old. Although he developed a precocious interest in philosophy, his interest later shifted toward education, and he dedicated his studies to practical pedagogical problems. Opposing the theories of Immanuel Kant (q.v.), he developed his own system of psychology which he taught at the universities of Königsberg and Gottingen. Herbart held a dynamic conception of the mind and agreed with the pedagogical methods of Johann Pestalozzi (q.v.) and Friedrich Froebel (q.v.), which were based on experience rather than on formal instruction. He used the term "apperception" to indicate conscious mental content, which he believed is achieved when the strongest ideas drive other ideas out of the field of consciousness. Herbart is regarded as the originator of scientific pedagogy founded on psychology.
Bibliography: Davidson, J. 1906. *A new interpretation of Herbart's psychology.*

HERCULES. *See* HERACLES.

HERDER, JOHANN GOTTFRIED VON (1744-1803). A German philosopher and poet. He was acquainted with Johann Wolfgang von Goethe (q.v.), who helped him to obtain several official positions at the court of Weimar. Herder believed that mankind evolved according to a divine plan, which he described in his *Ideas for a Philosophy of the History of Mankind* (1784-1791). He felt that cultural evolution and the environment, which he believed were closely related, influenced man's history. He approached the understanding of human nature by postulating the unity of psychological functions with the soma. This approach has caused him to be considered an early follower of dynamic psychology.
Bibliography: Clark, R. T. 1955. *Herder: his life and thought.*

HEREDITARY NATURE OF CRIME, THE. A book published in Great Britain in 1870. It was written by J. B. Thomson (1810-1873), resident

surgeon of the general prison for Scotland in Perth. Thomson stated that "the business of Prison Surgeons must always be with mental diseases" and that "the treatment of crime is a branch of psychology." He believed that criminality was hereditary and that criminals belonged to a distinct class, had peculiar physical and mental characteristics, and frequently suffered from epilepsy (q.v.), insanity and other mental diseases. He also argued that criminality was incurable, which, according to him, proved "its hereditary nature."
Bibliography: Sanders, W. B., ed. 1976. *Juvenile delinquency.*

HERING, EWALD (1834-1918). A German physiologist. Opposing the theories of Hermann Helmholtz (q.v.) he studied the problems of visual space perception and developed a theory of color vision. He also wrote about memory (q.v.), which he regarded as a universal biological principle through which organic matter recapitulates its past history. According to him sensations depend on consciousness.
Bibliography: Alexander, F. G., and Selesnick, S. T. 1966. *The history of psychiatry.*

HERMAPHRODITUS. The son of Hermes and Aphrodite in Greek mythology (q.v.). The nymph Salmacis so loved him that she was granted union with him in one body, and all those who bathed in the fountain dedicated to her acquired male and female characteristics in the same body. The idea of double sexuality is found in a number of ancient Greek cults and marriage customs. Oriental androgynous cults are older and reflect the same idea.
Bibliography: Licht, H. 1971. *Sexual life in ancient Greece.*

HEROD AGRIPPA II (A.D. 27-100). A Jewish king of Chalcis. He never achieved his political ambitions and failed to become king of Judea. Although Mosaic law condemned incest (q.v.), Herod lived with his sister Berenice and openly acknowledged their relationship. After the fall of Jerusalem they went to Rome, and Berenice became the mistress of Titus (A.D. 40?-81), conqueror of Judea, thus providing Agrippa with more reasons for his bitterness.
Bibliography: Jordan, R. 1974. *Berenice.*

HERODOTUS (c.484-c.425 B.C.). A Greek historian, sometimes referred to as the "Father of History." His histories contain many descriptions of abnormal behavior such as the story of Cleomenes (q.v.) whose madness Herodotus attributed to either divine punishment or excessive drinking. He also described cauterization (q.v.) of the head, which was used by the Libyans to prevent epilepsy (q.v.).
Bibliography: Myres, J. L. 1953. *Herodotus: father of history.*

HEROD THE GREAT (c.73 B.C.-4 B.C.). A king of Judea. His life was a remarkable demonstration of homicide and sadism (q.v.). On his accession

to the throne, he massacred every member of the Hasmonaean family. In 30 B.C. he executed the high priest Hyrcanus. In 29 B.C. he murdered his second wife Mariamne (q.v.). In 28 B.C. his mother Alexandra suffered the same fate. He later executed three of his sons. He was of a paranoid (*see* PARANOIA) disposition. He had ten wives and fourteen children. In the New Testament there is an account of the massacre of the Innocents at Bethlehem (Matt. 2. 16), which is attributed to him.
Bibliography: Gross, W. J. 1968. *Herod the great.*

HEROIN. An ester of morphine (q.v.), which in turn is derived from opium (q.v.). It was discovered in 1898 by Heinrich Dreser (q.v.). At first it was believed to be less addictive than morphine and was used to treat morphine addiction, but by 1902 it was recognized as a dangerous and habit-forming drug (q.v.).
Bibliography: Morton, J. F. 1977. *Major medicinal plants.*

HEROPHILUS OF CHALCEDON (c.335-280 B.C.). A Greek physician and founder of an early school of medicine in Alexandria. He and Erasistratus (q.v.) are considered the originators of neuroanatomy. Both Celsus (q.v.) and Tertullianus (q.v.) report that Herophilus dissected live animals. In opposition to Aristotle (q.v.), who considered the heart (q.v.) the center of everything, he recognized the brain as the central organ of the nervous system. Herophilus gave the first clear description of the ventricles of the brain. He is remembered now for his description of the confluences of the sinuses and the chorioid plexuses.
See also BRAIN, CONCEPTS OF.
Bibliography: Phillips, E. D. 1973. *Greek medicine.*

HERPESTIS MONNIERA. Thyme-leaved gratiola, a creeping annual plant found in marshy grounds in Pakistan and India. It is used in Eastern medicine for the treatment of epilepsy (q.v.) and of insanity.

HERRICK, ROBERT (1591-1674). An English clergyman and poet. His poetry was sensuous, but the many mistresses he wrote about were mostly imaginary. His descriptions of the rural rites of the time contain an almost pagan awareness of the worship of the soul. His poem *The Mad Maid* (1648) deals with insanity.
Bibliography: Nevius, B. 1963. *Robert Herrick.*

HERRISON HOSPITAL. A mental hospital in Dorset, England. The name is derived from the land on which it stands, which in the twelfth century had belonged to Terri Haereng (later corrupted to Herrison). The first asylum for the area had been founded at Forston by Francis John Browne in 1827, who offered his mansion, seven acres of land, and a large sum of money for an "asylum for thé benefit of pauper lunatics." Following the conversion of the mansion, the asylum was opened in 1832 with sixty-five patients. After many extensions, it was transferred to a new building at Herrison in 1863.

HERVEY DE SAINT-DENIS, MARIE JEAN LÉON (1823-1892). A French man of letters and a lecturer in Chinese language and literature. Beginning when he was thirteen years old, he recorded the dreams (q.v.) of nineteen hundred and forty-six nights over a period of twenty years. In 1867 he published anonymously a book entitled *Dreams and the Means to Direct Them*. It recorded his own dream experiences and how he had trained himself to master the content of his dreams. It also presented a survey of previous dream theories. Sigmund Freud (q.v.) quoted the book and lamented the fact that he had never been able to obtain a copy of it, because of its rarity.
Bibliography: Ellenberger, H. F. 1970. *The discovery of the unconscious.*

HESELTINE, PHILIP ARNOLD (1894-1930). An English composer, better known under the pseudonym Peter Warlock. He was a great admirer of Frederick Delius (q.v.) and a friend of D. H. Lawrence (q.v.). His music was Elizabethan in style. He committed suicide (q.v.) by gas poisoning, following a life of emotional discord.
Bibliography: Gray, C. 1934. *Peter Warlock: a memoir of Philip Heseltine.*

HESSE, HERMANN (1877-1962). A German novelist and poet. Because he was a pacifist, he emigrated to Switzerland at the beginning of World War I and became a Swiss citizen in 1923. He underwent a Jungian analysis and had some treatment from Carl G. Jung (q.v.) himself. His novels involve the struggle of the individual for an integrated and harmonious life. In his *Demian* (1919) he used analytic psychology to study incest (q.v.). Other works dealt with withdrawal from the world and aspects of man's nature. His language is sensuous and full of sensitivity and understanding. He was awarded the Nobel Prize for literature in 1946.
Bibliography: Boulby, M. 1967. *Hermann Hesse: his mind and art.*

HICKOK, LAURENS PERSEUS (1798-1888). An American clergyman and philosopher, professor of mental and moral philosophy at Union College in New York. He may have been the first to develop psychology as a science in the United States. In 1849 he published *Rational Psychology*, which contains an historical introduction that covers philosophical concepts from Aristotle (q.v.) to Immanuel Kant (q.v.) before proceeding to a discussion of a general theory of perception, which he called "sense psychology," understanding, and reason. In 1854, he published a second book, *Empirical Psychology*, which in its last revision was subtitled *The Human Mind as*

Given in Consciousness. In this volume, he advocated a classification of the "facts of mind" as they "come within everyman's own experience."
Bibliography: Harms, E. 1972. America's first major psychologist, Laurens Perseus Hickok. *J. Hist. behav. Sci.* 8:120-23.

HIGGINS, GODFREY (1773-1833). An English archaeologist and magistrate. In 1813 William Vickers appeared before him accused of assault. Higgins found him insane and sent him to York Lunatic Asylum (q.v.) in spite of the pleas of Vicker's wife, who feared that he would be mistreated there. Some months later she again appealed to Higgins to release her husband, who was now ill from starvation and general mistreatment. Higgins investigated the case, and his investigation led to a wider inquiry into the management of the York Asylum and eventually to improved conditions there and in other hospitals. His enormous correspondence with Samuel Tuke (q.v.) shows how they joined forces to promote the interests of the insane.
Bibliography: Tuke, S. 1813. Reprint 1964. *Description of the retreat.*

HILDEGARD OF BINGEN, SAINT (1098?-1179). A German Benedictine nun, founder and abbess of the convent of Rupertsberg. She practiced medicine and wrote on medical matters, including normal and morbid psychology. She discussed insanity, frenzy, despair, obsession (q.v.), anger, and idiocy (*see* IDIOT). In her writings, she noted that "when headache and migraine and vertigo attack a patient simultaneously, they render a man foolish and upset his reason. This makes many people think that he is possessed of a demon, but that is not true." Saint Hildegard disregarded Galenic (*see* GALEN) tradition and attributed the black bile (q.v.) that was believed to cause melancholy (*see* MELANCHOLIA) not to humoral imbalance but rather to the serpent's breath that had contaminated Adam at the time of his fall. Thus, for her, melancholy was a universal affliction, rather than the temporary sickness of an individual.
Bibliography: Walsh, J.J. 1920. *Medieval medicine.*

HILL, OCTAVIA (1838-1912). An English social reformer. Both her parents were prominent public service figures, who supported industrial reforms, lending libraries, and further education for the working classes. When Octavia was fourteen years old, the family lost its considerable fortune, and she was forced to earn her own living. Her inclination for social work was encouraged by John Ruskin (q.v.), her former teacher and close friend, and led to the establishment of organized relief for poor families. Her approach included an assessment of the family, social rehabilitation, and consideration of housing, and education.
Bibliography: Moberley-Bell, E. M. 1942. *Octavia Hill.*
Thomson Hill, W. 1956. *Octavia Hill.*

HILL, ROBERT GARDINER (1811-1878). An English physician. He was house surgeon at the Lincoln Asylum (q.v.), where he experimented with

nonrestraint methods, lived among the patients, and advocated moral treatment. In his book *Total Abolition of Personal Restraint in the Treatment of the Insane*, published in 1839 he wrote that "in a properly constructed building, with sufficient number of suitable attendants, restraint [q.v.] is never necessary, never justifiable, and always injurious." He was also the proprietor of several private establishments for the mentally ill, including a house at Shilling Thorpe, Lincolnshire, that previously had belonged to Francis Willis (q.v.).
Bibliography: Hunter, R., and Macalpine, I. 1963. *Three hundred years of psychiatry*.

HILL, THOMAS (?-1599). An English writer. Among his works are two of interest to the behavioral sciences. One entitled *The most pleasante Arte of the Interpretation of Dreames* was published in London in 1567 and was successful enough to warrant further editions. In it certain events and objects appearing in dreams (q.v.) were interpreted as symbols of the dreamer's unconscious wishes and anxieties. In the other book, which was published in 1571 and entitled *The Contemplation of Mankinde, containing a singular discourse after the Art of Physiognomie, on all the members and partes of man.* . . . the author attempted a comparison between physical and psychological characteristics.
Bibliography: Hunter, R., and Macalpine, I. 1963 *Three hundred years of psychiatry*.

HILL FOLK, THE. The members of two American families living in a small town in western Massachusetts. Both families were the subject of an investigation on feeblemindedness and heredity, a fashionable field of study in the early 1900s. The investigation hoped "to show how crime, misery, and expense may result from the union of two defective individuals."
See also EUGENICS.
Bibliography: Danielson, F. A., and Davenport, C. B. 1912. *The Hill folk: report on a rural community of hereditary defectives.*

HIP. An abbreviation of the term "hypochondria" (q.v.), which was used in reference to depression. Hence "hipped" meant depressed.
Bibliography: 1978. *Brewer's dictionary of phrase and fable.*

HIPÓLITOS. Members of a religious order founded in Mexico in the sixteenth century by Bernardino Alvarez (q.v.). They were dedicated to the care of the sick, especially the mentally ill, who were treated in San Hipólito Hospital (q.v.), which was founded by Alvarez. They adopted a brown habit. In 1700, Pope Innocent XIII (1655-1704) officially recognized the order, which then became known as the Religious Order of Saint Hyppolitus.
Bibliography: Rumbaut, R. D. 1970-1971. Bernardino Alvarez: new world psychiatric pioneer. *Am. J. Psychiat.* 127:1217-221.

HIPPIES. Unconventional young people. The term was first used by young people in California in 1966 and 1967. By 1968 the movement had begun to evaporate. The cult featured a philosophy of love and peace, rejection of material property, a tendency to take drugs (q.v.), communal life styles, libertarian sexual behavior, and an unconventional style of dress that included beads, bells, flowing dresses, and long hair.

HIPPOCRATES OF COS (460–377 B.C.). A contemporary of Socrates (q.v.) and the most famous of the Greek physicians. Little is known about him. Probably none of the works ascribed to him are authentic, but his methods and doctrine are known through the works of others. He introduced principles of scientific medicine based upon observation of logic and denied the influence of spirits and demons in the production of diseases. He was a proponent of the humoral theory (q.v.), which he believed was due to wrong proportions of phlegm, blood, and black and yellow bile (q.v.). Considering the brain to be the major gland he believed that wisdom, understanding, and moral judgment were found there, and he held humidity of the brain responsible for madness. "Depravement of the brain arises from phlegm and bile; those mad from phlegm are quiet, depressed and oblivious; those from bile excited, noisy and mischievious." He recognized three forms of mental disorder: phrenitis (delirium), mania (excitement without fever), and melancholia (qq.v.) (chronic mental disturbances). He also mentioned hysteria (q.v.), which he considered to be a woman's disease. He briefly discussed the Scythian disease (q.v.) and thought that epilepsy (q.v.) was due to brain dysfunction (due to excess of phlegm in the brain) and hereditary in nature. It was particularly liable to occur if the wind was from the south for then the brain was more humid than usual. He also believed that the interpretation of dreams (q.v.) could be useful and treated mania with the root of the mandrake (q.v.)

Bibliography: Jones, W.H.S., trans. 1923, *Hippocrates. the medical works.* Sigerist, H. E. 1933. *Great doctors.*

HIRING OF LUNATICS. In Elizabethan times lunatics (q.v.) often were hired from asylums (q.v.) to provide entertainment at social functions. A chorus of lunatics appears in the tragedy *The Changeling* (q.v.) by Thomas Middleton (1570?-1627) and William Rowley (1585?–?1642).

HIRSCHFELD, MAGNUS (1868–1935). A German physician. He promoted the study of the psychological and sociological aspects of human sexual behavior. He was a homosexual transvestite and, thus, wrote subjectively on transvestism. He also wrote on intermediate sexual states and sexual pathology, as well as conducting statistical inquiries on homosexuality (q.v.). He was responsible for popularizing the term "homosexuality," which was coined by Károly Mária Benkert. Hirschfeld believed that the difference between the sexes was a matter of degree and advocated tolerance toward sexual deviants. In 1899 he became the editor of the *Yearbook of Inter-*

mediate Sexual States to which Sigmund Freud (q.v.) and Auguste Forel (q.v.) contributed articles. He also founded the World League for Sexual Reform.
Bibliography: Ellis, A., and Abarbanel, A., eds. 1961. *The encyclopaedia of sexual behaviour.*

HIS, WILHELM (1831-1904). A Swiss neurologist active in the field of the developmental analysis of the nervous system. His discoveries necessitated the introduction of new concepts and he coined the terms *dendrite, neurite, neuroblast,* as well as other words that are now familiar. In 1886 he began to work for the foundation of the Brain Commission, which, in 1908, established the Central Institute for Brain Research in Amsterdam, the Netherlands. He contributed to anthropology with his book *Crania Helvetiae,* which was written in 1864 in collaboration with Ludwig Rütimeyer (1825–1895). He lived and worked most of his rather Spartan life in Leipzig. When human remains were found there in a local churchyard he was asked to identify them. He confirmed that they were the remains of Johann Sebastian Bach (1685–1750).
Bibliography: Haymaker, W. and Schiller, F. 1970. *The founders of neurology.* 2d. ed.

HISTORY OF RASSELAS, PRINCE OF ABYSSINIA, THE A philosophical romance by Samuel Johnson (q.v.). It was written in 1759, a month after his mother's death, to pay for her funeral expenses. It depicts the prince's disillusionments in his quest for happiness, and it is said to be autobiographical.
Bibliography: Grange, K. M. 1962. Dr. Samuel Johnson's account of a schizophrenic illness in Rasselas (1759). *Med. Hist.* 6: 162-68.

HITCH, SAMUEL (1800-1881). A British physician. He put into practice his progressive ideas on the management of the insane at the Gloucester Lunatic Asylum (q.v.). He introduced trial leave, parole, female nurses in male wards, and self-governing units. In 1841 he was one of the founders and the first secretary of the Association of Medical Officers of Asylums and Hospitals for the Insane (q.v.).
Bibliography: Hunter, R., and Macalpine, I. 1963. *Three hundred years of psychiatry.*

HITLER, ADOLF (1889-1945). An Austrian-born German dictator. As a youth he was interested in art and thought that he would become a great artist. This delusion (q.v.) caused him to neglect other school subjects and disregard examinations with predictably disastrous results. His failures in school caused him to hate intellectuals. After dropping out of high school and twice failing the admission examinations for the academy of art, he lived by doing odd jobs. Most of his time was spent in political argument. At the

start of World War I, he joined the Bavarian army and rose no higher than corporal. After the failure of the "Beer Hall Putsch" in 1923, he was imprisoned for his political activities, and, while in prison, he dictated his book *Mein Kampf*, which expresses his brutal opportunism, his contempt for people, and his fanaticism. He became chancellor of Germany in January 1933 and by March 1933 was in absolute power. During World War II, the United States Office of Strategic Services commissioned a psychological report on Hitler, who emerged from it as an hysterical (*see* HYSTERIA) psychopathic (*see* PSYCHOPATHY) personality, given to rages, swings of mood, and perverted sexual practices. He married his mistress, Eva Braun (1912–1945), in his Berlin bunker, and after the ceremony they are believed to have committed suicide.
Bibliography: Langer, W. 1973. *The mind of Adolf Hitler.*

HITSCHMANN, EDWARD (1871-1957). An Austrian physician. Paul Federn (q.v.) introduced him to Sigmund Freud (q.v.). He became interested in "pathographies," biographies written from the medical and psychological point of view, and investigated, using statistical questionnaires, the sexual life of healthy people. His psychoanalytic studies of literary personalities led him to believe that traumatic experiences in childhood often act as a creative stimulus and that the father is of great significance in the destiny of an individual. In 1938, fleeing from the Nazis, he went to London, and in 1940, he emigrated to Boston, Massachusetts, where he worked at the Psychoanalytic Institute.
Bibliography: Alexander, F.; Eisenstein, S.; and Grothjan, M., eds. 1966 *Psychoanalytic pioneers.*

HITZIG, EDUARD (1838-1907). A German neurologist. He experimented with electrical stimulation of the brain and demonstrated the localization of the motor areas in the brain cortex.
Bibliography: Haymaker, W., and Schiller, F. 1970. *The founders of neurology.* 2d. ed.

HOBBES, THOMAS (1588-1679). An English philosopher. He opposed supernatural explanations of phenomena and advocated deductive methods of inquiry. His psychology was based on sense perception and he believed that the instinct for preservation and the need to seek pleasure and avoid pain regulated all psychological phenomena. He originated the doctrine of association, dependent on the temporal sequence in which sensations are perceived, and appreciated the influence of emotion on memory (q.v.). According to him, men were basically antisocial and needed coercion to live peacefully. Hobbes greatly influenced the doctrine of economic determinism

and a scientific approach to legislation. His principal works include *Human Nature* (1650) and *Leviathan* (1651).
Bibliography: Watkins, J.W.N. 1965. *Hobbes's system of ideas.*

HOBBIDIDANCE. A malevolent spirit. One of the five fiends that tormented the madman, Poor Tom, in William Shakespeare's (q.v.) *King Lear* (4.1).

HOBGOBLIN. A mischievious sprite. The term is used also to indicate an object that inspires superstitious fear.
Bibliography: 1978. *Brewer's dictionary of phrase and fable.*

HOBHOUSE, LEONARD TRELAWNEY (1864-1929). An English philosopher and sociologist. He studied the anthropological and psychological aspects of society and believed that biological and spiritual development in man occur simultaneously. Of his many works, *Mind in Evolution* (1901) is the most relevant to psychology.
Bibliography: Ginsberg, M., and Hobson, J. A. 1931. *L.T. Hobhouse: his life and work.*

HOCCLEVE, THOMAS. *See* OCCLEVE, THOMAS.

HOCH, AUGUST (1868-1919). A Swiss psychiatrist. He emigrated to the United States and, after various appointments, became director of the Psychiatric Institute of the New York State hospitals and professor of psychiatry at Cornell University. He emphasized the need to assess the premorbid personality of a patient in order to arrive at an accurate diagnosis. He believed that dementia praecox (q.v.) was related to hereditary and environmental factors and encouraged hospitals to keep case histories for research purposes.
Bibliography: Zilboorg, G. 1941. *A history of medical psychology.*

HOCHE, ALFRED (1865-1943). A German psychiatrist who performed research in the field of organic disorders of the nervous system. He asserted that psychoanalysis (q.v.) was not a scientific approach but rather a form of "magical medicine" that produced cures because of the attention lavished on the patients by the physicians.
Bibliography: Ellenberger, H. F. 1970. *The discovery of the unconscious.*

HOEFER, WOLFGANG (1614-1681). A physician at the Viennese court. In his *Hercules Medicus* (1657) he described the cretins (*see* CRETINISM) found in the Austrian Alps and offered diagnostic criteria for their condition.
Bibliography: Kanner, L. 1964. *A history of the care and study of the mentally retarded.*

HOFFMANN, ERNST THEODOR WILHELM (*or* AMADEUS) (1776-1822). A German composer and romantic (*see* ROMANTICISM) writer. He

altered Wilhelm to Amadeus in honor of Wolfgang Amadeus Mozart (1756–1791). His parents separated, and left him to be brought up by relatives. He was nervous and moody. When he was already married and in his mid-thirties, he fell in love (q.v.) with one of his pupils, a young girl with a beautiful voice. Her family married her to an elderly drunkard, and Hoffman, in a state of hopeless passion, idealized her in his writings. His work displays his fascination with magnetism (q.v.), which he regarded as a kind of possession (q.v.) of one person by another. Although his life was shortened by alcoholism (q.v.), he wrote two novels and some fifty short stories mostly about somnambulism (q.v.), double personality, delusions (q.v.), and other psychological states. He is the central figure in the opera *The Tales of Hoffman* by Jacques Offenbach (1819-1880).
Bibliography: Negus, K. 1965. *E.T.A. Hoffmann's other world.*

HOFFMANN, FRIEDRICH (1660-1742). A German professor of medicine at the University of Halle and physician to Frederick the Great (q.v.). He was the leader of the iatromechanical school and believed that disease was caused by the presence of an undefined substance that produced spasms if overabundant and exhaustion if deficient. Treatment was designed to make the patient calmer or more energetic, as required, by drugs (q.v.) composed of various chemicals. He regarded melancholy (*see* MELANCHOLIA) as the first degree of mania (q.v.).
Bibliography: Zilboorg, G. 1941. *A history of medical psychology.*

HOFFMANN, HEINRICH (1809-1894). A German physician and author of children's books. He was in charge of the psychiatric hospital in Frankfurt-on-Main, where he founded the first department specifically for emotionally disturbed children. Under the pseudonym of Reimerich Kinderlieb he wrote and illustrated *Struwwelpeter* (1847), the story of "shock-headed Peter," a horrid unkempt boy with straw-like hair, nails that were never cut and dirty hands. In the nineteenth century *Struwwelpeter* was considered a good moral tale for teaching children the dire consequences of disobedience, and it was translated into several languages. In more recent years it has been regarded as psychologically harmful to young readers.

HOFFMANN, JOHANN (1857-1919). A German neurologist. He observed that in hemiplegics snapping of the index or ring finger produces flexion of the thumb because of organic brain lesion. This phenomenon now is known as the Hoffmann's sign.
Bibliography: 1969. *Garrison's history of neurology*, ed. L. C. McHenry.

HOFFMANN, MORITZ (1622-1698). A German anatomist and botanist. In 1662 he suggested that melancholia (q.v.) could be cured by blood transfusion (q.v.), rather than bleeding (q.v.).
Bibliography: Zilboorg, G. 1941. *A history of medical psychology.*

HOFMANN, ALBERT (1906-). A Swiss chemist. In 1943, while experimenting with lysergic acid diethylamide (LSD) (q.v.), a derivative of rye (q.v.) ergot (q.v.), he accidentally sniffed the substance and discovered that it was a potent hallucinogen.

Bibliography: Alexander, F. G., and Selesnick, S. T. 1966. *The history of psychiatry.*

HOGAR DE BENEFICENCIA DE SAN JUAN. The first mental hospital in Puerto Rico. It was founded in 1844.

Bibliography: Leon, C. A., and Rosselli, H. 1975. Latin America. In *World history of psychiatry*, ed. J. G. Howells.

HOGARTH, WILLIAM (1697-1764). An English painter, engraver, and satirist. Many of his subjects illustrate his condemnation of eighteenth-century customs and practices. His famous series *The Rake's Progress* (q.v.) includes a scene in Bedlam (q.v.) that indicates the attitudes of patients and visitors. The engraving *Gin Lane* is a blistering commentary on alcoholism (q.v.).

Bibliography: Jarrett, D. 1976. *The ingenious Mr. Hogarth.*

HOLBACH, PAUL HENRI DIETRICH, BARON D' (1723-1789). A French materialistic philosopher. He opposed religious doctrine and held enlightened views on suicide (q.v.). In 1770 he wrote *Le Système de la Nature* in which he denied the existence of God, presented intellect and sensibility as functions of matter, and stated that the end of mankind is happiness.

Bibliography: Wickwar, W. H. 1935. *Baron d'Holbach: a prelude to the French Revolution.*

HOLBEIN, HANS, THE YOUNGER (1497-1543). A Bavarian historical artist and court painter to Henry VIII (1491-1547). He illustrated Desiderus Erasmus' (q.v.) *Praise of Folly* (q.v.) and Thomas More's (q.v.) *Utopia* (1516). He was said to be a dissolute man, given to drinking, unable to maintain a good relationship with his family, and spending little time with his wife and children. Yet when he died, his will included provision for two illegitimate children.

Bibliography: Wittkower, R., and Wittkower, M. 1963. *Born under Saturn.*

HÖLDERLIN, JOHANN CHRISTIAN FRIEDRICH (1770-1843). A German poet and writer. He was orphaned as an infant. After qualifying in theology, he refused to enter the church and became a children's tutor. He hoped to be helped by Johann Schiller (q.v.) but found him too overwhelming. His great passion for Susette Gontard, whose children he tutored, inspired much of his poetry, but his romance ended abruptly when he quarreled with her husband. His first nervous breakdown occurred when he was asked to preach in the private chapel of a new employer. From 1806 on, he was regarded as an incurable schizophrenic (*see* SCHIZOPHRENIA).

After a spell in the asylum at Tubingen in 1808, he was boarded out (*see* BOARDING-OUT OF MENTAL PATIENTS) with a cabinetmaker until his death.
Bibliography: Ryan, L. J. 1962. *Friedrich Hölderlin*.

HOLERGASIA. A term introduced by Adolph Meyer (q.v.). It indicates a complete lack of integrated mental activity.

HOLLAND, HENRY (1788-1873). A fashionable English physician. Among his patients were Queen Caroline, William IV (1765-1837), Queen Victoria (1819-1901) and Prince Albert. His lucrative practice allowed him to indulge in his passion for travel. In 1817, after observing patients affected by pellagra (q.v.) in Italy, he wrote a paper describing the severe mental disorders that could result from it and that often led to dementia or suicide (q.v.).
Bibliography: Holland, H. 1817. On the pellagra, a disease prevailing in Lombardy. *Medico-Chirurgical Transactions*. 8:317-48.

HOLLOWAY, THOMAS (1800-1883). A Cornish patent medicine vendor. He worked in the family's grocery shop in Penzance, Cornwall, England, but his ambition and drive eventually made him a wealthy man. He relentlessly advertised himself and the pills and ointments that he sold. When he heard Lord Anthony Shaftesbury speak on the need for a semicharitable middle-class asylum (q.v.), he was so impressed that he decided to make the construction of such an asylum his life work. Holloway Sanatorium (q.v.) was the result of his generosity. He applied his business acumen and his genius for advertisement to its creation. He insisted that it should be built in red brick so that it could be seen by the maximum number of people and chose a site between two railway lines for the same reason. He died a few months before it was finished.
Bibliography: Anon. 1933. *The story of Thomas Holloway*.

HOLLOWAY SANATORIUM. An English hospital for mental disorders opened in 1887 at Virginia Water in Surrey. Funds for it were provided by Thomas Holloway (q.v.) on the advice of Lord Anthony Shaftesbury (q.v.).
Bibliography: Anon. 1933. *The story of Thomas Holloway*.

HOLLY HOUSE. A private asylum (q.v.) in the Hoxton district of London. It was founded in 1792 by John Burrows and continued after his death in 1799 by his widow Mrs. Esther Burrows and his son George William Burrows. James Parkinson (q.v.) was its visiting physician. By 1819 it housed 118 private patients. Holly House was probably the best of the Hoxton madhouses (q.v.).
Bibliography: Parry-Jones, W. Ll. 1972. *The trade in lunacy*.

HOLMES, SIR GORDON MORGAN (1876-1965). A British physician and neurologist, born in Dublin, Ireland (q.v.). In 1911 he and Henry Head

(q.v.) were the first to describe the concept of body-image, or the mental idea each person has of his own body. He developed a test for ataxia that demonstrates the loss of cerebellar control on the coordination of movements. Some of the functions of the thalamus were also elucidated by him.
Bibliography: Critchley, M. 1979. *The divine banquet of the brain.*

HOLMES, OLIVER WENDELL (1809-1894). An American doctor and poet. In 1870 he wrote a paper entitled "Mechanism in Thought and Morals" in which he described a number of automatic, unconscious mechanisms that caused him to be uncertain of the existence of free choice. He, therefore, thought the theory of moral irresponsibility was questionable and elaborated on this idea in a paper in 1875 entitled "Crime and Automatism."
Bibliography: Bowen, C. D. 1948. *Yankee from Olympus.*

HOLMES, SHERLOCK. A fictional detective in the stories of Sir Arthur Conan Doyle (q.v.). He was endowed with amazing mental qualities and represented as an eccentric individual with peculiar mannerisms. He would take repeated doses of cocaine (q.v.) but was never addicted to it, reflecting the then common belief that the drug was not addictive. Holmes was modeled in part on Dr. Joseph Bell (1837-1911), an eminent Edinburgh surgeon and one of Doyle's teachers. He often suggested to Doyle problems for Holmes to solve.
Bibliography: Doyle, A. C. 1952. *The complete Sherlock Holmes.*

HOLST, FREDRIK (1791-1871). A Norwegian physician. He was interested in mental disorders and persuaded the Norwegian parliament to investigate the condition of the mentally ill. A commission, established in 1824, recommended the creation of four mental hospitals.
Bibliography: Retterstøl, N. 1975. Scandinavia. In *World history of psychiatry*, ed. J. G. Howells.

HOLT, EDWIN BISSELL (1873-1946). An American psychologist who taught at the universities of Harvard and Princeton. An erudite and versatile man, he believed that the key to the explanation of mind was to be found in the study of behavior. Among his works are *The Concept of Consciousness* (1914) and *Animal Drive and the Learning Process* (1931).
Bibliography: Boring, E. G. 1950. *A history of experimental psychology.*

HOLY DISEASE. The ancient belief that some diseases were caused by gods. Hippocrates (q.v.) in the treatise *On the Sacred Disease* asserted that no maladies, including insanity and epilepsy (q.v.), were holy diseases but rather they were all natural phenomena. Plato (q.v.), however, believed that a form of insanity was a gift of the gods, whose divine breath could inspire prophets and grant them a knowledge of the future. Aretaeus of Cappadocia (q.v.), and Caelius Aurelianus (q.v.) also believed in holy delirium (q.v.). The belief that the insane are divinely protected and have special powers of clairvoyance has been common in many cultures at various times.

HOLY GHOST HOUSE. A name given to houses established for the poor and the sick in Sweden and Finland in the sixteenth century. During the Reformation, they usually were founded in monasteries that had been confiscated. In 1551 King Gustavus I (q.v.) founded a Holy Ghost House at Danviken, near Stockholm. Since he was interested especially in the care of the mentally ill, this institution may have sheltered them from its beginnings. In the eighteenth century it had an annexe that was used as a madhouse and was then the only institution in Sweden capable of accommodating a large number of mental patients. At Åbo (Turku) (q.v.), Finland, a Holy Ghost house existed as early as 1396.
See also ASYLUMS.
Bibliography: Retterstøl, N. 1975. Scandinavia. In *World history of psychiatry*, ed. J. G. Howells.

HOLY TRINITY HOSPITAL. A medieval hospital in Salisbury, England. It was established in the fourteenth century to care for the physically ill and women in childbirth, but it also received mad people, the "furiosi." It may have been one of the first hospitals in England to admit the mentally ill.
Bibliography: Walsh, J. J. 1920. *Medieval medicine.*

HOLY WELLS. Wells believed to have curative powers. Originally associated with water deities, they became associated with saints and holy men during the Middle Ages (q.v.). The mentally ill were often taken in pilgrimage to them, and they would bathe or drink the miraculous waters. Such wells have existed in many countries. In Thailand, for example, the well of Phran Boon Larng Nuer (q.v.) is still believed to have curative properties. In Scotland several wells and springs were dedicated to Saint Fillan, and in Wales they were often dedicated to Saint Winifred and Saint David. In Ireland Glen-na-Galt (q.v.) was a famous place of healing.
See also KHALUNE-ARSHAN SPRING, LLANDEGLIA, SAINT FILLAN POOL, SAINT MAREE WELL, SAINT NUN'S POOL, SAINT RONAN'S WELL, SAINT ROSAMUND'S POND, and SAINT WINIFRED'S WELL.

HOME, DANIEL DUNGLAS (1833-1886). A Scottish spiritualistic medium (q.v.). He became famous for his seances during which pianos and heavy furniture would float about and musical instruments would play by themselves. He was adopted by an aunt in America but was asked to leave because mysterious rappings disturbed her home when he was present. It was believed that he could fly in and out of windows and was immune to fire burns. Robert Browning (q.v.), who attended his seances wrote a poem

about him entitled *Sludge the Medium* in 1864. He performed in the presence of many European sovereigns, but he was expelled from Rome after he was accused of witchcraft (q.v.). In 1871 Sir William Crookes, (1832-1919), a distinguished physicist, conducted experiments with Home in full light and was convinced of his powers.
Bibliography: Home, Mrs. Daniel Dunglas. 1888. *D. D. Home: his life and mission.*

HOMER. Greek poet. He is said to have lived between the twelfth and eighth century B.C., and he is believed to have written The *Iliad* and the *Odyssey* (q.v.). These works contain many references to madness, which in the Homeric tradition was manifested by unusual behavior, as well as delusions (q.v.) and hallucinations (q.v.). Madness was believed to be a holy disease (q.v.) that was sent by the gods as either a gift or a punishment. The *Odyssey* also contains a mention of nepenthes (q.v.), a drug, which was added to the wine offered to Helen's guests to relieve their sorrows.
Bibliography: Bowra, C. M. 1972. *Homer.*

HOMME MACHINE. A term introduced by René Descartes (q.v.) to indicate the mechanical essence of man, whom he regarded as a physicomathematical apparatus.
Bibliography: Zilboorg, G. 1941. *A history of medical psychology.*

HOMOSEXUALITY. Sexual relations between members of the same sex. The term, a Latin root with a Greek prefix, was coined in 1869 by the Hungarian writer Károly Mária Benkert (who changed his name to Kertbeny in 1848), and was popularized by Magnus Hirschfeld (q.v.). "Uranism" (q.v.) another term for the same concept, was coined by Karl H. Ulrichs (1825-1895) but fell into disuse. Homosexuality was recognized and regarded as normal in many ancient cultures. This may have been due to the preponderance of males over females, to the lower life expectancy of women, or to the practice of female infanticide (q.v.) in societies in need of warriors. Homosexuality, which was influenced by the Dorians, who migrated into the Greek peninsula in the eleventh century B.C., was widely practiced in some Greek states. The Dorians were inclined to sexual relations between men because they entered the country in bands of warriors. Greek literature and art abound in examples of love not only between men but also between women, although the Athenian democracy did not wholly approve of it. The Romans also were tolerant of homosexuality. Christianity brought a reversal of attitudes. Homosexuality is mentioned as evil in the Bible (q.v.) (Genesis 19: 5-8) and in Leviticus (20:13) in which the punishment for a man "who lie with mankind" was death. In England, for example, anal intercourse was punishable by death from the time of Henry VIII (1491-1547) until 1828, and the last such sentence was carried out in 1811. Following the Wolfenden Report (q.v.) the law on homosexuality in England

was amended in 1967 to allow homosexual behavior in private between consenting adult males. Lesbianism (q.v.) was never a punishable offence. Famous male homosexuals include Frederick the Great, Peter Tchaikovsky, William Somerset Maugham, Thomas E. Lawrence, Oscar Wilde, and Yukio Mishima (qq.v.). Among the women there were Vita Sackville-West, Virginia Woolf, Margaret Radclyffe Hall, and the Ladies of Llangollen (qq.v.). See also DORIAN LOVE.
Bibliography: Bullough, V. L. 1977. *Sexual variance in society and history.*

HONEY. At Trapezos (q.v.), an ancient city in Asia Minor, the honey collected from the box tree was said to have a particularly strong smell that would drive some men mad but would cure epilepsy (q.v.). Aristotle (q.v.) mentioned it in his list of substances to be used in the treatment of epilepsy.
Bibliography: Whitwell, J.R. 1936. *Historical notes on psychiatry.*

HONT, ALFRED D' (1845-1900). A Belgian magnetizer (*see* MAGNETISM). He assumed the name of Donato. During his stage performances, he was said to heal sick people by magnetism. Riots and hysteria (q.v.) were not uncommon at his performances. He demonstrated the part played by imitation in hypnotic phenomena, and the term "donatism" (q.v.), denoting a particular type of hypnosis dependent on imitation, is derived from his name.
Bibliography: Ellenberger, H. F. 1970. *The discovery of the unconscious.*

HOOD, SIR WILLIAM CHARLES (1824-1870). A British physician. He was the proprietor and physician of a private asylum, known as Fiddington House, in Devizes. In 1851 he became the first medical superintendent of the Colney Hatch Asylum (q.v.) the county asylum for Middlesex, and instituted there a ward for boys under the age of fifteen. The following year he was appointed resident medical superintendent of Bethlem Royal Hospital (q.v.), and he set about transforming the hospital from an asylum for the poor and insane into a mental hospital for private patients. In 1862 he left Bethlem Royal Hospital and became Lord Chancellor's visitor in Lunacy. He was also treasurer for Bethlem and Bridewell (q.v.). In his book, entitled *Suggestions for the Future Provision of Criminal Lunatics* and published in 1854, he suggested many improvements in the provisions for the criminally insane. In 1868 he was knighted for his "services to psychological medicine and practice." Overwork is said to have undermined his health, and he died of pleurisy at the age of forty-five.
Bibliography: Hunter, R., and Macalpine, I. 1974. *Psychiatry for the poor.*

HOOKE, ROBERT (1635-1703). An English philosopher and scientist. He was a founding member of the Royal Society (q.v.). Following the Great Fire of London in 1666, he was appointed surveyor of that city, an office "by which he got a great estate," according to John Aubrey (q.v.). He

designed the new Bethlem Royal Hospital (q.v.) at Moorfields and the College of Physicians. He also advanced microscopy as a method for research. His book *Micrographia* was published in 1665.
Bibliography: Espinasse, M. 1956. *Robert Hooke.*

HOOLIGAN. A rough individual or a member of a street gang. The term is derived from the Hooligans, members of a nineteenth-century Irish family notorious for their lively pranks.
Bibliography: Weekley, E. 1968. *Etymological dictionary of modern English.*

HOOTON, ERNEST ALBERT (1887-1954). An American anthropologist. Some of his investigations on criminology attempted to prove that certain physiognomic characteristics could be found in criminals and that they were linked to organic inferiority and primitivism. It was an attempt to correlate personality with facial features.
Bibliography: Hooton, E. A. 1939. *Crime and the man.*

HOP. A perennial climbing vine. In its wild state it is usually found in damp hedges and thickets. It is used commercially for making beer. It is used also in herbal medicine as an hypnotic and an analgesic. An infusion of its leaves is used by gypsies to soothe the quarrelsome and calm fretful infants, as well as to control excessive sexual desires. Pillows stuffed with hops are believed to induce sleep and prevent nightmares (q.v.). In nineteenth-century America, the hop was prescribed as a sedative and an hypnotic. A tincture of it was used in the treatment of delirium tremens (q.v.), nervous irritation, and anxiety.
Bibliography: le Strange, R. 1977. *A history of herbal plants.*

HÔPITAL GÉNÉRAL. A general hospital founded in Paris in 1656 by an edict of Louis XIV (1638-1715). It was an institution for beggars, abandoned children, cripples, delinquents, mental defectives, and the lunatics (q.v.). The inmates, about 6,000 in number, were kept out of sight and spent most of their day in idleness. Those citizens of Paris who were caught giving alms to street beggars were fined four livres, and the revenue from these fines went to the Hôpital Général.
Bibliography: Galdston, I., ed. 1967. *Historic derivations of modern psychiatry.*

HOPKINS, MATTHEW (? - 1646). An English lawyer and the son of a Suffolk clergyman. As he could not make a living in the town of Ipswich, he moved to Manningtree in Essex, during the Civil War. In this tense wartime atmosphere, witch-hunting prospered, and he became witch finder general. He developed special, cruel techniques, such as sleep deprivation (q.v.), to obtain confessions, and several hundred people were brought to trial and hanged in Suffolk and Norfolk. By charging enormous fees for his

investigations, Hopkins became rich. Eventually his integrity was questioned, and he retired to Manningtree, where he died of tuberculosis (q.v.) within a year.
Bibliography: Robbins, R. H. 1959. *Encyclopedia of witchcraft and demonology.*

HORMIC PSYCHOLOGY. A term referring to the theory put forth by William McDougall (q.v.) in his *Introduction to Social Psychology* (1908). It saw no incompatibility between a nervous-energy view of mind and life and a doctrine of final courses. McDougall held that all activity has a purpose and a goal as well as a basis in instinct. Furthermore, according to him, every instinct had an emotional counterpart and social life, and responses developed from basic instincts.
Bibliography: Flugel, J. C. 1945. *A hundred years of psychology.*

HORNBOSTEL, ERICH VON (1877-1936). A German scientist and experimental psychologist. He believed in the unity of the senses and asserted that certain qualities apply to all the senses. He was particularly interested in the psychology of music and was in charge of the Phonogram Archiv, a record collection of primitive music that was begun by Carl Stumpf (q.v.).
Bibliography: Boring, E. G. 1950. *A history of experimental psychology.*

HORNEY, KAREN (1885-1952). A German psychoanalyst. In 1932, after about twelve years of psychoanalytic (*see* PSYCHOANALYSIS) work in Berlin, she emigrated to the United States. Horney was interested in feminine psychology and denied the theory of penis-envy, asserting that it was unlikely that half the human race was dissatisfied with its sex. She replaced the concept of libido (q.v.) with that of culture and tried to show Sigmund Freud (q.v.) as a biologically orientated theorist. She also disagreed with the great emphasis placed on childhood experiences and asserted that the patient should be understood in terms of present-life situations and practical psychological realities, rather than theoretical abstractions.
Bibliography: Rubins, J. L. 1978. *Karen Horney: gentle rebel of psychoanalysis.*

HORSEBACK RIDING. A form of therapy sometimes advised in the treatment of hysterical (*see* HYSTERIA) diseases. In the seventeenth century, Thomas Sydenham (q.v.) thought that the ensuing shaking and tossing of the blood would help to invigorate body and spirits and would cause noxious matters to be dispersed. In the eighteenth century, both Bernard de Mandeville (q.v.) and Frances Fuller (q.v.) prescribed it. Mandeville advised two hours on horseback for hysterical young girls, and Fuller, who recommended it in his *Medicina Gymnastica* (1705), noted that it was important to match horse and rider.
Bibliography: Leigh, D. 1961. *The historical development of British psychiatry.*

HORSLEY, SIR VICTOR ALEXANDER HADEN (1857-1916). A British pioneer in experimental and neurological surgery. He was a brilliant man, appreciative of the arts and often aggressive and dogmatic. He passionately opposed the use of alcohol and tobacco. His experiments with the thyroid gland led to the use of thyroid extract in the treatment of cretinism (q.v.). He died of heatstroke in Mesopotamia, while serving with the British Army.
Bibliography: Haymaker, W., and Schiller, F. 1970. *The founders of neurology*. 2d. ed.

HORTEGA, PIO DEL RIO (1882-1945). A Spanish anatomist. His name is linked to histological discoveries, which at first were not made known because of the antagonism of his chief, Santiago Ramon y Cajal (q.v.), who actually dismissed him. His studies on and his classification of brain tumors were published in a series of papers.
Bibliography: Haymaker, W., and Schiller, F. 1970. *The founders of neurology*. 2d. ed.

HORTUS SANITATIS. An herbal compiled in the fifteenth century from the works of older writers. The earliest edition, which was printed in Mainz, Germany, in 1491, was edited by Johan von Kaub or Cube. It contained many descriptions, as well as woodcut illustrations, of plants used in the treatment of mental disorders, including mandragora (q.v.).
Bibliography: Arber, A. 1970. *Herbals: their origin and evolution*.

HOSPITALISM. A term first used by Emelyn Lincoln Coolidge (q.v.) in 1909 to describe a condition developed by children hospitalized for long periods. The children studied were said to be apathetic and lacked resilience.
Bibliography: Coolidge, E. L. 1909. *Care of infants who must be separated from their mothers because of some especial need on the part of the child*. Papers and discussions of the American Academy of Medicine, Conference on Prevention of Infant Mortality.

HOSPITALLERS. Originally, people who provided accommodation for pilgrims. From this practice developed the Knights Hospitallers, or the Knights of St. John at Jerusalem (c.1048). Later they were called after the locations of their institutions, thus, the Knights of Rhodes (1310) and the Knights of Malta (1529). They originally were soldiers; but since the end of the eighteenth century they have been dedicated to the care of the physically and mentally ill in many hospitals.
Bibliography: 1978. *Brewer's dictionary of phrase and fable*.

HOSPITAL OF BONIFAZIO. An Italian hospital for the mentally ill. It was opened in Florence in 1788, after the Grand Duke Pietro Leopoldo

(1747-1792) had introduced legislation for the insane. For the first time, mental patients in Florence were not hospitalized with patients suffering from venereal and skin diseases. The hospital's first superintendent was Vincenzo Chiarugi (q.v.), who introduced humanitarian regulations, minimized restraint (q.v.), and advocated recreation for the patients.
Bibliography: Mora, G. 1959. Vincenzo Chiarugi (1759-1820) and his psychiatric reform in Florence in the late eighteenth century. *J. Hist. Med. and Allied Sci.* 14: 424-33.

HOSPITAL OF INCURABLE FOOLS, THE. The title of the English translation of *L'Hospidale de Pazzi Incurabili,* written in 1586 by a learned Italian monk, Tomaso Garzoni (q.v.). The volume was divided into discourses on the various types of mental illness. Garzoni's classification was based on moral criteria tempered by Galenic (see GALEN) theory. He recognized psychopathic (*see* PSYCHOPATHY) disorders, alcoholism (q.v.), delusions (q.v.) of grandeur, melancholia (q.v.), dementia, and feigned insanity (q.v.) as well as other disorders. In spite of the beliefs of the time, he did not mention demonaic possession (q.v.). The book was translated into English in 1660 and into French in 1620.
Bibliography: Garzoni, T. 1586. Reprint. 1953. *L'ospidale de pazzi incurabili.*

HOSPITAL OF SANTA DOROTEA. A religious institution dedicated to the care of the mentally ill. It was established in Florence, Italy, in the seventeenth century.
Bibliography: Mora, G. 1975. Italy. In *World history of psychiatry,* ed. J. G. Howells.

HOSPITALS AND ASYLUMS OF THE WORLD. A four-volume work and portfolio by Sir Henry Charles Burdett (q.v.). It was published in London in 1891 through 1893. It deals with the history, administration, and planning of a large number of hospitals and asylums (q.v.) throughout the world. The author personally visited many of the institutions or acquired his descriptions by correspondence with those in charge of them.
Bibliography: Burdett, H. C. 1891. *Hospitals and asylums of the world.*

HOT DRINKS. Jean Esquirol (q.v.), perhaps thinking of the English habit of drinking tea, wondered whether hot drinks were one cause of the great number of suicides (q.v.) observed in England.
Bibliography: Esquirol, J.E.D. 1845. Reprint. 1965. *Mental maladies: a treatise on insanity.*

HÔTEL-DIEU, L'. The oldest hospital in Paris. It was founded in 656 by Saint Landri bishop of Paris. Like its modern counterpart, it was situated near the cathedral of Notre-Dame. Up to the 16th century, the clergy cared for the inmates, the aged and the sick-poor, relying for funds on the charity of benefactors, among whom was Louis IX. After 1660, a decree of the Paris Parliament ordered that it should provide special accommodations "for the confinement of mad men and women," who until then had been kept with the vagabonds and the criminals also sheltered in the hospital. During the French Revolution the name was temporarily changed to Mason de l'Humanité and many of the patients were transferred to Bicêtre (q.v.) under the care of Philippe Pinel (q.v.).

Bibliography: Burdett, H. C. 1891. *Hospitals and asylums of the world.*

HOUDINI, HARRY (ERICH WEISS) (1874-1926). An American conjuror, famous for his daring escapes. He was the son of a self-styled Hungarian rabbi. At the age of twelve, Houdini ran away from home. When he was fourteen years old, he read the memoirs of the French magician Jean Eugène Robert Houdin (1805-1871), and was so impressed by them that he assumed Houdin's name and based his life on him. When he was thirty-three years old, however, the ambiguity of his feelings toward this father figure prompted him to write an attack on his hero entitled *The Unmasking of Robert-Houdin* (1908). He was pathologically attached to his mother, symbolically enthroning her, pouring gold pieces in her lap, listening to her heart beat, and contemplating suicide (q.v.) when she died. He married, but his behavior remained childlike, and he was so dependent on his wife that she washed his ears daily for thirty-three years. He recoiled from sexuality and from any form of behavior that did not meet his strict moral code. His personality was full of contradictions. When he died, the Library of Congress inherited his extensive collection of books on magic, one of the most complete and valuable in the world.

Bibliography: Meyer, B. C. 1976. *Houdini: a mind in chains: a psychoanalytic portrait.*

HOULLIER, JACQUES (HOLLERIUS) (?-1562). A French medical writer. He believed that mental disorders were natural phenomena and rejected the theory of demoniac possession (q.v.).

Bibliography: Calmeil, L. J. 1845. *De la folie considérée sous le point de vue pathologique, philosophique, historique et judiciarre.*

HOWARD, HENRY, EARL OF NORTHAMPTON (1540-1614). An English Roman Catholic and one of the most learned nobles of the sixteenth century. In 1583 he wrote a book condemning judicial astrology (q.v.) and witchcraft (q.v.) in England. In consequence he was sent to prison.

Bibliography: 1900. *The dictionary of national biography.*

HOWARD, JOHN (1726-1790). A sheriff of Bedford County, England. In 1780 he inspected the prisons in Europe, as well as all those in England and Ireland. He found that most of the prisons contained some insane

individuals. Their plight so impressed him that he dedicated the rest of his life to prison reform and to the establishment of separate wards for the insane in hospitals.
Bibliography: Goshen, C. E. 1967. *Documentary history of psychiatry.*

HOWE, SAMUEL GRIDLEY (1801-1876). An American physician. His sympathies were always with the oppressed as evidenced by his assistance to both the Greeks and the Poles in their struggle for independence. He was interested in blind and deaf children and gave some of them homes in his own house until the establishment of the Perkins Institute for the Blind (q.v.) in Boston. He served as director of it from 1832 until 1876. His experience with feebleminded blind children led to his work with the mentally retarded. Howe devised a classification that distinguished between idiots, fools, and simpletons. After an extensive survey of the condition and number of idiots in the United States he obtained the establishment of training facilities and schools for them. Oliver Wendell Holmes' (q.v.) memorial tribute to him reads in part:

> He touched the eyelids of the blind,
> And lo, the veil withdrawn,
> As o'er the midnight of the mind
> He led the light of dawn.

See also MASSACHUSETTS SCHOOL FOR IDIOTIC AND FEEBLE MINDED CHILDREN.
Bibliography: Deutsch, A. 1949. *The mentally ill in America.*

HOWITZ, F. (1828-1912). A British physician. In the 1890s he and others carried out experiments with the thyroid gland. The experiments led to the use of dry extract of thyroid for the treatment of mental retardation.
See also HORSLEY, SIR VICTOR ALEXANDER HADEN.
Bibliography: Kanner, L. 1964. *A history of the care and study of the mentally retarded.*

HOXTON MADHOUSES. Private asylums (q.v.) in the Hoxton district of London. The name "Hoxton" was once synonymous with "lunacy" in England because for 300 years the London district was notorious for its private asylums. In the latter part of the seventeenth century and early part of the eighteenth century nearly all London's private lunatics were accommodated in Hoxton. An 1819 assessment of certified lunatics in private madhouses showed that 544 out of 1,551 certified lunatics were inmates in Hoxton madhouses. Three of the madhouses were within a few hundred yards of each other: Whitmore House (q.v.), Holly House (q.v.), and Hoxton House. John Warburton, the proprietor of Whitmore House, also had two large private madhouses in Bethnal Green and supplied male keepers

from Whitmore House for George III (q.v.). Charles Lamb (q.v.) and his sister Mary (q.v.) were at one time patients in the Hoxton houses.
Bibliography: Morris, A. D. 1958. *The Hoxton madhouses*.

HUARTE DE SAN JUAN, JUAN (JUAN DE DIOS) (c.1530-1592). A Spanish physician. His work represents an early attempt to combine physiology with psychology. In 1575 he wrote a book entitled *Examen de Ingenios (Probe of the Mind)*, which was translated into many languages and greatly influenced contemporary beliefs. He did not speculate on the nature of the soul but rather emphasized personality differences. Huarte devised aptitude tests and wrote on how to insure greater intelligence in children and how to choose a marriage partner. He considered a warm climate (q.v.) to be important in furthering appropriate behavior and intelligence and claimed diet (q.v.) also could influence mental health.
Bibliography: Goshen, C. E. 1967. *Documentary history of psychiatry*.

HUA THO (c. 190-265 A.D.). A famous Chinese surgeon, reputed to have discovered the use of anaesthetics. He offered to cure the headache of the emperor Ts'ao Ts'ao by trepaning (*see* TREPANATION) his skull, but the emperor declined. He repeated his offer to a famous warrior, who misunderstood his good intentions, accused him of attempted murder, and had him beheaded.
Bibliography: Wong, K. Chi-Min, and Wu Lien-Teh. 1936. *History of Chinese medicine*.

HÜBERTZ, JEANS RASMUSSEN (1794-1855). A Danish physician. He was a pioneer in reforms in the treatment of the mentally ill. He advocated improvements in the national mental health services and the establishment of more mental hospitals. In 1855, Hübertz founded a service for the mentally retarded.
Bibliography: Retterstøl, N. 1975. Scandinavia. In *World history of psychiatry*, ed. J. G. Howells.

HUFELAND, CHRISTOPH WILHELM (1762-1836). A German physician and professor of pathology at the universities of Jena and Berlin. He advocated better provisions for public health and considered mental health to be a community problem. He introduced the term "dipsomania" (q.v.).
Bibliography: Zilboorg, G. 1941. *A history of medical psychology*.

HUGHES, HOWARD ROBARD (1905-1976). An eccentric American businessman, aircraft designer, and film producer. He was born to an immense fortune and was probably the richest man in the world. He was an orphan by the time he was eighteen years old, and his parents' early death made him dread germs. Living in a perpetual state of anxiety, he insisted that everything should be wrapped in paper tissue and that all windows should be sealed. He became addicted to codeine because he could not bear the slightest pain. His entourage of greedy hangers-on brought about his physical and mental collapse. He died of malnutrition, weighing less than ninety pounds.

Bibliography: Barlett, D. L., and Steele, J. B. 1979. *Empire: the life, legend and madness of Howard Hughes.*

HUGH OF LINCOLN, SAINT (c.1140-1200). A Carthusian monk, born in Avalon, near Grenoble, in Burgundy. In 1175 the English king Henry II (1133-1189) chose him as bishop of Lincoln. It is recorded that he was asked to bless a man under the influence of demonaic possession (q.v.) — probably a case of epilepsy (q.v.) or acute psychosis (q.v.)—who was kept tied by his head, hands, and feet to large stakes. The victim was gnashing his teeth, grimacing, and rolling his eyes, but, according to the chronicle, he regained his senses when Hugh blessed him with water and salt.

Bibliography: Rubin, S. 1974. *Medieval English medicine.*

HUGH OF LUCCA (BORGOGNONI, UGO) (?-c.1258). An Italian physician. He served as a military surgeon during the crusade to Syria and Egypt. His experience on the battlefield led him to believe that a large part of the brain could be removed without much functional loss. He was the father and teacher of Theodoric (q.v.) through whom we know of his work.

Bibliography: Pagel, W. 1959. *Symposium: Medieval and Renaissance contributions to the knowledge of the brain and its functions.*

HUGO, VICTOR MARIE (1802-1885). A French poet, novelist, and dramatist. He is perhaps the greatest figure in French literature. His childhood was spent traveling between Corsica, Italy, and Spain, as his father was a general in the army of Napoleon I (q.v.). In 1812, his parents separated, and he lived with his mother in Paris. In 1822, he married Adele Foucher whom he had known since childhood. She was the cause of the break between Victor Hugo and Charles Augustin Sainte-Beuve (1804-1869) for Sainte-Beuve fell passionately in love with her. Hugo endured a period of deep depression after the death of his favorite daughter and her husband in 1843. After the revolution of 1848, he entered political life and became an eloquent defender of liberty, but his political ambitions did not come to fruition. He was banished from France by Napoleon III (q.v.) and lived in exile in Jersey and Guernsey accompanied by his family, his lifelong mistress Juliette Drouet, and a few friends. During this period, he became interested in spiritualism (q.v.). His son Charles probably acted as the medium (q.v.), and Hugo came to believe that spirits were dictating poems to him. In 1870, after the fall of the second empire, he returned to Paris, where he was a legend, and eventually he was elected senator of the third Republic. After his death his

body lay in state under the Arc de Triomphe, guarded by cuirassiers carrying torches. It was then taken to his burial place in the Pantheon on a pauper's hearse, as he had wished. Of his many works, the most famous are *Notre Dame de Paris* (1831), *Les Misérables* (1862), *Les Travailleurs de la Mer* (1866) and *Quatre-vingt-treize* (1873). They lack humor, but they are a sensitive comment on human failings and social conditions. He was Pierre Janet's (q.v.) favorite author.
Bibliography: Maurois, A. 1966. *Victor Hugo and his world*, trans. O. Bernard.

HULL, CLARK L. (1884-1952). An American psychologist. His early years, which were spent on a farm, were marred by poor health, but eventually he managed to complete his education at the University of Wisconsin. He remained there as a professor until he moved to Yale University. He was interested in the theory of learning and wrote a book on hypnosis (*see* HYPNOTISM) and suggestibility in 1933 that was based on his experiments. His belief in behaviorism (q.v.) led to investigations into the possibility of replacing certain human capacities with robots.
Bibliography: Hull, C. L. 1943. *Principles of behavior*.

HUMAN SKIN BELTS. Belts made of human skin, usually obtained from the corpses used in anatomical demonstrations. They were believed to have therapeutic virtues and were worn by women during childbirth, by epileptics (*see* EPILEPSY), and by those suffering from hysteria (q.v.). Thomas Bartholin (1616-1680), a famous Danish physician, was among those who made and prescribed these belts.
Bibliography: Scherz, B., ed. 1969. *Historical aspects of brain research in the seventeenth century*.

HUME, DAVID (1711-1776). An English philosopher and historian. He developed an interest in philosophy as a youth, and, after abandoning his studies of law and a brief business venture, he went to France, where he spent three years with the Jesuits. When he returned to England, he had completed his most famous work *A Treatise on Human Nature*, which was published between 1739 and 1740 in three volumes. The first volume deals with "Understanding," the second with "The Passions," and the third with "Morals." Hume was a restless individual. He was driven by an urge to write but checked by his own high standards. He was sensitive, ambitious, and self-critical, yet in constant need of reassurance and approval. His philosophy of skepticism was based on the theory that all human knowledge is imperfect because it is acquired through the senses and based on subjective experience. In his "Essay on Suicide and Immortality" written in 1777, he explained that he considered suicide (q.v.) a duty in certain circumstances. At different periods during his life, Hume was a librarian, a secretary to a general, a diplomat, a politician, and a companion to a wealthy but insane

marquis. He gained success and recognition in the last thirty years of his life. In 1765 he offered refuge to Jean Jacques Rousseau (q.v.) in England but quarreled with him when Rousseau displayed his paranoia (q.v.).
Bibliography: Stroud, B. 1977. *Hume.*

HUMORAL THEORY. The term "humor" is derived from the Latin *humor*, meaning moisture. The humors were believed to be composed of four elements: fire (q.v.), air, earth, and water, which imparted hot, cold, dry, and wet qualities: hot + dry = fire; hot + moist = air; cold + dry = earth; cold + moist = water. A balance of these qualities represented harmony and health. This theory was attributed to Empedocles (q.v.) and was developed (probably by Hippocrates [q.v.]) into a more sophisticated concept of humors in which permutations of the four qualities, which were translated into bodily terms, produced health or disease. The four elements were: hot + moist = blood; cold + moist = phlegm; hot + dry = choler (q.v.) or yellow bile, cold + dry = melancholia (q.v.) or black bile (q.v.). This theory, which was then further expanded by Galen (q.v.) was still current in the Middle Ages (q.v.) and even later. Physical and mental qualities called "complexions" or "temperaments," were believed to be determined by the humors. A predominance of black bile, for example, was said to produce a melancholic individual, while yellow bile produced a choleric individual. Some items of diet (q.v.) were believed to cause an increase in one or other of the humors, hence treatment focused on restoring the balance by administering suitable correctives and avoiding offending foods. Astral bodies, the seasons, and other natural phenomena were also believed to influence the humoral balance. The application of the humoral theory in psychiatry can be found in *A Treatise of Melancholie* (q.v.) by Timothy Bright (q.v.) and *Anatomy of Melancholy* (q.v.) by Robert Burton (q.v.).
Bibliography: Cumston, C. G. 1968. *An introduction to the history of medicine.*

HUMORS. *See* HUMORAL THEORY.

HUMPHREYS, MILTON WYLIE (1844-1928). An American scholar and teacher. He undertook detailed research on the development of language in children.
Bibliography: Humphreys, M. W. 1880. *A contribution to infantile linguistics.*

HUMPHRY, ROGER (fl. 1757). An American soldier. In 1757 he killed his mother while "delirious and distracted." He was tried, found to be insane, and therefore acquitted. His father was ordered to keep him near

his home in a special "small place" to be erected and maintained at public expense.
See also ASYLUMS, ONE MAN.
Bibliography: Deutsch, A. 1949. *The mentally ill in America.*

HUNAYN IBN ISHAQ (JOHANNITIUS ONAN, or ONEIN) (809-850). A Nestorian physician, the son of a Christian Arab druggist. He settled in Bagdad and translated ancient Greek textbooks into Syrian for Harun al-Rashid (q.v.), who paid him in gold pieces equalling the weight of the volumes translated. Aristotle, Hippocrates, and Galen (qq.v.) thus became known to the Arabs and influenced their medical tradition.
Bibliography: Elgood, C. 1951. *A medical history of Persia and the eastern caliphate.*

HUNDT, MAGNUS (1449-1519). A professor of medicine at Leipzig. His book *Anthropologium* (q.v.) contains a scheme of the brain in which common sense, imagination (q.v.), rationalization, and memory (q.v.) are allocated to the frontal lobes, midbrain, and cerebellum, or to the four ventricles corresponding to these parts. He was the first to use the term "anthropology" to mean the knowledge of man.
Bibliography: Clarke, E., and Dewhurst, K. 1972. *An illustrated history of brain function.*

HUNTER, ALEXANDER (1729-1809). A British physician and agriculturist, considered an authority on the subject of asylum construction and administration. He was consulted about the building of Leicester Infirmary and the reorganization of hospitals for pauper lunatics in France. He felt that an asylum should not be built as a part of a general hospital and should be located in the country. His opinions led to the locating of mental hospitals in isolated areas of the countryside in the nineteenth century. He was physician to the York Lunatic Asylum (q.v.), which was investigated after his death. The investigation revealed that Hunter had neglected the interests of the patients in favor of his own. He invented a valueless "powder," which was sold in large quantities in the north of England as a "sovereign remedy to cure the distempered brain."
Bibliography: Hunter, R., and Macalpine, I. 1963. *Three hundred years of psychiatry.*

HUNTER, JOHN (1728-1793). A British surgeon and anatomist born in Scotland. He was the founder of surgical pathology. As a youth he went to London to assist his famous brother, William Hunter (1718-1783). He was rough and passionate, spent much of his free time in brothels and taverns, yet he was a deeply dedicated worker and a surgical genius. Hunter was well aware of the influence of emotions on physical ailments and knew that anger could precipitate an attack of the angina pectoris from which he suffered. He died after a particularly stormy board meeting at Saint George's

Hospital in London. He had been contradicted by a colleague and had left the room in an attempt to control his temper, but the effort so taxed his circulation that he collapsed. He was buried in Westminster Abbey.
Bibliography: Dobson, J. 1969. *John Hunter.*

HUNTER, WALTER S. (1889-1954). An American psychologist and a leader in the behavioristic approach to psychology. He suggested the term "anthroponomy" for the study of behavior in man, which he regarded as more important than the study of his mental functions.
Bibliography: Boring, E. G. 1950. *A history of experimental psychology.*

HUNTINGTON, GEORGE (1851-1916). An American physician. He was the son and the grandson of physicians who had lived and worked in East Hampton, Long Island, where hereditary chorea had been endemic for several generations among families of English immigrants. In 1872 he became the first clinician to give a detailed description of this progressive hereditary chorea, which is characterized by irregular movements and speech disorders leading to dementia. It is now known as Huntington's chorea.
Bibliography: Bruyn, G. W. 1968. Huntington's chorea: historical, clinical and laboratory synopsis. In *Handbook of clinical neurology*, ed. P. J. Vinken et al.

HURLER'S DISEASE. A lipid disturbance affecting bone, cartilage, skin, and such like. It leads to such peculiar deformities that it has also been called gargoylism (q.v.) . It was first described by Charles Hunter (1872-1955), but its name is derived from Gertrud Hurler, a German pediatrician, who described it in greater detail in 1919.
Bibliography: Hunter, C. 1917. A rare disease in two brothers. *Proc. roy. Soc. Med.* 10: 104-16.

HURONS. Group of North American Indian Tribes. In the 1890s a Jesuit missionary, Father Raguenau reported that they believed disease to be caused by nature, magic (q.v.), or unfulfilled wishes, which could be either known or unconscious. If the unfulfilled wishes of the sick person were not known, they were found by divination (q.v.), for fulfillment was believed to bring about a return to health. It was regarded as the duty of the community to gratify the sick person's wishes, and thus a sick person could acquire wealth at the expense of others, who in turn could become sick.
Bibliography: Ellenberger, H. F. 1970. *The discovery of the unconscious.*

HURRY OF THE SPIRITS. Another term for madness. It was used in the eighteenth century. The expression was quoted by William Battie (q.v.) in his *A Treatise on Madness* (q.v.), which was published in 1758.

HUSCHKE, EMIL (1797-1858). A German anatomist. His studies of cerebral location contributed to brain anatomy. In 1854 he published a book, *Schädel, Him und Seele des Menschen und der Thieve nach alter, Geschlecht und Race* that contained the first photograph of the brain.
Bibliography: Clarke, E., and Dewhurst, K. 1972. *An illustrated history of brain function.*

HUSSERL, EDMUND (1859-1938). A German philosopher and founder of the phenomenological school of philosophy. His influence on existentialism (q.v.) can be seen through his pupil Jean-Paul Sartre (q.v.), and through Otto Binswanger (q.v.), who realized that phenomenology also could be applied to clinical psychiatry.
Bibliography: Husserl, E. 1890. *Logische untersuchungen.*

HUTCHISON, ROBERT (1871-1960). A British pediatrician. He was one of the first pediatricians to include child psychiatry (q.v.) in his work.
Bibliography: Hutchison, R. 1904. *Lectures on the diseases of children.*

HUXLEY, ALDOUS LEONARD (1894-1963). An English novelist. He studied medicine, but a disease of the eyes prevented him practicing it. A member of a brilliant family, he turned to writing. At first he satirized the pretentious and artificial society of the 1920s, as in *Crome Yellow* (1921). Later he became bitter and depressed, and his search for spiritual values led to an interest in occultism, which was reflected in his *Eyeless in Gaza* (1936). It also led to his association with the Ramakrishna mission in Hollywood. He was morbidly preoccupied with the dangers of scientific progress, and his concern is shown in his best-known book *Brave New World* (1932) in which he depicts a repulsive scientific utopia (q.v.). With increasing pessimism he took refuge in mysticism and, as a short cut to it, mescaline (q.v.). His experiences of mescaline intoxication are described in *The Doors of Perception* (q.v.).
Bibliography: Brander, L. 1970. *Aldous Huxley.*

HUYGENS, CHRISTIAN (1629-1695). Dutch physicist, astronomer, and musician. His wide field of interests covered the study of man and his mental faculties. He referred to the animal spirits (q.v.), which he regarded as the vital energy, or the *vis viva* (q.v.), on which all human functions depended.
Bibliography: Bell, A. E. 1947. *C. Huygens and the development of science in the seventeenth century.*

HYE WAY TO THE SPYTTEL HOUSE. A work by the English author and printer Robert Copland (fl.1508-1547), which was written around 1536. He stated the only thing that could save the husband of a nagging wife from an attack of madness would be a bed in the Royal Hospital of Saint Bartholomew (q.v.) or in "Bedlem," Bethlem Royal Hospital (q.v.).

We have chambers purposely for them
Or else they should lodge in Bedlem.
Bibliography: Copland, R. 1930. *Hye way to Spyttel House*, ed. A. V. Judges.

HYGEIA. In Greek mythology (q.v.) she was the daughter of Aesculapius (q.v.). Like him, she was considered a divinity of health. She is represented holding a cup from which a serpent drinks.
Bibliography: 1961. *Everyman's clinical dictionary*, ed. John Wasmington.

HYPNOS. In Greek mythology (q.v.), the winged god of sleep. He was represented carrying a horn from which he poured a sleep-bringing liquid and a branch with which he would touch the foreheads of the tired to induce sleep.
Bibliography: Hammond, N.G.L., and Scullard, H. H., eds. 1973. *The Oxford classical dictionary*.

HYPNOTISM. The term is a shortened version of the word "neurypnology" (q.v.), which was coined by James Braid (q.v.) to replace mesmerism (q.v.) and magnetism (q.v.). Braid first used it in 1842 in his *Satanic Agency and Mesmerism Reviewed*, a pamphlet written in answer to an attack by the Reverend H. McNeile of Manchester. References to the practice of hypnotism have been found in ancient Egyptian, Grecian, and Roman works. A bas-relief found in a tomb in Thebes has a scene that depicts the hypnotizing of a man. The Ebers papyrus (q.v.) also mentions practices similar to those later employed to produce hypnotic states. Asclepiades (q.v.) treated manic patients by inducing a lethargic sleep similar to somnambulism (q.v.) in them. The Roman emperor Vespasian was said to have curative powers that he could exercise through hypnotism. Many early oracles (q.v.), mystics, and prophets imparted their advice while in a state of trance that was self-induced by various means; for instance, the monks of Mount Athens would stare fixedly at their umbilicai. These phenomena were considered supernatural until the idea of a magnetic fluid that could affect the mind was introduced. At first magnets (q.v.) were believed to be vital in producing the phenomena, but toward the end of the eighteenth century they were discarded as the idea that magnetism was related to a personal quality, or "fluid" emanating from the operator, arose. This belief was advanced further by Franz Mesmer (q.v.). In the nineteenth century the phenomena of hypnosis were investigated scientifically, and hypnotism gained followers among eminent psychiatrists. The work of Pierre Janet (q.v.) and many of his contemporaries contributed to its progress toward a form of psychological treatment that considered the unconscious (q.v.). Dynamic psychiatry (q.v.) developed from this approach, which was used for a while by Sigmund

Freud, Alfred Adler, and Carl Jung (qq.v.). It opened the way to a better understanding of psychic phenomena.

Bibliography: Tinterow, M. M. 1970. *Foundations of hypnosis: from Mesmer to Freud*.

HYPOCHONDRIA (or HYPOCHONDRIASIS). A term applied to a preoccupation with ill-defined physical symptoms that are often accompanied by depression and anxiety. It is derived from the Greek term meaning "below the cartilage," especially that of the breast-bone. The hypocondrium acquired the same role as the uterus (q.v.). The noxious fumes arising from the bowels, liver (q.v.), spleen (q.v.), or the mesentery were said to produce the same symptoms as those arising from the uterus. The *Oxford English Dictionary* claims that the surgeon Thomas Gale (1507-1587) first used the term in English in 1563. Gottfried Smoll may have been the first to write at length on hypochondria in 1610. He divided the disorder into hypochondria of the spleen, hypochondria of the mesentery, and hypochondria "phantasticae" (of the imagination [q.v.]). Robert Burton (q.v.) divided melancholia (q.v.) into three kinds, one of which he called "hypochondriacall melancholy." He also referred to the subdivisions (hepaticke, splenaticke, mesariacke) devised by André du Laurens (q.v.). In 1633 John Hawkins (q.v.) wrote the first book on the subject, *Hypochondriac Melancholy*, which was followed by many treatises on the same theme. Thomas Sydenham (q.v.) became aware that hysteria (q.v.) extended to both sexes but avoided the term as it linked it to the uterus. He preferred to use the term "hypochondria" when the disorder occurred in males. Bernard de Mandeville (q.v.) discussed both in *A Treatise of the Hypochondriack and Hysterick Passions* in 1711. The remedies for the complaint were many and as haphazard as the concept of the disease. John Wesley (q.v.) in his *Primitive Physic, or an Easy and Natural Way of Curing Most Diseases* (1791), prescribed cold baths, or "an ounce of quicksilver every morning, and ten drops of Elixir of Vitrol in the afternoon, in a glass of cold water." From the medical field, the term spilled into literary works; Laurence Sterne (q.v.) wrote that the hypochondriac was like "a miser who amasses treasures which he has no heart to enjoy," thus giving a new slant to the term. In 1822, a new and narrower meaning of morbid preoccupation with imaginary complaints were given to the term by Jean Pierre Falret (q.v.) in his book *De l'Hypochondrie et du suicide*. A number of authors, however, continued to equate hypochondria with a form of insanity, before Falret's meaning was accepted.

Bibliography: Fisher-Homberger, E. 1970. *Hipochondrie*.

"HYPOCHONDRIACK, THE." The title of a column written by James Boswell (q.v.) for the *London Magazine*. He used the term in the eighteenth-

century sense of depressive in reference to the melancholic (see MELAN-CHOLIA) subject matter of his column.
Bibliography: Bailey, M., ed. 1951. *Boswell's column.*

HYSSOP. *Gratiola,* also known as *Gratia Dei* (grace of the Lord) because of its value as a medicinal herb. It is usually found on dry banks and among ruins and rocks. It is mentioned in the Bible (q.v.) for use in treatment of many diseases, including nervous disorders and epilepsy (q.v.). David (q.v.) praised it and asked to be given it: "Purge me with hyssop, and I shall be clean." (Ps. 51: 7.) Large doses of an infusion of its roots produce vomiting followed by purging (q.v.), both of which were considered beneficial in the treatment of insanity.
Bibliography: le Strange, R. 1977. *A history of herbal plants.*

HYSTERIA. A term derived from the Greek word for the uterus (q.v.). Since antiquity, disorders of the uterus were considered responsible for a group of symptoms that were called "hysterical". Hysteria, therefore, came to be considered a disorder unique to women until Thomas Sydenham (q.v.) demonstrated its presence in males. The dramatic nature of symptoms made those affected easy prey to superstitions and accusations, including accusations of demonaic possession (q.v.) and witchcraft (q.v.). The link between hysteria and sexuality (q.v.) has remained in the doctrines of psychoanalysis (q.v.), but its manifestations are now called "conversion symptoms."
See also MASS HYSTERIA.
Bibliography: Veith, I. 1965. *Hysteria: the history of a disease.*

HYSTERICAL CONVERSION. The term "hysterical conversion" and the concept it covers were introduced into psychiatry by John Ferriar (q.v.) in 1795 in his *Medical Histories and Reflections.* The term implies that psychic energy is transformed into physical energy and so causes physical symptoms. The term "conversion" was reintroduced to psychiatry by Sigmund Freud (q.v.) in 1894 in *The Definite Neuropsychosis.*
Bibliography: Freud, S. 1976. *The complete psychological works.*
Hunter, R., and Macalpine, I. 1963. *Three hundred years of psychiatry.*

I

IAGO. A character in the play *Othello* by William Shakespeare (q.v.). He is a psychopath, who is completely selfish and has no use for "love and duty." In the original Italian source, Iago killed Desdemona with a stocking filled with sand.
Bibliography: Orgel, S. 1968. Iago *Am. Imago.* 25:258-73.

IBSEN, HENRIK (1828-1906). A Norwegian dramatist and poet. The family was reduced to near poverty when his parents lost their wealth in a business venture. At the age of sixteen, he was apprenticed to an apothecary, as he could not afford to study medicine. The frustration and unhappiness of these early years never left him and are reflected in his dramas, which often include doctors ministering to sick minds. He possessed a penetrating insight into the psychological conflicts found within the family and within society. His plays, dealing with such social issues as marriage, corruption, venereal disease, government, man's delusions of superiority, and mental disorders, caused the critics to assert that they were studies in insanity best fitted for the lecture room in Bedlam (q.v.). Among his works are the verse dramas *Brand* (1866) and *Peer Gynt* (1867) and the plays *A Doll's House* (1879), *Ghosts* (1881), *Rosmersholm* (1886), *The Lady from the Sea* (1888), *Hedda Gabler* (1890), and *The Master Builder* (1892). Insanity and its causes are recurrent themes throughout them. A series of severe strokes toward the end of his life so destroyed his memory, that he could not even remember the alphabet.
Bibliography: Meyer, M. 1974. *Ibsen.*

ID. A term first used by Georg Groddeck (q.v.). Sigmund Freud (q.v.) borrowed it from him and used it to indicate that part of the personality that is inherited and unconscious.
Bibliography: Freud, S. 1923. *The ego and the id.*

IDEAL AND NOTIONAL INSANITY. *See* INSANITY, IDEAL AND NOTIONAL.

IDÉES FIXES. A term used by Pierre Janet (q.v.) to describe the mental state of neurotic (see NEUROSIS) individuals and their inner conflict with reality.
Bibliography: Janet, P. 1924. *Neuroses et idées fixes.*

IDELER, KARL WILHELM (1795-1860). A German psychiatrist, and chief of the Charité (Berlin) (q.v.) for twenty-eight years. His work, inspired by Georg Stahl (q.v.) led the way to a new approach to the treatment of mental disorders by focusing attention on psychopathology. He emphasized the emotional life of the patient and believed that ungratified instinctual drives could lead to a breakdown of personality. To him, insanity was in part hereditary and in part "the fairytale-like poetry of a boundless craving of the heart," or man's flight into fantasy when reality becomes unbearable. He firmly believed in psychotherapy (q.v.) even for psychosis (q.v.) but did not discard emetics and salves.
Bibliography: Kraepelin, E. 1962. *One hundred years of psychiatry.*

IDIOT. A term derived from the Greek *idios*, meaning "isolated and solitary," and conveying the observation that a man deprived of intellect is set aside from the rest of the community. In the modern context, the term is employed to indicate the lowest grade of feeblemindedness resulting in an Intelligence Quotient not over approximately 25.
See also IMBECILE.

IDIOT SAVANT. A term that indicates a feebleminded individual who has remarkable talents in one or more directions, for example, in the areas of memory (q.v.), mimicry, calculation or music. Blind Tom, for example, could play two tunes on the piano simultaneously, and Gottfried Mind (q.v.) was so clever at painting cats that he was called the "Katzen-Raphael."
Bibliography: Barr, M. W. 1904. *Mental defectives.*

IDIOTS' CAGE. An iron cage used in the Middle Ages (q.v.) and even as late as the eighteenth century to display idiots (q.v.) and insane patients. The cage was placed in public squares for the entertainment of the citizens. Such a cage was used in Brno, Czechoslovakia, until 1770 (see Plate 6).
Bibliography: Vencovsky, E. 1975. Czechoslovakia. In *World history of psychiatry,* ed. J. G. Howells.

IDRIS. A giant prince in Welsh mythology (q.v.). According to legend, his chair is hewn in the rock at the top of Cader Idris, a mountain in mid-Wales. It is said that any man who spends a night sitting in it will either go mad or become a poet endowed with supernatural inspiration.
Bibliography: Bord, J., and Bord, C. 1976. *The secret country.*

IK. A dying African tribe that lives in the mountains near the borders of Uganda and Kenya. After years of nomadic life, they were forced to settle

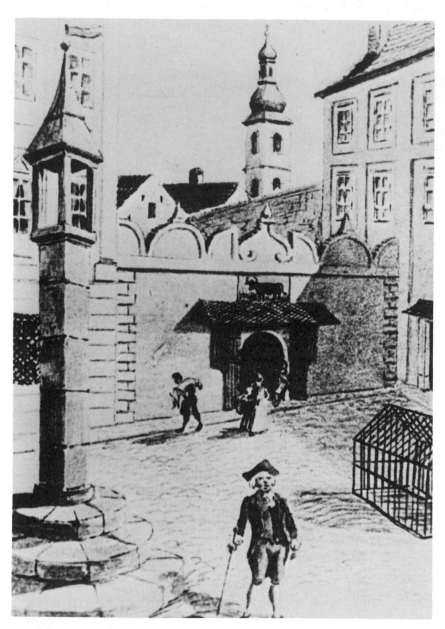

6. IDIOT'S CAGE FOR EXHIBITING THE INSANE. The display of the insane was sometimes taken to extremes. The cage on the right was used for exhibiting the insane in eighteenth-century Czechoslovakia. By courtesy of the Department of Medical Illustration, Ipswich Hospital.

in a given territory and to become farmers. The poor soil, droughts, and their inexperience led to a struggle for survival in which the strongest members of the tribe exploited, neglected, and destroyed the weak. Children, old people, and the sick were abandoned, deprived of food and shelter, and denied love, an emotion completely lost by the tribe. Morality and acceptable behavior degenerated under the stress and were replaced by bitterness, degradation, and a complete lack of feeling. A child seeking affection from his parents was regarded as mad.

Bibliography: Turnbull, C. M. 1972. *The mountain people.*

IKARA. A Swiss patient of Maxmilian Bircher-Benner (q.v.). Her vivid reminiscences conveyed the impression that she had led a previous life in a prehistoric era. Bircher-Benner believed that she had recorded her story during the two years she spent in his sanitorium in Zurich, Switzerland.

Bibliography: Bircher-Benner, M. 1944. *Der menschenseele not, erankung und gesundung.*

ILLNESSES OF THE WIND. In ancient China (q.v.) the winds that swept the valleys of the Yellow River were believed to be responsible for headaches and mental diseases, which consequently were termed "illnesses of the wind."

Bibliography: Kiev, A., ed. 1968. *Psychiatry in the Communist world.*

IMAGINATION. The ability to form a mental image of something not present or not thought of before. Human imagination has been a subject for discussion and speculation since antiquity. Aristotle (q.v.) believed it to be a combination of intellect and sensory perception. Francis Bacon (q.v.) thought that the imagination had "great power to hurt" but could also help in restoring health. The more advanced of his contemporaries regarded witches (*see* WITCHCRAFT), devils, and other unexplained phenomena as tricks of the imagination. John Cotta (q.v.) wrote that charms and incantations (q.v.) could produce cures "in the person imaginant and confident of receiving help." Defects of imagination, reason, and memory (q.v.) were considered the major factors in the diagnosis of insanity. Ludovico Muratori's (q.v.) treatise, which was entitled *On the Power of Human Imagination* (1740), discussed dreams (q.v.) and such pathological expressions of the imagination, as visions, ecstasy (q.v.), and phobias (q.v.). In 1750 Peter Shaw (q.v.) wrote that "many Diseases arise from a perverted Imagination; and some of them are cured by affecting the Imagination only." Franz Mesmer (q.v.) opened the door to therapeutic techniques that used and abused imagination and suggestion.

IMAGO. 1) A term introduced into psychoanalysis (q.v.) by Carl Jung (q.v.). It referred to his concept of primordial images. 2) A journal founded in 1912 by Hans Sachs (q.v.) and Otto Rank (q.v.) for the publication of psychoanalytically orientated papers on literature, art (q.v.), and mythology (q.v.). Sigmund Freud's (q.v.) *Totem and Taboo* was published as an article in its first issue. A new *American Imago* was founded by Sachs in 1939. 3) The title of a novel by the Swiss writer Carl Spittaler (1845-1924) in which a young poet projects his image of the woman he loves onto a person who is quite different in reality. The novel, published in Jena in 1906, was popular with the psychoanalysts of the time.

IMBECILE. A term derived from the Latin *imbecillitas*, meaning "weakness" and used for any form of feebleness. It later became associated with weakness of the mind to a degree less severe than idiocy.
See also IDIOT.

IMHOTEP (fl. c. 2980-2950 B.C.). An Egyptian sage, magician (*see* MAGIC), architect, and probably the first of all physicians. He was physician to Zoser, (2980-2950 B.C.), a pharaoh of the third Dynasty. He was deified in 525 B.C. and venerated as a god of medicine. A temple of healing, in which incubation sleep (q.v.) was practiced, was established in Memphis (q.v.) in his honor.
Bibliography: Sigerist, H. E. 1933. *Great doctors.*

IMMACULÉE CONCEPTION, L'. The title of a series of five essays written by André Breton (q.v.) and Paul Éluard (1895-1952). The series was published in Paris in 1930. The two authors, founding members of surrealism (q.v.), deliberately imitated in their writings the expressions of mental disorder as found in acute mania (q.v.), delusional states (*see* DELUSIONS), general paralysis of the insane (q.v.), schizophrenia (q.v.) and feeblemindedness.
Bibliography: Gaunt, W. 1973. *The surrealists.*

IMMERSION. An early form of therapy for mental disorders. In medieval times immersion in holy wells (q.v.) and natural pools was used as a form of therapy for mental disorders. In some parts of the world this practice lingered into the eighteenth century. In Scotland, for example, mental patients were still being immersed in Saint Fillan's pool (q.v.) in the eighteenth century. Sudden immersion in cold water was also used in the eighteenth and nineteenth centuries as a form of shock therapy. A refinement was to place the patient in a box perforated with air holes and keep him under water until air bubbles ceased to rise; he was then brought out and revived.
See also BATH OF SURPRISE, BOWSENNING, DUCKING, and WATER THERAPY.
Bibliography: Zilboorg, G. 1941. *A history of medical psychology.*

IMPOTENCE. Sexual impotence in all cultures and at almost all times has been the subject of superstitious opinions and practices. It has been attributed to divine punishment, malevolent spirits, curses (q.v.) and witchcraft (q.v.).

The *Malleus Maleficarum* (q.v.) claimed that it and other sexual disorders were caused by witchcraft. Johann Weyer (q.v.) reported in his *De Praestigiis Daemonum* (q.v.) some of the superstitions connected with impotence and the remedies then used. It was believed, for example, that writing a magic (q.v.) formula on virginal parchment and chanting a psalm of David (q.v.) over it seven times before laying it on the affected parts would cure the problem. In the nineteenth century, Pierre Janet (q.v.) regarded impotency as a symptom of neurosis (q.v.), rather than a cause of it. Sigmund Freud (q.v.) and psychoanalysis (q.v.) have further highlighted the problems of sexual inadequacy.

IMPRINTING. A term coined in 1939 by the ethologist Konrad Lorenz (q.v.) to describe an early form of learning found in some animals, particularly ducks. He found that some animals would follow and become attached to the first moving object that caught their attention at birth. The same phenomenon had been described in 1873 by Douglas Spalding (q.v.), an English naturalist. In the sixteenth century, Thomas More (q.v.) alluded to the idea of imprinting in his book *Utopia*:

They breed vast numbers of chickens by a most extraordinary method. Instead of leaving the hens to sit on the eggs, they hatch out dozens at a time applying a steady heat to them—with the result that when the chicks come out of the shells, they regard the poultryman as their mother, and follow him everywhere!
Bibliography: Sluckin, W. 1965. *Imprinting and early learning*.

INCANTATIONS. Spoken or chanted magic (q.v.) formulas. They are found in the history of all civilizations. Some special incantations were believed to cure mental disorders. The monotony of repetition, as well as the powerful suggestion attached to them, often caused trance-like states. During the transition from pagan rites to Christian ceremonies, the words of various pagan incantations were adapted to Christianity, and the intercession of the Mother of God or of certain saints was requested. Medieval manuscripts often contain examples of incantations. The herbals often list incantations to be used in conjunction with certain herbal remedies or while gathering the plants.
Bibliography: Sigerist, H. E. 1977. *A history of medicine*. Vol. 1.

INCEST. Sexual intercourse between persons of kinship or affinity in a degree that prohibits marriage. Some ancient societies openly practiced incest. It was permitted in ancient Japan, Peru, and Egypt (q.v.). Egyptian members of the royal family could marry only blood relatives. Most societies, however, have regarded incest as a serious crime. The early Christians condemned it, and the first individual to be excommunicated from the church was a Corinthian found guilty of incest. Cases of incest are found frequently in mythology (q.v.); for example, Zeus killed Uranus, his father, and married Gaea, his mother. The most famous example is the Greek classic, Oedipus (q.v.), and it was from *Oedipus Rex* by Sophocles (q.v.) that Sigmund Freud (q.v.) derived the term "Oedipus complex." There are also biblical examples of incest. In the Old Testament, Lot is seduced by his daughters after leaving Sodom. Throughout history, incest has been a recurrent theme in literature. William Shakespeare made incest the central theme of *Hamlet*, (q.v.) and *Rosmersholm* by Henrik Ibsen (q.v.), so admired by Freud, also deals with the subject. Famous writers accused of incestuous relationships include Lord Byron (q.v.) and William Wordsworth (q.v.).

INCUBATION. The practice of sleeping within the precincts of a temple to be cured of illness. It was most common among the Egyptians, Greeks, and Romans, but it also existed in other parts of the world. It was most widely employed in the temples of Aesculapius (q.v.). In these temples, patients were encouraged to make whatever offerings they could to the god, and sometimes they slept in the skins of the animals they had sacrificed. Before entering the inner part of the temple they were purified by bathing and anointing, they had to abstain from certain foods or follow a period of fasting (q.v.). Weakened, sometimes drugged, and subjected to powerful suggestion, the patients experienced dreams (q.v.) during which the god gave them advice about treatment or cured them in their sleep. The dreams were sometimes interpreted by the priests, and the cures obtained were recorded in votive inscriptions. A somewhat facetious description of a typical experience is found in Aristophanes' (q.v.) *The Plutus*.
Bibliography: Stubbs, S.G.B., and Blight, E. W. 1931. *Sixty centuries of health and physick.*

INCUBUS. A male demon said to seduce women during their sleep. A succubus (q.v.) was a female demon who seduced men in their sleep. As early as Aristotle (q.v.), it was realized that the incubus was, in reality, a form of mental disorder in which dreams (q.v.) are accompanied by a feeling of suffocation, and impending death and followed by fear and exhaustion on awakening. Caelius Aurelianus (q.v.) postulated that the disorder was a form of epilepsy (q.v.), and many held that it led to insanity. Arnold of Villanova (q.v.) combined demonology with Galenic (*see* GALEN) humoral theory (q.v.) and claimed that the presence of warm humors attracted the devil, who was more likely to enter the body, especially at night, as he liked warmth. Johann Weyer (q.v.) firmly stated that it was not a devil but a sickness that caused the symptoms of oppression and terrifying dreams. He was refuted by Jean Bodin (q.v.). The Inquisition (q.v.) relied heavily on the belief in incubi, and the *Malleus Maleficarum* (q.v.) related many instances of incubi sleeping with witches (*see* WITCHCRAFT). Later medical writers blamed imbalance of diet (q.v.) for the incubus, and it began to disappear from classifications of mental disorders.

INDEX LIBRORUM PROHIBITORUM. A list of books prohibited by the Roman Catholic Church. The list was begun as early as the fifth century by Gelasius who served as pope from 492 to 496. The first formal Index was published by Pope Paul V (1552-1621) in the sixteenth century through the offices of the Inquisition (q.v.). Many works that denied demonaic possessions (q.v.) and affirmed insanity as a sickness were listed in the Index. The enlightened writings of Johann Weyer (q.v.), for example, were banned, and, until the beginning of the twentieth century, Catholics were not allowed to read them.

INDIAN HEMP DRUGS COMMISSION. A commission set up in 1893 to report on all aspects of the cultivation, preparation, distribution, consumption, and effects of cannabis sativa (q.v.) in India. The report covered the years 1893 to 1894 in seven volumes and concluded that there was not enough evidence to believe that Indian hemp (cannabis) caused insanity, as believed at the time. The commission recommended controlling its production and placing some restrictions on it, but they rejected the proposal that it should be completely prohibited.

INDIAN PENNYWORT. Hydrocotyle asiatica. The plant is common in Pakistan and is abundant in damp localities in Bengal. In small doses it acts as a stimulant; in large amounts it is a narcotic. It is used in Eastern medicine for a host of disorders, including epilepsy (q.v.) and insanity. One or two leaves every morning may be prescribed for stuttering, and a powder, made from the dried leaves and mixed with milk, is used sometimes to improve memory (q.v.).
Bibliography: le Strange, R. 1977. *A history of herbal plants.*

INDIVIDUAL PSYCHOLOGY. A doctrine developed by Alfred Adler (q.v.) around 1912. At first it was a form of psychoanalysis (q.v.) that tried to correct feelings of inferiority. Many aspects of it were linked to the philosophy of Friedrich Nietzsche (q.v.).
See also PSYCHOLOGY.
Bibliography: Bottome, P. 1957. *Alfred Adler: apostle of freedom.*

INFANCY. The first five years of life. Until the nineteenth century, high infant mortality made this period of little concern to psychiatrists, although a few pediatricians did offer advice on infant mental health. In the nineteenth century attitudes toward infancy began to change. Jean Esquirol (q.v.) believed the period of infancy was free from insanity, but he added, "jealousy sometimes poisons the sweet enjoyments of early life, and produces a true melancholy with delirium. Some children, jealous of the tenderness and caresses of their mother, become pale and emaciated, fall into a state of marasmus and die." The twentieth century has seen the establishment of branches of psychology and psychiatry dedicated to the treatment of deviations from normality in infancy and to the understanding of the mental and emotional development during that period.

Bibliography: Esquirol, J.E.D. 1845. Reprint. 1965. *Mental maladies: a treatise on insanity.*
Howells, J. G., ed. 1979. *Modern perspectives in the psychiatry of infancy.*

INFANTICIDE. The killing of an infant. History and mythology (q.v.) record many instances of infanticide during ritual sacrifices. Greek mythology offers many examples of infanticide by parents; Kronos and Medea being the most famous. The biblical slaughter of the innocents is an example of mass infanticide. An ancient practice prescribed the enclosing of a child in the foundation of a building (now symbolically represented by the laying of the foundation stone). Eskimos destroyed all children with congenital anomalies. As twins were considered abnormal, they also were killed. Mohave Indians killed all half-breed infants at birth. Many cultures killed a proportion of female babies. This practice survived in China (q.v.) until the 1880s.

Bibliography: Piers, M. W. 1978. *Infanticide: past and present.*

INFERIORITY COMPLEX. A sense of personal inferiority. Pierre Janet (q.v.) described a feeling of inferiority that he called *sentiment d'incomplétude.* Alfred Adler (q.v.) further developed this concept, which he termed "inferiority complex."

Bibliography: Roazen, P. 1974. *Freud and his followers.*

INGENIEROS, JOSÉ (1877-1925). An Argentinian psychiatrist, philosopher, and sociologist. He was influenced by Auguste Comte (q.v.) and Herbert Spencer (q.v.) and applied the theories of positivism (q.v.) to criminology, education, and sociology. In 1907 he founded the Buenos Aires Institute of Criminology. It was the first such institute in South America. He also founded the journal *Archivas de Psiquiatria y Criminologia,* which was the first psychiatric periodical in South America. Of his several works, *El Hombre Mediocre,* published in 1913, was the most influential. Other books include works on simulated insanity, biological psychology and on psychopathology in art (q.v.).

Bibliography: Leon, C. A., and Rosselli, H. 1975. Latin America. In *World history of psychiatry,* ed. J. G. Howells.

INHIBITORY INSANITY. *See* INSANITY, INHIBITORY.

INK BLOTS. A projective technique developed by Hermann Rorschach (q.v.) after fourteen years of experimentation. The shapes of the ink blots stimulate the patient's thoughts and fantasies from which an assessment of the patient's condition is made. The ink blot findings were first published by Rorschach in 1921 in a volume entitled *Psychodiagnostik*.

INNER SENSES. Mental faculties so called by Robert Burton (q.v.) because he thought that they were "within the brain pan." He recognized three inner senses: common sense, fantasy, or imagination (q.v.), and memory (q.v.). The first, common sense, was the most important and, according to him, resided in the forepart of the brain. It allowed for judgment. Fantasy, in the middle of the brain, examined what was provided by common sense, retained and recalled old experiences and made up new images. During sleep fantasy was free to "conceive strange, stupend, absurd shapes"; in melancholics (*see* MELANCHOLIA) it produced "monstrous and prodigious things" and in artists it was overactive. Memory, sited at the back of the brain, recorded the experiences brought in by the senses and permitted their recall.
Bibliography: Burton, R. 1621. Reprint. 1964. *The anatomy of melancholy*.

INNOCENT IV (?-1254). A pope continuously engaged in struggles with Frederick II (q.v.). Innocent's efforts to smother free thinking gave impetus to the Inquisition (q.v.), which became well established under his papacy.
Bibliography: Gontard, F. 1964. *The popes*, trans. A. J. Peeler and E. F. Peeler.

INNOCENT VIII (1432-1492). A pope. In 1484 he appointed Johann Jacob Sprenger (q.v.) and Heinrich Kraemer (q.v.) as inquisitors and charged them to find, prosecute, and destroy those people who "unmindful of their own salvation and straying from the Catholic Faith, have abandoned themselves to devils, incubi [*see* INCUBUS], and sucubi [*see* SUCCUBUS] and by their incantations [q.v.], spells, conjurations, and other accursed charms and crafts [commit] enormities and horrid offences." He followed these appointments with the appointment of Tomas de Torquemada (q.v.) as grand inquisitor of Spain.
Bibliography: Gontard, F. 1964. *The popes*, trans. A. J. Peeler and E. F. Peeler.

INN SIGNS. Tom O'Bedlam (q.v.) was a common signboard displayed by inns and taverns in England from the seventeenth century. Such a sign could be seen in Redbourne, a village in Hertfordshire. One side of the sign depicted "Mad Tom in Bedlam" and the other "Tom at Liberty."
Bibliography: O'Donoghue, E. G. 1914. *The story of Bethlehem Hospital*.

INQUISITION. A tribunal of the Roman Catholic Church, formally established by Pope Gregory IX (q.v.), in 1233. It became more firmly established and feared under Innocent IV (q.v.) and was most active under Innocent VIII (q.v.), who appointed Johann Sprenger (q.v.) and Heinrich Kraemer (q.v.) as inquisitors in 1484. The Inquisition sought to identify, persecute, and exterminate heresy and witchcraft (q.v.) as well as smother any form of free thinking that might be regarded as heretical. The official textbook of the Inquisition was the *Malleus Maleficarum* (q.v.). In the seventeenth century the influence of the Inquisition began to diminish as scientists started to defend their ideas and intellectual integrity against the demand for blind obedience to the dictates of the church.

Bibliography: Turbeville, A. S. 1926. *Medieval heresy and the Inquisition.*

INSANE OFFENDERS ACT. British legislation resulting from Lord Thomas Erskine's (q.v.) defense of James Hadfield (q.v.) in 1800. The act stated that those judged criminally insane should be "detained during His Majesty's pleasure." Previously those acquitted on the grounds of insanity were often set free. Due to the speed in which the act was passed, no place of detention for the criminally insane was available until 1816, when a ward for them was established in Bethlem Royal Hospital (q.v.).

Bibliography: Walker, N. D. 1968. *Crime and insanity in England.*

INSANE POOR, LEGISLATION IN ENGLAND. Until 1744, the only legal provisions for the insane poor in England concerned custodial care for the violent insane who were too dangerous to be left free. In 1744 a new law empowered two justices to order the arrest of pauper lunatics found wandering aimlessly. In 1808 a law was enacted that provided for the construction of public lunatic asylums (q.v.). Few counties complied with the law, and where asylums were established, they were poorly managed. In 1845 the commissioners in lunacy (q.v.) were empowered to inspect asylums. In 1853 a more stringent act made provisions for pauper lunatics compulsory for every county; a further measure, in 1868, provided that chronic lunatics transferred from an asylum to a workhouse should continue to be listed as patients on the books of the asylum. Finally, in 1874, a small government grant was given to all asylums.

See also COUNTY ASYLUMS, INSPECTION OF MADHOUSES, LENZIE ACT, VAGRANT ACT, and WYNN ACT.

Bibliography: Howells, J. G., and Osborn, M. L. 1975. Great Britain. In *World history of psychiatry*, ed. J. G. Howells.

INSANIA. The Latin term from which the term "insanity" is derived. It was first used by Celsus (q.v.) in the third book of his *De Re Medicina*. Cicero (q.v.) thought that insania was different from furor (q.v.). The "insanus," according to him, was emotionally ill but intellectually capable of understanding, while the "furious" could not be held responsible for his actions and was truly mad.

See also FEIGNED INSANITY; GENERAL PARALYSIS OF THE INSANE; INSANITY, ABORTIVE; INSANITY, IDEAL AND NOTIONAL; INSANITY, INHIBITORY; INSANITY, MORAL; INSANITY, PARALYTIC; and INSANITY, PUERPERAL.

INSANITY, ABORTIVE. Carl Westphal (q.v.) referred to obsessional (*see* OBSESSION) states as "abortive insanity."
Bibliography: Zilboorg, G. 1941. *A history of medical psychology.*

INSANITY, ARTIFICIAL. Daniel H. Tuke (q.v.), referring to the techniques of James Braid (q.v.), called hypnotism (q.v.) "artificial insanity." In 1866 he wrote a paper entitled "Artificial Insanity or Braidism," which was published in the *Journal of Mental Science.*
Bibliography: Tuke, D. H. 1892. *A dictionary of psychological medicine.*

INSANITY, IDEAL AND NOTIONAL. Two categories in Thomas Arnold's (q.v.) classification of mental disorders. He identified ideal insanity as a disorder of ideas and notional insanity as abnormal conceptualization.
Bibliography: Arnold, T. 1782-1786. *Observations on the nature, kinds, causes and prevention of mental disease.* 2 vols.

INSANITY, INHIBITORY. A term introduced by Daniel H. Tuke (q.v.) to indicate a disorder in which there is lack of the social and moral inhibitions that allow man to function in society. According to him, a psychopathic (*see* PSYCHOPATHY), asocial individual would suffer from inhibitory insanity.
Bibliography: Tuke, D. H. 1892. *Dictionary of psychological medicine.*

INSANITY, MORAL. A nineteenth-century concept of what is now called "emotional illness." The term was introduced by James C. Prichard (q.v.), who was the first to describe it as an illness in its own right. Daniel H. Tuke (q.v.) defined it in his dictionary as: "A disorder which affects the feelings and affections, or what are termed the moral powers, in contradistinction to those of the understanding or intellect." Tuke's lengthy list of international references at the end of the entry indicates that the pre-Freudian physicians of the time were preoccupied by this condition.
Bibliography: Tuke, D. H. 1892. *A dictionary of psychological medicine.*

INSANITY, PARALYTIC. A term for general paralysis of the insane (q.v.) introduced in 1838 by Jean Parchappe (q.v.) to emphasize the connection between the general paralysis and the softening of the cortex.
Bibliography: Parchappe, J.B.M. 1838. *Recherches sur l'encephale.*

INSANITY, PUERPERAL. Postpartum psychosis (q.v.). The earliest recorded clinical description of postpartum psychosis may be that quoted by Hippocrates (q.v.) in the third book of *On Epidemics.*
Bibliography: Semelaigne, A. 1869. *Études historiques sur l' aliénation mental dans l'antiquité.*

INSPECTION OF MADHOUSES. In the eighteenth century public unrest over the state of asylums (q.v.) in England, led to the passage of an act in

468 / INSTINCTS, THEORY OF

1774 that directed the Royal College of Physicians to appoint five members who were to inspect and license madhouses within London and an area of seven miles round it. In other districts magistrates were similarly empowered. In the nineteenth century the commissioners in lunacy (q.v.) were established to inspect asylums throughout England and Wales.
See also INSANE POOR, LEGISLATION IN ENGLAND.
Bibliography: Letchworth, W. P. 1889. *The insane in foreign countries.*

INSTINCTS, THEORY OF. A theory developed by Sigmund Freud (q.v.) following his work in 1905 on the sexual instincts and the ego instincts. According to Freud an instinct is a primal trend or urge that cannot be resolved.
Bibliography: Freud, S. 1905. *Three essays on the theory of sexuality.*

INSTITUTE FOR THE CARE AND EDUCATION OF IDIOTS. The first large German institution for the feebleminded. It was opened by C. W. Saegert in Berlin in 1845.
Bibliography: Ireland, W. W. 1898. *Mental afflictions of children.*

INSTITUTE OF LIVING. A nonprofit American psychiatric hospital. It was chartered by the Connecticut State Medical Society in 1822 and has been in continuous operation in Hartford since that year. Charles Dickens (q.v.) visited the institute in 1842 during his visit to the United States and he reported on it in his *American Notes and Pictures from Italy.*
See also HARTFORD RETREAT.
Bibliography: Braceland, F. J. 1972. *The Institute of Living: The Hartford Retreat, 1822-1972.*

INSTITUTION OF FEEBLEMINDED YOUTH. An American institution founded in Columbus, Ohio, following a legislative enactment on April 17, 1857. In 1881 a disastrous fire destroyed a large part of it, but no lives were lost. Its first superintendent was Dr. A. Doren (q.v.).
Bibliography: Kanner, L. 1964. *A history of the care and study of the mentally retarded.*

INTELLIGENCE TEST. Tests for the measurement of intellectual ability. The first tests were devised by Francis Galton (q.v.) in the 1880s. Later intelligence tests were developed by James Cattell, Alfred Binet, and Theodore Simon (qq.v.) as well as others.
Bibliography: Peterson, J. 1926. *Early conceptions and tests of intelligence.*

INTERACTIONISM. René Descartes (q.v.) postulated that mind and body interacted and that the point of contact between them was sited in the pineal

gland, which he regarded as the locus of the soul. This school of thought came to be known as "interactionism."
Bibliography: Kemp Smith, N. 1953. *New studies in the philosophy of Descartes.*

INTERNATIONAL COMMITTEE FOR MENTAL HYGIENE. An organization founded in Washington, D.C., in 1930 through the efforts of Clifford W. Beers (q.v.). Its first president was Dr. William A. White (q.v.).
Bibliography: Deutsch, A. 1949. *The mentally ill in America.*

INTERNATIONAL CONGRESS OF PSYCHIATRY. The first International Congress of Psychiatry was held in Paris, France, in 1950.
Bibliography: Galdston, I. ed. 1967. *Historic derivations of modern psychiatry.*

INTERNATIONAL PSYCHOANALYTICAL ASSOCIATION. A central organization of psychoanalysts. It was founded in 1910 at the Second International Congress of Psychoanalysis in Nuremberg, Germany. The founders of the association were a small group of followers of Sigmund Freud (q.v.).
Bibliography: Sulloway, F. J. 1979. *Freud: biologist of the mind.*

INTERPERSONAL THEORY. A therapeutic approach based on the importance of understanding the interactions between people as the key to understanding personality problems. It was developed by Harry Stack Sullivan (q.v.) in 1953.
Bibliography: Sullivan, H. S. 1953. *The interpersonal theory of psychiatry.*

INTROVERT TYPE. One of the psychological types in the classification devised by Carl Jung (q.v.).
See also EXTROVERT TYPE.
Bibliography: Jung, C. G. 1923. *Psychological types,* trans. H. G. Baynes.

INTUITION TYPE. Carl Jung (q.v.) recognized four function types in his classification. They were linked to intuition, feeling, thinking, and sensation.
See also SENSATION TYPE and THINKING TYPE.
Bibliography: Brome, V. 1978. *Jung: man and myth.*

INVERNESS MADHOUSE. A madhouse existing near a bridge in Inverness, Scotland until the nineteenth century. Houses for lepers (*see* LEPROSY) and the insane were often placed near bridges and the main roads out of towns to allow the inmates to beg alms from passing travelers. Robert Gardiner Hill (q.v.) described the Inverness Madhouse as follows:

At Inverness, between the second and third arches of the old bridge, built in 1685, there is a dismal vault, used first as a jail and afterwards as a mad-house. This appalling place of durance, where the inmates were between the constant hoarse sound of the stream beneath, and the occasional trampling of feet and rattling of wheels overhead, existed as late as 1815, and is said not to have been abandoned till its last miserable inmate, a maniac, had been devoured by rats.

Bibliography: Letchworth, W. P. 1889. *The insane in foreign countries.*

IRELAND, WILLIAM WETHERSPOON (1832–1909). A Scottish physician and a descendent of John Knox through his paternal grandmother. His wide range of interests included art, psychology and literature. He bacame assistant surgeon to the East India Company and during the siege of Delhi in 1857 (about which he subsequently wrote a history) he was severely wounded. He lost one eye, was retired by the company, and spent ten years recuperating. In 1889 he was well enough to accept the office of medical superintendent of the Scottish National Institute for Imbecile Children. In 1880, Ireland established a private home for mentally retarded children. He wrote on mental disorders in children and on idiocy (*see* IDIOT). His book *On Idiocy and Imbecility* (1877) was considered the first systematic textbook on the subject and contained a new classification comprising twelve subdivisions of retardation: 1) genetous idiocy; 2) microcephalic idiocy; 3) eclampsic idiocy; 4) epileptic (*see* EPILEPSY) idiocy; 5) hydrocephalic idiocy; 6) paralytic idiocy; 7) traumatic idiocy; 8) inflammatory idiocy; 9) sclerotic idiocy; 10) syphilitic (*see* SYPHILIS) idiocy; 11) cretinism (q.v.) 12) idiocy by deprivation. In 1898 he published *The Mental Afflictions of Children: Idiocy, Imbecility and Insanity.* He also was interested in the psychological study of famous people and wrote essays on many of them, including Mohammed, Martin Luther, Joan of Arc, and William Blake (qq.v.), among others. One book, which was entitled *Through the Ivory Gate* (1889), was devoted to Emanuel Swedenborg (q.v.).

Bibliography: Ireland, W. W. 1885. *The blot upon the brain.*

IRELAND. Superstition dominated the treatment of mental disorders and the mentally ill in Ireland, as in other countries, for many centuries. Incantations (q.v.), exorcism (q.v.), prayers, holy wells (q.v.), and special herbs were all part of the treatment, which was administered more frequently by clerics than by doctors. One superstition held that lunatics, if left to wander, would spontaneously congregate in a valley called Glen-na-galt (q.v.). It was Jonathan Swift (q.v.) who founded the first asylum (q.v.) for the insane in Ireland. It was known as Saint Patrick's Hospital (q.v.) and opened in Dublin in 1745. It and four houses of correction remained the only places that would receive lunatics until 1810, when the government ordered an inquiry. The inquiry resulted in the appropriation of a building in Dublin, which was adapted to serve as an asylum for the whole of Ireland. Known

as the Richmond District Lunatic Asylum (q.v.), it opened in 1815 and was the first public asylum in Ireland.
Bibliography: Tuke, D. H. 1882. *History of the insane in the British Isles.*

IRENE. A patient of Pierre Janet (q.v.). He made her the subject of one of his classic case histories. She was admitted to the Salpêtrière (q.v.) at the age of twenty-three, suffering from hallucinations, (q.v.), amnesia (q.v.), somnambulism (q.v.), and hysterical (*see* HYSTERIA) crises. The symptoms had appeared after the death of her tuberculotic (*see* TUBERCULOSIS) mother, whom she had nursed. Janet treated her with hypnotism (q.v.), during which suggestion and mental stimulation were employed.
Bibliography: Janet, P. 1904. L'amnésie et la dissociation des souvenirs. *Journal de psychologie* 1: 28-37.

IRIS. A tuberous plant. Celsus (q.v.) recommended an ointment made from it for cases of mental disorders. The ointment was to be rubbed into the scalp of the patient and the treatment repeated until successful.
Bibliography: Celsus. *De Medicina,* trans. by W. G. Spencer, 1935-38.

IRISH, DAVID (fl. 1700). An unqualified practitioner. He kept a private madhouse at Guildford in Surrey, England, and publicized it in 1700 in a booklet entitled *Lavamen Infirmi: or, Cordial Counsel to the Sick and Diseased.* The book was plagiarized from more learned works, especially Timothy Bright's (q.v.) *Treatise of Melancholie* (q.v.). Irish promised to cure the curable, while the "not curable, he will take them for term of life, if paid quarterly. . . ." The madhouse remained in his family for at least a century.
See also ADVERTISING.
Bibliography: Parry-Jones, W. Ll. 1972. *The trade in lunacy.*

IRMA. A patient of Sigmund Freud (q.v.). On the night of July 23 or 24, 1895, Freud had a dream (q.v.) about Irma. On waking, he immediately made notes about what he had dreamed and subsequently analyzed the content of his dream in detail. This interpretation was the first he undertook and became the prototype of dream analysis.
Bibliography: Freud, S. 1900. *The interpretation of dreams.*

IROQUOIS INDIANS. North American Indian tribe found in the northeastern part of the United States. Dream analysis was part of their cultural pattern. They regarded dreams (q.v.) as "windows of the soul" and believed that unconscious wishes could be expressed in dreams.
Bibliography: Wallace, A. 1959. The institutionalization of cathartic and control strategies in Iroquois religious psychotherapy. In *Culture and mental health,* ed. M. Opler.

IRRITABILITY. A kind of automatic response to stimuli, which Francis Glisson (q.v.) attributed to all tissues, particularly nerve tissue. The theory

of irritability was widely expanded by John Brown (q.v.) and Albrecht Von Holler (q.v.) in the eighteenth century and continued to influence psychiatric thought in the nineteenth century.
Bibliography: Brown, J. 1780. *Elementa medicinae.*

ISABELLA OF PORTUGAL (1428?-1496). The second wife of John II (1405–1454) of Castile. She was the mother of Queen Isabella the Catholic of Spain. Left a widow at twenty she became melancholic, (*see* MELANCHOLIA) and then insane. She was said to have transmitted insanity to her granddaughter, Joanna of Castile (q.v.), who in turn was held responsible for the insanity of Don Carlos (q.v.). Isabella was kept in solitary confinement in the castle of Arevalo for forty years.
Bibliography: Chapman, E. C. 1918. *A history of Spain.*

ISHTAR. Babylonian and Assyrian goddess of love and war. She appears in many myths of the Near and Middle East. Although she was the goddess of erotic love, she was also vengeful, irritable, possessive, and extravagant. Tammuz, her husband, rejected her love and accused her of turning her lovers into beasts. Ritual prostitution was a part of her rites.
Bibliography: Benét, W. R., ed. 1965. *The reader's encyclopedia.*

ISIDORE OF SEVILLE, SAINT (560?-636). A Spanish scholar. He became archbishop of Seville in 600. He wrote a treatise on medicine that followed the traditions of Hippocrates (q.v.) and Galen (q.v.). He believed that melancholy (*see* MELANCHOLIA) was caused by black choler (q.v.), which was more apt to form during cold (q.v.), dry weather (q.v.). In this way, he drew a relationship between the seasons and melancholy. In his *Etymologies*, an encyclopedia, he tried to distinguish between the mentally ill with no intellect (*amens*) and those who retained part of their understanding (*demens*). Fatua (q.v.) is also mentioned by him.
Bibliography: MacKinney, L. C. 1937. *Early medieval medicine.*

ISIS. An Egyptian goddess identified with the moon (q.v.). She was consulted in cases of illness and was believed to advise on treatment through revelations.
Bibliography: Cerný, J. 1952. *Ancient Egyptian religion.*

ISOLATION. Jean Esquirol (q.v.) thought that isolation was beneficial in the treatment of insanity. Believing that new surroundings would produce new sensations and thus break the chain of ideas that bothered the patient, he recommended isolating the patient from familiar surroundings and having

him cared for by strangers. He noted that foreigners were more often cured than local residents because the latter were not sufficiently isolated.
Bibliography: Esquirol, J. E. D. 1845. Reprint 1965. *Mental maladies: a treatise on insanity.*

ISOLDE (ISEULT). Heroine of the Tristan (q.v.) and Isolde legend that appears in the short verse romance *Tristan* written by Gottfried von Strassburg around 1250. When Tristan dies, Isolde, overcome by grief, also dies. She thus serves as an early example of psychosomatic death. In 1865 Richard Wagner (q.v.) composed *Tristan and Isolde* based on the legend. It gives a powerful and dramatic rendering of the emotions felt by the dying Isolde, who has willed her own death.
Bibliography: Harewood, ed. 1969. *Kobbe's complete opera book.*

ITARD, JEAN MARIE GASPARD (1774-1838). French physician. He specialized in the training of deaf-mutes and, following his experiences with the wild boy of Aveyron (q.v.), pioneered the systematic training of the mentally retarded. Itard could not accept that the boy, who was found living alone and far removed from all human contacts, was ineducable and set about turning him "from savagery to civilization, from natural life to social life." He believed that the child's condition was the result of social and educational neglect and isolation. Although he was not wholly successful, Itard's efforts were a positive contribution to the understanding and management of mental defectives. Less well known is his description, written in 1825, of the case of the Marquise de Dampierre, who, from the age of seven until her death at the age of eighty-five, suffered from jerking tics and involuntary vocalization of obscene epithets. This was the first description of a condition that was later investigated by Georges Gilles de la Tourette (q.v.) and eventually named after him.
Bibliography: Lane, H. 1977. *The wild boy of Aveyron.*

IVAN IV, VASILIEVICH (IVAN THE TERRIBLE) (1530–1584). A czar of Russia. He was brought up among violence and bloodshed. He was three years old when his father died. His mother, who may have been poisoned, died when he was eight years old. He came to believe that force provided the only means of survival. An anxious, irritable, ruthless, and cruel man, he enjoyed watching animals and people tortured and put to death. After the death of his first wife in 1560, he ruled Russia by terror, alternating between fits of religion and mysticism and periods of sadism (q.v.). Although he was married six more times, none of his later wives exercised the same good influence on him as his first wife had. During a quarrel he killed his

son Ivan with his own hands, and it was said that this event led to his death by sorrow.
Bibliography: Vipper, R. 1947. *Ivan Grozny.*

IVY, GROUND. *Glechoma,* an aromatic perennial, common in many countries. The leaves of ground ivy were believed to have curative properties in cases of mental disorders. John Wesley (q.v.) thought that melancholia (q.v.) could be cured by the juice of ground ivy taken twice a day. He also advised rubbing the head several times a day with vinegar (q.v.) in which ground ivy leaves had been infused. The following prescription was one of his:

Boil juice of ground ivy with sweet oil and white wine juice into an ointment. Shave the head anointed therewith, and chafe it in, warm, every other day for three weeks; bruise also the leaves and bind them on the head, and give three spoonfuls of the juice warm every morning.

In the United States in the nineteenth century, the ground ivy was believed to be beneficial in hypochondria (q.v.) and monomania (q.v.).
Bibliography: le Strange, R. 1977. *A history of herbal plants.*

IWAKURA HOSPITAL. A psychiatric hospital near Kyoto, Japan. Its origin is linked with the legend of Princess Daiunji (q.v.), the daughter of the emperor Sanjo II, who reigned in the eleventh century. She was cured of her melancholia (q.v.) by drinking the water from the holy fountain of a temple at Iwakura. The temple became famous as a place for treatment of the mentally ill, and the village around it provided family care (q.v.) for the temple's visitors. The first hospital there was built in 1884, and its staff continued the tradition by supervising the care of patients housed in the surrounding inns and cottages. After 1950 the Japanese government made it illegal for mental patients to be treated outside of hospitals, therefore the Iwakura system of care was discontinued. A new, Western-style hospital was built in 1953.
Bibliography: Greenland, C. 1963. Family care of mental patients. *Am. J. Psychiat.* 119:1000.

IXTAB. The goddess of suicide (q.v.) in Mayan culture. She was also called "the lady of the rope." According to Mayan culture, those who died by their own hand were sacred and their souls went to a special heaven of their own.
Bibliography: Van Hagen, V.W. 1970. *El mundo de los Mayas.*

J

JACINTH (*or* HYACINTH). A gem, a variety of zircon. In the Middle Ages (q.v.), it was believed to avert depression. Marbodius (1037-1125), bishop of Rennes, wrote that it dispelled sadness and "vain suspicions" (paranoia [q.v.]). Albertus Magnus (q.v.), in his *Book of Secrets*, wrote that "it maketh strangers sure, and acceptable to their guests. And it provoketh sleep for the coldness of it."
See also PRECIOUS STONES.
Bibliography: Evans, J. 1922. *Magical jewels*.

JACKSON, JOHN HUGHLINGS (1835-1911). One of the most important British neurologists. His work was greatly influenced by Charles Brown-Sequard (q.v.). Jackson's early education left him without a classical background or an appreciation of the arts, and his reading was limited to thrillers and Westerns, which he tore into two parts, and carried in his jacket pockets. As soon as each page was read, it was discarded. If he borrowed a book, he was likely to return it with the relevant pages torn out. Because he was a poor speaker and a poor writer, his ideas were slow to be recognized but eventually greatly influenced his followers. In 1862 Jackson joined the staff of the newly founded National Hospital for the Paralysed and Epileptic in Queen Square, London. In 1865 he married his cousin, Elizabeth Dade, who died in 1876 of cerebral thrombophlebitis, which caused frequent focal seizures. This particular type of epilepsy (q.v.) was first described by him and now is known as Jacksonian epilepsy. The death of his wife left him inconsolable, and for the remainder of his life he kept her place set at the dinner table. His last years were made more lonely by deafness. He became vague and absentminded and suffered from vertigo. The concept of levels

of evolution of the nervous system was formulated by him. In *Factors of Insanity* he listed the positive symptoms of psychosis (q.v.).
Bibliography: Jackson, J. H. 1932. *Selected writings.*

JACK THE CLIPPER. A term first used in Chicago, Illinois, in reference to a man who clipped off the hair of many girls in the space of several years. The term now indicates any individual with a morbid urge to cut off women's hair.
Bibliography: Hinsie, L. E., and Campbell, R. J. 1960. *Psychiatric dictionary.*

JACK THE RIPPER. The assumed name of an individual who committed a number of brutal murders in the East End of London between 1888 and 1889. His victims were all prostitutes. It was postulated that he was a physician, suffering from epilepsy (q.v.).
Bibliography: Knight, S. 1976. *Jack the Ripper: the final solution.*

JACOB, SARAH (1857-1869). A Welsh country girl. She became nationally famous for her assertion that she could live without food or drink. Her hysterical (*see* HYSTERIA) assertions convinced her parents, and many people joined in the delusion (q.v.). Organized guides met visitors at the trains and conducted them to the farm at Lletherneuadd. There they were confronted by the strange sight of the little girl, who was dressed as a bride, wreathed with flowers, and propped up in a bed surrounded by gifts. Eventually the medical press and the *Times* became involved in the controversy. When four nurses from Guy's Hospital were sent to the Welsh village to watch over her, it became apparent that, unable to get food by subterfuge, she would starve. Still believing in "the miracle" of her fast (*see* FASTING), her parents forbade that she should be given food, and she died.
Bibliography: Cule, J. 1967. *Wreath on the crown: the story of Sarah Jacob, the Welsh fasting girl.*

JACOBI, CARL WIEGANT MAXIMILIAN (1775-1858). A German physician. He was medical superintendent of the Siegburg Asylum, which was near Bonn. Jacobi asserted that no psychology was necessary to understand and treat insanity, which he regarded as an organic disorder of the brain. He advocated classifying mental patients into categories according to the "degree of influence which their disease has over their moral and social behaviour" and according to the type of treatment they required. He translated into German *Description of the Retreat* by Samuel Tuke (q.v.) and combined it with a copy of his own book on the construction of asylums (q.v.).
Bibliography: Jacobi, M. 1834. *On the construction and management of hospitals for the insane,* trans. J. Kitching.

JACOPONE DA TODI (1230?-1306). An Italian poet and mystic. As a young man he practiced law but left himself enough free time to lead a very

gay life. He had been married for a year when his beautiful wife died, after the room in which they were dancing with a crowd of young friends collapsed. It was discovered that under her rich gown she was wearing a penitent's hair shirt. The discovery so affected Jacopone that he turned away from society and entered a convent, where he passionately extolled the need for penance and preached against vice, especially among the clergy. His works are filled with mysticism and a desire for suffering is epitomised in one of his poems in which he asks the Lord to send him ill health. He begs for no less than twenty-two different diseases, the more painful the better, and hopes that they will culminate in a hard death, that his remains will be devoured by a wolf, and that they will be reduced to dung among thorns and rocks.
Bibliography: Underhill, E. 1919. *Jacopone da Todi: poet and mystic.*

JAENSCH, ERICH R. (1883-1940). A German psychologist and pupil of Georg E. Müller (q.v.). He was particularly concerned with problems of visual perception in the representation and perception of space and eidetic imagery. He tried to establish a closer link between philosophy and psychology.
See also BASEDOWOID TYPE and TETANOID TYPE.
Bibliography: Jaensch, E. R. 1941. *Zur Eidetik und Integrationstypology.*

JAGUNÇOS. A Brazilian Indian tribe converted to a mystical form of religion by Antonio Conselheiro during the 1890s. Conselheiro's teachings were found by the government to be disruptive, and he and his followers were prosecuted. They preferred to die fighting rather than to compromise with the government—an example of religious suicide (q.v.).
Bibliography: Fedden, G. R. 1938. *Suicide.*

JAKOB, ALFONS MARIA (1884-1931). A German neurologist. His work covered various aspects of degeneration in the central nervous system, including neurosyphilis. He described a disease entity that was distinguished by mental deterioration and disorders of the pyramidal and extrapyramidal system. The condition is now known as Jackob-Creutzfeldt's disease, as another German neurologist, Hans Gerhald Creutzfeldt (1885-1964) also contributed to its elucidation. Jakob's laboratory in Hamburg became a center of interest for neurologists of many countries.
Bibliography: Haymaker, W., and Schiller, F. 1970. *The founders of neurology.* 2d. ed..

JAKOBSSTAD. The site of the first institution in Finland for the feebleminded. It was founded in 1876 by M. K. Lundberg.
Bibliography: Barr, M. W. 1904. *Mental defectives.*

JAMES I OF ENGLAND, VI OF SCOTLAND (1566-1625). The son of Mary Queen of Scots (1542-1587) and Lord Henry Darnley (1545-1567).

In 1603 on the death of Elizabeth I, James succeeded to the English throne. He believed in witches but distinguished between them and those suffering from "melancholique humours." He opposed the views of Johann Weyer (q.v.) on witchcraft (q.v.) and refuted *The Discovery of Witchcraft* (1584) by Reginald Scot (q.v.) in a volume entitled *Daemonologie in the Forme of a Dialogue* (q.v.). He ordered all copies of Scot's book to be burned. In 1605, he wrote a report on Anne Gunter (q.v.) whom he had personally examined. He found her to be sick with love (q.v.), rather than "bewitched." Although James encouraged the belief in witches, he promoted the medical examination of those accused of witchcraft who prior to then had been scrutinized by the church only. Mayerne (q.v.), the royal physician, wrote that the king suffered from "terrifying insomnia" and hallucinations (q.v.), he was easily moved, melancholic (*see* MELANCHOLIA), and given to bouts of wrath. Other recorded symptoms suggest that he was probably a victim of porphyria (q.v.).
Bibliography: Wilson, D. H. 1956. *James VI and I.*

JAMES III (1451-1488). Son of James II of Scotland. He became king at the age of nine. Unbalanced and easily influenced by others, his extravagances and vagaries alienated the loyalty of his people. He invited the Danish astrologer-physician Andrew Alaman to Scotland, and Alaman's astrological (*see* ASTROLOGY) prediction that the king would die at the hands of a member of his own family caused James to become even more suspicious and paranoid (*see* PARANOIA).
Bibliography: Mackenzie, A. M. 1935. *The rise of the Stewarts 1329-1513.*

JAMES V (1512-1542). A king of Scotland. After the death of his first wife, he married Mary of Guise (1515-1560). The uncertain tenor of their marriage took a turn for the better when Mary produced two sons, but they both died in infancy. It was thought at the time that their unexpected deaths were due to the sins of their father being visited upon them. The king, who was already bowed by political troubles and prone to collapse in moments of stress, became depressed and predicted that he would die before the end of the year, although he seemed quite healthy. As he lay in the sickroom at his favorite palace, he was told of the birth of a daughter, Mary, the future queen of Scots, but he was so disappointed that the child was not male that he sank deeper into his melancholy (*see* MELANCHOLIA) and died within a week.
Bibliography: Hay, D. 1955. *The letters of James V.*

JAMES, HENRY (1843-1916). An American writer and the son of a distinguished philosopher. James was given an unorthodox education augmented by long journeys through Europe. Believing that his writings were not understood by Americans and after various absences from the United

States, he settled in Britain in 1876. His novels pioneered psychological realism and an awareness of the social conflicts between the New World and the Old. His novel *The Turn of the Screw*, which was first published in 1898, is of special psychiatric interest. It is a horror story concerning a governess whose behavior accurately mirrors the symptoms of temporal lobe epilepsy (q.v.), a syndrome described by John Hughlings Jackson (q.v.) in the journal *Brain* (q.v.) about a year before James wrote the novel. Fredrick Macmillan, the publisher of *Brain*, was also James' publisher, and it is possible that they discussed Jackson's papers, or the latter may have been directly acquainted with James and helped him. It is also theorized that James derived the framework of the story from the case of two children allegedly possessed (*see* POSSESSION) by the spirits of bad servants. James himself wrote that he heard the story during a dinner conversation with the archbishop of Canterbury.
Bibliography: Edel, L. 1977. *Life of Henry James*.

JAMES, WILLIAM (1842-1910). An American philosopher and psychologist. His father was a famous philosopher and his brother, Henry James (q.v.), a famous writer. William James developed a theory of behavior based on the belief that instincts and their linked emotions were hereditary. He regarded the mind and mental processes as subordinate to the organism as a whole in the struggle for survival. As early as 1875, James organized courses in physiological psychology (q.v.) that were supported by facilities for experiments at Harvard University. In 1890, after twelve years of hard work and much ill health, he completed his *Principles of Psychology* in which he expanded his famous theory of emotions that he had originally propounded in 1884. During the terrible earthquake of 1906 he was in San Francisco and later wrote about his experience and feelings at that time in "On Some Mental Affects of the Earthquake." James is regarded as America's senior psychologist. Among his works are *Talks to Teachers* (1899); *The Varieties of Religious Experience* (1902); *Pragmatism* (1907) and *The Meaning of Truth* (1909). Pierre Janet (q.v.) was greatly influenced by him.
Bibliography: Watson, R. I. 1963. *The great psychologists*.

JAMES-LANGE THEORY OF EMOTION. *See* EMOTION, THEORY OF.

JANET, PIERRE (1859-1947). A French psychiatrist. Born in Paris, where he lived most of his life, he came from an intellectual upper middle-class family. As a child he experienced the hardships of war during the siege of Paris by the Germans. He was a shy and solitary adolescent, who went through a period of deep depression, culminating in a religious crisis from which he emerged as an agnostic. In 1881, at the age of twenty-two he became a professor of philosophy. His second teaching appointment was at the Liceum of Le Havre, and it was there that he began to do psychiatric

research at the local hospital. He also began to collect material for a thesis on certain aspects of hallucinations (q.v.) and became interested in hypnotism, (q.v.). In 1885 he published the results of his experiments with Léonie (q.v.). His paper brought him fame, but he realized that he could not undertake more research in psychopathology without a degree in medicine. He received his doctorate in 1889, with a thesis entitled *L'autotisme psychologique*, which went into several editions. It was on the basis of this thesis that he later claimed to have formulated the concept of the unconscious (q.v.) before Sigmund Freud (q.v.). In 1890 Janet, at the invitation of Jean Martin Charcot (q.v.) became the director of the psychological laboratory (q.v.) at the Salpêtrière (q.v.). Although Charcot died three years later, his influence left a permanent mark on Janet. Janet tried to unify academic and clinical psychology and his original interest in hysteria (q.v.) and hypnotism developed into a wider interest in human behavior as a whole. He developed a theory of obsessive ideas (idée fixe [q.v.]) and further developed the concepts of neurasthenia (q.v.) and psychasthenia (q.v.) based on the belief of psychic weakness. He was so careful about divulging material concerning his patients he stipulated in his will that the files of over 5,000 patients should be burned at his death. By the time of his death he had seen two world wars that had considerably changed Europe. He is buried in the cemetery of Bourg-la-Reine, Paris.
Bibliography: Altschule, M. D. 1976. *The development of traditional psychopathology.*

JANSSENS, ABRAHAM (1575-1632). A Flemish painter. He was an impetuous man, who was often overwhelmed by the consequences of his actions. He married a beautiful girl and produced a large brood of children, but the worry of providing for them reduced him to melancholy (*see* MELANCHOLIA), which in turn prevented him from working. He would stroll aimlessly around Antwerp, listless and depressed until his friends restored him to fleeting good humor.
Bibliography: Wittkower, R., and Wittkower, M. 1963. *Born under Saturn.*

JARKMAN. A sixteenth-century term for a beggar clever enough to pretend insanity and to forge official documents allowing him to beg. It was a corruption of Abraham-man, or Abraham-men (q.v.).
Bibliography: 1978. *Brewers dictionary of phrase and fable.*

JARRETT, MARY C. The American social worker who originated the designation "psychiatric social worker." In 1913 she was appointed director of social work at the Boston Psychopathic Hospital. With the help of Elmer Southard (q.v.) she systematized case-history taking and the training of psychiatric social workers.
Bibliography: Gray, F. P. 1938. *The open mind: Elmer Ernest Southard 1876-1920.*

JARVIS, EDWARD (1803-1884). An American physician. His studies of medical statistics, particularly in relation to insanity made him famous. He

investigated the causes of mental illness and tried to determine whether or not its incidence was related to civilization and industrial development. Jarvis was a keen reformer of mental institutions. In 1843 he opened a private asylum (q.v.) in his own home.
Bibliography: Grob, G. N. 1978. *Edward Jarvis and the medical world of nineteenth-century America.*

JASPER. A gem. Galen (q.v.) believed that it protected its wearer from lethargy and epilepsy (q.v.). It was also believed to offer protection against phantasms and witchcraft (q.v.).
See also PRECIOUS STONES.
Bibliography: Evans, J. 1922. *Magical jewels.*

JASPERS, KARL THEODORE (1883-1969). A German philosopher and psychiatrist. The work of Friedrich Nietzsche (q.v.), particularly in the field of instincts, was one of the major influences in shaping his thoughts. His writings contributed to a better understanding of psychopathology, and his individual approach to the interpretation of morbid phenomena greatly influenced orthodox psychiatric practice. He was professor of philosophy at Heidelberg University from 1921 until 1948, except for the years between 1936 and 1945, when the Nazis forbade him to teach. In 1948 he went to Basle, Switzerland, as professor of philosophy.
Bibliography: Jaspers, K. 1962. *General psychopathology*, trans. J. Hoening and M. Hamilton.

JASTROW, JOSEPH (1863-1944). An American psychologist born in Poland. His interest turned from psychophysics to experimental psychology (q.v.). In 1888, he was appointed professor of psychology at the University of Wisconsin, where he opened a laboratory. His work included research in telepathy (q.v.), the occult, spiritualism (q.v.), hypnotism (q.v.), deception, and the dreams (q.v.) of the blind.
Bibliography: Jastrow, J. 1900. *Fact and fable in psychology.*

JEALOUSY. In his *Anatomy of Melancholy* (q.v.), Robert Burton (q.v.) referred to jealousy as a precipitating factor and a cause of depression. Nineteenth-century British psychiatrists considered jealousy in its medico-legal implications. Both D. H. Tuke (q.v.) and Henry Maudsley (q.v.) wrote about it in these terms. In France, Jacques Moreau de Tours (q.v.) wrote a book entitled *De la folie jalouse* (1877) in which he discussed jealousy as a form of insanity. In Germany, Richard von Krafft-Ebing (q.v.) also studied jealousy, especially in alcoholics (*see* ALCOHOLISM). Karl Jaspers (q.v.) and Emil Kraepelin (q.v.) recognized two types of jealousy: one, a morbid process in neurosis (q.v.) and another, a form of paranoia (q.v.) in a disintegrating personality. At various times and by different schools of psychiatry (q.v.) jealousy has been thought to be a part of a disorder or a disorder in its own right. Delusions (q.v.) of jealousy have been called the Othello syndrome by J. Todd and K. Dewhurst.

Bibliography: Todd, J. and Dewhurst, K.. The Othello syndrome, a study of the psychopathology of sexual jealousy. 1955. *J. Nerv. Ment. Dis.* 122, 367-74.

JEKYLL and HYDE. *See* THE STRANGE CASE OF DR. JEKYLL AND MR. HYDE.

JELLIFFE, SMITH ELY (1866-1945). An American psychiatrist and neurologist. He began his professional career as a botanist who was a collector of facts and well versed in many fields, particularly in medical history, pharmacology, and biology. Jelliffe became interested in the evolution of mental development and realized the connections between physical and psychological phenomena. His work in this field gained for him the title of "father of psychosomatic medicine [q.v.] in America." He helped to forge a closer link between psychoanalysts and university psychiatrists and freely disseminated ideas of Sigmund Freud (q.v.).

Bibliography: Jelliffe, S. E. 1939. *Sketches in psychosomatic medicine.*

JENNER, EDWARD (1749-1823). An English physician and pupil of John Hunter (q.v.). He originated the vaccination against smallpox. Jenner lost both parents early in life and was given to depression. He wrote of himself: "I have been through life, almost from the earliest period of my recollection, haunted by melancholy."

Bibliography: Fisk, D. 1959. *Doctor Jenner of Berkeley.*

JENNINGS, HERBERT SPENCER (1868-1947). An American naturalist. He was particularly interested in animal behavior and genetics. According to him, even the simplest organisms displayed behavior that could be modified. From his work in this area, he concluded that consciousness was inherent in all animal life and that behavior depended on the mind rather than on simple physiochemical reactions.

Bibliography: Jennings, H. P. 1904. *Behavior of the Lower Organisms.*

JEPSON, GEORGE (1745-1836) *and* **JEPSON, KATHERINE** (1797-1822). Husband and wife and the superintendent/apothecary and matron of the York Retreat (q.v.). George Jepson was a weaver, who had taught himself some medicine. Katherine Jepson (née Allen) had had previous nursing experience at Brislington House (q.v.). They worked at the Retreat for

twenty-six years and they introduced various forms of humane nursing. They are regarded as the originators of systematic mental nursing in England.
Bibliography: Hunter, R., and Macalpine, I. 1963. *Three hundred years of psychiatry*.

JEREMIAH. A prophet of the Old Testament. He was disliked and persecuted for his defeatism. His name has come to be used to indicate a depressed individual who sees the future as hopeless.
Bibliography: 1978. *Brewer's dictionary of phrase and fable*.

JEROME, SAINT (c.340-420). A Christian ascetic (q.v.) and scholar, born in Stridon on the border of Dalmatia. In 386 he went to a monastery in Bethlehem and devoted his time to study and writing. He formulated regulations for the monks and enjoined them to care for the sick and the mentally ill. He was hostile to science and vowed never to read pagan books.
Bibliography: Kelly, J.N.D. 1976. *Jerome*.

JERUSALEM. A hospital for mental patients existed in Jerusalem as early as A.D. 491.
Bibliography: Burdett, H. C. 1891. *Hospitals and asylums of the world*.

JESSEN, PETER WILLERS (1793-1875). A German physician. In 1857 he and Johannes Friedrich von Esmarch (q.v.) suggested that syphilis (q.v.) was the essential cause of general paralysis of the insane (q.v.).

JET. A black semiprecious stone. In ancient times lapidaries attributed anaesthetic properties to it. It also was believed to protect those who wore it from spells, illusions, and enchantments.
See also PRECIOUS STONES.
Bibliography: Evans, J. 1922. *Magical jewels*.

JEU DE LA FEUILLÉE, LE. A French play by Adam de la Ahlle (c.1240-1288), it was first performed in 1262. Among its characters is a madman who suffers from delusions (q.v.) of grandeur and persecution mania (q.v.). Reflecting the popular image of a madman in France at that time, he is depicted as noisy, restless, and destructive. A monk attempts to cure him through the use of holy relics but fails, and the patient is sent home to a regime of rest and quiet, which reflects the popular treatment of the time.

JEWELL, JOHN (1522-1571). An English theologian and bishop of Salisbury. He was deeply involved in the religious controversies of the sixteenth century. One of his sermons, given in the presence of Queen Elizabeth I (1533-1603) asked for a more stringent execution of the laws against witchcraft (q.v.). Bishop Jewell maintained that he had seen innumerable examples of the witches' work that caused the Queen's subjects to pine away. Ac-

cording to his description, "'their colour fadeth, their flesh rotteth, their speech is benumbed, their senses are bereft."
Bibliography: Sitwell, E. 1962. *The queens and the hive.*

JOAN (POPE) (fl. 853-855). A legendary character and example of transvestism in the Middle Ages (q.v.). According to the legend, her name was Giliberta. She assumed male dress to follow her lover, who was a monk. When he died, she continued her deception, studied theology, and went to Rome, where she was eventually elected pope after the death of Pope Leo IV (800?-855). It was said that her true identity was discovered when she gave birth to a child during a religious procession. She was thrown into a dungeon and died there. The story first appeared in the thirteenth century in the writings of the Dominican Étienne de Bourbon.
Bibliography: von Döllinger, J.J.I. 1872. *Fables respecting the popes of the Middle Ages.*

JOANNA OF CASTILE (1479-1555). Also known as Juana la Loca, Joanna the Mad. She was the eldest daughter of Ferdinand (1452-1516) and Isabella of Castile (1451-1504). She became queen of Castile and Aragon and the mother of Charles V (q.v.), the Holy Roman emperor from 1519 to 1556. When she was seventeen years old, she married Philip the Fair of Burgundy (1478-1506) an unfaithful husband. Her jealousy (q.v.) drove her to the edge of madness, and she became totally deranged when he died. She had him dressed in his regalia and seated on a throne as if he were alive. When the corpse was embalmed, she refused to be separated from it and rushed across Spain with the coffin. She would stop occasionally to check that the body was still in the coffin, and she would not allow any woman near it. One night, finding that her train had stopped in a convent of nuns, she would not rest there and insisted that they should continue the macabre journey in a storm. In 1509 she was confined to the castle of Tordesillas, where she lived in melancholic squalor with the embalmed corpse of Philip close by. She died there, after forty-nine years of insanity. In death she remained close to her husband, they are buried together in the Chapel Royal in Granada, next to Ferdinand and Isabella. Joanna's great-grandson, Don Carlos (q.v.) was said to have inherited her insanity.
Bibliography: Hume, M. 1906. *Queens of old Spain.*

JOAN OF ARC, SAINT (1412?-1431). A French national heroine, born in Domrémy, France. At the age of thirteen she began to have visual and auditory hallucinations (q.v.) that frequently involved the archangels Michael and Gabriel. Under the influence of their voices, she dressed as a soldier and led the French army to raise the siege of Orléans. Her assurance and confident bearing seemed extraordinary to many people. Captured by the Burgundians and sold to the English, she was tried for witchcraft (q.v.)

and heresy. She was condemned and burned at the stake. Her unusual behavior has prompted many explanations. It has been suggested that she suffered from Menière Disease, that she was a transvestite hysteric (*see* HYSTERIA), an epileptic (*see* EPILEPSY), and a royal bastard among other things.
Bibliography: Grayeff, F. 1978. *Joan of Arc: legends and truth.*

JOÂO DE DEUS (SAINT JOHN OF GOD) (1495-1550). Not to be confused with Juan de Dios Huarte (q.v.). He was a Portuguese shepherd and soldier whose real name was Juan Ciudad Duarte. His mother died of grief, and his father retired to a monastery while he was on a crusade. Feeling guilty for these events, he became depressed and restless and traveled from place to place. He finally settled in Granada (q.v.), and, while there, heard a sermon about Saint Sebastian, which left him extremely agitated, crying for mercy for his sins. His behavior was such that he was sent to an asylum (q.v.) where he was flogged and mistreated. On his release, he began to help the sick and the poor and to speak for a more humane treatment of the insane. He founded two hospitals and the religious order of the Hospitallers of Saint John of God, which is still dedicated to the treatment of the mentally and physically ill. When he died, the city of Granada gave him a noble funeral and grandeés of Spain carried his coffin. He is the patron saint of the sick, hospitals, nurses, and in Ireland, of alcoholics.
Bibliography: McMahon, N. 1959. *The story of the hospitallers of Saint John of God.*

JOCASTA. The legendary queen of Thebes. Her husband Laius ordered her to destroy their child because it had been prophesied that he would be killed by his son. The child, named Oedipus (q.v.), was abandoned but survived and grew to manhood unaware of his identity. He killed Laius in a quarrel and married his widow. When the truth was revealed Oedipus gouged out his eyes in shame, and Jocasta hanged herself. Sigmund Freud (q.v.) used the legend in his theory of incestuous (*see* INCEST) wishes, hence the terms "Oedipus complex" and "Jocasta complex," referring to the sexual attachment of sons and mothers.
Bibliography: Sophocles. *Three Theban plays*, trans T. H. Banks.

JOFFROY, ALEXIS (1844-1908). A French neurologist and psychiatrist. He studied general paralysis of the insane (q.v.) as it related to syphilis (q.v.) but did not agree that the two were linked. He argued that syphilis was widespread in Africa, but paralysis was not, and therefore the two could not be connected. To further his argument, he pointed out that mercury (q.v.) did not prevent or cure general paralysis but did help in cases of syphilis.
Bibliography: Fourner, A., and Raymond, F. 1905. *Paralysis général et syphilis.*

JOFRÉ, JUAN GILABERT (1350-1417). A Spanish monk. After he had obtained his legal degree, he was so moved by deep religious feelings that he joined the religious order of the Mercedarians whose purpose was the ransoming of slaves and prisoners of war from the Arabs. While preaching their cause in Valencia to raise funds, Jofré came across a crowd of people who were mocking and mistreating a lunatic (q.v.). He took the poor man under his protection, and his next sermon was a plea for the establishment of a hospital for the insane. Jofré received help from a wealthy citizen named Lorenzo Salom, and eventually enough funds were raised for the establishment of a hospital "for the innocent ones," the insane. Thus the Sancta Maria dels Inocents (q.v.) was founded in Valencia in 1409 and was one of the first psychiatric hospitals in the Western world. (See Plate 7.)
Bibliography: Rumbaut, R. D. 1971-1972. The first psychiatric hospital in the Western world. *Am. J. Psychiat.* 128:1305-309.

JOHANNITIUS ONAN *or* **ONEIN.** *See* HUNAYN IBN ISHAQ.

JOHN XXI (c.1210-1277). The name assumed by Petrus Hispanus (q.v.) on his election as pope in 1276. The only pope who was a physician.

JOHN OF GADDESDEN (c.1280-1349). An English physician and clergyman. He practiced medicine in Oxford and London. When he was appointed court physician to Edward II (1284-1327), he became the first English medical man to receive such an appointment to an English monarch. Around 1314, he wrote a compendium of medicine entitled *Rosa Medicinae*, or *Rosa Anglica*, which was a mixture of Arab folk remedies and superstition. In it he discussed frenesis, mania (q.v.), folly, melancholia (q.v.), and epilepsy (q.v.). He relied on the humoral theory (q.v.) and thought that melancholia was caused by an excess of black bile (q.v.) while corrupt humors caused mania. He attributed epilepsy to a lesion in the upper part of the head and treated it by diet (q.v.), purging (q.v.), and regulating the daily life of the patient. He also devised a mixture of soporific herbs to promote deep sleep during surgical operations. Gaddesden kept most of his remedies secret in order to enhance the physician's status. Albrecht von Haller (q.v.) called him "an empiric, full of superstition, obviously untrained, a lover and eulogist of quack medicines, greedy of gain, an expert in kitchen-lore." Geoffrey Chaucer (q.v.), who may have met him at court, ranked him among the greatest physicians, which reflected the opinion of his times.
Bibliography: Cholmeley, H. P. 1912. *John of Gaddesden and the* Rosa Medicinae.

JOHN OF SALISBURY (c.1115-1180). An English philosopher and divine, famous for his scholarship. He was a pupil of Pierre Abelard (q.v.) in Paris and a friend of Thomas à Becket (1118-1170), whose murder in the cathedral

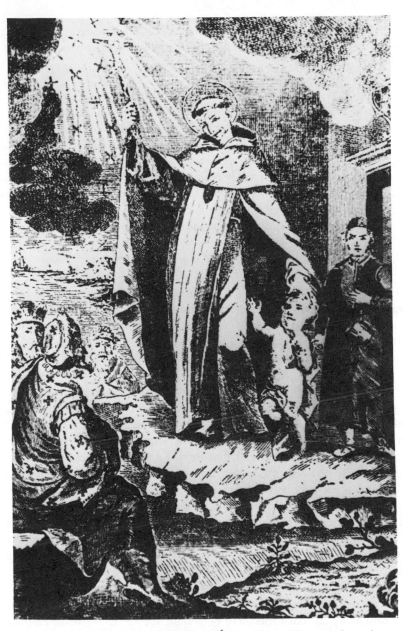

7. FATHER JUAN GILABERT JOFŔE, in an old engraving, shown
with all his attributes: the halo of sanctity, the miraculous shower of
crosses, ships for the redemption of captives, a foundling, and, behind him,
the mental hospital he founded and a mental patient in characteristic garb
of two colors, the left and right sides of the tunic contrasting. By courtesy
of the Department of Medical Illustration, Ipswich Hospital.

of Canterbury he witnessed. He disliked excess, advocated tolerance, and asserted that the devil had no power to cause mental disorders.
Bibliography: Webb, C. C. J. 1909. *John of Salisbury.*

JOHNSON, JAMES (1777-1845). A British physician born in Ireland. He was physician extraordinary to William IV (1765-1837). Johnson was proprietor, editor, and almost sole writer of the monthly *Medico-Chirurgical Journal.* He was the author of a number of books and in one of them, *Change of Air and the Pursuit of Health* (1831), he described a disease that he believed was caused by stress brought about by the Industrial Revolution. He thought that the English were particularly prone to it because they were overworked, did not exercise enough, and lived in a polluted atmosphere. The only remedy he could suggest was travel (q.v.) abroad and a period of rest every year.
Bibliography: Johnson, J. 1831. *Change of air and the pursuit of health.*

JOHNSON, MARY (?-1647). A colonial American woman who lived in Connecticut. She was the first victim of a law that was enacted in 1642 and demanded the death penalty for any man or woman found guilty of witchcraft (q.v.).
Bibliography: Taylor, John M. 1908. *Witchcraft delusion in colonial Connecticut.*

JOHNSON, SAMUEL (1709-1784). An English author, born in Lichfield, the son of a bookseller. His childhood was marred by his parents' continuous conflicts, which left him with a permanent dislike of parental authority and may explain the support he gave to James Boswell (q.v.) during the latter's disagreements with his father. Johnson was a precocious child, who could read at the age of two, and had an extraordinarily retentive memory (q.v.). When he was three years old he was taken to London to be touched for the King's evil (scrofula [q.v.]) by Queen Anne; his family believed that the bad humor of his wet nurse was responsible for his disease. He was deaf in his left ear, almost blind in his left eye, and of a generally weak disposition. At twenty-six, he married a widow twenty-three years older than himself. Johnson was a gloomy man; Boswell, his biographer, mentions the "dejection, gloom and despair which made existence a misery." When he was depressed he had to abandon study and meditation. With great insight he once told Boswell that "melancholy people are apt to fly to intemperance which gives a momentary relief but sinks the soul much lower in misery." Advising a friend who was going on a journey for his health, Johnson wrote, "Cast away all anxiety, and keep your mind easy. . . .with an unquiet mind, neither exercise, nor diet, nor physick can be of much use." He kept a lamp burning by his bedside so that he could read at anytime during the night to disperse the phantoms in his mind. Like his father, he was an hypochondriac

(see HYPOCHONDRIA) and considered himself perpetually on the borderline between sanity and insanity. Many of his writings, especially his *Lives of the Poets* (1779-1781) show a deep understanding of emotional problems. Author of poems, articles, essays, and political commentaries, he is best remembered for his *Dictionary of the English Language* which was published in 1755. His fame, however, is mostly due to Boswell's well-known biography *The Life of Dr. Johnson* (1791).
Bibliography: Bate, W. J. 1978. *Samuel Johnson.*

JOKES. In 1897 Sigmund Freud (q.v.) began to work on a study of jokes, after noticing a similarity between them and dreams (q.v.). His interest had been aroused by Theodor Lipps (q.v.), *Komik and Humor*, and he investigated the subject in depth. The result was his book *Jokes and Their Relation to the Unconscious* (1905), which reflects many aspects of life in Vienna at that time.
Bibliography: Freud, S. 1905. *Der Witz und seine Beziehung zum Unbewussten.*

JOLLY, FRIEDRICH (1844-1904). A German psychiatrist. He conducted research on memory (q.v.), hallucinations (q.v.), aetiology of mental disorders, and the treatment of the insane in hospitals.
Bibliography: Zilboorg, G. 1941. *A history of medical psychology.*

JONES, ERNEST (1879-1958). A British psychoanalyst, born in Wales. As a child he suffered from nightmares (q.v.), which were attributed to the horrific tales his Welsh nanny told him, and vertigo, which he later tried to conquer by climbing mountains. His admiration for the doctor who came to deliver his two sisters, prompted him to study medicine, and he graduated at the age of twenty-one. He became interested in the unconscious (q.v.) and its relationship to sexual instincts. In 1908 he met Sigmund Freud (q.v.) and from that date he became a key figure in psychoanalysis (q.v.), which he introduced to the English-speaking countries. He remained a close and faithful friend of Freud and wrote a biography of him in three volumes between 1953 and 1957. Jones was disliked, however, by many of his fellow psychoanalysts, who were suspicious of his motivations. His psychoanalytical technique was somewhat rigid, and in his early years especially, he often got into difficulties with the sexual fantasies of his female patients. Between 1926 and 1929, he successfully defended psychoanalysis before an official committee of the British Medical Association. Jones also played a major part in helping Freud and his family to leave Vienna. In 1939 he delivered Freud's funeral address, at the request of Freud's family.
Bibliography: Davis, T. G. 1979. *Ernest Jones 1879-1958.*

JONES, JOHN (1645-1709). An English physician. In 1700 he wrote a book entitled *The Mysteries of Opium Reveal'd* in which he described the effects of opium (q.v.). He was aware of the possibility of addiction to it

and described withdrawal symptoms, which include "great and even intolerable distresses, anxieties, and depression of spirit."
Bibliography: Jones, J. 1700. *The mysteries of opium reveal'd.*

JORDEN, EDWARD (1569-1632). A British physician. He was the author of *A Briefe Discourse of a Disease Called the Suffocation of the Mother.* Published in 1603, it was the first English book on hysteria (q.v.). Jorden tried to explain the effects of witchcraft (q.v.) as the effects of nervous disorders connected with the uterus (q.v.). The volume was an attempt to counteract *Daemonologie In the Forme of a Dialogue* (q.v.) by King James I of England and VI of Scotland (q.v.). Jorden was one of the first physicians to give expert evidence in a witchcraft trial. He appeared in the case of Mary Glover (q.v.) in 1602 and later declared Ann Gunter (q.v.) to be hysterical rather than possessed (*see* POSSESSION) by the devil.
Bibliography: Hunter, R., and Macalpine, I. 1963. *Three hundred years of psychiatry.*

JOSEPH P. KENNEDY, JR., MEMORIAL FOUNDATION. A foundation established in 1946 in the United States to assist research in mental retardation and promote the treatment, care, and education of the mentally retarded. It was named after the elder brother of President John F. Kennedy (1917-1963). The Kennedy family developed an interest in mental retardation when it was discovered that one of their daughters was retarded.

JOSEPHSON, ERNST (1851-1906). A Swedish artist. Following repeated disappointments, he is said to have become psychotic (*see* PSYCHOSIS) at the age of thirty-seven. His paintings, poetry, and interest in spiritualism (q.v.) became involved in his delusional (*see* DELUSION) system. He believed that his room was the entrance to heaven and that his own function was to examine the arriving souls before admitting them to the presence of God. He would draw their pictures, interview them, and forgive their sins according to his judgment. His long illness followed an uncertain course with occasional periods of remission.
Bibliography: Millner, S. L. 1948. *Ernst Josephson.*

JOURNAL DE PSYCHOLOGIE. A French journal of psychology founded by Pierre Janet (q.v.) and his friend Georges Dumas in 1904. Most of Janet's articles were published in it.

JOURNAL OF APPLIED PSYCHOLOGY. A journal founded in the United States by Granville Stanley Hall (q.v.) in 1915.

JOURNAL OF GENETIC PSYCHOLOGY. A journal of psychology, originally called *Pedagogical Seminary.* It was founded in 1891 by Granville

Stanley Hall (q.v.). It was the second journal of psychology founded in the United States. The first was the *American Journal of Psychology* (q.v.) .

JOURNAL OF INSANITY. See AMERICAN JOURNAL OF PSYCHIATRY.

JOURNAL OF PSYCHO-ASTHENICS. See AMERICAN JOURNAL OF MENTAL DEFICIENCY.

JOURNAL OF PSYCHOLOGICAL MEDICINE AND MENTAL PA-THOLOGY. The first British psychiatric journal. It was founded in London by Forbes B. Winslow (q.v.) in 1848. Competition from *The Asylum Journal* (q.v.) forced it to include articles on medical politics, literature, and science. In 1861 its name was changed to *The Medical Critic and Psychological Journal*, and it continued publication until 1863. The original name was resumed in 1875, when L.S.F. Winslow, the son of the founder, revived it and continued its publication for another eight years.

JOURNALS BY PATIENTS. In some mental hospitals journals are published by the patients, who contribute articles, undertake the editing, and see to the printing. Early examples are the *Retreat Gazette*, the *Asylum Journal, Excelsior*, the *Opal, Moonbeams*, and *New Moon* (qq.v.). Bibliography: Deutsch, A. 1949. *The mentally ill in America.*

JOYCE, JAMES AUGUSTINE ALOYSIUS (1882-1941). An Irish novelist and poet, born in Dublin and educated by the Jesuits. His father was an improvident and a drunkard, unable to care for and support his wife and ten children. Joyce was for a time, like his father had been, a medical student in Dublin, but the narrow bigotry of Catholicism in Ireland so exasperated him that he left Dublin for Paris, after begging the fee for the trip from friends. He returned twice to Ireland, but most of his life was spent on the Continent where he suffered poverty and ill health. He wandered about Europe with a Dublin chambermaid, whom he eventually married in 1931. His writings show insight and compassion for the failings of men and a deep understanding of the many aspects of personality. His most famous novel, *Ulysses* (1922) presented a new structure in writing. It relied on a subtle form of communication and at times used what he called "the interior monologue," or stream of consciousness. Carl Jung (q.v.) wrote an article about *Ulysses* but did not understand the work and thought that it did not matter whether it was read back to front. Jung even failed to see its obvious connection with the *Odyssey* (q.v.). Some authorities have felt that Joyce's *Ulysses* and *Finnegans Wake* were expressions of schizophrenic (*see* SCHIZOPHRENIA) writing. Joyce did consult Jung about his daughter, Lucia, who was said to be insane. Jung believed that she was schizophrenic, "drowned" in the unruly sea of thoughts on which her father "floated." Bibliography: Cixous, H. 1976. *The exile of James Joyce*, trans. S. A. J. Purcell.

JUAN DE DIOS. See HUARTE DE SAN JUAN, JUAN, and JOÃO DE DEUS.

JUDAS ISCARIOT. A disciple of Jesus. Judas' guilt over his betrayal of Jesus to the Romans caused him to commit suicide (q.v.): "he went and hanged himself" (Matt. 27: 5.) According to the Acts (1: 16-20), his mode of suicide was not by hanging, but by throwing himself off a rock.

JUKES. The fictitious name given to an American family studied in 1875 by Richard L. Dugdale (q.v.). H. Estabrook also studied the family in 1915. Several generations of this family, including some 2,820 persons, were eventually screened in a genetic investigation into mental deficiency. Mental defect was regarded as mostly hereditary and pauperism, criminality, and other social problems were linked with it. The studies on the Jukes and other genetic studies caused widespread public anxiety about mental deficiency, which was believed to be a menace to civilization.
See also EUGENICS, HILL FOLK, NAM KALLIKAK FAMILY.
Bibliography: Dugdale, R. L. 1875. *The Jukes, a study in crime, pauperism, disease, and heredity.*
Estabrook, A. H. 1915. *The Jukes in 1915.*

JUNG, CARL GUSTAV (1794-1864). A Swiss physician, grandfather of the psychiatrist Carl G. Jung (q.v.). He was a colorful figure, charming and impulsive. He was a successful physician in Basel, Switzerland, as well as a writer and a dramatist. It was rumored that he was an illegitimate son of Johann Wolfgang von Goethe (q.v.). He married three times and had thirteen children, not all of whom gave him joy. He became interested in mentally deficient children and in 1857 established a home for them.
Bibliography: Steiner, G. 1965. *Erinnerangen au Carl Gustav Jung.*

JUNG, CARL GUSTAV (1875-1961). A Swiss psychiatrist. Until he was nine, he was an only child whose grandfather, Carl Gustav Jung (q.v.), and father were physicians. When he was twelve years old, he thought that he was two different people, himself and an old man living in the eighteenth century. After a head injury, he began to suffer from fainting spells, but some of them were self induced so that he could stay away from school. They disappeared when he overheard his father remarking that he might be an epileptic (*see* EPILEPSY). Until late adolescence he was frequently depressed. As a young man he became interested in philosophy and later developed an interest in psychology and psychiatry. In 1902, after receiving

his medical degree, he worked under Eugen Bleuler (q.v.) at the Burghölzli Hospital (q.v.) in Zürich, Switzerland. In 1903, he married Emma Rauschenbach, an exceptional woman, who became his disciple and collaborator. Sigmund Freud (q.v.) once referred to Jung's early work on word association (q.v.) as "the first bridge between experimental psychology and psychoanalysis." Jung also advanced the idea that dementia praecox (q.v.) could be a psychosomatic disorder of the brain and therefore within the scope of psychoanalysis. When he met Freud in 1907, their meeting lasted for thirteen uninterrupted hours. Jung did much to publicize the psychoanalytic movement in Switzerland, which Freud appreciated. Later, however, Freud viewed him with a certain suspicion because he believed him to be a possible rival. This may explain why Freud's autobiography contains no mention of Jung. Jung strongly disagreed with Freud's psychoanalytic libido (q.v.) theory. Jung's publication of *Psychology of the Unconscious* in 1912 signified the formal break between the two men. Myths, legends, and stories from the classics had always interested Jung, who connected them with dreams (q.v.), primitive mentality, and what he called the "collective unconscious," around which he built his own system of analytical psychology. With the development of this theory, he founded a rival school to Freud's. He was interested in the future of the psyche (q.v.) as well as in its past. The terms "introvert" (q.v.) and "extrovert" (q.v.) were introduced by him around 1900. As well as a psychiatrist, he was also a painter and a sculptor. Following a cardiac infarction in 1944, Jung was seriously ill and became obsessed (*see* OBSESSION) with the thought that his doctor would die in his place, which indeed happened. Jung died in Zürich, during a spectacular thunderstorm; his favorite tree was struck by lightning two hours after his death.
Bibliography: Brome, V. 1978. *Jung: man and myth*.

JUNG-STILLING, JOHANN HEINRICH (1740-1817). German physician and writer. He was also known by his original name Heinrich Jung and his pseudonym Heinrich Stilling. His work was pervaded by a mysticism that reflected his deep religious feelings. In his novel, *Theobald oder die Schwarmer*, published in 1785, he wrote about a young girl, who was so deeply depressed that no doctor could cure her. She was cured eventually by a kindly clergyman, who encouraged her to talk about her troubles, counseled her, and brought about her union with the man she loved. The novel serves as an early example of psychotherapy (q.v.). Jung-Stilling is better known for his five-volume autobiography entitled *Heinrich Stillings Jugend* (1777-1804), a religious counterpart of Jean Jacques Rousseau's (q.v.) *Confessions* (q.v.). It was edited by Johann Wolfgang von Goethe (q.v.) and presented a valuable picture of mid-eighteenth century life.
Bibliography: Günther, H. R. 1948. *Jung-Stilling: ein Beitrag zur Psychologie des Pietismus*.

JUNOT, ANDOCHE (1771-1813). A French general. He was created Duc d'Albrantes by Napoleon I (q.v.) in 1807 for his services during the invasion of Portugal. He was a dashing and impetuous individual, who was nicknamed "La Tempête." Self-assertion, or perhaps loneliness, caused him to say, "Moi, je suis mon ancêtre" ("Me, I am my ancestor"). After Napoleon's defeat in Russia, Junot was made the scapegoat (q.v.) and sent to govern Illyria. He was said to have become insane, but it seems more likely that he became deeply depressed because of the events around him, including an extravagant wife. He tried to commit suicide (q.v.) by throwing himself out of a window while visiting his father in Dijon, but he survived with a broken leg, which necessitated amputation. He then tore off the bandages and died a week later.

JURAMENTADO. A Spanish term literally meaning "cursed." It is used to indicate an acute disorder that is similar to amok (q.v.). The affected individual works himself into a frenzy that often leads to extreme aggression and, in turn, is followed by amnesia (q.v.). The trance-like state may be caused by a severe emotional shock or may be precipitated by rituals involving incantations (q.v.) and music. It is usually found among Malayans.
Bibliography: Goldenson, R. M. 1970. *The encyclopedia of human behavior.*

JURIEU, PIERRE (1637-1713). A French Protestant theologian. In 1686 his prophecies of the fall of the Roman Catholic Church and the end of the persecutions of the Huguenots were circulated throughout France and soon gave rise to an epidemic of hysteria (q.v.). Children uttered prophecies, and whole crowds of people were seized with paroxysms of sobbing and fell into convulsions.
See also CAMISARDS.
Bibliography: Ducasse, A. 1946. *La guerre des Camisard.*

JUSTINE (fl.1850-1894). A French woman. She was a patient of Pierre Janet (q.v.) and suffered from a morbid fear of death and cholera. In 1894, he treated her by hypnosis (*see* HYPNOTISM), and his observation of this patient led to the development of his theory of idées fixes (q.v.).
Bibliography: Janet. P. 1894. Histoire d'une idee fixe. *Revue Philosophique,* 37: 121-68.

JUSTINE AND JULIETTE. A book originally published in French in 1791 under the title *Justine; ou les Malheurs de la vertu.* It was written in prison by the Marquis de Sade (q.v.) and described various cruel sexual perversions.
Bibliography: Marquis de Sade. 1791. *Justine; ou les malheurs de la vertu.*

JUVENAL (DECIMUS JUNIUS JUVENALIS) (A.D. 60?-?140). A Roman poet. He was famous for his biting satire on the public morals and manners of his time. He was an acute observer who could depict vividly the fears, pleasures, joys, and sorrows of his fellow men. He described dementia as follows:

Worse by far than all bodily hurt is dementia: for he who has it no longer knows the names of his slaves or recognises the friend with whom he has dined the night before, or those whom he has begotten and brought up.

He also observed that goitre was found among inhabitants of the Alps and invented the maxim "mens sana in corpore sano" ("a healthy mind in a healthy body").
Bibliography: Highet, G. 1962. *Juvenal the satirist.*

JUVENILE PSYCHOPATHIC INSTITUTE. An organization in Chicago, Illinois, founded by William Healy (q.v.) in 1909. Its purpose was to investigate and rehabilitate young delinquents. In 1917 it became the Illinois Juvenile Psychopathic Institute, and, in 1920, its name was again changed to the Illinois Institute for Juvenile Research. In addition to investigating delinquency, it undertook research projects in biochemistry, and neurology, as well as developmental studies and routine psychological testing.
Bibliography: Deutsch, A. 1949. *The mentally ill in America.*

K

KAAN, HENRICUS. A Russian physician. In 1844 he wrote in Latin *Psychopathia Sexualis* in which he described sexual deviation. The book antedated by forty-two years the more famous work of Richard Von Krafft-Ebing (q.v.).
Bibliography: Ellenberger, H. F. 1970. *The discovery of the unconscious.*

KAFKA, FRANZ (1883-1924). An Austrian novelist, born in Prague, Czechoslovakia, of Jewish parents. His childhood was blighted by a strained family atmosphere which was later reflected in his novels. He was a hypersensitive and introspective man, who was deeply attached to his dominant father and, later, to Dora Dymant, with whom he briefly experienced happiness in a desperate love affair, when he was already dying of tuberculosis (q.v.). Influenced by Søren Kierkegaard (q.v.), Kafka wrote of a world of despair and aimlessness in which futility pervaded everything and hope seldom appeared. Reality and irreality are described by him in a dream-like way, sharpened by humor. His characters, like himself, stray in a bewildering world. His most famous novels, which were published posthumously, are *The Trials* (1925) and *The Castle* (1926). Many of his unfinished works were later published by his friend Max Brod (1884–1968).
Bibliography: Kafka, F. 1935–1937. *Collected works*, ed. M. Brod.
Sokel, W. 1964. *Franz Kafka.*

KAHLBAUM, KARL LUDWIG (1828-1899). A German psychiatrist. Inspired by the approach of the time, which gave more importance to clinical observation of the course of the disease rather than the search for its cause, he attempted to devise a nosology of mental disorders based on definite clinical entities. He believed that all symptoms could be divided into groups, each containing a certain type of abnormal behavior, which he called a "symptom complex." In 1874, he introduced and described the term "ca-

tatonia" (q.v.). He also introduced the terms "verbigeration" (q.v.) and "cyclothymia" (q.v.).
Bibliography: Kahlbaum, K. L. 1874. Reprint 1973. *Catatonia* 1973.

KALAMAZOO, MICHIGAN. The first American farm colony for the chronic and harmless insane was founded in Kalamazoo in 1883. It was based on the "village" principle of construction, which Dr. Richard Hills superintendent of the Ohio Lunatic Asylum (q.v.) in Columbus, Ohio, had advocated in 1863.
Bibliography: Deutsch, A. 1949. *The mentally ill in America.*

KALAWOUN HOSPITAL. A general hospital in existence in Cairo, Egypt, in the fourteenth century. One of its four sections was dedicated to mental disorders. Because it received contributions from wealthy citizens, it was able to provide excellent care for its patients and even cared for discharged patients until they had obtained gainful employment. In subsequent centuries the hospital deteriorated, and its services were restricted to the inpatient care of the mentally ill. At the beginning of the nineteenth century, it closed down completely. Patients were transferred first to Azbakeya Hospital and, after another move, were housed in an old disused royal palace at Abbasia in 1880. The palace, which had been damaged by a fire, was painted yellow, and the hospital became known as "the yellow palace."
See also AL-MANSUR, CAIRO LUNATIC ASYLUMS, and EGYPT.
Bibliography: Baasher, T. 1975. The Arab countries. In *World history of psychiatry*, ed. J. G. Howells.

KALE. *Brassica oleracea acephala*, a plant now cultivated for culinary use. Originally it grew wild along the shores of the Black Sea and some parts of Europe. The Greeks set great store by it and used it for its medical properties especially as a remedy for nervous disorders and to improve memory.
Bibliography: de Baïracli Levy, J. 1974. *The illustrated herbal handbook.*

KALI. The goddess of death, destruction, and disease in Hindu mythology (q.v.). Her cult frequently includes animal sacrifice. She is represented with skulls round her neck and corpses hanging from her ears and is described as "beautiful and terrible." The Thugs (q.v.) sacrificed their victims to her.
Bibliography: Renou, L. ed. 1961. *Hinduism.*

KALLIKAK FAMILY. The fictitious name given by Henry Goddard (q.v.) to a New Jersey family that was the subject of a genetic study in 1912. The pseudonym is a fusion of two Greek words meaning "good" and "bad," and was used to denote the two lines of descendants of an American Revolutionary soldier. The soldier fathered children of two women, one of whom was a feebleminded servant girl and the other, a "respectable" girl of good family. The descendants of the first union were mostly poor, antisocial, and mentally subnormal, while the children of the second union were respected and useful members of society. The study purported to prove that feeblemindedness, which Goddard believed was hereditary, was the main source of most social problems.

See also EUGENICS.

Bibliography: Goddard, H. H. 1912. The Kallikak Family.

KALLMANN, FRANZ J. (1897–1965). A German-born psychiatrist and geneticist. He worked under Karl Bonhoeffer (q.v.) and studied psychoanalysis (q.v.) at the Psychoanalytic Policlinic (q.v.) in Berlin. In 1928 he was appointed director of the neuropathology laboratories for the psychiatric hospitals in Berlin, but by 1936 the political situation in Germany caused him to emigrate to the United States. In 1938, his completed manuscript was translated into English and was published under the title of *The Genetics of Schizophrenia* in the United States. As professor of psychiatry at Columbia University in New York, Kallmann's approach to mental disorders influenced many young psychiatrists. After his studies on the occurrence of schizophrenia (q.v.) in twins, he came to believe that schizophrenia had a strong hereditary aetiology. He also investigated the genetics of behavior disorders and manic-depressive psychoses (q.v.).

Bibliography: Kallmann, F. J. 1953. *Heredity in health and mental disorder.*

KALMUC IDIOCY. A type of idiocy (*see* IDIOT) named after a Mongolian tribe because of the facial features accompanying it. The first clinical description of the symptoms was presented in a lecture in Edinburgh in 1875 by J. Fraser. A. Mitchell followed with an account of sixty-two patients with similar features.

See also MONGOLISM.

Bibliography: Fraser, J. and Mitchell, A. 1876. Kalmuc Idiocy: report of a case with autopsy and notes on 62 cases. *J. ment. Sci.* 22: 161-62; 169-79.

KALYB. A legendary baby-snatcher. She was said to have kidnapped Saint George from his nurse and kept him as her own child. She serves as an early example of the ambivalent feelings children have for their foster mothers for it is said that Saint George imprisoned her in a rock where spirits tore her apart, although he owed his special gifts to her.

Bibliography: Marcus, G. J. 1929. *Saint George of England.*

KAMA. The god of love in Hindu mythology (q.v.). He is the husband of Rati, the personification of voluptuousness. He was burnt to cinders by Shiva for awakening thoughts of passion in him while he was engaged in

penance, but he was later reborn. The legend reflects the unresolved conflict between asceticism and physical gratification.
Bibliography: Renou, L. ed. 1961. *Hinduism.*

KAMADA, HO (1754–1821). A Japanese philosopher who is considered to be the first Japanese psychologist. He organized a system of Oriental psychology that was free from European and American influences.
Bibliography: Misiak, H. and Sexton, V. S. 1966. *History of psychology.*

KAMA-SUTRA. An erotic Indian work, probably dating from the first century A.D. It was compiled by the sage Vatsyayana and was regarded as a textbook on the "science of love" (Kama-sutra) because it described various techniques in the art of erotic love (q.v.). Modern studies in human sexual behavior have revived interest in it.
Bibliography: Burton, R. and F. F. Aburthnot trans. Reprint 1963. *Kama Sutra.*

KAMSIM. A violent humid wind. It was believed to be one of the causes of insanity among Egyptians. Jean Esquirol (q.v.) mentioned it in his *Mental Maladies.*
See also WINDS.
Bibliography: Esquirol, J.E.D. 1845. Reprint 1965. *Mental maladies: a treatise on insanity.*

KANDINSKY, VIKTOR CHRISANFOVICH (1825-1889). A Russian psychiatrist. Together with Clérambault (q.v.) his name is associated to a syndrome of paranoid (*see* PARANOIA) ideas in which the patient feels that his mind is controlled by another person or an external power. The syndrome is now known as the Kandinsky-Clérambault Syndrome—first described by both workers in 1890.

KANKAKEE HOSPITAL. A state mental hospital in Illinois. When it opened in 1879, Kankakee Hospital pioneered a new type of hospital architecture in the United States. The hospital consisted of cottages grouped around a central building. Each group of cottages accommodated about one hundred patients.
Bibliography: Deutsch, A. 1949. *The mentally ill in America.*

KANNER, LEO (1894–1981). A psychiatrist, born in Austria. His research on childhood autism (q.v.), which he regarded as a form of schizophrenia (q.v.) that is closely linked to early mother-child relationships, has contributed greatly to the field of child psychiatry (q.v.). He has also written works on mental retardation and folklore (q.v.). As the undisputed leader of child psychiatry, he did much to establish child psychiatry as a specialty, and his book *Child Psychiatry* (1945) has been a standard work for many years.

Bibliography: Kanner, L. 1945. *Child psychiatry.*
———. 1969. Autistic disturbances of affective contact. In *Modern perspectives in international child psychiatry*, ed. J. G. Howells.

KANT, IMMANUEL (1724–1804). A German philosopher, the son of a Prussian soldier of Scottish ancestry. He was born and educated in Königsberg, Germany, and lived, worked, and died there, never moving more than forty miles from it. He never married, and the pattern of his life was so predictable that the inhabitants of Königsberg set their watches by his walks. Unlike his writings, his lectures often were humorous and witty. His philosophy took shape in his *Critique of Pure Reason*, which was published in 1781. It was based on the principle that reason is absolute. Knowledge depends upon the senses and upon understanding, which, in turn, depend upon space and time. According to Kant, man's knowledge is limited by his inability to conceive of limited or unlimited space and time. He believed that mental health resulted from a good adjustment to the environment, which he felt primitive man had achieved. Kant wrote that "the only feature common to all mental disorders is the loss of common sense (*sensus communis*) and the compensatory development of a unique, private sense (*sensus privatus*) of reasoning." Because he was interested in the classification of mental disorders, his *Anthropologie* (q.v.) contained an improvised semiology and classification of insanity. It, however, ignored the wholeness of man. Kant maintained that the field of psychopathology did not belong to medicine but rather belonged to philosophy. According to him, the germ of insanity developed at the same time as the germ of procreation, that is at puberty. He reached this erroneous conclusion because he had never observed any children afflicted with mental disorders and, therefore, thought that they did not develop them. His theory, however, provides an example of his own principle that an individual will reach false conclusions when his premises are false, even if his thinking is correct, or, conversely, when his premises are correct, but his thinking is incorrect. In his old age he suffered from nightmares (q.v.), hallucinations (q.v.), and disorders of memory (q.v.). His intellect disintegrated, and his last few months were depressing to himself and to his friends.

Bibliography: Goldman, L. 1971. *Immanuel Kant*, trans. R. Black.

KAPPERS, CORNELIUS ARIËNS (1877–1946). A Dutch neurologist. In 1908 he became the director of the Central Institute for Brain Research in Amsterdam. After twenty-one years of research there, in 1929 he was offered the chair of comparative neuroanatomy at the University of Amsterdam. In

his later years, after visits to China (q.v.) and to Syria, he became interested in anthropology.
Bibliography: Haymaker, W., and Schiller, F. 1970. *The founders of neurology*. 2d. ed.

KASTHOFER, KARL (1777–1853). A Swiss forester. He noticed that cretinism (q.v.) was common in the valleys of the Alps but did not occur in the mountains. This observation prompted him to postulate that the condition would improve in the mountains, and he offered to Johann Jakob Guggenbühl (q.v.) forty acres of land near Interlaken, which was more than 4,000 feet above sea level. The institution of Abendberg (q.v.) was built on this land. Kasthofer also advocated the substitution of colonies situated at high altitudes for prisons and almshouses.
Bibliography: Kanner, L. 1964. *A history of the care and study of the mentally retarded*.

KAT. *Catha edulis Forskal*, a psychoactive shrub. In ancient Arabia (*see* ARABS), it was used as a remedy for depression because of its euphoric and stimulant properties. Arab mystics using it would attain states of ecstasy (q.v.), which were attributed to supernatural intervention. In the Yemen the chewing of kat leaves is still common.
Bibliography: Baasher, T. 1975. The Arab countries. In *World history of psychiatry*, ed. J. G. Howells.

KATERINA IVANOVNA. A character in *The Brothers Karamazov* (q.v.) by Fyodor Dostoevsky (q.v.). She is evil, tenacious, and sado-masochistic. It has been said that she was modeled on his companion, Apollinariya Suslova, who served as a model for subsequent "infernal" women in his novels.
Bibliography: Dostoevsky, F. 1880. *The brothers Karamazov*, trans. C. Garnett. 1979.

KATHERINA. The heroine of William Shakespeare's (q.v.) comedy *The Taming of the Shrew*. She is known to be a stubborn scold. Petruchio, who finally tames her through marriage (q.v.), forbids her to eat burnt meat, which, in Shakespeare's time, was believed to influence moods by producing choler (q.v.), one of the humors (q.v.).

KATTADIYAS. Special folk doctors in the traditional medicine of Sri Lanka (formerly Ceylon). Those believed to be possessed (*see* POSSESSION) by evil spirits are taken to the kattadiyas, who drive the devils away by chanting mantras from sacred books.

KATZ, DAVID (1884–1953). A German experimental psychologist and a pupil of Georg Müller (q.v.). In 1911 he wrote a phenomenological study

on color perception entitled *Die Erscheinungsweisen der Farben*. He also investigated the phenomena involved in touch.
Bibliography: Boring, E. G. 1950. *A history of experimental psychology.*

KAULBACH, WILHELM VON (1805–1874). A German painter with a keen sense of drama. Among his works is a vivid drawing of a group of the insane.
Bibliography: *The Oxford companion to art.* 1970. ed. H. Osborne.

KAVAN, ANNA (1901–1968). A writer born in France but living mostly in England or California. She changed her name from Helen Ferguson to Anna Kavan by deed poll. Perhaps in an attempt to suppress the unhappiness of her early life, which she blamed on her wealthy mother, Kavan became a heroin (q.v.) addict. In *World of Heroes* she explained that she "was always afraid of falling back into that ghastly black isolation of an uncomprehending, solitary, over-sensitive child." Her behavior was so erratic that on one occasion she hurled a roasted fowl across the table at a guest. Many of her stories were written during periods of mental illness. *Asylum Piece*, which was published in 1940, describes her experiences in various Swiss and English clinics. During World War II, she worked as a researcher for an American military psychiatric unit. She possessed an exceptional insight into mental disorders and hallucinations (q.v.), which was reflected in her paintings of bizarre subjects and her novels. *Ice* (1967) has the quality of a nightmare (q.v.) with disturbing images of an endless journey to certain extinction. When she was found dead in 1968, a syringe of heroin was in her hand.
Bibliography: Kavan, A. 1940. *Asylum piece and other stories.*

KAWABATA, YASUNARI (1899–1972). A Japanese writer and winner of the Nobel Prize for literature in 1968. His childhood was punctuated by losses. His parents died when he was a year old; his only sister was separated from him and died in childhood; his grandmother died when he was seven years old; and his grandfather died when he was sixteen years old. Acutely conscious of his loneliness, he longed for close, warm relationships. He lived in a fantasy world dominated by the past and was such a firm believer in spirits that he would talk aloud to them. His writings reflect his rebellion against the Japanese literature of the 1920s, as well as his wish to create beauty and describe the pathos of human life. He helped to establish a number of young Japanese writers, including Yukio Mishima (q.v.). He finally committed suicide (q.v.) in his room overlooking the mountains and the ocean.
Bibliography: Kawabata, Y. 1970. *The complete works of Kawabata Yasunari.*

KEAN, EDMUND (1787?–1833). An English actor. He was noted for his psychological interpretations of the characters of Othello, King Lear, and

Richard III (qq.v.). He was an alcoholic (*see* ALCOHOLISM) and led such a dissolute life, that it resulted in the breakdown of his physical and mental health.
Bibliography: Disher, M. W. 1950. *Mad genius: a biography of Edmund Kean.*

KEATS, JOHN (1795-1821). An English poet. His father was a livery stable keeper, who died when his son was eight years old. As a child, Keats showed more than normal aggression, for he was constantly involved in fights. He was apprenticed to an apothecary-surgeon, Thomas Hammond, whose lack of skill put many student's off surgery. To ease the dreariness of his life, Keats turned to poetry. His first published poem, *Ode to Solitude* (1816) occurred when he was twenty-one years old. His first volume of poetry, entitled *Poems* (1817), and his *Endymion* (1818), which are now regarded as classics of English literature, were viciously attacked by critics in 1818, just as his personal life was beset by misfortune: his younger brother Tom (1799–1818) was dying of tuberculosis (q.v.) and his relationship with Fanny Brawne (1800-) was causing him unhappiness. His well-known poem *Lamia* (1820) was based on a story from the *Anatomy of Melancholy* (q.v.) Keats died in Rome of tuberculosis, which he had contracted while nursing his brother. His poem *Ode to a Nightingale* is a supreme description of depression and loneliness.

> Forlorn! the very word is like a bell
>   To toll me back from thee to my sole self!
> Adieu! the fancy cannot cheat so well
>   As she is fam'd to do, deceiving elf.
> Adieu! adieu! thy plaintive anthem fades
>   Past the near meadows, over the still stream,
>   Up the hill-side; and now 'tis buried deep
>   In the next valley-glades:

Bibliography: Gittings, R. 1968. *John Keats.*

KELLER, JOHANN (1830-1884). A Danish theologian and founder of institutions for deaf-mutes (*see* DEAF-MUTISM), mental defectives, and idiots (q.v.). His first school was opened in a broken-down building in 1856 but subsequent institutions were so well established that on his death the Danish government took them over, leaving only a school for feebleminded children under the control of his son Christian, who continued the work.
Bibliography: Kanner, L. 1964. *A history of the care and study of the mentally retarded.*

KELLEY, EDWARD (1555-1595). An English alchemist (*see* ALCHEMY) and medium (q.v.). He was accused of digging up the dead in order to

question them. He also was involved with John Dee (q.v.) in crystal gazing and the search for the philosopher stone (q.v.). His ears were cut off as punishment for his practices and he always wore a black skull cap to hide this mutilation. His crystallomancy at the court of Rudolph II (1552-1612) of Germany brought him rich rewards but eventually led to his imprisonment and cost him his life when he tried to escape.
Bibliography: Salgado, G. 1977. *The Elizabethan underworld.*

KELLY, GEORGE ALEXANDER (1905-1967). An American psychologist. He evolved a system of psychology based on personal constructs. He was also a member of the original Committee on Training in Clinical Psychology, which was established by the American Psychiatric Association (q.v.) in 1947.
Bibliography: Kelly, G. A. 1955. *Psychology of personal constructs.*

KELVIN, SIR WILLIAM THOMSON (1824-1907). A British mathematician and physicist, born in Belfast. He serves as an outstanding example of exceptional intelligence. He was a child prodigy and a mathematical genius (q.v.). When he was just over ten years old he matriculated at the University of Glasgow. In 1846 he was elected professor of natural philosophy there and during his long life made incomparable contributions to the field of physics.
Bibliography: Thompson, S. 1910. *Life of Kelvin.*

KENDROP CONVENT. A convent in Germany. It was the scene of an epidemic of demoniac possession (q.v.) among the nuns in the sixteenth century. The event is an example of communicated hysteria (q.v.).
Bibliography: Esquirol, J.E.D. 1865. Reprint. 1965. *Mental maladies: a treatise on insanity.*

KENTIGERN, SAINT (c. 518-603). Apostle of Strathclyde Britons in Scotland and bishop of Glasgow. His touch was said to heal the mentally disordered.
Bibliography: Stevenson, W. 1874. *The legends of Saint Kentigern.*

KENTUCKY LUNATIC ASYLUM. An American mental hospital established in 1822 by a legislative act. It provided accommodation for 200 lunatic, maniac, or otherwise dangerous patients. Those that were "quiet and peaceable" were boarded out (*see* BOARDING-OUT OF MENTAL PATIENTS) as before. Physical restraint (q.v.) was frequently used on the excuse that the function of the asylum (q.v.) was to confine violent patients, rather than to treat them. Around 1826 this policy was changed and moral treatment was instituted.
Bibliography: Deutsch, A. 1949. *The mentally ill in America.*

KEPLER, JOHANNES (1571-1630). A German astronomer, born in Württemberg. His revolutionary laws of planetary motion laid the foundation

for modern astronomy. He changed the concept of *anima* (q.v.), or soul, to that of *vis*, or force, thus advancing a less mystical interpretation of psychological phenomena in man.
Bibliography: Armitage, A. 1966. *John Kepler.*

KERES. In Greek mythology (q.v.), the ghosts of the dead. They were usually associated with evil intentions toward the living. The ghost of a murdered person was thought to have the power to cause insanity in the murderer. The Keres were represented as birds of prey.
Bibliography: Harrison, J. 1955. *Prolegomena to the study of Greek religion.*

KERLIN, ISAAC N. (1834-1893). An American physician whose work was in the field of mental retardation. He introduced occupational training for mental defectives at the Pennsylvania Training School for Feebleminded Children. He believed in sterilization (q.v.) of mental defectives and obtained parental permission to perform this procedure on many patients. Kerlin was one of the founders of the Association of Medical Officers of American Institutions for Idiots and Feebleminded Persons, which later became the American Association of Mental Deficiency (q.v.).
Bibliography: Kanner, L. 1964. *A history of the care and study of the mentally retarded.*

KERN, KARL FERDINAND (1814-1868). A German physician. He began his career as a teacher. After teaching deaf-mutes (*see* DEAF-MUTISM), he became interested in the training of mental defectives and studied medicine. He advocated special schools for retarded children and lectured on educational methods designed for them.
Bibliography: Kanner, L. 1964. *A history of the care and study of the mentally retarded.*

KERNER, ANDREAS JUSTINUS (1768-1862). A German physician and minor poet. He was the son of a civil servant in Württemberg. The local asylum was next to his house, and from his home he could see the tower in which Faust (q.v.) was reputed to have conducted his experiments in magic (q.v.). As a child he suffered from a nervous ailment and was treated by magnetism (q.v.), which led to his interest in Franz Mesmer (q.v.) and mesmerism (q.v.). He used mesmerism and exorcism (q.v.) to treat those patients suffering from what he called "demonic-magnetic" disease. His most famous patient was Friedericke Hauffe (q.v.) whose story he wrote in 1845. In 1857 he published *Klecksographien*, a collection of ink-blots and the verses they had inspired in him. It was from this collection Hermann Rorschach (q.v.) developed his ink-blot tests in 1921.
Bibliography: Straumann, H. 1928. *Justinus Kerner und der Okkultismus in der deutschen Romantik.*

KESURUBAN. A seance-like performance practiced in Indonesia. Advice about an illness and the formula for the needed medication are revealed to the believers through a medium. Often the prescription is burned, and the ashes swallowed.

Bibliography: Kline, N. S. 1963. Psychiatry in Indonesia. *Am. J. Psychiat.* 119:809-15.

KHALUNE-ARSHAN SPRING. A sacred spring located between Outer Mongolia and China (q.v.) near the hills of the Great Khingan mountains. Its water was said to have curative properties. Buddhist priests acted as healers and supervised the treatment of the sick, who had traveled to the spring from Mongolia, Tibet, China, and Siberia. Their methods of treatment included mystical procedures with great suggestive power. Harmless water snakes, sacred to the Mongols, were kept round the pool, which was in the shape of a reclining giant. Pilgrimages to the spring continued well into the twentieth century.

See also HOLY WELLS.

Bibliography: Kourennoff, P. M., and St. George, G. 1970. *Russian folk medicine.*

KHLYSTY. A secret Russian religious sect of the eighteenth century. It believed that God was reached through sexual orgies. Meetings began with the singing of hymns by candlelight. As the candles burned low, the participants would dance until they were seized by a frenzy that culminated in indiscriminate sexual acts, regardless of age or of consanguinity. Grigori Rasputin (q.v.) was said to have been a member of the sect.

Bibliography: Fülöp-Miller, R. 1928. *Rasputin: the holy devil.*

KHONS. An ancient Egyptian god. He was said to have the power of curing those who had been driven insane by demonaic possession (q.v.). An Egyptian stele in the Bibliotheque Nationale in Paris, describes how he cured a princess of the Twentieth Dynasty.

Bibliography: Zilboorg, G. 1941. *A history of medical psychology.*

KIBBUTZ. Collective farm settlements in Israel. The first was founded in 1902 in the Jordan Valley. By 1960 about 5 percent of the country's population lived in kibbutzim. Because both parents work, children live in children's houses during the day. The early start of the day also makes it more convenient for the children to sleep in the children's houses. Some experts, including Bruno Bettelheim in his *Children of the Dream* (1969), regard this custom as detrimental to the child's psychological welfare. Others have pointed to its advantages. They have claimed that parents who have worked all day are free to give their children undivided attention in the evenings. As in orthodox forms of child care, parents of the kibbutzim spend their free day with their children.

Bibliography: Miller, L. 1969. Child rearing in the kibbutz. In *Modern perspectives in international child psychiatry*, ed. J. G. Howells.

KIERKEGAARD, SØREN AABYE (1813-1855). Danish theologian and philospher. His early life was depressed and lonely, reflecting the attitudes

of his gloomy family. He was a joyless figure, who was often mocked by the gay citizens of Copenhagen. Kierkegaard believed that man had become too involved in trying to understand the universe and had neglected the understanding of himself and his personal relationship with God. He attacked the worldliness of orthodox religion, and his philosophy, based on the thesis that subjectivity is truth, found no followers during his lifetime. In the twentieth century, however, he is regarded as the forerunner of existentialism (q.v.). His premature death was said to be due to overwork.
Bibliography: Thompson, J. 1973. *Kierkegaard.*

KIESER, DIETRICH GEORGE (1779-1862). A German physician and medical writer. He was a pupil of Franz Mesmer (q.v.). His concept of the polarity and oscillation of psychological forces foreshadowed the twentieth-century belief that psychological conflict is one cause of mental disorder.
Bibliography: Kieser, D. G. 1855. *Elemente der Psychiatrik.*

KIESOW, FRIEDRICH (1858-1940). A German psychologist who worked under Wilhelm Wundt (q.v.) in his laboratory at Leipzig. He established the existence of four qualities of taste: sweet, sour, salt, and bitter. He also undertook research in the field of tactile sensations.
Bibliography: Boring, E. G. 1950. *A history of experimental psychology.*

KIMULUE. A psychosexual disorder recognized by medicine men in the Diegueno Indian tribes of California. Those afflicted lose interest in life, become apathetic, and are troubled by unusually vivid sexual dreams (q.v.). If convulsions are a part of the symptomatology, the disorder is called *echul.*
Bibliography: Goldenson, R. M. 1970. *The encyclopaedia of human behavior.*

KIND, KARL FRIEDRICH (1825-1884). A German physician, son-in-law of Karl F. Kern (q.v.). He left teaching to acquire the medical qualifications that would enable him to care for mental defectives. In 1868 he became director of the school for retarded children at Langenhangen, Hanover. His work was dedicated to institutional reforms.
Bibliography: Kanner, L. 1964. *A history of the care and study of the mentally retarded.*

KINDERGARTEN. German for "garden of children." The term indicates the system of teaching through play that was initiated by Friedrich Froebel (q.v.) in 1837. He opened the first kindergarten in Bad Blankenburg, Germany.
Bibliography: Alexander, F. G., and Selesnick, S. T. 1966. *The history of psychiatry.*

KING, ALBERT FREEMAN AFRICANUS (1841-1914). An Anglo-American gynecologist and professor of obstetrics. He believed that hysterical (*see* HYSTERIA) women had a dual personality: "a reproductive ego" and a "self-preservative ego." According to him, the denial of the reproductory functions was responsible for hysteria. He also believed that hysteria was more common in spring and summer, especially among women leading a leisurely life. King was in the theater when Abraham Lincoln (q.v.) was assassinated and attended to him.

Bibliography: King, A.F.A. Hysteria. 1891. *Am. J. Obstetr.* 24.

KINGSLEY, CHARLES (1819-1875). An English clergyman and novelist. He was an active exponent of Christian socialism and thought that the church should be vigorously involved in social action for the working classes. Uncharacteristically for a Victorian (q.v.) clergyman brought up in a puritanical household, he developed a voracious sexual appetite for his future wife, Fanny Grenfell, and showered her with erotic messages accompanied by even more erotic drawings that represented either the two of them in a naked embrace, or the unfortunate girl naked and subjected to torture. Guilt about these expressions of his feelings made him insist on severe penance for both of them, including fasting (q.v.), flagellation (q.v.), and lying naked on cold floors. They eventually married and were said to be happy, although he remained a highly nervous man, often ill from overexertion and prone to nervous breakdowns. He wrote numerous books and articles, which were collected in twenty-eight volumes between 1879 and 1881 but his best remembered work is *The Water Babies* (1863).

Bibliography: Chitty, S. 1974. *The beast and the monk: a life of Charles Kingsley.*

KING'S TOUCH. A healing rite during which a king or queen "lays hands" on the ill to bring about a cure. Based on the power of suggestion, the rite originated in France with Robert the Pious in the tenth century and was introduced into England by Edward the Confessor (q.v.) in the eleventh century. Scrofula (q.v.) was known as the King's evil because it was the disease commonly treated by the royal touch. Gold coins or medals were issued to the sick as a kind of admission token. Charles II (1630-1685) of England was said to have touched nearly 100,000 people. The last English sovereign to practice it was Queen Anne (1665-1714). In 1712, she touched Samuel Johnson (q.v.), without success.

Bibliography: Block, M. 1973. *The royal touch: sacred monarchy and scrofula in England and France.*

KINSEY, ALFRED CHARLES (1894-1956). An American zoologist and biologist. He is known for his work in the field of human sexual behavior. In 1948, with W. B. Pomeroy and C. E. Martin, he published *Sexual Behavior of the Human Male.* He followed this with *Sexual Behavior of the Human Female* written in 1953 with W. B. Pomeroy, C. E. Martin and P. H. Gebhard. These works have provided the impetus for further research in psychosexology.

KIPLING, JOSEPH RUDYARD (1865-1936). An English novelist and poet, born in Bombay, India. When he was six years old his parents, who were visiting England from India, left him in lodgings in Southsea near Portsmouth, preparing him for the separation. The woman who looked after him beat him constantly and took his books, his only consolation, away from him. It was six years before his mother realized the situation and, returning from India, removed him from the home. He never forgot the unhappy experience, which he wrote about in *Baa, Baa, Black Sheep*. His works, despite being full of action, reveal a flight into an imaginary world where man is in constant combat with dangerous external forces. The children's stories *Jungle Book* (1894) and *Just So Stories for Little Children* (1902) are perhaps the best remembered of his numerous works.
Bibliography: Mason, P. 1975. *Kipling*.

KIRCHER, ATHANASIUS (1602-1680). A German Jesuit, scholar, and mathematician. He spent most of his life in Rome. Kircher is considered a precursor of Franz Mesmer (q.v.) and hypnotism (q.v.) because in 1667 he published a book entitled *Magneticum Naturae Organum, de Triplici-Naturae Magnete, Inanimato, Animato, Sensitivo* in which he claimed many phenomena that seemed mysterious could be explained in terms of magnetic (*see* MAGNET) rays. According to him, feelings, such as love, hate, and friendship depended on two kinds of magnetic activity: sympathic, or good, and antipathic, or bad. Kircher is credited with the first recorded experiment in hypnotism.
Bibliography: Tinterow, M. M. 1970. *Foundations of hypnosis: from Mesmer to Freud*.

KIRCHHOFF, THEODOR (1853-1922). A German psychiatrist and historian of psychiatry. According to him, people who were accused of witchcraft (q.v.) were suffering from epilepsy (q.v.) or from senile dementia.
Bibliography: Kirchhoff, T. 1912. Geschicte der Psychiatrie. In *Handbuch der Psychiatrie*, ed. Aschaffenburg.

KIRKBRIDE, THOMAS STORY (1809-1883). An American psychiatrist, born of Quaker (q.v.) parents. For forty-three years he was superintendent of the Pennsylvania Hospital (q.v.), the first psychiatric hospital in the United States. He advocated a special type of architecture for mental hospitals and in 1854 wrote a volume entitled *On the Construction, Organization, and General Arrangements of Hospitals for the Insane* (q.v.). His plan became a model for hospital building. He promoted moral therapy and the abolition of restraint (q.v.) and stressed the importance of properly

trained nursing staffs that were carefully selected and well paid. He believed that "insanity should be classed with other diseases . . . every individual who has a brain is liable to insanity, precisely as every one who has lungs is liable to pneumonia. . . ." He also thought that poor mental patients should be the responsibility of the state. Kirkbride was one of the original thirteen founders of the American Psychiatric Association (q.v.).
Bibliography: Bond, E. D. 1947. *Dr. Kirkbride and his mental hospital.*

KIRKPATRICK, CLIFFORD (1898-). An American sociologist and a pioneer in mental testing. His work includes research in family functioning, intelligence and migration, and dating behavior.
Bibliography: Kirkpatrick, C. 1955. *The family: as process and institution.*

KIRSCHMANN, AUGUST (1860-1932). A German psychologist. He was a pupil of Wilhelm Wundt (q.v.) at his Leipzig laboratory and worked with him on experiments concerning color contrast.
Bibliography: Flugel, J. C. 1965. *A hundred years of psychology.*

KLAESI, JAKOB (fl. early twentieth century). A Swiss psychiatrist. Many of his concepts were similar to those of Alfred Adler (q.v.). Klaesi believed that neurosis (q.v.) resulted from the clash between egoistic instincts, which he called *cratophorous* instincts, and social instincts, or *aristophorous* instincts. In the early 1920s he introduced a new type of prolonged sleep treatment (q.v.) in which sleep was induced by sedatives. He argued that rest would relieve the brain inflammation that had produced excitement.
Bibliography: Klaesi, J. 1937. *Vom seelischen Kranksein: Vorbeugung und Heilen.*

KLAGES, LUDWIG (1872-1956). A German philosopher and psychologist. He is considered the founder of graphology (q.v.) as a science, as well as the founder of expressive psychology. He regarded Friedrich Nietzsche (q.v.) as the true founder of modern psychology. In his main work *Der Geist als Widersacher der Seele* (the intellect as antagonist of the soul) he discussed conflicts, divided personality, drives, and other aspects of normal and abnormal psychology.
Bibliography: Muller, R. 1971. *Das Verzwistete Ich: Ludwig Klages und Sein Philosophisches Hauptwerk Der Geist als Widersacher der Seele.*

KLEIN, MELANIE (1882-1960). An Austrian child psychoanalyst who settled in England in 1926. She believed that oedipal (*see* OEDIPUS) hostility could begin in early infancy and consequently introduced new concepts into child analysis to counteract the infantile aggressive impulses that later produce neurosis (q.v.). She also conducted research in childhood depressive and schizoid (*see* SCHIZOPHRENIA) states and originated a school of psy-

choanalysis (q.v.) based on object theory. It emphasizes the need for children to resolve their ambivalence toward the mother and the breast.
Bibliography: Klein, M. 1932. *Psychoanalysis of children*, trans. A. Strachey.

KLEIST, HEINRICH VON (1777-1811). A German dramatist, poet, and novelist. As a young man he abandoned a career in the army to study philosophy because he hoped to control his destiny through a better informed mind. After reading the works of Immanuel Kant (q.v.), he decided that perfect knowledge was unattainable and turned to writing. In 1811, after the *Berliner Abendblätter*, which he contributed to and edited, had been suppressed, Kleist became despondent and poverty-stricken. He committed suicide (q.v.) on the shore of the Wannsee with a woman he had met earlier and who was likewise depressed. Ernest Jones (q.v.) wrote a paper dealing with his suicide entitled "On Dying Together."
Bibliography: March, R. 1954. *Life of Heinrich von Kleist*.

KLEMM, GUSTAV OTTO (1883-1939). A German psychologist and pupil of Wilhelm Wundt (q.v.). He conducted research in the fields of apperception of spatial relations, racial psychology, oscillation of attention, and localization of sounds. He later turned his attention to the psychology of work.
Bibliography: Murchison, C., ed. 1936. *A history of psychology in autobiography*. vol. 3.

KLUGE, CARL ALEXANDER FERDINAND (1782-1844). A German physician. He was so convinced of the existence of animal magnetism (q.v.) that he wrote a textbook about it in 1811 entitled *Versuch einer Darstellung des animalischen Magnetismus als Heilmittel*. He thought that an individual went through six degrees of somnambulism (q.v.) as he passed from the waking state to sleep and, eventually, to perception of past or future events. According to him, individuals in a state of deep trance could communicate with people living far away. Because he was a distinguished and respected physician, his opinions influenced many, and they carefully followed his instructions on how to magnetize patients.
Bibliography: Ellenberger, H. F. 1970. *The discovery of the unconscious*.

KLÜVER, HEINRICH (1897-). A German psychologist. He pursued postgraduate studies in the United States and held several distinguished positions in research and teaching. He has written on neuropsychology, behavior mechanisms, psychopharmacology, and genetic psychology. He also described the behavioral changes that occur following the removal of

temporal lobes in monkeys. These changes are known now as the Klüver-Bucy syndrome. He also invented a new method of staining nerve tissue.
Bibliography: Klüver, H. 1933. *Behaviour Mechanisms in Monkeys.*

KNIGHT, HENRY M. (1827-1880). An American physician. He pressed for better facilities for the care of the mentally retarded in Connecticut. An inquiry conducted on his initiative into the number of mentally retarded in the state revealed that they were "as numerous as the insane, eight times as numerous as the deaf and dumb, and more than twice as many as the blind." Knight turned his own home in 1858 into an institution for the mentally defective and dedicated himself to their care and education. After a long struggle, his work was recognized. In 1861 his institution became the Connecticut School for Imbeciles. Knight was appointed superintendent of it and better premises were provided. The school remained in existence until 1917, when a new training school was opened.
Bibliography: Kanner, L. 1964. *A history of the care and study of the mentally retarded.*

KNIGHT, PAUL SLADE (1785-1846). A British physician and naval surgeon. In 1816 he became the medical superintendent and manager of the Lancaster County Lunatic Asylum. He published his clinical observations in 1827 in a book entitled *Observations on the Causes, Symptoms, and Treatment of Derangement of the Mind, Founded on an Extensive Moral and Medical Practice In the Treatment of Lunatics.* He asserted that "deranged intellect" was "a corporeal disorder," but "religion and the passions" were responsible for the characteristics of the disease. To investigate the aetiology of insanity he devised a questionnaire to be filled in by doctors and relatives of the patients, but he also emphasized the importance of examining the patient, rather than relying upon the statements by the family. Although he personally designed instruments of restraint (q.v.) to be used in his hospital, he advocated music therapy (q.v.). In 1824, Knight was dismissed from his post, after he was accused of embezzling asylum property.
Bibliography: Knight, P. S. 1827. *Observations on the causes, symptoms, and treatment of derangement of the mind, founded on an extensive moral and medical practice in the treatment of lunatics.*

KNOWLE HOSPITAL. A mental hospital in Hampshire, England, opened in 1852. The staff lives in an eighteenth century house, which is listed as a building of historic interest. In 1883, an extension to accommodate four hundred patients was completed, using the labor of Russian prisoners of war from the Crimea.

KOFFKA, KURT (1886-1941). A German psychologist and a pupil of Carl Stumpf (q.v.). He enlarged the concepts of the Gestalt psychology (q.v.),

and, in 1921 he became one of the founders of *Psychologische Forschung* (q.v.). His article "Perception: An Introduction to Gestalt Theory," written for the American *Psychological Bulletin*, was a definite statement of the new movement. It was considered quite controversial by those American psychologists, who favored the Gestalt School of Psychology. In 1927, Koffka settled in the United States, and in 1932 he was given a professorship at Smith College in Massachusetts, which he retained until his death.
Bibliography: Koffka, K. 1935. *Principles of Gestalt psychology.*

KOHLER, WOLFGANG (1887-1967). A German psychologist, born in Estonia. At the start of World War I he was caught on the Spanish island of Tenerife, where he was studying the animals of the ape station. Unable to return to Germany, he continued his studies and conducted experiments on the visual discrimination of apes and chickens. His work on perception and insight contributed to the development of Gestalt psychology (q.v.). In 1920, he published *Die physischen Gestalten in die Ruhe und im stationärem Zustand*, which resulted in his appointment to the chair of philosophy of the University of Göttingen.
Bibliography: Kohler, W. 1926. *Gestalt psychology.*

KO HUNG. A famous Chinese physician and medical writer of the fourth century A.D. Relating the achievements of early physicians, he stated that Thai Tshang Kung (205-150 B.C.) "used to cut open skulls of patients and arrange their brains in order."
Bibliography: Brothwell, D., and Sandison, A. T. 1967. *Diseases in antiquity.*

KOKOSCHKA, OSKAR (1886-1980). An Austrian painter and writer. As an exponent of expressionism (q.v.), he became famous for his revealing psychological portraits, which were said to lay bare the souls of his subjects. His work often has depicted human agony and despair. Some of his posters and lithographs were regarded as shocking.
Bibliography: Hoffman, E. 1947. *Kokoschka: life and work.*
Kokoschka, O. 1974. *My life,* trans. D. Britt.

KOLLER, CARL (1857-1944). A German physician. In 1884, Sigmund Freud (q.v.) mentioned to him that cocaine (q.v.) numbed the tongue. The remark led Koller to use cocaine as a local anesthetic in eye operations. To Freud's bitterness, Koller claimed the discovery as his own.
Bibliography: Sulloway, F. J. 1979. *Freud: biologist of the mind.*

KÖLLIKER, RUDOLF ALBERT VON (1817-1905). A Swiss physician. He greatly contributed to the field of neurology (q.v.) by anticipating the neuron theory. He taught until he was eighty-five years old, and even after retiring wrote many papers of outstanding clarity. He was one of the first

to recognize the genius Santiago Ramon y Cajal (q.v.), who paid tribute to his scientific acumen, his rectitude and his modesty. Kölliker traveled widely, enjoyed hunting and mountain climbing, and included yodeling in his many accomplishments.
Bibliography: Haymaker, W., and Schiller, F. 1970. *The founders of neurology*. 2d. ed.

KÖNIG, ARTHUR (1856-1901). A German psychological physicist. His work was mostly in the field of color vision and its problems. He was a supporter of Hermann Helmholtz (q.v.) and published his work on optics, adding a bibliography on vision of 8,000 titles.
Bibliography: Boring, E. G. 1950. *A history of experimental psychology*.

KORAN, THE. The sacred book of Islam, which contains the revelations made to Mohammed (q.v.) by the angel Gabriel. It was transmitted orally until 651 A.D. when the caliph Uthman (c.574-656) ordered it written, following the deaths of the best Koran reciters on the battle field. The Koran, like the Bible (q.v.), contains passages of psychiatric interest. It mentions, for example, the interpretation of dreams (q.v.), the prohibition of suicide (q.v.), alcohol, and all narcotics, the changes of behavior brought about by evil spirits, and sexual deviations. The Koran emphasizes human relationships and the responsibilities, duties, and moral principles that govern them. It also considers the emotional aspect of illness and urges a kindly attitude toward those who are weak of understanding, "maintain them for the same, clothe them, and speak kindly unto them." Mohammed's plea to be delivered of the "mischief of the moon," is a reference to epilepsy (q.v.), which was believed to worsen during a full or new moon.
Bibliography: Arberry, A. J. 1964. *The Koran interpreted*.

KORDIAKOS. A term used in the Talmud (q.v.) to describe a syndrome that followed excessive drinking of new wine. It was characterized by mental confusion, dizziness, and odd behavior. The disorder was recognized as acute but distinguished from insanity. Those affected were considered to be temporarily unable to make decisions. A diet of red, lean meat was the contemporary treatment. The commentary on kordiakos is accepted now as one of the earliest descriptions of delirium tremens (q.v.).
Bibliography: Hankoff, L. D. 1972. Ancient descriptions of organic brain syndrome: the "kordiakos" of the Talmud. *Am. J. Psychiat.* 129: 233-36.

KORO. An anxiety state related to a fear of castration. It is found among the inhabitants of southern China (q.v.) and the Malay Archipelago. Those affected believe that the penis is receding into the abdomen. The organ is often tied to a stick, or friends and relatives may help to clamp it into a box

in an effort to prevent its disappearance, which they believe would cause death.
Bibliography: Wittkower, E. D. 1968. Transcultural psychiatry. In *Modern perspectives in world psychiatry*, ed. J. G. Howells.

KORSAKOV, SERGEI SERGEIEVICH (1853-1900). A Russian psychiatrist and neurologist. He is considered one of the founders of Russian psychiatry. In 1887 he described the mental and neurological symptoms usually caused by chronic alcoholism (q.v.). He called the syndrome *cerebropathia psychica toxemica* (q.v.), now known as Korsakov's syndrome. He also is acknowledged to have established the concept of paranoia (q.v.). Korsakov believed in the nonrestraint of mental patients and the need for them to receive more personal attention. He advocated family care (q.v.) and initiated a system of boarding out (q.v.) under medical supervision, on farms. He devised a classification of mental diseases. In 1890 he founded the Moscow Society of Neuropathologists and Psychiatrists.
Bibliography: Haymaker, W., and Schiller, F. 1970. *The founders of neurology*. 2d. ed.

KOZHEVNIKOV, ALEKSEI YAKOVLEVICH (1836-1902). A Russian neurologist. After studies abroad, he returned to Russia to teach neuropathology and became Moscow University's first professor of nervous and mental diseases. He founded a neurological clinic in Moscow with a museum attached to it, which he financed himself. He also tried to reform the conditions for mental patients throughout Russia. In the field of neurology, he described familial spastic diplegia and a form of epilepsy (q.v.) subsequently associated with his name.
Bibliography: Haymaker, W., and Schiller, F. 1970. *The founders of neurology*. 2d. ed.

KRABBE, KORUD H. (1885-). A Danish neurologist. In 1934 he described familial infantile diffuse sclerosis, now known as Krabbe's disease. He also demonstrated that cerebral vascular malformations are often the cause of meningeal hemorrhages.

KRAEMER, HEINRICH (1430-1505). A German Dominican monk. In collaboration with Johann Jacob Sprenger (q.v.), he wrote a book on witchcraft (q.v.) entitled *Malleus Maleficarum* (q.v.). Kraemer was an unpopular and dreaded figure during his investigations of heresy. The faculty of theology at the University of Cologne did not endorse his work unanimously, notwithstanding a papal bull by Innocent VIII (q.v.) ordering it, but he and Sprenger persisted and in 1486 obtained the official support of Maximilian I (1459-1519) King of the Romans and future Holy Roman emperor. As inquisitor, Kraemer was responsible for causing the death of many deluded, sick people who had been accused of witchcraft and heresy.

Bibliography: Turberville, A. S. 1920. Reprint 1964. *Mediaeval heresy and the inquisition.*

KRAEPELIN, EMIL (1856-1926). A German psychiatrist and professor of psychiatry at the universities of Dorpat, Heidelberg in 1891 and Munich in 1903. He became interested in psychiatry as a medical student and even then believed that mental disorders were caused by such physical traumas as poisons, head injuries, or fevers. His theory of organic causes remained unchallenged until the 1920s. He studied according to the natural history method, following the course of the disease from its beginning to its termination. He systematized the classification of mental disorders into cause, symptomatology, course, final stage, and pathological anatomical findings and introduced new nosological concepts. He divided mental diseases into the two classes devised by Paul Moebius (q.v.): exogenous and endogenous. In 1896, he introduced the concept of dementia praecox (q.v.), which grouped together catatonia, hebephrenia, and paranoia (qq.v.). In 1899, he introduced a concept of manic-depressive insanity as a distinct disease entity. Kraepelin believed mental illness to be predetermined and basically incurable, and, therefore, placed his faith in prevention. Tragically, this belief greatly influenced German psychiatry during the Nazi regime, when mental patients were ruthlessly destroyed or sterilized in an effort to eradicate mental illness. The first edition of Kraepelin's *Textbook of Psychiatry* was published in 1883. The book was subsequently revised many times and translated into several languages. The English translation made a considerable impact on the American classification of mental disorders. The Wolf-man (q.v.), Sigmund Freud's (q.v.) famous patient, originally had been in Kraepelin's care for several years.

Bibliography: Kraepelin, E. 1904. *Lectures on clinical psychiatry.*

KRAFFT-EBING, RICHARD VON (1840-1902). A German neurologist and president of the Viennese Neurological Society. By experiments with paralytics whom he had inoculated with luetic material, he was able to prove a definite relationship between syphilis (q.v.) and general paralysis of the insane (q.v.). He also worked in the field of forensic psychiatry and described sexual aberrations in a book, first published in 1886, entitled *Psychopathia Sexualis.* The terms "masochism" (q.v.) and "sadism" (q.v.) were introduced by him in this book, which nearly caused the cancellation of his honorary membership in the Medico-Psychological Association (q.v.). In 1897, speaking at the international congress in Moscow, he coined the phrase "civili-

zation and syphilization," a premonition of future trends that would link mental pathology with ways of life.
Bibliography: Krafft-Ebing, R. 1897. *A textbook of mental diseases.*

KREMERS, BARBARA. A young girl from the town of Unna, Germany. Her psychological malingering was investigated by Johann Weyer (q.v.) in 1574. She was believed to be able to survive without eating. Weyer brought her to his own house where her fasting (q.v.) was discovered to be a fraud. Encouraged by Weyer and his family, Kremers showed a good appetite and was soon cured of her other hysterical (*see* HYSTERIA) symptoms of lameness in her legs and twisted arms. Weyer described this case in a booklet published in 1577 and entitled *De Lamiis Liber: Item de Commentitiis Jejuniis* (on alleged fasting).
Bibliography: Zilboorg, G. 1941. *A history of medical psychology.*

KRETSCHMER, ERNST (1888-1964). A German psychiatrist. He studied the physical appearance of psychiatric patients and tried to correlate body build and constitution with psychiatric disorders. He distinguished four main types: athletic (q.v.) (similar to a gorilla) and the least prone to mental illness; asthenic (q.v.) (similar to a chimpanzee) and more prone to schizophrenia (q.v.); pyknic (similar to an orang-outang) and dysplastic (intermediate type). He also developed a classification of cycloid and schizoid disorders that ranged from depression to mania (q.v.). Although his theories have not been widely accepted, his concepts have stimulated a number of investigations on the same lines. Kretschmer was president of the German Society of Psychotherapy but resigned his post in 1933 when Adolf Hitler (q.v.) wanted the society to adapt its concepts to the Nazi philosophy and expel its Jewish members.
Bibliography: Kretschmer, E. 1921. *Körperbau und charakter.*

KREUGER, IVAR (1880-1932). Swedish financier and industrialist. Even as a child he showed such psychopathic (*see* PSYCHOPATHY) traits as a complete inability to distinguish right from wrong, lack of guilt at his dishonesty, and pride in his undisputed ability to cheat. He had a brilliant mind, which he used to defraud other people. Kreuger developed an international monopoly in the match industry and was involved in vast financial enterprises that lent money to various governments in return for industrial concessions. In 1929 his enterprises collapsed revealing one of the greatest frauds in history. Three years later he committed suicide (q.v.) in Paris. It has been suggested that some of his behavior can be explained as a result of general paralysis of the insane (q.v.).
Bibliography: Shaplen, R. 1961. *Kreuger, genius, and swindler.*

KREUTZER SONATA. A famous sonata for piano and violin by Ludwig van Beethoven (q.v.). Leo Tolstoy (q.v.) wrote a novel so entitled, which

is a psychological study of the pathological jealousy (q.v.) that is aroused in a husband while his wife plays the sonata. The main character is a psychologist of sorts and a man of intellect but also a supreme egotist, who tells of his life and the love in his marriage that is turning to hatred. Jealousy, suspicion, and murder are part of the story, which Tolstoy used to plead for easier laws for the dissolution of unhappy marriages.
Bibliography: Tolstoy, L. 1889. *The Kreutzer Sonata.*

KRIES, JOHANNES VON (1853-1928). A German physiologist and experimental psychologist. His work dealt with the physiology of vision. He elaborated the "duplicity theory," which holds that the cones of the retina are responsible for vision in bright light and the rods of the retina are responsible for vision in twilight. In 1886 he wrote a book on the theory of probabilities, but his major work, published in 1882, was *Die Gesichtesempfindungen und ihre Analyse.*
Bibliography: Boring, E. G. 1950. *A history of experimental psychology.*

KRIS, ERNST (1901-1957). A German psychologist, who settled in the United States. He attempted to apply the principles of ego psychology in psychoanalytic (*see* PSYCHOANALYSIS) practice. In his studies of artists, he introduced the concept of regression in the service of the ego. In the light of this concept, he commented on the artistic creations of psychotics (*see* PSYCHOSIS) and on the psychology of creative processes.
Bibliography: Kris, E. 1952. *Psychoanalytic explorations in art.*

KRISHABER, MAURICE (1836-1883). A Hungarian-born French physician. His work included research in the field of nervous diseases. He described a form of anxiety neurosis (q.v.), which he termed cerebro-cardiac neuropathia (q.v.). He noted that patients suffering from it had sleep disorders, palpitations, and dizziness with an overall feeling of acute anxiety that was not related to any specific cause.
Bibliography: Krishaber, M. 1873. *De la nérveopathie cérébro-cardiaque.*

KRONOS (CRONUS). In Greek mythology (q.v.), the son of mother Earth and Uranus, whom he castrated. He married his sister Rhea and swallowed their children to escape the prophesy that they would dethrone him. According to the myth, the youngest son Zeus was saved by his mother and banished Kronos. Sigmund Freud (q.v.) used the legend in one of his papers illustrating fear of the father, but he mistakenly assumed that Zeus had castrated Kronos.
Bibliography: Schneck, J. M. 1968. Freud and Kronos. *Am. J. Psychiat.* 125:692-93.

KRUEGER, FELIX (1874-1948). A German psychologist. He was a pupil of Wilhelm Wundt (q.v.) and worked at Wundt's Leipzig laboratory. He

later became its director. Krueger founded a school of psychology based on the concept of entirety of the mind and the recognition of the various influences upon its development. It was referred to as the school of *Ganzheits Psychologie*, or totality psychology. Krueger believed that cultural factors and social conditions should be considered in the total assessment of the individual's development; therefore his work was not limited to laboratory experiment but included observation of cultural customs and institutions.
Bibliography: Misiak, H., and Sexton, V. S. 1966. *History of psychology.*

KUAN-TZU. A Chinese work compiled in about 300 B.C. It mentions that institutions for the insane existed in China as early as 1150 B.C.
Bibliography: Wong, K. Chi-Min and Wu, Lien-Tu. 1932. *History of Chinese medicine.*

KUBIE, LAWRENCE S. (1896-1973). An American psychiatrist. His family had wanted him to become a lawyer, but, after a short time of studying economics and political science, he turned to medicine. In 1950 he wrote a lucid exposition of psychoanalysis (q.v.), entitled *Practical and Theoretical Aspects of Psychoanalysis.* For the last fourteen years of his life he worked and taught at the Sheppard and Enoch Pratt Hospital (q.v.), where a library named after him is housed.

KUBLA KHAN. One of the best poems of Samuel T. Coleridge (q.v.). He composed it in 1797 on waking from a sleep induced by opium (q.v.). According to him, the verses came to him during sleep, and he had only to write them down. While doing this, he was interrupted by a visitor and later found that the interruption had driven from his memory (q.v.) the remainder of the poem.
Bibliography: Coleridge, E. H. ed. 1912 *Complete poetical works.* 2 vols.

KUDA-KEPANG. The terms *kuda*, horse, and *kepang*, bamboo, refer to a phenomenon observed in Indonesia. A boy and a girl are paid to gyrate to monotonous music and the snapping of a whip. After some hours they appear to fall into a state of trance. In this condition they are able to chew and spit out all kinds of objects, including light bulbs, without any apparent damage to their mouths.
Bibliography: Kline, N. S. 1963. Psychiatry in Indonesia. *Am. J. Psychiat.* 119:809-15.

KUFFNER, KAREL (1858-1939). A Czech physician. He became chief of the Charles University department of psychiatry in Prague. His *Textbook of Psychiatry*, published in 1897, was the first of its kind in Czechoslovakia. In it he introduced a new nosology that became the basis of psychiatric terminology in his country. His approach was materialistic, for he believed

that mental disorders were caused by defective brain development or diseases of the nervous system. In 1926 he was one of the early workers to offer a clinical description of schizophrenia (q.v.).
Bibliography: Vencovsky, E. 1975. Czechoslovakia. In *World history of psychiatry*, ed. J. G. Howells.

KULESHOVA, ROSA. A contemporary Soviet woman. Her capacity to perceive colors and read ordinary print by touch was investigated by Russian psychologists in the 1960s. A report of their observations was published in 1963 in *Soviet Psychology and Psychiatry*.
See also DERMO-OPTICAL PERCEPTION (DOP).
Bibliography: Goldenson, R. M. 1970. *Encyclopedia of human behavior*. vol 1.

KÜLPE, OSWALD (1862-1915). A Russian-born psychologist. His family was of German origin. While studying in Leipzig, he met Wilhelm Wundt (q.v.), who changed the course of his studies from history to philosophy and experimental psychology (q.v.). Külpe contributed to this branch of psychology with his work on such higher mental processes as will and thought. He conducted his investigations at the laboratory of Würzburg, where he developed a school of imageless thought. He later became interested in psychology as it relates to medicine and received an honorary medical degree from the University of Giessen. In his *Grundriss der Psychologie*, (Outline of Psychology) published in 1893, he defined psychology as the science of "the facts of experience" and believed that "the first truly complete systematic psychology comes from Aristotle."
Bibliography: Misiak, H., and Sexton, V. S. 1966. *History of Psychology*.

KUMYSS. A Tartar term for fermented mare's milk, which was introduced into Russia by the Mongols at the time of their invasion. Their strength and endurance was attributed to the fact that during long marches they were sustained by mare's milk and horse blood, which they drank directly from a neck vein of the animal. It was drunk in great quantities as a form of intensive therapy for a multitude of physical and mental disorders. Kumyss curative centers were scattered throughout the steppes in the Volga plains. The centers attracted patients from all walks of life until horse breeding declined after the Russian Revolution.
Bibliography: Kourennoff, P. M., and St. George, G. 1970. *Russian folk medicine*.

KUO, Z. Y. (1898-   ). A Chinese animal psychologist. He emphasized the importance of the environment. Kuo attacked the concept of instincts and purposive behavior with such success that the term "instinct" was seldom heard in some psychological departments. His research led to the introduction of behaviorism (q.v.) in China (q.v.).

Bibliography: Kuo, Z. Y. 1924. A psychology without heredity. *Psychological Review*, 31:427-51.

KUO YU. A Chinese classic written around 100 B.C. It contains a classification of mental disorders. Among its practical suggestions is a list of suitable occupations for various categories of the physically and mentally handicapped.

Bibliography: Chin, R., and Chin, Al-li S. 1969. *Psychological research in Communist China.*

KUSSMAUL, ADOLF (1822-1902). A German physician. In 1877 he investigated and described a form of voluntary mutism (q.v.) in the insane (now known as Kussmaul's aphasia) and introduced the term "word blindness" to describe aphasia. He is remembered also for introducing a systematic procedure in the collection of data for research.

Bibliography: Schmidt, J. E. 1959. *Medical discoveries: who and when.*

L

LACLOS, PIERRE AMBROISE FRANÇOIS CHODERLOS DE (1741-1803). A French army officer. He was the author of an epistolary novel entitled *Les Liaisons Dangereuses*, which was first published in 1782. The protagonist of the novel recounts the various immoral ways he has used to seduce young girls. Laclos hoped to educate by illustrating the villainy of the professional seducer. He had considerable psychological insight and underlined the fact that to seduce and corrupt an honest young woman, she first must be made to lose respect for her mother and hence for herself.
Bibliography: Versini, L. 1968. *Laclos et la tradition*.

LACORDAIRE, JEAN BAPTISTE HENRI (1802-1861). A French theologian and Dominican preacher. His 'Conférences' at Notre Dame in Paris made him famous. At a time when the church was dubious of magnetism (q.v.), he asserted his belief in it in a sermon delivered in 1846. He stated that magnetism consisted of "natural but irregular forces" used by God to oppose the materialism of the times.
Bibliography: Sheppard, L. 1964. *Lacordaire*.

LACTANTIUS, LUCIUS CAELIUS FIRMIANUS (c.240-c.320). A Christian writer, brought up in Africa. He was tutor to the son of Constantine the Great (288?-337). In his *Divinarum Institutionum Libri Septem* he described the ways in which demons affect the viscera and, through them, the human mind. He also reported the belief that anger was linked with the gallbladder, fear with the heart (q.v.), joy with the spleen (q.v.), and sexual pleasure with the liver (q.v.).
Bibliography: Chadwick, H. 1967. *The early church*.

LACTATION. For centuries suppression of lactation after childbirth was considered a cause of insanity in women. As late as the nineteenth century, it was believed that the suppressed milk found its way to the brain. As it was already known that emotional and physical shocks could also cause the suppression of milk, particular care was exercised to protect nursing women. In ancient Rome a crown was placed over the entrance of the house to signify that no malevolent intrusion was allowed.

Bibliography: Esquirol, J.E.D. 1845. Reprint. 1965. *Mental maladies: a treatise on insanity.*

LADD, GEORGE TRUMBULL (1842-1921). An American psychologist. After graduating in theology, he spent ten years in the ministry and then taught mental and moral philosophy at Bowdoin College in Maine. In 1881 he began to teach physiological psychology at Yale University in Connecticut and established the Yale laboratory of psychology in 1892. His book *Elements of Physiological Psychology*, written in 1887, synthetized the literature relevant to that field and underlined the importance of the nervous system. His interest in both theology and psychology helped to unite the trends of the old and new psychology in the United States. He was the second president of the American Psychological Association (q.v.).

Bibliography: Misiak, H., and Sexton, V. S. 1966. *History of psychology.*

LADY CHICHESTER HOSPITAL. The first English hospital to provide inpatient treatment for nervous disorders in their early stages. Founded in 1905 by Dr. Helen Boyle (q.v.), it was an ordinary dwelling house located in the middle of the town of Brighton. Its first patients were women and girls on the point of a breakdown, who, without the hospital, would have been sent to traditional asylums (q.v.) and certified insane. In 1920 it moved to its present larger premises in Hove, Sussex.

Bibliography: Hingston, C. L. April 1955. The jubilee of the Lady Chichester Hospital, Hove, Sussex. *The Medical Women's Federation J.*

LAEHR, HANS HEINRICH (1820-1905). A German psychiatrist. In 1872 he described the first known case of morphine (q.v.) addiction in a paper published in the *Allegemeine Zeitschrift für Psychiatrie.* He also compiled a vast bibliography of psychiatry, neurology, and psychology. The work was comprised of two large volumes and included thousands of items covering the period from 1459 to 1799.

Bibliography: Laehr, H. 1899. *Die literatur der Psychiatrie, Neurologie und Psychologie von 1459-1799.* 2 vols.

LAFAYETTE, MARIE JOSEPH DU MOTIER, MARQUIS DE (1757-1834). A French reformer, statesman, and officer. He never knew his father and seldom saw his mother, who died when he was thirteen years old. He was brought up by his grandmother and aunts. He married when he was sixteen years old, and three years later he went to America. It was during this time that George Washington (1732-1799) became his father figure.

Lafayette was particularly attracted to secret societies and strange sects. He became interested in Franz Mesmer (q.v.) and his work and subscribed to a fund for the formation of a society whose members would share in Mesmer's so-called secrets and spread his teaching. Mesmer also asked Lafayette to introduce his work to Washington. Lafayette's mastery in handling crowds was extraordinary. He would address his listeners as "children" even as a young man and easily managed to create a benevolent impression.
Bibliography: Gottschalk, L. R. 1935. *Lafayette comes to America.*

LAFONTAINE, CHARLES (1803-?). A French magnetizer (*see* MAG-NETISM). He claimed he was a member of the aristocracy of France and early in life had left his family to become an actor. After accidentally hypnotizing (*see* HYPNOTISM) a woman, he became a magnetizer. He gave demonstrations in theaters and had a successful private practice that attracted patients from several countries. His performances often caused riots that had to be quelled by the police. He was believed to be so powerful that he could visit taverns of low repute without fear of robbery. It was during his visit to England in 1841 that James Braid (q.v.) saw his performance in Manchester and became interested in magnetism. Lafontaine also wrote an autobiography of great interest.
Bibliography: Lafontaine, C. 1886. *Mémoires d'un magnétiseur.*

LA FONTAINE, JEAN DE (1621-1695). A French poet and fabulist. He never liked the routine of steady work and spent most of his dissipated life supported by wealthy patrons. In 1658 he abandoned his wife and child and lived in the household of Madame de La Sablière, one of his patrons. Although he was warmhearted and sincere, he was also feckless, frivolous, inconstant in his affections, and weak in his resolution. His *Contes et Nouvelles en Vers* (1664-1674) offended some of his contemporaries, and he disavowed them in 1692 when he experienced a religious conversion following a serious illness. His handling of characters and situations shows a deep psychological understanding of human nature.
Bibliography: Vianey, J. 1939. *La psychologie de La Fontaine.*

LAGERLÖF, SELMA OTTILIANA (1858-1940). A Swedish novelist. She was very pious and experienced recurrent feelings of guilt, starting from childhood. Her anxiety was sometimes so great that she had hallucinations (q.v.) of horrible and frightening old women. Her writing reflected her emotional state and often depicted harsh and cruel figures, especially stepmothers and witches (*see* WITCHCRAFT). Of her many works *Marbacka* (1922) and *The Diary of Selma Lagerlöf* (1937) are autobiographical.
Bibliography: Wägner, E. 1942-1943. *Selma Lagerlöf.* 2 vols.

LAGNEIA FUROR. A term introduced by John Mason Good (q.v.) to denote erotomania (q.v.).
(*See also* ALUSIA, APHLEXIA, ECPHRONIA, and EMPATHENIA.)

LAGUNA, ANDRES DE (1499-1560). A Spanish physician and personal physician to the Emperor Charles V (q.v.). Unlike Andras Vesalius (q.v.) his opinions regarding the essence of man's soul followed the teachings of Plato (q.v.), but to the concepts of a rational and a sensuous soul he added a vegetative soul. Regarded as the Spanish Galen, he greatly influenced medicine in his country.
Bibliography: Lopez Ibor, J. J. 1975. Spain and Portugal. In *World history of psychiatry*, ed. J. G. Howells.

LAI. In Chinese folklore (q.v.), a spirit that haunted the imperial harem in the twelfth century A.D. It was represented as a headless, shapeless thing that was covered with shining hair. Sometimes it laid in the beds of the concubines, who then would dream that someone was sleeping with them. Its concept is similar to that of the incubus (q.v.) in Western culture.
Bibliography: Veith, I. 1975. The Far East. In *World history of psychiatry*, ed. J. G. Howells.

LAKE OF PSYCHOLOGY. The name under which Lake Zürich in Switzerland came to be known during the 1920s. The name was derived from the number of psychologists who attended the Burghölzli Hospital (q.v.), the Institute of Applied Psychology, and other training institutions in the area.

LAMARCK, JEAN BAPTISTE DE (1744-1829). A French naturalist. He believed that an animal's form could be modifed through the animal's effort to adapt to its environment and that these acquired modifications could be inherited by its progeny. Lamarck's theories paved the way for Charles Darwin's (q.v.) theory of evolution. Darwin derived from him the theory of transmission of acquired characteristics. Neuropsychiatrists found in his theories a confirmation of the belief that behavioral deterioration could be inherited.
Bibliography: Cannon, H. G. 1960. *Lamarck and modern genetics*.

LAMB, LADY CAROLINE (1785-1828). An English novelist and the wife of William Lamb, Lord Melbourne (1779-1848), prime minister to Queen Victoria (1819-1901). She was a restless, reckless exhibitionist (*see* EXHIBITIONISM), who lacked restraint and craved continuous excitement. She formed an association with the poet Byron (q.v.), who soon tired of her outbursts and neurotic (*see* NEUROSIS) demands. After Byron's death, her behavior so deteriorated that her husband was forced to divorce her. It was

said that the shock of her unexpected meeting with Byron's funeral cortege permanently affected her mind.
Bibliography: Jenkins, E. 1932. *Lady Caroline Lamb*.

LAMB, CHARLES (1775-1834). An English writer. He had a lonely childhood in a tense household; his mother's and father's temperaments caused frequent clashes that were aided by the presence of an aunt, Sarah Lamb, a suspicious and resentful person. The stutter that Lamb developed probably deprived him of a university education. His schoolmaster at Christ's Hospital, the Reverend James Boyer, was a sadistic individual, who would cane the boys in a blind rage. In 1795 Lamb spent six weeks in one of the Hoxton madhouses (q.v.). In 1796, his sister Mary Ann Lamb (q.v.) attacked their father and murdered their mother. Lamb was obliged to take charge of the situation and look after her as her guardian for the remainder of his life. The tragedy deeply affected him and may have led to his frequent bouts of heavy drinking and smoking. He suffered from what he described as "a sad depression of spirits and a most unaccountable nervousness." He shared his life with his sister, and the two of them adopted an orphaned girl named Emma Isola whom they tenderly loved. The last nine years of his life were very sad: Mary's insanity had fewer periods of remission, and, after many moves, they settled in isolation in the country. His alcoholism (q.v.) worsened, and his behavior became more eccentric. The final blow was the death of his beloved friend Samuel T. Coleridge (q.v.).
Bibliography: Howe, W. D. 1973. *Charles Lamb and his friends*.

LAMB, MARY ANN (1764-1847). An English writer and elder sister of Charles Lamb (q.v.). In 1796 she stabbed her overbearing mother to death in a state of fury. She was found temporarily insane and by order of the Coroner's Court, placed in a private asylum, Fisher House (q.v.). She was later placed in Charles' custody, and brother and sister lived together. Her madness had periods of remission, during which her behavior was more orderly than her brother's. At these times she was able to collaborate with him and indeed to comfort him in his own depression. During acute episodes of derangement she again was confined in private asylums (q.v.) or had a nurse to look after her at home. Even when she was well, she was conscious of her illness, for she wrote to a friend, "a perception of not being in a sane state perpetually haunts me." Her brother died while she was deeply deranged, and she survived him for thirteen years.
Bibliography: Howe, W. D. 1973. *Charles Lamb and his friends*.

LA METTRIE, JULIEN OFFRAY DE (1709-1751). A French physician and philosopher. After abandoning a career in the church, he gained his degree in medicine at the age of fifteen. His materialistic views were expressed in his *Histoire Naturelle de l'Âme* (1745), which he wrote following his

experiences during a fever. He had discovered that his thinking power was affected by his physical condition and concluded that thought depends upon the mechanical action of the brain. His materialism, which was considered atheistic as it stated that the only pleasures were those of the senses and that the soul died with the body, caused such protest that he had to flee from France. Frederick the Great (q.v.) gave him asylum in Germany, where he continued to write. Equating the mind with the soul, he arrived at the concept of man-machine, which he then expounded in his *L'Homme Machine* in 1748. His later works were on the concept of pleasure and the art of enjoying life through physical love and other hedonistic (*see* HEDONISM) pursuits. He was said to have died of overeating at the age of forty-one.
Bibliography: Boissier, R. 1931. *La Mettrie.*

LAMIA. In Greek and Roman mythology (q.v.), she was a female demon. As queen of Libya, she had been loved by Jupiter. Juno, consumed with jealousy (q.v.), had destroyed her children and thus caused her insanity. Lamia revenged herself on all children she met by enticing and devouring them. In Africa, the Lamiae were half-woman and half-serpent creatures, who were said to entice men and then devour them. In the Middle Ages (q.v.) Lamiae was another term for witches (*see* WITCHCRAFT). Robert Burton (q.v.) tells of them in his *Anatomy of Melancholy* (q.v.), and John Keats (q.v.) wrote a poem entitled *Lamia* (1820), based on Burton's story.
Bibliography: Lawson, J. C. 1910. *Modern Greek folklore and ancient Greek religion.*

LANCELOT. A knight of the Round Table in the Arthurian legends. Lover and champion of Queen Guinevere, he was driven to madness by her jealousy (q.v.). The legends describe how he was restrained and treated until he recovered his sanity.
Bibliography: Chrétien de Troyes. *Arthurian romances*, trans. W. W. Comfort.

LANCRE, PIERRE DE (?-1630). A French demonologist. He wrote about sorcery and described states of hallucination (q.v.) and delusion (q.v.) consistent with severe mental illness. In 1613 he wrote *Tableau de l'inconstance des mauvais anges et démons*, which was followed by *L'incrédulité et mécréance du sortilège plainement convaincué* in 1622. He believed in the power of the devil and advocated that all those suspected of witchcraft (q.v.) should be put to death.
Bibliography: Semelaigne, R. 1930. *Les pionniers de la psychiatrie française.*

LAND FOR ASYLUMS. In the nineteenth century there was a reform movement to provide mental patients with industrial and agricultural work. In England it was proposed that county asylums should have a minimum of one acre of land for every ten patients. The provision of land for asylums (q.v.) was considered so important that the first issue of *The Asylum Journal* (q.v.), published on November 15, 1853, contained an article entitled *On the Acreage of Land Attached to County Asylums* and written by Dr. John Thurnam, (q.v.) when he was medical superintendent (1850-73) of the Wiltshire County Asylum, Devizes, England.

LANDRY, JEAN BAPTISTE OCTAVE (1826-1865). A French physician. He was the first to describe an acute ascending paralysis (now known as Landry's paralysis) that spreads from the lower limbs to the bulbar and respiratory muscles. His description opened the doors to a new field of research. Despite his many accomplishments—he was an excellent violinist, an expert dancer and singer, a sportsman, and a geologist—he was compelled to run a hydrotherapy establishment for the treatment of nervous disorders. Jean Martin Charcot (q.v.) was at his bedside when he died of cholera, which he had contracted while helping the poor in an epidemic.
Bibliography: Haymaker, W., and Schiller, F. 1970. *The founders of neurology*. 2d. ed.

LANDSEER, SIR EDWIN HENRY (1802-1873). An English painter, famous for his animal studies. He began to paint as a child and exhibited his work at the Royal Academy when he was only thirteen years old. His output was enormous. Using both hands simultaneously, he could draw two different subjects. In the latter part of his life, his mental and artistic powers declined. It is said that he died insane, suffering from general paralysis of the insane (q.v.). Among his best known works are the *Monarch of the Glen* (1851) and the bronze lions in Trafalgar Square, London, at the foot of Nelson's Column.
Bibliography: Lennie, C. 1976. *Landseer the Victorian paragon*.

LANE, HOMER T. (1875-1925). An American reformer in the field of juvenile delinquency. He began by organizing a club in Detroit, Michigan, for street corner gangs, and eventually he directed a home for young delinquents. He pioneered self-government and became an authority on the subject. Personal difficulties, including a love affair with a young teacher, brought about his resignation. He emigrated to England where he founded a colony, the Little Commonwealth, in Dorset for delinquent children. Again, his naïve failure to protect his reputation resulted in accusations of improper behavior, and an inquiry resulted in the closure of the colony in 1918. More difficulties arose in 1925, when he was accused of extorting money from a wealthy psychotic (*see* PSYCHOSIS) woman. He left England for Paris and died there a few months later. His belief that children need love, respect,

and freedom, rather than coercion, to learn, has been expounded by his disciples David W. Wills and Alexander S. Neill (q.v.).
Bibliography: Wills, D. W. 1964. *Homer Lane: a biography.*

LANGE, CARL GEORGE (1834-1900). A Danish physician and psychologist. Almost simultaneously with William James (q.v.), he developed a theory of emotion (known as the James-Lange theory) that was based on the belief that emotion depends on the experience of bodily and physical changes involving the viscera and the muscular system. These changes, according to Lange, follow the perception of an exciting fact.
See also EMOTION, THEORY OF.
Bibliography: Lange, C. G. 1885. *Om Sindsbevoegelser.*

LANGE, JOHANN (1485-1565). A German physician. He rejected traditional methods of diagnosis based on theory and adopted observation as the basic principle in his clinical practice. Even so, he believed that some diseases were caused by supernatural phenomena. In describing the autopsy of a man who had committed suicide (q.v.), Lange claimed that the various objects found in his stomach, including four knives, bits of iron and a bunch of hair, were put there by the devil. Similarly, he claimed that a patient who had vomited nails and needles was bewitched. His *Epistolae Medicinae*, a collection of his medical observations, was published in 1554.
Bibliography: Zilboorg, G. 1941. *A history of medical psychology.*

LANGERMANN, JOHANN GOTTFRIED (1768-1832). A German physician, son of simple peasants. His doctoral dissertation was the first in Germany on a psychiatric subject. It was entitled *De Method Cognoscendi Curandique Animi Morbos Stabilienda* (1797), (on the methods of recognizing and curing lasting mental illnesses) and in it he discussed the methods of diagnosis and treatment of mental disorders. Although he wrote nothing else in this field, he devoted himself to the treatment of the mentally ill and displayed an unusually enlightened attitude toward their care. He believed that many physical disorders had a psychological aetiology and totally rejected the belief that mental illness was caused exclusively by damaged nervous systems. He divided patients into "curable" and "incurable" groups. In 1805 he founded a mental hospital in Germany, Saint Georg Insane Asylum, in Bayreuth, where his humanitarian approach was put into practice.
Bibliography: Zilboorg, G. 1941. *A history of medical psychology.*

LANGLAND (or LONGLAND), WILLIAM (LONG WILL) (1330?-?1400). An English poet, author of *The Vision of William Concerning Piers the Plowman*, an alliterative allegorical poem reflecting the thoughts and ways of life in fourteenth-century England. Langland roamed about the

country with beggars and wandering lunatics, his own reason also waxing and waning. In his poem he exorted his fellow men to give shelter and protection to the "lunatic lollers, who are God's minstrels and merry-mouthed jesters."
Bibliography: Salter, E. 1962. *Piers Plowman: an introduction.*

LANGLEY, JOHN NEWPORT (1852-1925). An English physiologist. In 1898 he introduced the term "autonomic nervous system," and his work greatly contributed to the mapping of its pathways.
Bibliography: Haymaker, W., and Schiller, F. 1970. *The founders of neurology.* 2d. ed.

LANTERNISTES. In seventeenth-century France, members of what would become the Société des Sciences. This group gathered together after the day's work was done, and discussed scientific topics with an open mind and great impartiality. They were so respected for their rectitude that occasionally parliament would seek their advice. François Bayle (q.v.), a member of the group, was consulted in a case of presumed witchcraft (q.v.) that occurred in Toulouse. The term "Lanternistes" was derived from the lanterns they carried to their meetings. In 1729, the group became known as the Société des Sciences.

LAO-TZU (*or* **LAO-TZE**) (c.604-531 B.C.). A Chinese philosopher and founder of Taoism, a liberal religion. In Taoism, man abjures all striving and the principle of righteousness, or right conduct, is considered all important. Ceremonies and rituals are discouraged. The teachings of Lao-Tzu provided the basis of later Chinese psychology and contain elements similar to existentialism (q.v.).
Bibliography: Watts, A. 1976. *Tao: the watercourse way.*

LAPINLAHTI HOSPITAL. The first mental hospital in Finland to be especially constructed for mental patients. It was opened in 1841, following a governmental inquiry into the care of the mentally ill. Its first superintendent was Dr. L. A. Fahlander. The hospital is now the psychiatric clinic of Helsinki University.
Bibliography: Retterstøl, N. 1975. Scandinavia. In *World history of psychiatry*, ed. J. G. Howells.

LAPIS ARMENIACUM. *See* ARMENIAN STONE.

LAPIS LAZULI. A deep blue, violet, or greenish blue semiprecious stone. In antiquity it was believed to have many curative properties. The Egyptians made much use of it and thought that it possessed mystical qualities. The Greeks and the Romans employed it in the treatment of epilepsy (q.v.) and

believed that it could dispel melancholy (*see* MELANCHOLIA). It was also used as a remedy for sterility. Unstable individuals were reputed to be unable to keep it in their possession for long.
See also PRECIOUS STONES.
Bibliography: Hodges, D. M. 1972 *Healing gems.*

LARVATUS (*or* LARVARUM PLENUS). A popular term in pre-Christian Rome. It referred to the "bewitched" or the mentally ill, who were considered full of *larvae* (specters).
Bibliography: Zilboorg, G. 1941. *A history of medical psychology.*

LASÈGUE, ERNEST CHARLES (1816-1883). A French physician. He studied persecution mania (q.v.) and published his observations in 1852. The syndrome subsequently became known as Lasègue's disease. In 1877 in collaboration with Jules Falret (q.v.), he described a mutually induced, contagious neurosis (q.v.) that they termed *folie à deux* (q.v.).
Bibliography: Lasègue, C., and Falret, J. 1877. La folie à deux (ou folie communiquée). *Ann. med.-psychol.* 18: 321. English trans. R. Michaud. 1964. *Suppl. Am. J. Psychiat.* 121: No. 4.

LASHLEY, KARL SPENCER (1890-1958). An American physiological psychologist. He is best known for his work on the localization of brain functions. Although he was essentially a behaviorist, he studied the functioning of the total organism, rather than particular stimuli and responses to them. He also contributed to the study of color vision, conditioning instinct, sex, and learning and heredity. The jumping technique for rats was invented by him. Lashley was professor of neuropsychology at Harvard University from 1935 to 1955. In 1929 he was president of the American Psychological Association (q.v.).
See also LASHLEY'S PRINCIPLE OF EQUIPOTENTIALITY.
Bibliography: Goldenson, R. M. 1970. *The encyclopedia of human behavior.*

LASHLEY'S PRINCIPLE OF EQUIPOTENTIALITY. A principle propounded by Karl S. Lashley (q.v.). It asserts that the whole of the cortex, except for the motor and sensory areas, can participate in any learned performance.
Bibliography: Lashley, K. S. 1929. *Brain mechanisms and intelligence.*

LASSAIGNE, AUGUST (1819-?). A French magnetizer. He began his career as a conjuror and became interested in magnetism (q.v.) during a performance in which a young girl, Prudence Bernard (q.v.) was hypnotized (magnetized). He married Bernard, who proved to be a natural somnambulist (*see* SOMNAMBULISM) and together they went on tour giving public performances. In his memoirs he described their experiences, his belief that his wife had a divine mission similar to that of Joan of Arc (q.v.), and the way in which the state of their relationship could improve or lessen his power to magnetize her.

Bibliography: Lassaigne, A. 1851. *Memoirs d'un magnetiseur, contenant la biographie de la somnambule Prudence Bernard.*

LATAH. A hysterical (*see* HYSTERIA) disorder prevalent among Malay women. The predominant symptoms are hypersuggestibility, imitative behavior, and repetition of obscene phrases. It is usually precipitated by a sudden and unexpected event, although an attack may be induced by teasing.

Bibliography: Yap, P. M. 1952. The latah reaction: its pathodynamics and nosological position. *J. Ment. Sci.* 98: 515.

LATHROP, JULIA CLIFFORD (1858-1932). An American social worker. She was a member of the advisory committee on child welfare and became the first director of the Children's Bureau (q.v.), which was established by President William Howard Taft (1857-1930) in 1912.

Bibliography: Addams, J. 1936. *My friend, Julia Lathrop.*

LAUDANUM. The name given by Paracelsus (q.v.) to a supposedly miraculous drug that he carried in the hollow pommel of his sword. Among its ingredients were gold and pearls. The term later was used to indicate an opiate, and it is likely that the "arcanum" of Paracelsus also contained some opium (q.v.). In the seventeenth century, Thomas Sydenham (q.v.) prescribed alcoholic tincture of opium with saffron (q.v.) for many disorders, and it was this mixture that was listed in the pharmacopoeia as laudanum. Thomas de Quincey (q.v.) in his *The Confessions of an English Opium-Eater* (q.v.) gave a vivid description of laudanum addiction and withdrawal symptoms. Other famous addicts include George Crabbe (q.v.) and Samuel Coleridge (q.v.). In the nineteenth century laudanum was implicated in many sensational murder trials.

Bibliography: Matthews, L. G. 1963. *History of pharmacy in Britain.*

LAUGHING GAS. The popular name for nitrous oxide. In the nineteenth century, its exhilarating properties were exploited by many people, who indulged in sniffing the gas to the point of intoxication. Laughing gas parties were common, and both Samuel Coleridge (q.v.) and Robert Southey (q.v.) not only took part in them but also described the effects of the gas. John Scoffern, in a book entitled *Chemistry No Mystery* (1839), provided more details about the parties at which "old and young, rich and poor" joined together expecting great fun. According to him, the party-goers sometimes would become so excited that fights would develop, and young men would take unheard-of liberties with the ladies. He also reported that chemists

engaged in the preparation of the gas would often experience "whimsical distortion of features."
Bibliography: Scoffern, J. 1839. *Chemistry no mystery.*

LAURENS, ANDRÉ DU (1560?-1609). A French physician, physician to Henry IV (1553-1610) of France and Marie de Medici (1573-1642). He was professor of medicine and chancellor of Montpellier University. The works of Galen (q.v.) and Avicenna (q.v.) were well known to him, and his own writings reviewed some of the issues discussed by them, such as the cerebral localization of reason, memory (q.v.), and imagination (q.v.). He was a follower of the humoral theory (q.v.) and regarded an excess of melancholic humor as the cause of mental disorders. He believed that the insane should be shown compassion although they were "the torment and the scourge of the doctor." In 1599 Richard Surphlet translated his work into English under the title *A Discourse of the Preservation of the Sight: of Melancholike Diseases; of Rheums, and of Old Age.*
Bibliography: Hunter, R., and Macalpine, I. 1963. *Three hundred years of psychiatry.*

LAURUS NOBILIS (TRUE LAUREL). A small tree with fragrant leaves, widely cultivated in Europe and Asia. In the East its seeds and fruits were used in the treatment of hysteria (q.v.). In Greek and Roman times it was the tree dedicated to Apollo (q.v.) and Aesculapius (q.v.), the god of medicine. It was believed to protect against disease and witchcraft (q.v.).
Bibliography: Leyel, C. F. 1949. *Hearts-ease.*

LAUSANNE, DE. *See* SARRASIN DE MONTFERRIER.

LAUTRÉAMONT, COMTE DE (1846-1870). Pseudonym of Isidore Lucien Ducasse, a French poet born in Montevideo, Uruguay. He is said to have suffered from mental disorder, which is reflected in his delirious (*see* DELIRIUM) and horrifying writings. His epic *Les Chants de Maldoror*, posthumously published in 1890, was a source of inspiration for surrealism (q.v.), and, therefore, he is regarded as the father of the surrealist movement. The work, which tells of Maldoror's hatred of mankind, contains descriptive passages reminiscent of hallucinatory (*see* HALLUCINATION) experiences and nightmares (q.v.).
Bibliography: Blanchot, M. 1973. *Lautréamont et Sade.*

LAVATER, JOHANN KASPAR (1741-1801). A Swiss clergyman and spiritual adviser. He believed that facial features could be correlated to normal and abnormal mental characteristics. He is considered the founder of physiognomy (q.v.), which he defined as the "science or knowledge of the correspondence between the external and the internal man." As a healer he combined physiognomy with mesmerism (q.v.). He expounded his ideas

in *Physiognomische Fragmente* which was first published in 1758 and translated into English in 1789 under the title *Essays on Physiognomy.*
Bibliography: Janensky, C. 1928. *J. C. Lavater.*

LAVOISIER, ANTOINE LAURENT (1743-1794). A French chemist, who clarified many essentials of body chemistry. In 1784 he became a member of a commission appointed by the French government to investigate magnetism (q.v.) and its curative effects. Franz Mesmer (q.v.) refused to be investigated, and the commission had to be content with observing magnetism as practiced by his pupil, Charles Deslon (q.v.). They concluded that Mesmer's claims of having discovered a new physical fluid were unfounded and that magnetic treatment could be harmful.
Bibliography: Cochrane, J. A. 1931. *Lavoisier.*

LAWRENCE, DAVID HERBERT RICHARDS (1885-1930). An English novelist. His mother, better educated than his hard-drinking, coal-miner father, fought to keep him out of the mines and to provide him with an education. His childhood was spent in an atmosphere of continuous quarreling between his parents. As he grew older his mother's love became even more demanding and stifling. As an adult, he was an almost pathological egoist and displayed contempt for common humanity. His vivid descriptions of emotions, passions, and sexual encounters were considered obscene, and an exhibition of his paintings in London was closed by the police on the grounds of indecency. His dream was to establish ideal communities, in which people would live without laws or money and mate freely. In 1912 Lawrence eloped with Frieda von Richthofen, a German aristocratic but slatternly woman, wife of a Nottingham professor. His marriage to her in 1914 gave him the opportunity to practice at least one of the things he preached — wife-beating. Their anticonflict attitudes during World War I forced them to leave England and travel abroad. This long perigrination provided Lawrence with a source of material for his writings, although he often exploded against the countries visited. He called Sardinians, for example, "dirty disgusting swine" and compared the temples of Ceylon to "decked-up pigsties." After the war, Lawrence became firmly convinced of the decline of Western culture and advocated racism and anti-democratic attitudes. He recommended that children should remain illiterate and that the masses should be led by the higher classes. Lawrence's fight against ugliness and materialism left him angry and confused. The feelings and thoughts he expressed in his works, however, cover a wide range of human behavior.
Bibliography: Sagar, K. 1980. *The life of D. H. Lawrence.*

LAWRENCE, THOMAS EDWARD (LAWRENCE OF ARABIA) (1888-1935). British author, soldier, and archeologist, born in North Wales. He

was an illegitimate child. His father's wife was so lacking in charm that she was referred to as "the Vinegar Queen." Her husband preferred the children's nanny to his wife and eventually left her and his five daughters, changed his name to Lawrence, and set up house with the nanny, by whom he had five sons. To hide their irregular union, they led an isolated life that was intensely religious and proper. T. E. Lawrence was not allowed to mix with other children. When he discovered from a school mate that his parents were not married, he was shocked by the hypocrisy of their life and horror stricken at the strength of their physical relationship. Later in life he conceived an intense revulsion to physical love. His ambivalent feelings about himself were demonstrated in his need to be liked which strongly contrasted with his self-consciousness. He expressed these feelings quite clearly: "The craving to be famous, and the horror of being known to like being known. . . .There was my craving to be liked — so strong and nervous that never could I open myself friendly to another." In 1922 he enlisted in the air force under the name of Ross. When his identity was discovered in 1923, he enrolled in the tank corps, but in 1925 he rejoined the air force, using the name Shaw, which he legally adopted in 1927. His account of the exploits that had made him a legendary figure in the Middle East was entitled *The Seven Pillars of Wisdom* and was privately printed and circulated in 1926. His real personality and motivations have remained obscure despite his own writings and many speculative works about him.
Bibliography: Stewart, D. 1977. *T. E. Lawrence.*

LAWRENCE, SIR WILLIAM (1783-1867). A British physician. He was an exponent of the theory of evolution and vigorously defended his teachings against those contemporaries who accused him of propagating corrupting ideas. He firmly believed that mind disease was brain disease and that physical remedies, such as purging (q.v.), vomiting, and bleeding (q.v.) were the only effective treatments for it. He regarded psychotherapy (q.v.) with scorn and contempt. As surgeon to Bethlem Royal Hospital and Bridewell (qq.v.) he was able to observe the insane closely.
Bibliography: Hunter, R. and Macalpine, I. 1963. *Three hundred years of psychiatry.*

LAYCOCK, THOMAS (1812-1876). A British physician. He believed that psychology was an integral part of medicine because, according to him, the nervous system and the functions of the mind could be explained in terms of evolution and of body and mind relations. He also believed that the brain had an unconscious functional activity, which he claimed he had been the first to demonstrate both in health and in insanity. In 1855 Laycock originated the first course on medical psychology and mental diseases at the

University of Edinburgh in Scotland. John Hughlings Jackson (q.v.) was one of his pupils.

Bibliography: Laycock, T. 1860. *Mind and brain: or the correlations of consciousness and organisation.*

LAZARETTO *or* **LAZAR HOUSE.** A hospital for lepers. The term was derived from the biblical Lazar, the patron saint of lepers (*see* LEPROSY) and poor men, or, possibly, from the first isolation place for travelers who had been in contact with plague, built in 1464, in Pisa, Italy, near the church of St. Lazar. As the incidence of leprosy declined, some lazar houses were used to shelter beggars, the indigent sick, and the mentally ill. Thus, many asylums originated in lazar houses.

See also ABÖ (TURKU).

Bibliography: Mercier, C. A. 1915. *Leper houses and mediaeval hospital.*

LEAD POISONING. Lead poisoning is known to damage the brain and produce abnormal behavior. In nineteenth-century Scotland the vapor of lead produced in mining was accepted as a cause of insanity in lead miners. The popular term for this disorder was "mill-reeck" (q.v.). Painters were another group who often showed symptoms of lead poisoning. In modern times children living in areas with high lead in the environment have been found to be hyperkinetic.

Bibliography: Waldron, H. A., and Stöffen, D. 1974. *Subclinical lead poisoning.*

LEAR. A legendary king of Britain and the subject of a play by William Shakespeare (q.v.). Shakespeare borrowed the subject from the *Chronicals* of Raphael Holinshed (?-c.1580) but described Lear as senile and harassed into madness by the machinations of his daughters Goneril and Regan. The play contains many passages of psychological interest, descriptions of abnormal behavior caused by anxiety, destructive emotions and the effect of stress on the heart. A description of feigned insanity (q.v.) displays the Tudor view of the mentally ill.

Bibliography: Howells, J. G. and Osborn, M. L. 1973. King Lear — a case of senile dementia. *Hist. Med.* 5: 30-31.

LEAR, EDWARD (1812-1888). An English painter and writer. He was the product of his mother's twentieth pregnancy and suffered from bronchitis and asthma, as well as epilepsy (q.v.). It was possible for him to have as many as eighteen seizures in a single day. His life was dominated by his illness. As a child half-blind without glasses, he was frightened by what he thought he saw around him. A grotesquely large nose added to his unhappiness, and he considered himself hideous. Four of his sisters died within four months, but his favorite, Ann, survived to care for him during his adolescence. He never married and was sexually maladjusted. Although he

was given to depression and irritability, his works, for example, *A Book of Nonsense* (1846) and *The Owl and the Pussycat* (1871), are known for their absurd humor, fantasy, and whimsical attitude toward life.
Bibliography: Lehmann, J. 1977. *Edward Lear and his world.*

LEATHER CAPS. A special headdress for epileptic (*see* EPILEPSY) patients to prevent them injuring themselves during seizures. Sir John Bucknill (q.v.), editor of the *Asylum Journal* (q.v.), described it in the journal's first issue in 1853: "For epileptics a ring is made of chamois leather to surround the head; it is stuffed with horsehair so that the ring is flattened like a marrow quoit; the whole is covered with grey serge which passes over the vertex and converts the affair into a by no means ill-looking cap."

LEAVESDEN ASYLUM. An English asylum (q.v.) near London. In 1870, following the dictates of the 1867 Metropolitan Poor Act, the Metropolitan Asylum Board opened two large establishments in Leavesden and Caterham. The ugly three-storied constructions were designed to accommodate 1,500 patients in three enormous wards, one on each floor. These asylums were to receive those paupers who were legally classified as "chronic, harmless, lunatic, idiot or imbecile", but, because of the acute lack of facilities throughout the country, they were obliged to accept mental patients of all categories and, for the first two years, of all ages. After the first two years children were moved out.
See also CATERHAM ASYLUM and INSANE POOR, LEGISLATION IN ENGLAND.
Bibliography: Ayres, G. M. 1971. *England's first state hospitals and the metropolitan asylums board, 1867-1930.*

LEBLANC, MARIE-ANGELIQUE (1721?-?). The name assumed by a girl found in 1731 in Sogny, France. She was approximately ten years old when she was found, and presumably she had been living in the wild from birth. She fed on the birds, frogs, and fish, that she caught, and her behavior was that of a wild animal. After her capture, she was placed in the care of some nuns who taught her to speak. She became the target of much curiosity by famous people interested in the question of whether heredity or nurture was more important in determining behavior. In 1755 Charles-Marie de la Condamine wrote an account, entitled *Histoire d'une Jeune Fille Sauvage Trouvée dans les Bois a l'Âge de Dix Ans.*
See also FERAL CHILD.
Bibliography: Malson, L. 1972. *Wolf children.*

LE BON, GUSTAVE (1841-1931). A French physician and sociologist. He maintained that a crowd has a "collective soul" that is subjected to the will of the leader in the same way that the mind of a hypnotized (*see* HYPNOTISM) individual is subjected to the hypnotist. According to Le Bon, a rational and well-behaved individual, acting in a group, could lose his critical sense and his inhibitions and become aggressive and immoral. His theory appealed to the educated public, who found in it an explanation for many sociological problems. Sigmund Freud (q.v.) utilized the theory in *Group Psychology and the Analysis of the Ego* (1920).

Bibliography: Le Bon, G. 1895. *La psychologie des foules.*

LE CAMUS, ANTOINE (1722-1772). A French philosopher and author. In 1753 he wrote a book entitled *Médecine de l'Esprit* in which he discussed his belief that body and soul influence each other in sickness. He offered advice on how to preserve a state of good mental functioning in order to maintain bodily health and how to correct mental dysfunction when it was present.

Bibliography: Semelaigne, R. 1930. *Les pionnieres de la psychiatrie Française.*

LEÇONS DU MARDI. The regular Tuesday afternoon lectures held at the Salpêtrière (q.v.) by Jean Martin Charcot (q.v.). Following the lectures, a small circle of distinguished visitors were invited to evening soirées at his house in the Boulevard St. Germain. On occasions, his guests included the Emperor of Brazil, the Bey of Tunisia, the Grand Dukes of Russia, as well as famous writers, politicians and physicians.

Bibliography: Guillain, G. J. 1959. *Charcot, his life, his work,* trans. by P. Bailey.

LEE, NATHANIEL (1653?-1692). An English dramatist. After studying at Cambridge University, he moved to London. He was handsome, clever, and a good elocutionist with a pleasant voice, but despite these qualities failed as an actor because of his nervous disposition. He turned to writing dramas and collaborated with John Dryden (q.v.) in 1679. Lee was said to have a prodigious thirst, and many stories about his drinking and extravagance circulated in the taverns of London. In 1684, he became insane and was confined in Bethlem Royal Hospital (q.v.) under the care of Dr. Edward Tyson (q.v.). It was said that the cause of his illness was excessive drinking. He was released in 1689 but suffered a relapse in the following year. He managed to escape from his keepers and died of alcoholism (q.v.) at an early age. Lee's best known tragedy is *The Rival Queens*, first performed in 1677, but he wrote many other works, even when hospitalized. His experiences in Bethlem Royal Hospital were reflected in a poem entitled *Caesar Borgia*. William Hogarth (q.v.) commemorated him in the last plate of his series entitled *The Rake's Progress* (q.v.) by showing the letters LE scratched on the wall of a ward of Bethlem Royal Hospital.

Bibliography: Ham, R. G. 1969. *Otway and Lee.*

LEECHBOOK. A collection of herb-remedies and folk medicine. Some collections date from the Anglo-Saxon period. Leechbooks often contained

descriptions of mental disorders and suggested treatments using herbs, bleeding (q.v.), and anointing. It was believed that epilepsy (q.v.) could be forestalled by drinking one's own urine for nine days. The *Leech Book of Bald*, one of the earliest to survive, belonged to Bald (c. 900-950) an early physician; it was written down by a scribe called Cild. Its material is so arranged that it starts by discussing the head and its ailments and gradually works down to the feet. *Leechdoms, Wortcunning, and Starcraft of Early England* was transcribed into modern English by the Reverend Thomas Oswald Cockayne (1807-1873) and published in 1865. It consisted of a series of medical manuscripts written by unknown authors in the tenth and eleventh centuries. There are within it references to the treatment of insanity through herbs, salves, and baths (q.v.). Demoniac possession (q.v.) was distinguished from insanity. The Saxon medical practices reflected in the leechbooks were mixed with Roman practices, some of which came from Greek sources. Leechbooks continued to be compiled in the latter part of the Middle Ages (q.v.).
Bibliography: Dawson, W. R. 1934. *A leechbook.*

LEECHES. Elongated worms furnished with sucking discs. They were widely used in early medicine. When applied to the side of the head, they were believed to be beneficial in the treatment of mental disorders.

LEFT-HANDEDNESS. According to Cesare Lombroso (q.v.), left-handedness was not only one of the signs of mental degeneration but also, paradoxically, a sign of genius (q.v.). Among the great men who were left-handed, he cited Michelangelo (q.v.) and Leonardo da Vinci (q.v.).
Bibliography: Lombroso, C. 1888. *The man of genius.*

LEG-LOCKS. Heavy iron hobbles, linked by a ring. Until the middle of the nineteenth century, they were used to restrain violent patients in asylums (q.v.).
Bibliography: Leigh, D. 1961. *The historical development of British psychiatry.*

LE GRAS, LOUISE DE MARILLAC (1591-1662). French founder of the religious order of Sisters of Charity in France. In 1645 she undertook the care of the insane in special institutions called Les Petites Maisons (q.v.) and organized a body of nurses specially trained for this work.
Bibliography: : Zilboorg, G. 1941. *A history of medical psychology.*

LEHMANN, ALFRED (1858-1921). A Danish psychologist, and pupil of Wilhelm Wundt (q.v.). He worked in the field of "expression" methods in relation to feelings. He looked at mental phenomena from the point of view

of energy. Lehmann was director of the Copenhagen psychological laboratory (q.v.).
Bibliography: Flugel, J. C. 1945. *A hundred years of psychology.*
Lehmann, A. 1912. *Grundzüge der Psychophysiologie.*

LEIBNIZ, GOTTFRIED WILHELM (1646-1716). A German philosopher and mathematician. He attempted to reconcile religion and science and believed in a "pre-established harmony." In his system of philosophy he held a psychological view of the world; he created the theory of monads in which each monad was an irreducible entity, or life force, that reflected the world from its own point of view. The theory of psychophysical parallelism evolved from these ideas. As well as emphasizing the determinism limiting human choice, Leibniz also emphasized the existence of subconscious (q.v.) mental states, or "unclear perception." His greatness and intellectual influence was not recognized until after his death. The word "dynamic" was coined by him in relation to mechanics. Alfred Adler (q.v.) leaned toward his concepts.
Bibliography: Russell, B. 1961. *A critical exposition of the philosophy of Leibniz.*

LEIDESDORF, MAX (1818-1889). An Austrian psychiatrist and professor of psychiatry in Vienna. Sigmund Freud (q.v.) worked for some weeks at his clinic. Leidesdorf was cautious about accepting the claims made by Jean Martin Charcot (q.v.) and subsequently by Freud in regard to hysteria (q.v.). In 1865 Leidesdorf published his main work, entitled *Treatise of Mental Diseases*, which was preceded by a survey of the history of psychiatry. He was essentially a somatologist and his contributions were mostly in the field of the anatomy of the nervous system.
Bibliography: Ellenberger, H. F. 1970. *The discovery of the unconscious.*

LEJEUNE, JEROME JEAN (1926-   ). A French geneticist. He was the first to discover chromosomal aberrations in man and those chromosomal abnormalities that lead to mongolism (q.v.).
Bibliography: Lejeune, J.; Turpin, R.; and Jerome, H. 1965. *Les cromosomes humains.*

LELOYER, PIERRE (1550-1634). A French demonologist. In his journeys through France, Italy, and Morocco he saw many insane people whom he regarded as sick, rather than possessed. He described the conditions he had observed in a four-volume work entitled *Spectres*, published in 1588. In it a whole chapter was dedicated to visual and auditory hallucinations (q.v.), which Leloyer regarded as phenomena brought about by "corrupted senses." Despite these views, he still believed that the devil could cause abnormal behaviour by occupying the body of its victims, or using his art to make them believe that they were animals.
Bibliography: Zilboorg, G. 1941. *A history of medical psychology.*

LEMNIUS (or LEMMENS), LIÉVEN (1505-1568). A Dutch physician and theologian. He believed that those accused of witchcraft (q.v.) and those

said to be possessed (*see* POSSESSION) by the devil were sick and would respond to treatment. He derived his methods of treatment from the writings of Hippocrates (q.v.) and Galen (q.v.) and based them on the humoral theory (q.v.). He tried to describe abnormal psychological phenomena from factual observation. Lemnius thought that climate (q.v.) and geographical position could affect physical and mental health and that "humours, not evil spirits, cause diseases: even the power of speaking in unknown tongues is not due to possession, but to latent memories."
Bibliography: Lemnius, L. 1553. *Occulta naturae miracula.*

LEMOYNE, FRANÇOIS (1688-1737). A French painter. He was an ambitious man, always anxious lest others should do better than himself. He was irritable and prone to headaches. After the death of his wife, he became increasingly depressed and fascinated by thoughts of suicide (q.v.). When his friends decided to arrange treatment for him, he became suspicious and fearful that they were plotting to send him to prison. He locked himself in his room and stabbed himself to death, silently plunging the sword into his body no less than nine times.
Bibliography: Wittkower, R., and Wittkower, M. 1963. *Born under Saturn.*

LENIN, NIKOLAI (1870-1924). The pseudonym of Vladimir Ilych Ulyanov, Russian revolutionary leader. He came from a close, warm and friendly family. The enormous stress imposed on him by his revolutionary activities and his later political position was on the whole exceptionally well withstood by him. The only symptom of anxiety that seems to have existed was his almost chronic insomnia and occasional headaches. It was through the help of Lenin that Ivan Pavlov (q.v.) received funds for his research. In 1922 Lenin suffered an attack of hemiplegia. Although he recovered and partially resumed work, episodes of the same disorder recurred with varying severity until his death from respiratory paralysis two years later. A postmortem examination showed considerable brain damage, yet he had retained a powerful intellect to the end. His brain was extensively studied by Russian anatomists in a specially founded Institute. In his *Philosophical Notebooks*, Lenin emphasized his theory that psychic life is a reflection of reality. He was an exponent of dialectical materialism.
Bibliography: Fisher, L. 1964. *The life of Lenin.*

LENZIE ACT. The popular name given in Scotland to the Lunacy Act (1857) enabling poor-law authorities to continue to provide accommodation for the insane under license of the commissioners in lunacy (q.v.). In 1875 the Barony Parochial Asylum, in Woodilee, Lenzie, became the first institution to use this Act to continue to provide asylums for paupers. The institution that they built was considered one of the finest in Great Britain.

Located ten miles from Glasgow, it had a liberal policy and abolished restraint (q.v.) and locked doors from the very beginning.
See also INSANE POOR, LEGISLATION IN ENGLAND.
Bibliography: Letchworth, W. P. 1889. *The insane in foreign countries.*

LEONARD, SAINT. Possibly a French hermit of the sixth century. Little is known about him. He was regarded in the Middle Ages as the patron saint of prisoners and lunatics, and both gave to him their chains as votive offerings when they were freed or cured.
Bibliography: Bonser, W. 1963. *The medical background of Anglo-Saxon England.*

LEONARDO DA VINCI (1452-1519). Italian Renaissance artist, scientist, and engineer. He was an illegitimate child who was raised in his father's household. From an early age he refused to allow anyone to enter his room, including the members of his own family. He was a very detached man who was capable of objective observation and utter aloofness. He wrote in his notes that the painter should remain solitary, avoid disappointments by not hoping for things difficult to achieve, have no friends in order to preserve his wholeness, and keep a calm mind. According to him, "intellectual passion drives out sensuality." He was a perfectionist; Giorgio Vasari (1511-1574), in his biography, remarked that he searched "for excellence above excellence and perfection above perfection." In many instances, Leonardo was decidedly odd; he became a vegetarian, asserting that those who eat meat were "sepulchre for other animals"; his house was full of contraptions to startle his visitors; many of his notes were in mirror writing. In his youth he was denounced for homosexual (*see* HOMOSEXUALITY) practices, but the letter accusing him to the administrators of justice in Florence was anonymous and he was acquitted. However, he did take into his house a beautiful young boy, Gian Giacomo de'Caprotti, spent much money on him and was seldom parted from him until, 26 years later, the youth died. Freud (q.v.) wrote an essay on Leonardo (Leonardo da Vinci: A Study in Psychosexuality, 1933), in which he gave great importance to his illegitimacy and to some doubtful childhood memories, which provided psychoanalytically oriented speculations as to his probable homosexuality. His anatomical studies include naturalistic illustrations of the brain drawn from models injected with wax.
Bibliography: Zubov, V. P. 1968. *Leonardo da Vinci*, trans. D. H. Krous.

LÉONIE (fl 1885). A young woman who was the subject of a series of experiments in hypnotism (q.v.) conducted by Pierre Janet (q.v.) in 1885. He first met her in Le Havre and found her easily hypnotized even at a distance. Janet's paper describing his experiments was presented to the Société de Psychologie Physiologique in Paris. It provoked great interest, and many distinguished people traveled to Le Havre to meet Léonie. Later, Janet

found that Léonie had been hypnotized in the past, and her present trances were repeat performances.
Bibliography: Janet, P. 1885. Note sur quelques phénomènes de somnambulisme. 1885. *Bulletins de la societé de psychologie physiologiques.* 1: 24-32.

LEOPARDI, CONTE, GIACOMO (1798-1837). An Italian poet known as the poet of despair. His childhood was so miserable that he later wrote no man would agree to return to childhood if he had to go through the same anxieties and fears. Both his parents were austere, cold, and authoritarian individuals. His mother carried her religious convictions to extremes: she rejoiced in the death of children, even her own, as she believed that they had escaped sin and gained heaven. She never missed an opportunity to point out their faults to her children and to take away from them even the smallest degree of confidence that they developed. Leopardi was equally unfortunate in his nurses, who terrified him with frightening tales. He suffered from poor health all his life, was asthmatic, unable to sleep, and often overcome by depression. He had various romantic attachments but, as he said, he searched for a phantom, for "the woman who cannot be found." He was desperately lonely; he wrote to his brother: "I need love, love, love, fire, enthusiasm, life: the world does not seem made for me." In a prayer to the Persian god of evil, he asked "not for riches nor love . . I ask for . . . death."
Bibliography: Origo, I. 1953. *Leopardi: a study in solitude.*

LE PLAY, PIERRE GUILLAUME FRÉDÉRIC (1806-1882). A French engineer and sociologist. The basic concepts of social economics were first announced by him and rested on his assertion that human happiness can be sought in social and moral development as well as in political and economic factors. He studied social phenomena from the point of view of human nature and regarded the family as the basic unit of society. His methods of observation depended on concrete evidence of life in the community and influenced, among others, the work of Charles Booth (1840-1916) on social conditions and poverty.
Bibliography: Le Play, P.G.F. 1871. *L'organisation de la famille.*

LEPOIS, CHARLES (1563-1633). A French medical writer. He isolated the clinical syndrome of postpartum psychosis (q.v.) after observing that some women develop mental disorders following childbirth. He thought that the disorders were caused by excess of dark humors (q.v.). He also believed that hysteria (q.v.) was not a condition exclusive to women and that its aetiology could be found in the brain, rather than in the uterus (q.v.).
Bibliography: Zilboorg, G. 1941. *A history of medical psychology.*

LEPROSY. An endemic chronic disease, frequently producing deformities. It is probable that syphilis (q.v.) and some of its manifestations occasionally

were confused with leprosy. When leprosy began to disappear, the Lazar houses (q.v.) frequently were converted into asylums (q.v.) for incurables and madmen.
Bibliography: Zambaco, D. A. 1914. *La lèpre, à travers les siècles et les contrées.*

LERMONTOV, MIKHAIL YUREVICH (1814-1841). A Russian poet. He was an only child. The death of his mother when he was three years old provoked a legal battle between his wealthy maternal grandmother and his father for his custody. He was placed in his grandmother's custody and received an extensive private education. At the age of twenty-three he wrote a poem on the death of Alexander Pushkin (q.v.) which brought him literary fame and the displeasure of the czar. He was exiled briefly to the Caucasus. His dissipated life was one long courtship with death. In the Hussars, he behaved with suicidal (*see* SUICIDE) abandon and fought duels in which he deliberately missed his opponents. He finally practically arranged his own death by provoking the duel that ended his life. In a poem entitled *A Dream*, written a few months before this last duel, he foresaw and longed for death. Many elements of Lermontov's life were similar to those of Sigmund Freud's (q.v.) patient, the Wolf Man (q.v.)., who strongly identified with him.
Bibliography: Mersereau, J. 1962. *Mikhail Lermontov.*

LESBIANISM. Female homosexuality (q.v.). The term is derived from Lesbos, a Greek island. The poetess Sappho (q.v.), who is believed to have indulged in homosexual practices, lived there most of her life. Famous lesbians include Vita Sackville-West, Virginia Woolf, Margaret Radclyffe Hall, and the Ladies of Llangollen (q.v.).
Bibliography: Rowse, A. L. 1977. *Homosexuality in history.*

LETCHWORTH VILLAGE. A colony for mental defectives established in 1909 in Thiells, New York. It was originally a custodial institution known as the Eastern New York Custodial Asylum, but it later lost much of its institutional atmosphere and became one of the best projects of its kind. It is located in a pleasant area and closely resembles an ordinary village.
Bibliography: Deutsch, A. 1949. *The mentally ill in America.*

LETHARGY. A term derived from the Greek word for drowsiness. Jean Martin Charcot (q.v.) and his followers regarded lethargy as the first stage of hypnotic (*see* HYPNOTISM) sleep. According to them, it was followed by catalepsy and somnambulism (q.v.).

L'ÉTOILE DU NORD. The title of an opera comique by Giacomo Meyerbeer (1791-1864). It tells the story of Peter the Great (q.v.), who falls in love with a girl from the Finnish village he visits in disguise. The opera has

a "mad scene" and ends with the heroine's restoration to sanity. It was first produced in Paris in 1854.
Bibliography: 1979. *Phaidon book of the opera.*

LEUBUSHER, R. (1821-1861). A French physician. He is credited with the observation that it is important for the mentally ill patient to understand that he is ill. This concept later developed into what is now known as "insight."
Bibliography: Zilboorg, G. 1941. *A history of mental psychology.*

LEURET, FRANÇOIS (1797-1851). A French physician and psychiatrist. He was a pupil of Jean Esquirol (q.v.) and became chief physician of Bicêtre (q.v.). Although he was quite modern in his belief that overwhelming impulses could be responsible for criminal acts, his treatment for hallucinations (q.v.) was not. It included pouring cold water for hours, over the head of the patient seated in a bath (q.v.). After this treatment, the patient was asked not to mention his hallucinations again unless he wished to undergo more douching. Most patients preferred to remain silent. Leuret regarded the douche (q.v.) as physical treatment and considered the cautionary interview with the patient afterward to be "moral medicine" (q.v.).
Bibliography: Leuret, F. 1834. *Psychological fragments on insanity.*
————1840. *On the moral treatment of insanity.*

LÉVI-STRAUSS, CLAUDE (1908-   ). A French anthropologist born in Brussels. His approach to the study of man is based on the belief that all human thoughts contain some logic, hence myths too have a logical basis. According to him, modern dynamic psychiatry has many concepts that can be identified in primitive medicine. His theories were later developed into the concept of structuralism.
Bibliography: Leach, E. 1970. *Lévi-Strauss.*

LEVITICUS. A book of the Old Testament containing the basic Jewish laws. A passage within it states that witches (*see* WITCHCRAFT) or those possessed (*see* POSSESSION) by an evil spirit should be put to death: "Any man or woman among you who calls up ghosts or spirits shall be put to death." The passage was used for centuries to justify persecution of the mentally ill who were not recognized as such and, therefore, retarded the advancement of psychiatry.
Bibliography: *Leviticus* 20: 27.

LÉVY-BRÜHL, LUCIEN (1857-1939). A French sociologist, ethnologist, and psychologist. His pioneer work on the primitive mind has influenced contemporary psychology and advanced the study of ethnology. He argued that the thinking of primitive people is based on mysticism as well as "pre-

logical" concepts and that their understanding of natural causes is made difficult by the cultural traditions of their society.
Bibliography: Lévy-Brühl, L. 1935. *The supernatural and nature in primitive mentality.*

LEWES, GEORGE HENRY (1817-1878). A British critic and author. He wrote the first book in English on physiology (*Physiology of Common Life* [1859-60]), advanced the study of neurology and wrote plays and novels as well as a life of Johann Wolfgang von Goethe (q.v.). His attitude to psychology was based on positivistic (*see* POSITIVISM) logic and a mixture of physiology and sociology. According to him, the mind was a unit similar to the body and possessed many elements that could be logically separated despite their common factors. He believed that there was a place for introspection in psychology but that it could not be the sole basis of a scientific approach. He expressed this view in his four-volume work entitled *Problems of Life and Mind*, which was published between 1874 and 1879. Lewes met Mary Ann Evans (George Eliot, [q.v.]) in 1850 and soon, despite his marriage, they were joined in an informal union that lasted until his death.
Bibliography: Haight, G. S., ed. 1954-1959. *The George Eliot letters.*

LEWIN, KURT (1890-1947). A German psychologist. In 1932, when he emigrated to the United States, he was already well known following his studies on association and motivation. He devised a conceptual system of psychology known as vector psychology, that used mathematical and topological terms to describe the behavior of the individual in his "life space" and the group dynamics occurring in society. Because his emphasis remained on motivation, his work is linked to behaviorism (q.v.). A collection of his writings appeared in English in 1935 in a volume entitled *A Dynamic Theory of Personality*. It was followed in 1936 by *Principles of Topological Psychology*.
Bibliography: Marrow, A. J. 1969. *The practical theorist: the life and work of Kurt Lewin.*

LEWIS, AUBREY (1900-1975). A British psychiatrist born in Australia. He was Jewish and religious but never visited Israel. Intellectuality was used as a protection for his shyness. Of outstanding erudition and intelligence, anxiety prevented him from embarking on the unpopular and hazardous road of real creativity. He destroyed ideas with wisdom and purpose but rarely rebuilt. He taught by threat and only those who survived could learn. When relaxed he had great charm and had a real capacity for communication with the unthreatening patient. Lewis was essentially kindly with a great sense of moral purpose, the highest standards, and an immense and endearing sense of humor. After World War II, he became the architect of the clinical

and teaching program at the Institute of Psychiatry, the Maudsley Hospital, London.
Bibliography: Lewis, A. 1967. *The state of psychiatry.*

LEWIS, MATTHEW GREGORY (1775-1818). An English novelist nicknamed the "Monk." In a poem entitled *The Maniac* Lewis described the fearful appearance of a madman, his glaring eyes and his screams which make the person hearing them fear for his own sanity. The supernatural, the gruesome, and the horrible often dominated his writings, especially his *Ambrosio, or the Monk*, published in 1796, and *Tales of Terror*, published in 1799.
Bibliography: Peck, L. F. 1962. *A life of Matthew G. Lewis.*

LIBIDO. The term was first employed in a psychological sense by the Roman philosopher Cicero (q.v.). He used it to indicate violent desire, one of the four passions recognized by him; the other three were joy, fear and discomfort. In 1895, before fully developing his libido theory, or theory of instincts (q.v.) Sigmund Freud (q.v.) used the term in a paper entitled *On the Grounds of Detaching a Particular Syndrome from Neurasthenia under the Description "Anxiety Neurosis"*. Moritz Benedikt (q.v.) and others had previously used the term to describe sexual desire, or sexual instinct.
Bibliography: Ellenberger, H. F. 1970. *The discovery of the unconscious.*

LICENSED HOUSES. A term used in England in the nineteenth century to indicate those private establishments that had obtained a licence from the College of Physicians to provide custodial care, as well as some medical care for the mentally ill. The increase in population and the absence of public institutions caused a great demand for this type of establishment, which became a profitable business and fetched high prices when they changed hands. Many were run solely for profit, and the facilities they offered were deplorable. Some improvements were brought about after the College of Physicians appointed commissioners in lunacy (q.v.) to inspect them.
See also ASYLUMS.
Bibliography: Parry-Jones, W. Ll. 1972. *The trade in lunacy: a study of private madhouses in England in the eighteenth and nineteenth centuries.*

LICHTHEIM, LUDWIG (1845-1915). A German physician and pioneer of modern neurology (q.v.). In 1885 he published his study on the modalities of aphasia and described a form of subcortical aphasia in which the patient is unable to say a word, but can indicate the number of syllables it contains. The disorder became known as Lichtheim's disease. He was among the first to perform brain puncture to assist diagnosis.
Bibliography: Lichtheim, L. 1885. On aphasia. *Brain* 7: 433-84.

LIÉBEAULT, AMBROISE-AUGUST (1823-1904). A French psychiatrist. He was the twelfth child of a peasant family and had to struggle to become a doctor, but once established in a country practice he prospered and was loved by his patients, who called him "le bon pĕre Liébeault." As a student he had been intrigued by magnetism (q.v.) and had found that he could easily hypnotize his subject. As a fully qualified medical practitioner, he began to use magnetism in his practice. He offered it free of charge to his patients but charged them the usual fee for more orthodox methods. His therapeutic successes encouraged him to retire from practice to write a book on magnetism. The volume, entitled *Du Sommeil et des États Analogues, Considérés surtout au Point de Vue de l'Action de la Morale sur le Physique* was published in Paris in 1866, but it is said that it sold only one copy in ten years. Liébeault returned to his practice with even greater success than before. He practiced magnetism openly and on a large scale, despite the disapproval of his medical colleagues. Hippolyte-Marie Bernheim (q.v.) heard of him when he cured one of his patients of sciatica and, after observing his technique, became a convert and made Liébeault known and respected in academic medical circles. The Nancy school (q.v.) of hypnotism, although under the leadership of Bernheim, regarded Liébeault as its spiritual father because he understood and put into practice the influence of the mind on the body. The introduction of psychotherapy (q.v.) in the treatment of psychosomatic disorders can be credited to him. He is said to have hypnotized some 10,000 patients.

Bibliography: Ellenberger, H. F. 1970. *The discovery of the unconscious.*

LIÉGEOIS, JULES. A French lawyer. He assumed legal responsibility for the techniques used by the Nancy school (q.v.). Liégeois conducted experiments with individuals under hypnosis (*see* HYPNOTISM) in which he suggested that they perform acts of violence and provided them with mock weapons. His views on criminal suggestion caused much controversy, because he believed that a hypnotized individual could be persuaded to commit criminal acts for which they could not be held responsible.

Bibliography: Ellenberger, H. F. 1970. *The discovery of the unconscious.*

LIEPMANN, HUGO CARL (1863-1925). A German neurologist and psychiatrist, born in Berlin of a Jewish family. He collected twenty-six brains and their case histories and investigated the mechanisms involved in the thinking process. In 1900 he published a monograph that gave what is probably the first accurate description of apraxia and its variants. He also discovered that the left cortical hemisphere is dominant in right-handed persons. During his studies of alcoholic delirium (q.v.), he found that hallucinations (q.v.) could be artificially induced. It was suggested to him that he would receive an appointment to the University of Berlin, if he changed

his name and became a Protestant, but he refused. His high ethical standards were further demonstrated during World War I when he voluntarily rationed himself to the same quantity of food that was allocated to patients in the asylum where he worked; he lost sixty pounds during that time. He suffered from paralysis agitans, which forced him to give up his post and eventually led to his suicide (q.v.) by poison.
Bibliography: Haymaker, W., and Schiller, F. 1970. *The founders of neurology.* 2d. ed.

LIERNEUX. A colony for the insane in Belgium. It was begun in the Walloon district in the latter part of the nineteenth century. Patients were boarded out in families under the supervision of the government in a system similar to that of the Gheel Colony (q.v.).
(*See also* BOARDING-OUT OF MENTAL PATIENTS).
Bibliography: Letchworth, W. P. 1889. *The insane in foreign countries.*

LIEUTAUD, JOSEPH (1703-1780). A French physician, Fellow of the Royal Society, and first physician to Louis XV (q.v.) and Louis XVI (1754-1793). He realized that mind and body exercise a reciprocal influence on each other and stated that although this fact was increasingly recognized, its mechanisms and extent were still unknown. He wrote several works on anatomy and medical practice.
Bibliography: Zilboorg, G. 1941. *A history of medical psychology.*

LIEVENS (or LIEVENSZ), JAN (1607-1674). Dutch painter and engraver. He was a friend of Rembrandt (q.v.). His disorderly way of life was reflected in the management of his children. One of his sons was so unruly that his parents applied to the town authorities to castigate him or send him to prison. The children had so little faith in their father that they asked to be granted the right to refuse their inheritance in case it consisted solely of debts.
Bibliography: Wittkower, R., and Wittkower, M. 1963. *Born under Saturn.*

LIFE FORCE. A Hippocratic (*see* HIPPOCRATES) concept that postulates the existence of a psychological force bound to the body through the senses and the motor system but capable of functioning on its own, for example, when it produces dreams (q.v.) during sleep. Since Hippocrates others have elaborated the same idea in the fields of natural philosophy and medicine. Friedrich Hoffman (q.v.) and Georg Ernst Stahl (q.v.) introduced a similar concept in the seventeenth century. The eighteenth-century school of vi-

talism (q.v.) furthered the idea of a vital force and provided a stimulus for developments in the history of psychology and neurology.
Bibliography: Zilboorg, G. 1941. *A history of medical psychology.*

LIFE INSTINCTS. Tendencies of self-preservation and reproduction postulated by Sigmund Freud (q.v.). He later postulated a contrasting death instinct (q.v.).
Bibliography: Fenichel, O. 1945. *The psychoanalytic theory of neurosis.*

LIFE'S PRESERVATIVE AGAINST SELF-KILLING. A book written at the beginning of the seventeenth century by John Sym (q.v.) , an English clergyman. He had become worried by the increase in suicide (q.v.) and set out to combat it. He divided suicide into direct and indirect categories and discussed types and means of suicide, signs of depression leading to it, and preventive measures.
Bibliography: Fedden, H. R. 1938. *Suicide.*

LIGUORI, ALFONSO MARIA DI (SAINT ALPHONSUS) (1696-1787). An Italian Roman Catholic theologian and founder of a religious order, the Congregation of the Most Holy Redeemer. His writings profoundly influenced the attitudes toward the mentally ill. He classifed sinful acts into natural, such as rape and adultery, and unnatural, such as bestiality and sodomy; his work, although theologically orientated, provided a rudimentary framework for sexual pathology. His moral theology included the role of counseling.
Bibliography: Talleria, R. 1951-1952. *Life of St. Alphonsus Liguori.* 2 vols.

"LIKE SWEET BELLS JANGLED, OUT OF TUNE AND HARSH." A telling metaphor used by William Shakespeare (q.v.) in describing Hamlet's state of mind.
Bibliography: *Hamlet*, 3: i.

LILITH. A female demon, whose evil activities were carried out at night. Superstitions about her were current in some Jewish communities until the seventh century. She was also called Lamia (q.v.).
Bibliography: 1978. *Brewer's dictionary of phrase and fable.*

LILLIPUT. The land of minute people visited by Gulliver, the hero of Jonathan Swift's (q.v.) satire *Gulliver's Travels* (1726). The term "lilliputian hallucinations," a feeling that the surroundings have diminished in size, is derived from it.

LILY OF THE VALLEY. *Convallaria majalis*, a woodland plant with fragrant, bell-shaped white flowers. The flowers were used in the treatment

of many disorders, including nervous ailments, epilepsy (q.v.), and hysteria (q.v.) . It was believed to be a mild narcotic. Early herbalists believed that Apollo (q.v.) had given it to Aesculapius (q.v.), the god of medicine.
Bibliography: le Strange, R. 1977. *A history of herbal plants.*

LIMBUS OF FOOLS, *or* **PARADISE OF FOOLS.** A region where the souls of fools (q.v.) or idiots are received. The theologians of the Middle Ages (q.v.) decided that those who could not be held responsible for their actions, could not be punished in purgatory or received into heaven, therefore, they devised this solution.
Bibliography: 1978. *Brewer's dictionary of phrase and fable.*

LINCOLN, ABRAHAM (1809-1865). The sixteenth president of the United States. He came from a farming family; his father was almost illiterate, and his mother died when he was nine years old. He acquired a stepmother who loved him dearly. Lincoln was poorly educated and tried various jobs until he decided to study law. The deaths of his mother, a sister, and, eventually, two sons left him with an obsession (q.v.) about mortality. The sudden madness of a neighbor troubled Lincoln so much that he became prone to what he called "a profound melancholia," which during his presidency often compelled him to rest. He was also never fully free of insomnia and hypochondria (q.v.), which he called "the hypo." His wife, Mary Todd (1818-1882) was mentally unbalanced, and the marriage was not a happy one. She was declared insane in 1875, but later recovered enough to be considered able to handle her affairs.
Bibliography: Oates, S. B. 1978. *With malice to none: the life of Abraham Lincoln.*

LINCOLN ASYLUM, THE LAWN HOSPITAL. A mental hospital in Lincoln, England. It originally was built to provide accommodation and treatment for educated people of moderate means. It opened in 1820 with twelve patients, and its first senior physician was Edward Charlesworth (q.v.). From its inception it adopted a liberal policy and minimal restraint (q.v.). It encouraged patients to mix socially and to keep themselves occupied with suitable work. It was the first mental hospital in England to remove the shackles from patients.
Bibliography: Melton, B. L. 1969. *One hundred and fifty years at The Lawn, Lincoln.*

LINDA DI CHAMOUNIX. The title of an opera (q.v.) by Gaetano Donizetti (q.v.) composed in 1842. It has a famous mad scene. The story concerns Linda, a farmer's daughter, who is wrongly supposed by her father to be living an immoral life. The loss of her lover drives the girl mad. Later, hearing the voice of her lover, she recovers her wits: "Ah! tardai troppo . . . . O luce di quest' anima" [Act 1.].
Bibliography: Harewood, ed. 1969. *Kobbe's complete opera book.*

LINDSAY, WILLIAM LAUDER (1829-1880). A Scottish botanist and medical practitioner. He worked at the Perth Royal Mental Hospital (q.v.) in Perth, Scotland. In 1878 he published a book entitled *The Theory and Practice of Non-restraint in the Treatment of the Insane*. The volume is of interest because it continued the controversy over restraint (q.v.) that was begun much earlier in the century and demonstrated the persisting resistance to nonrestraint.
Bibliography: Lindsay, W. L. 1878. *The theory and practice of non-restraint in the treatment of the insane.*

LINGUITI, GIOVANNI MARIA (1773-1825). An Italian priest. In 1813 he became the first lay superintendent to the hospital for the mentally ill at Aversa (q.v.). The institution had been converted from a convent. Linguiti introduced enlightened and humanitarian measures, including moral medicine (q.v.) and occupational therapy (q.v.), that made the hospital well known throughout Europe. In 1812 he wrote a book entitled *Richerche sopra le Alienazioni Della Mente Umana* in which he gave his views about mental abnormalities.
Bibliography: Mora, G. 1975. Italy. In *World history of psychiatry*, ed. J. G. Howells.

LINNAEUS, CAROLUS (1707-1778). The Latinized name of the Swedish botanist and physician Carl von Linné. He was the son of a Lutheran minister and remained deeply religious all his life. He became quite fashionable as a physician, and his patrons included Gustavus III (1746-1792), whose murder provided the plot of Verdi's opera 'Un ballo in maschera'. Linnaeus' reputation rests mainly on his classification of plants, which provided a model for medical systems and awakened interest in description and classification. In 1758 he extended his taxonomy into the animal world and placed man in the order of primates with the designation of *homo sapiens*. Linnaeus divided mental disorders into ideal, imaginary and pathetic. He also listed ten cases of wild children raised by animals and coined the term "feral child" (q.v.). Aphasia was probably first described by him in 1745. Despite his successful career, he was often depressed and found little consolation in his five children and his wife, a poorly educated and domineering woman.
Bibliography: Blunt, W. 1971. *The complete naturalist: a life of Linnaeus.*

LINTON, RALPH (1893-1953). An American anthropologist. His work was influenced by Karl Abraham (q.v.) and Sigmund Freud (q.v.), and he applied psychoanalytic (*see* PSYCHOANALYSIS) concepts to the interpretation of cultural phenomena.
Bibliography: Linton, R. 1945. *Cultural background of personality.*

LIPPI, FILIPPO (c. 1406-1469). An Italian painter. His parents died when he was young, and his relatives arranged a monastic life for him. His behavior as a monk was less than saintly. When commissioned by the nuns of Saint Margherita Prato to paint a panel for their high altar, he noticed a particularly beautiful novice, Lucrezia, within the convent. He persuaded the nuns to let her pose for him and in no time ran off with her. Lucrezia, also orphaned in early life and handed over to the nuns by her family, bore him a son, Filippino, but church authorities insisted that they return to their religious life. They promised, candle in hand, to mend their behavior and to be chaste and obedient, but soon had a change of heart, escaped again, and started a veritable epidemic of young nuns absconding with their lovers. In 1461 he was released from his vows. Filippo Lippi caused further scandal by forging a signature and, in the words of Giorgio Vasari (1511-1574), scandalized people by "spending extraordinary sums on the pleasure of love, in which he continued to take delight to the very end of his life." The beautiful sacred images he painted reflected none of his irreverent behavior.

Bibliography: Wittkower, R., and Wittkower, M. 1963. *Born under Saturn.*

LIPPS, THEODOR (1851-1914). A German psychologist and pupil of Wilhelm Wundt (q.v.). He was a member of the school of act psychology (q.v.). In 1883 he published an important book *Grundtatsachen des Seelenlebens*, which covered all the concepts of the new psychology. His work on optical illusions and esthetics made him well known, but he perhaps is best remembered for his theory of empathy. Sigmund Freud (q.v.) was inspired to study jokes (q.v.) and their relation to the unconscious (q.v.) by Lipps' book *Komik und Humor* (1898).

Bibliography: Boring, E. G. 1950. *A history of experimental psychology.*

LISSAUER, HEINRICH (1861-1891). A German neurologist. He was the first to describe atypical general paralysis of the insane (q.v.) with aphasia and convulsions. His findings were published posthumously in 1901, and the condition has since been known as Lissauer's dementia paralytica. His name is also associated with the spinal cord (Lissauer's tract) because of his study of the fibers composing it.

Bibliography: Jablonski, S. 1969. *Illustrated dictionary of eponymic syndromes and diseases.*

LISZT, FRANZ (1811-1886). A Hungarian child prodigy, composer, and pianist. He made his debut when he was nine years old and began his career as a pianist in Vienna at the age of twelve. He was moody, easily upset, and unable to lead a stable life. He constantly moved from place to place, giving concerts, meeting musicians, and offering generous help to many of them. He was involved in numerous encumbering love affairs, including a short-lived but passionate one with Lola Montez (q.v.). Two relationships of a lasting nature were those with Countess Marie d'Agoult (1805-1876), who

gave him three children, between 1834 and 1844, and with Princess Caroline Sayn-Wittgenstein, his companion from 1848-1861. But, perhaps because of his ambivalent feelings towards women, he seems to have been glad to escape them all by turning to religious mysticism and becoming a lay priest.
Bibliography: Newman, E. 1934. *The man Liszt.*

LITHIUM CARBONATE. The alkali metal was discovered by the Swedish chemist John A. Arfvedson (1792-1841) in 1817, and lithium salts were first used in medicine in 1858 as a form of treatment for gout. Later, lithia tablets were prescribed for numerous disorders despite their toxic effects. The first mention of lithium in the treatment of affective disorders was made by John F. J. Cade in 1948. The first international lithium conference was held in New York in 1978.
Bibliography: Cade, J. F. 1978. Lithium—past, present, and future. In *Lithium in medical practice*, ed. F. N. Johnson and S. Johnson.

LITTLE HANS. Herbert Graf, general manager of Geneva's Grand Théâter. As a child he was the subject of one of Sigmund Freud's (q.v.) famous case histories under the pseudonym of Little Hans. He was the first child of Max Graf, a musicologist and a member of Freud's inner circle. Graf supplied Freud with material about the child's dreams (q.v.), fantasies, and conversations and then conducted the analysis himself under Freud's guidance. During the period of treatment, Hans and Freud met briefly once only. The child's phobia of horses eventually receded. Freud's theory of infantile sexuality was confirmed by Little Hans' story, which was also the first child analysis. The events reported in it revolved around the child's abnormal preoccupation with penises and horses, aided by the father's leading questions. Not surprisingly, the publication of the case history and Freud's theories met with great skepticism. When he was nineteen, Herbert Graf visited Freud and was warmly received by him.
Bibliography: Freud, S. 1909. *Analysis of a phobia in a five-year-old boy.*

LITTRÉ, (MAXIMILIEN PAUL) ÉMILE (1801-1881) French scholar and philologist. He studied medicine, but gave it up to earn money in journalism; he edited medical journals. He belonged to a French school of philosophy that believed the progress of science would advance the progress of the human mind. He applied positivism (q.v.) to the study of languages and believed that morality had an organic basis.
Bibliography: Littré, E. 1870. *Les origines organiques de la morale.*

LIVER. At various times and in various cultures, the liver has been linked to mental and emotional disorders. Avicenna (q.v.) believed that it, as well as the stomach (q.v.) and the spleen (q.v.), was one of the seats of melancholia (q.v.). In later periods the liver was associated with the passions, lust, love, and courage; several examples of this association can be found in the plays of William Shakespeare (q.v.). The contemporary term "he is yellow," meaning "he is a coward," may derive from the observation that severe stress can cause liver dysfunction and jaundice.

LIVER OF A DEAD ATHLETE. During the Middle Ages (q.v.) this was prized as a talisman (q.v.) against epilepsy (q.v.).
Bibliography: Fort, G. F. 1883. *Medical economy during the Middle Ages.*

LIVINGSTONE, DAVID (1813-1873). A Scottish missionary, explorer, and physician, born in Lanarkshire. He was only ten years old when he was sent to work in the cotton mills, where he worked for twelve years. In 1836 he began to study medicine, and in 1840 he passed the final examinations of the Faculty of Physicians and Surgeons of Glasgow, Scotland. In that same year he sailed for Africa and spent most of his life exploring, discovering, converting, and trying to eradicate the slave trade. He married in 1844 but in 1856 sent his wife back to England for five years. She felt the rejection keenly and consoled herself with laudanum (q.v.) and alcohol. He was subject to violent changes of mood in which periods of dynamism and euphoria were followed by despondency, gloom, and apathy. His symptoms have been attributed to inherited cyclothymia (q.v.), or manic depressive insanity. He died in an unsuccessful attempt to find the source of the Nile.
Bibliography: Ransford, O. 1978. *David Livingstone: the dark interior.*

LIZARD. The backbone of a lizard, after it had been stripped of its flesh by ants, was one of the many revolting substances forced on epileptics (*see* EPILEPSY) in the hope of curing them.
Bibliography: Esquirol, J.E.D., 1845. Reprint. 1965. *Mental maladies: a treatise on insanity.*

LLANDEGLA. A location in Denbighshire, Wales, possessing a holy well (q.v.). Until the nineteenth century, patients suffering from epilepsy (q.v.) would walk around the well three times, repeating the Lord's Prayer, throwing coins into the water, and bathing in it. The patient also was expected to carry a bird around the well with him. It then spent the night with the patient in the village church. If the cure was successful, the disease was supposed to have been transferred to the bird.
Bibliography: 1969. *Readers Digest*, ed. *Book of British birds.*

LLANGOLLEN, THE LADIES OF. Two Irish women, Eleanor Butler (1739-1829) and Sarah Ponsonby (1755-1831), famous for their eccentricity. In 1778 they eloped together and were disowned by their families. After various problems, they settled in Llangollen, Wales, where they became a living legend. Their cottage and the interesting garden that they created attracted many celebrities of the time, who came to admire their intellectual way of life and to speculate on the nature of their relationship. Eleanor Butler, the older of the two and the more dominant character, had been educated in a Catholic convent in France, where she had little contact with the opposite sex. Although her appearance and mannerisms were masculine, she was totally dependent upon her companion, who tenderly cared for her during regular attacks of migraine (q.v.), fainting fits, nightmares (q.v.), and periods of acute, and often justified, anxiety. Their intense relationship lasted a lifetime.

Bibliography: Mavor, E. 1971. *The ladies of Llangollen.*

LLOYD, CHARLES (1775-1839). An English poet. He was a friend of Samuel Coleridge (q.v.) and Charles Lamb (q.v.). In 1811, he began to suffer from morbid suspicions and delusions (q.v.). He was placed in an asylum (q.v.) in France near Versailles, where he spent the remainder of his life.

Bibliography: Winslow, L. F. 1898. *Mad humanity: its forms apparent and obscure.*

LOBB, THEOPHILUS (1678-1763). A British physician and clergyman. In 1734 he published a book on fevers (*Rational Methods of Curing Fevers*) in which he listed their various aetiological factors. Recognizing the influence of emotional factors in bodily disorders, he added to insufficient rest and poor diet (q.v.) "too much joy and too much grief."

LOBELIA. A plant found in tropical and temperate woodlands and moist places. One variety, which is known as Indian tobacco, was used by the Mapuche Indians of Chile as a cure-all and, more specifically, for the treatment of chorea and other nervous twitchings. They also smoked its leaves to provoke sleep. Some varieties of lobelia contain an alkaloid that has hallucinogenic properties.

Bibliography: Emboden, W. 1972. *Narcotic plants.*

LOBOTOMY. Surgical incision into a lobe of the brain. It is one of the last of a long chain of attempts to relieve mental disorders with surgical intervention. Some primitive forms of lobotomy have been used from earliest times. Primitive tribes used trepanation (q.v.); Greek and Roman surgeons made openings in the skull to release noxious vapors; and essentially the same principle held good in medieval times. In 1891 Gottlieb Burckhardt, a Swiss psychiatrist, evolved a technique in which a piece of cortex was removed with the aim of calming manic patients. The modern technique of

bilateral prefrontal lobotomy, or leucotomy, was first developed by Egas Moniz (q.v.) in 1935.
Bibliography: Moniz, E. 1936. *Tentatives opératoires dans le traitement de certaines psychoses.*

LOCHMANUR. A lake in the far north of Scotland. Until the nineteenth century the waters of Lochmanur were reputed to have curative properties. Lunatics were stripped and immersed three times in the lake on the stroke of midnight in the belief that they would regain their reason.
Bibliography: Letchworth, W. P. 1889. *The insane in foreign countries.*

LOCKE, JOHN (1632-1704). An English empirical philosopher and physician. His principles were based on the proposition that it was important to discover the extent of human understanding before answering philosophical questions. This concept led to his best-known work *Essay Concerning Human Understanding*, which was published in 1690. He believed that natural morality could be achieved by the surrender of personal power to a ruler. He opposed the doctrine of innate ideas postulated by René Descartes (q.v.) and developed the theory of association outlined by Thomas Hobbes (q.v.). According to Locke, man's mind is a *tabula rasa* (q.v.) at birth; ideas are acquired through the senses, which provide perception of objects and of feelings. These ideas are held together by association. The term "association of ideas" was suggested by him. His views provided a basis for further developments in the psychology (q.v.) of associations and the schools of thought derived from it. In distinguishing madness from idiocy (*see* IDIOT), he wrote, "madmen put wrong ideas together and so make propositions, but argue and reason right from them, but idiots make very few or no propositions and reason scarce at all." He was a champion of liberal principles and preached toleration in an age that found these concepts barely acceptable. He was, therefore, often out of favor. Because he systematically analyzed the human mind, he is regarded as a pioneer of experimental psychology (q.v.). Philippe Pinel (q.v.) often cited him.
Bibliography: Dewhurst, K. 1963. *John Locke: physician and philosopher.*

LOCK HOSPITALS. A term originally applied to lazarettos (q.v.) where the patients were shut in by means of locks. Many of these hospitals later were used for mental patients, who also were locked in.

LOCUSTA. A false nurse who harms those she should care for. The original Locusta was a poisoner of the first century A.D. She is believed to have been employed by Agrippina the Younger (q.v.) to murder Claudius (10 B.C.-54 A.D.) and certainly was hired by Nero (q.v.) to kill Britannicus (A.D. 41-

55). She was exposed and put to death during the reign of the emperor Galba (5 B.C.?-A.D.61).
Bibliography: Suetonius, G. *The Twelve Caesars*, trans. Robert Graves.

LODGE, SIR OLIVER JOSEPH (1851-1940). An English physicist. He published many reports of his investigations in the field of physics. He became interested in the study of psychic phenomena and the problem of communication with the dead. He believed that his dead son had been able to communicate with him, and in 1916 he wrote an account of these experiences entitled *Raymond, or Life and Death*.
Bibliography: Lodge, O. 1933. *My philosophy, containing final views on the ether of space*.

LOEB, JACQUES (1859-1924). A German zoologist and physiologist. He spent most of his life in the United States. He was the leader of the mechanistic movement in psychology. Loeb believed that animal behavior could be explained in physical and chemical terms and expounded these ideas into his theory of tropism (q.v.). According to him, consciousness is dependent on "associative memory," therefore only the lower animals are unconscious. His views were first published, in 1899, in a volume entitled *Vergleichende Gehirnphysiologie und vergleichende Psychologie*.
Bibliography: Loeb, J. 1912. *The mechanistic conception of life*.

LOEWENFELD, LEOPOLD (1847-1924). A German psychiatrist and sexologist. In 1897 he published a textbook of psychotherapy (q.v.) in which he advocated hypnotism (q.v.), suggestion, and psychic gymnastics. In the same book he formulated rules to regulate the patient-doctor relationship during therapy.
Bibliography: Loewenfeld, L. 1904. *Die psychischen zwangserscheinungen*.

LOEWI, OTTO (1873-1961). A German pharmacologist and professor of pharmacology at Graz. He later became a research professor of pharmacology at New York University. He demonstrated the chemical transmission of nerve impulses and conducted important experiments in this field with his friend Henry Dale (q.v.).
Bibliography: Haymaker, W., and Schiller, F. 1970. *The founders of neurology*. 2d. ed.

LOGOS. A Greek term used to describe a philosophical concept that at various times has been modified to mean "thought," the intelligent world-principle, divine thought, or wisdom.

LOHE, CONRAD WILHELM (1808-1872). A German clergyman and philanthropist. He founded many institutions for education, the propagation

of the Christian faith, and the care of the sick. In 1854, in a few rented rooms above an inn, he began to care for a mentally defective child. Within a year, he had eighteen defective children in his care and had to move to larger premises. He eventually founded a special institution for the care of the retarded.
Bibliography: Kanner, L. 1964. *A history of the care and study of the mentally retarded.*

LOLITA SYNDROME. The sexual attraction for very young girls by mature men. The term derives from the novel *Lolita* by Vladimir Nabokov (1899-1977) written in 1955. The theme of the novel is the passion of a middle-aged man for an adolescent "nymphet."
Bibliography: Nabokov, V. 1958. *Lolita.*

LOMBROSO, CESARE (1836-1909). An Italian criminologist and psychopathologist. At various times, he was a professor of legal medicine, psychiatry and finally criminal anthropology. He wrote prolifically in all these fields. Despite the many revisions and alterations that he made in his works and the continuous controversies over his views, he influenced the study of personality and initiated the compilation of pathographies or biographies emphasizing the psychopathology of the subject. He regarded genius (q.v.) as analogous to insanity and due to hereditary and generative factors. Lombroso believed that delinquency was linked with a particular physical and mental constitution and thus introduced the concept of "criminal type." He also fought for constructive treatment of criminals and limitations on the death penalty. He is regarded as the father of scientific criminology.
Bibliography: Kurella, H. 1910. *Cesare Lombroso: a modern man of science.*

LONDON CRIES. The calls of sellers of wares and skills in the streets of old London. Each cry was distinctive in words and tune. Beggars pretending to be inmates of Bethlem Royal Hospital (q.v.) had their own cry:

> Poor naked Bedlam, Tom's a-cold.
> A small cut of thy bacon or a piece of
>   thy Sow's side, good Bessie.
> God almighty bless thy witts.

Bibliography: Warwick, A. R. 1968. *A noise of music.*

LONDON, JACK (1876-1916). An American novelist. He left home at fourteen to escape poverty and traveled as a sailor and tramp, roaming as far as Japan. He was a convinced socialist, especially after his firsthand experience of conditions during the 1893 depression and a period in prison. To his own ideas he added concepts derived from Charles Darwin (q.v.) and anthropologists and produced numerous works in which he made dra-

matic use of his knowledge of human atavism and adaptability. His own way of life was disordered and extravagant, he drank excessively and eventually committed suicide (q.v.).
Bibliography: Stone, I. 1971. *Sailor on horseback.*

LONGFELLOW, HENRY WADSWORTH (1807-1882). An American poet. His first marriage ended after four years with the death of his wife in 1835; he projected his feelings in a prose romance entitled *Hyperion* (1839) in which the hero tries to forget his sorrows through travel. Longfellow married again and was widowed again when his second wife tragically burned to death. After this event he passed through a period of deep depression, which he tried to cure by hard work. Many of his writings reflect social conditions at the time and show his skill as a storyteller. Of particular interest to psychiatry is his poem *The Lunatic Girl*.
Bibliography: Wagenknecht, E. C. 1966. *Henry Wadsworth Longfellow: portrait on an American humanist.*

LONGHEADED. A term applied to shrewd individuals. The shape of the head was believed to indicate certain intellectual qualities. A long head was believed to show cleverness.

LORAIN, PAUL JOSEPH (1827-1875). A French physician. His name is associated with a condition (the Lorain syndrome) in which infantile traits including physical and mental underdevelopment persist into adolescence and adulthood.
Bibliography: Lorain, P. J. 1871. *Du feminisme et de l'infantilisme chez les tuberculeux.*

LORENZ, KONRAD ZACHARIAS (1903-   ). An Austrian ethologist. His numerous studies on animal behavior have earned him the title of "Father of Modern Ethology." His work is based on the concept that an animal's behavior is produced by adaptive evolution. According to him, conflict drives can be diverted before they become too harmful. Among his famous books are *King Solomon Ring* (1952) and *On Aggression* (1966). His work has influenced thinking on child development.
See also IMPRINTING.
Bibliography: Nisbett, A. 1976. *Konrad Lorenz.*

LORRY, ANNE CHARLES (1726-1783). A French physician. He became interested in neurology (q.v.) and wrote a treatise entitled *De Melancholia et Morbis Melancholicis* which was published in 1765. In it he discussed melancholia (q.v.) as a mental disorder of somatic aetiology and differentiated it into three forms: *melancholia nervosa*, dependent on material causes and characterized by spasms; *melancholis humoralis*, caused by an excess of black bile (q.v.); and a mixed form. He may have been the first clinician

to describe cataleptic somnambulism (q.v.), a form of catalepsy that leaves the patient with no memory (q.v.) of the attack.
Bibliography: Lorry, A. 1765. *De melancholie et morbis melancholicis.*

LOTUS-EATERS, *or* **LOTOPHAGI.** In Homer's (q.v.) *Odyssey* (q.v.), a people who lived on the lotus. When Ulysses' (q.v.) men ate the lotus they lost all memory (q.v.) of their homes and friends, became idle and lacked initiative. In historical times Lotus-eaters were found by the Greeks on the coast of North Africa. Alfred Lord Tennyson (q.v.) wrote a poem entitled *The Lotos-Eaters* (1842) on the same subject.
Bibliography: Homer. *Odyssey.* Book 9.

LOTZE, RUDOLPH HERMANN (1817-1881). A German physician, philosopher and psychologist. From early adolescence he was disposed towards philosophy and poetry and published works in both fields. At the age of twenty-seven he became professor of philosophy at Göttingen, where his lectures for the next thirty-seven years embraced psychology. His work included early investigations in the subconscious (q.v.) and the unconscious (q.v.). Opposed to materialistic interpretations of the human mind, Lotze's writings, undogmatic and meticulous, had considerable influence in the field of psychology during that period and strengthened the links between psychology and physiology. He developed a theory of space perception that led to the foundation of an empiristic school of thought on the subject.
Bibliography: Santayana, G. 1971. *Lotze's system of philosophy.*

LOUDUN NUNS. The Ursuline nuns of a small convent in Loudun, France. In the 1630s they figured in an epidemic of hysteria (q.v.) involving demoniac possession (q.v.), sexual and aggressive conflicts, and political intrigue. Father Urbain Grandier (1590-1634), the priest of Loudun, incurred the displeasure of the powerful Cardinal Richelieu (q.v.) and was accused of having bewitched the mother superior, Sister Jeanne des Agnes and some of the nuns. Convulsions and other forms of hysterical behavior were produced for the benefit of the exorcists (*see* EXORCISM) appointed by the cardinal. The mother superior swore that she and her nuns had been bewitched by Father Grandier, who had thrown roses over the convent wall and sent devils to possess them. Grandier was tried and found guilty. He was tortured and burned alive, although he had been promised the mercy of death by garrotting. Two of the friars who tortured him were subsequently haunted by guilt and became insane. Dr. Mannouri, whose false findings had helped Grandier's conviction, died in a horrible delirium (q.v.). The nuns became a tourist attraction and continued their assertion of demoniac possession even after Grandier's death. They gave public performances of incredible lewdness. Their behavior reverted to normal only after Cardinal Richelieu lost interest in the imposture and withdrew financial support from the con-

vent. Some three centuries later, Georges Gilles de la Tourette (q.v.), coauthored with Dr. Gabriel Legues a book entitled *Soeur Jeanne des Agnes* that was based on this episode of epidemic hysteria. One of Gilles de la Tourette's own patients closely emulated the hysterical mother superior and in a fit of paranoia (q.v.) shot him as he sat in his office.
Bibliography: Huxley, A. 1952. *The devils of Loudun.*

LOUIS XI (1423-1483). A king of France. He was ugly, fat, had a large head and, despite his undoubted intelligence, was superstitious and boorish in manners. He contracted an unhappy marriage with Margaret of Scotland (1425?-1445), daughter of James I (1394–1437) of Scotland. Until her death, she succeeded in keeping him reconciled with his father Charles VII (1403-1461), but after her death, Louis' quarrels with his father caused him to be exiled. He suffered from epilepsy (q.v.) and asked to be infected with "quartan fever," or malaria, as this was reputed to cure epilepsy. According to *The Anatomy of Melancholy* (q.v.), Louis was convinced that "everything did stink about him, all the odoriferous perfumes they could get would not ease him, but still he smelled a filthy stink."
Bibliography: Hare, C. 1907. *The life of Louis XI.*

LOUIS XIII (1601-1643). A king of France, the son of Henry IV (1553–1610) and Marie de' Medici (1573-1642). He suffered from poor health, was extremely shy, and stuttered. In an attempt to improve his morose disposition, he was purged 200 times in a single year. Despite being subjected to sexual stimulation from an early age, he became sexually inadequate and was nicknamed "The Chaste." He was given to fits of furious rage and responded to stress with psychosomatic symptoms.
Bibliography: Vaunois, L. 1936. *Vie de Louis XIII.*

LOUIS XV (1710-1774). A king of France. He succeeded to the throne when he was five years old. His behavior oscillated between extremes; one moment it was extravagant and dissolute, the next excessively pious. He enjoyed many mistresses but regaled them with readings of sermons. Sickness fascinated him, and he loved morbid discussions of symptoms. His favorite themes of conversation were death, graves, and corpses. He was a dedicated gambler, and nothing was allowed to interrupt his games of cards. When a guest suddenly died at his table, he ordered his removal and called for the next hand.
See also JEANNE ANTOINETTE POISSON, MARQUISE DE POMPADOUR.
Bibliography: Gooch, G. P. 1956. *Louis XV.*

LOURDES. A French town in the Hautes-Pyrénées. It is famous for the grotto in which Saint Bernadette (q.v.) had a vision of the Virgin in 1858. The local spring is reputed to have miraculous properties, and sick people

from all over the world are brought to it. Jean Martin Charcot (q.v.) investigated the mechanisms behind the cures and predicted that their understanding would advance psychiatric treatment.
Bibliography: Charcot, J. M. 1893. *La foi qui guérit.*

LOVAT, MATTEO (fl. 1800). A nineteenth-century Italian shoemaker. He wanted to enter the church but his poverty forced him to become a shoemaker. He was a religious fanatic and a melancholic (*see* MELANCHOLIA). In 1805 in Venice, he castrated himself and tried to commit suicide (q.v.) by crucifying himself, complete with crown of thorns, on a contraption that he had built for this purpose and had hung outside his window. He was discovered and saved but eventually died in an asylum (q.v.), possibly from self-starvation. Cesare Lombroso (q.v.) reproduces an "authentic" picture of the episode in his book *The Man of Genius* (1891). (See Plate 8).
Bibliography: Winslow, F. B. 1840. *Anatomy of suicide.*

LOVE. The Greeks, the Romans, and the Arabs considered romantic love to be a cause of mental disorders and referred to "amorous melancholy" as if it were a disease. Galen (q.v.) gave great importance to the "passions," which included love. Juan Vives (q.v.) described the changes in behavior and the drives brought about by love. Other medical writers in later periods also referred to love as a factor in mental disorders until it was wrongly equated with sexuality, and morbid erotism became the pivot of psychoanalytic theories.

LOVE-APPLE. The term by which the Spaniards referred to the tomato, which they discovered in South America. They believed it to be a powerful aphrodisiac. The mandragora (q.v.) was also known by this term because of the same properties.
Bibliography: 1978. *Brewer's dictionary of phrase and fable.*

LOVERS OF LYON. A term used to refer to an eighteenth-century young man called Faldoni and a beautiful girl. They decided to commit suicide (q.v.) when their marriage was opposed. They met in an empty chapel and fired each other's pistols by pulling the rose-colored ribbons they had attached to them. They died embracing on the altar steps. Their suicide became famous and caused a spate of imitators to take their own lives.
Bibliography: Fedden, H. R. 1938. *Suicide.*

LOWELL, JAMES RUSSELL (1819 1891). An American poet, writer, and diplomat. His democratic ideas were in contrast to his upbringing. Of in-

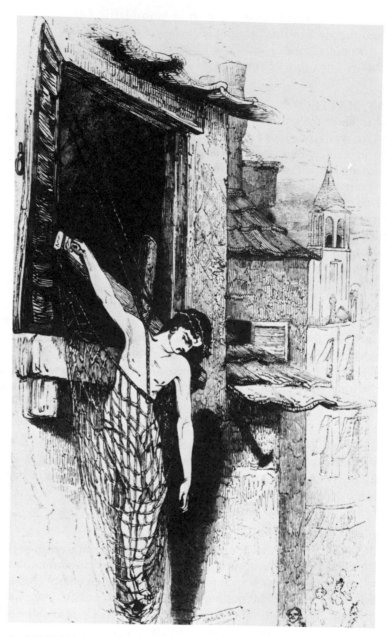

8. MATTEO LOVAT HANGING OUTSIDE HIS WINDOW AFTER
SELF-CRUCIFIXION in the contraption he had made for this purpose.
From H. R. Fedden, *Suicide*, 1838. By courtesy of the Department of
Medical Illustration, Ipswich Hospital.

terest to psychiatry is his poem *The Darkened Mind* in which he wrote about his mother, who was insane.
Bibliography: Norton, C. E., ed. 1894. *The complete writings of James Russell Lowell.*

LOWELL, ROBERT TRAILL SPENCE (1917-1977). An American poet and playwright. During World War II he refused to be classified a conscientious objector and was jailed. In 1940 he converted to Catholicism. His poems reflect his spiritual conflict and inner torture. Many of them are obsessively concerned with the history of his own family, his marriage, and his stressful mental state.
Bibliography: Fein, R. J. 1970. *Robert Lowell.*

LOW-LIFE, OR ONE HALF OF THE WORLD KNOWS NOT HOW THE OTHER HALF LIVE. A small book published anonymously in London in 1752, and reprinted three times between then and 1764. It described twenty-four hours in the life of London, Saturday night to Monday morning, by purporting to observe various people as they went about their business. The patients of Bethlem Royal Hospital (q.v.) are described as: "the unhappy patients at Bethlehem Hospital employed in breaking their wooden bowls, drawing figures with chalk on their partitions, rattling their chains, and making a terrible outcry occasioned by the heat of the weather having too great an effect upon their rambling brains." The nurses too are observed and the anonymous author describes how they take the best morsels from the food meant for the patients.
Bibliography: O'Donoghue, E. G. 1914. *The story of Bethlehem Hospital.*

LOWRY, LAWRENCE STEPHEN (1887-1976). An English painter. He frequently painted industrial scenes populated by a myriad of small figures. As a young man he retired into a world of his own to protect himself from his mother, who was so insensitive to his art that she was embarrassed when people bought his pictures. Yet, when she died, he was so grieved that he nearly lost his reason. Although he had many friends, he could not believe that they really cared about him and what he did. His emotions were kept under firm control, and he was often depressed. Lowry never married; his relationships with young girls were totally platonic. After his death, semi-erotic and brutal drawings of "Ann" were found, but the identity of the girl has remained a mystery.
Bibliography: Rohde, S. 1979. *A private view of L. S. Lowry.*

LOYOLA, SAINT IGNATIUS OF (1491-1556). Originally a Spanish soldier whose real name was Íñigo de Oñez y Loyola. He became converted to a life of service in the church in 1522 and in 1534 founded the Society of Jesus, which was approved by the pope in 1540. Loyola devised strict

spiritual rules on which the training of the Jesuits is still based and advocated meditation as a means of controlling emotion. His works, *Constitutions of the Order* and *Spiritual Exercises* have influenced the thinking and the lives of many people.
Bibliography: Young, W.J., trans. 1956. *St. Ignatius' own story.*

LSD. *See* LYSERGIC ACID DIETHYLAMIDE.

LUBBOCK, SIR JOHN (1834-1913). An English banker and politician. He is best known as a popular science writer, especially on archeology and entomology. In 1882 he published a book entitled *Ants, Bees, and Wasps* in which he described the social life of insects. It stimulated interest about the mind in animals and the study of instinct.
Bibliography: Lubbock, J. 1888. *Senses, instincts, and intelligence of animals.*

LUCAS, JAMES (1813-1874). An English eccentric, the son of a West Indian merchant. He was a well-educated man who became a hermit. Against his wishes and to his annoyance, he provided Charles Dickens (q.v.) with the model for Mr. Mopes in *Tom Tiddler's Ground* (1861). He never washed, slept on cinders, and became known as "the Hertfordshire hermit"; many famous people visited him.
Bibliography: Pope-Hennesy, U. 1968. *Charles Dickens.*

LUCETT, JAMES (fl. 1812). An Englishman who, with Delahoyde, claimed to have invented a "secret" process for the cure of insanity. They were able to interest a number of influential persons in their methods. The sons of George III (q.v.) personally organized trials on Bethlem Royal Hospital (q.v.) patients in the hope that the treatment, which consisted primarily of cold showers on the head of patients sitting in hot baths, would benefit their father. The trials proved that the claims of the two gentlemen were false. Eventually Delahoyde left England, and Lucett went to prison for debts. On his release, he wrote *An Exposition of the Reasons which have Prevented the Process for Relieving and Curing Idiocy and Lunacy and every Species of Insanity, from having been further Extended* (1815).
Bibliography: Macalpine, I., and Hunter, R. 1968. *George III and the mad-business.*

LUCIA DI LAMMERMOOR. The title of an opera by the Italian composer Gaetano Donizetti (q.v.). One of the most famous of operatic mad scenes appears in this opera. Lucia, who has been tricked into marrying Arturo rather than her lover Edgardo, loses her mind and stabs Arturo. As she imagines that she and Edgardo are about to be married, she sees an apparition coming between them, and she reenacts the scene of her rejection by Ed-

gardo. She promises to pray for Edgardo in heaven. She dies of her sorrow although this is not depicted on stage.
Bibliography: Harewood, ed. 1969. *Kobbe's complete opera book.*

LUCIANI, LUIGI (1840-1919). An Italian physiologist. He is known for his pioneer work in the field of cerebellar physiology. He studied the cerebellum by observing decerebelated dogs and monkeys that had been kept alive for over a year. He believed that the brain is a complex of overlapping areas that made exact localization of functions impossible. In 1878 he established the cortical pathogenesis of epilepsy (q.v.). He was the author of a *Treatise on Human Physiology*, first published in 1901 and translated into English in 1911.
Bibliography: Haymaker, W., and Schiller, F. 1970. *The founders of neurology.* 2d. ed.

LUCIE (fl.1880s). A patient of Pierre Janet (q.v.). At the age of nineteen, she suffered from fits of terror without apparent cause. Janet discovered through automatic writing that she had experienced a traumatic episode as a child and that a second personality, Adrienne, could remember the events and was frightened by them. Janet treated her by hypnotism (q.v.), automatic writing, and the use of a special rapport that made her particularly dependent on his suggestions. Lucie's case, which Janet published in 1886 is considered the first recorded cure by catharsis (q.v.).
Bibliography: Janet, P. 1886. Les actes inconscients et le dédoublement de la personnalité pendant le somnambulisme provoqué. *Revue Philosophique* 22:577-92.

LUCIUS JUNIUS BRUTUS (fl. c.520 B.C.). An early fool (q.v.). He simulated idiocy (*see* IDIOT) so well that the sons of the Roman king Tarquinius (534-510 B.C.) decided to take him with them on the return journey from Delphos to Rome so that he could amuse them.
Bibliography: Esquirol, J.E.D. 1845. Reprint. 1965. *Mental maladies: a treatise on insanity.*

LUCRETIUS (TITUS LUCRETIUS CARUS) (c.99-55 B.C.). Roman poet and philosopher. According to tradition, his wife Lucilla gave him a love potion that drove him mad and led to his suicide (q.v.) at the age of forty-four. His main poem, the result of a life's work, was *De Rerum Natura* in which he sought to explain that the course of the world was not dependent on divine intervention. In the same work he gave an excellent description of an epileptic (*see* EPILEPSY) attack. He wished to free mankind from its fear of the all powerful gods.
Bibliography: Lucretius. *De rerum natura*, trans. C. Bailey.

"LUDIBRIA FAUNORUM." A Latin expression, literally meaning the "games of the fauni." These spirits of the wood were said to make sport of human beings by driving them mad. Pliny the Elder (q.v.) called certain mental disorders "ludibria faunorum."

LUDWIG II OF BAVARIA (1845-1886). A Bavarian king. He so hated his mother, Mary of Hohenzollern, that he referred to her as "my predecessor's widow." She was blamed for having introduced madness into the family, but his paternal great-aunt, the Princess Alexandra of Bavaria (q.v.) was also said to have been insane and believed that she had swallowed a glass sofa. Ludwig was obsessed (*see* OBSESSION) with swans and the building of fantastic castles. His interest in the arts developed into a consuming passion that was beyond the limits of reason. Richard Wagner (q.v.) became his friend and the king delighted in impersonating heroes from Wagner's operas. Benedict Morel (q.v.) saw the king in 1867, was struck by his looks, and remarked that "future madness" could be seen in his eyes. By 1870 the whole of Bavaria was aware of his madness and his deteriorating physical appearance. He detested the company of others and so hated being seen that operas, performed in semidarkness, had to be arranged for him alone. A dining-table had to be constructed in such a way that it could be hoisted through the floor by invisible servants, and a screen was erected in front of him in the council chambers. He would sleep during the day, and read or wander about during the night, ill-treating servants and often condemning them to death (the sentences were ignored by his ministers). He suffered from delusions (q.v.), hallucinations (q.v.), insomnia, and periods of intense excitement. In 1886, Dr. Bernard Gudden (q.v.), superintendent of the asylum at Munich, was consulted about the mental health of the king. He diagnosed paranoia (q.v.) and arranged treatment for the king after the appointment of a regent. When Ludwig was told, he had Dr. Gudden and those agreeing with him arrested and ordered that "the skin should be torn from the traitors and they should be starved." They were, on all accounts, released after two hours and hastened to increase the distance between themselves and their sovereign. Ludwig, who had threatened to commit suicide (q.v.), was eventually captured and taken to a castle on the shore of Lake Starnberg with Gudden in clinical charge. Both king and physician were found drowned one evening, but there was insufficient evidence to reconstruct the facts. Otto (q.v.), the king's brother, was also insane but nevertheless succeeded him.
Bibliography: Blunt, W.J.W. 1970 *Dream king: Ludwig of Bavaria.*

LUDWIG, CHRISTIAN GOTTLIEB (1709 1773). A German philosophic physician and botanist. In a volume published in 1758 entitled *Institutiones medicinae clinicae,* he theorized that mania (q.v.) or melancholia (q.v.) could be caused by fantasy.

LUDWIG, KARL FRIEDRICH WILHELM (1816-1895). A German physiologist. His physiological studies included research on the role of the nervous system in circulation. Ivan Pavlov (q.v.) studied with him in Leipzig.
Bibliography: Haymaker, W., and Schiller, F. 1970. *The founders of neurology.* 2d. ed.

LUES DIVINA *and* **LUES DEIFICA.** Two of the many Latin terms for epilepsy (q.v.). Translated they mean respectively "divine plague" and "sacred plague" and reflect the belief that the disorder was sent by the gods. Those affected were believed to have the divine gift of prophecy.
Bibliography: Temkin, O. 1971. *The falling sickness.*

LUKE, SAINT. A Greek physician of Antioch. He was one of the Apostles who joined Saint Paul in missionary work. Luke is the author of the third gospel in which seven miracles are mentioned. Five of them are of a medical nature, and it is probable that the disorders were hysterical (*see* HYSTERIA). The cures may have been brought about by suggestion. He is the patron saint of doctors.
Bibliography: Luke, 7:11-17, 13:10-17; 14:1-6; 17:11-19; and 22:50-51.

LULLIUS, RAIMUNDUS (c.1232-1315). His name has many spellings. Lully, Lulio, Ramon Llull, and such like. He was a Spanish physician, theologian, and philosopher, known as "Doctor Illuminatus." As a youth he led a dissolute life, but in 1266 he experienced a religious conversion and became a missionary devoted to mysticism and study. He devised a mechanical contraption to solve all problems and acquire knowledge by the manipulation of fundamental notions. He is considered the father of modern logistic thought and influenced Gottfried Leibnitz (q.v.). He preached in France, Italy, and Africa and, according to tradition, was stoned to death for attempting to convert the Muslims. His novel *Blanquerna* described an ideal country.
Bibliography: Hillgarth, J. N. 1972. *Ramon Lull and Lullism in fourteenth-century France.*

LUNACY IN MANY LANDS. A book by George A. Tucker, an Australian psychiatrist and proprietor of private mental hospitals in Melbourne and later in Sydney. Beginning in 1881 when he needed a rest because of ill health he spent three and a half years visiting over 400 mental hospitals in Australia, as well as every state in the United States, every province in Canada, Tasmania, New Zealand, Hawaii, Europe, and Tunisia and Algiers in Africa. On the average, he visited two asylums (q.v.) a week. As well as his personal observations, the book contains some reports obtained by questionnaires rather than visits. Tucker drew a number of conclusions from his travels. He advocated that asylums should contain no more than 300 inmates

and that research of all kinds should be "made incumbant on the medical officers of every asylum." The book is a remarkable achievement that gives a realistic account of the state of mental hospitals in the latter part of the nineteenth century. It was first published by the government of New South Wales in 1887 and was 1,564 pages long.
Bibliography: Tucker, G. A. 1887. *Lunacy in many lands.*

LUNATIC. The term is derived from the Latin *luna*, meaning "moon," and reflects the widespread belief that the mind was affected by the moon (q.v.).

LUTHER, MARTIN (1483-1546). A German religious reformer and translator of the Bible (q.v.). His father was a miner. Both his parents were unloving and cruel, and both beat him so badly that sometimes they drew blood. When he was twenty-two years old, he had a vision during a thunderstorm and decided to become a monk. Despite his penetrating mind, he was superstitious and given to delusions (q.v.). He believed that mental defectives were the work of the devil and therefore should be destroyed. He once advised that a mentally retarded boy should be drowned. Similarly, the blind, the dumb, and the lame, according to him, should not receive medical treatment because they were possessed (*see* POSSESSION) by Satan. He once wrote: "The greatest punishment that God can inflict on the wicked is to deliver them over to Satan. There are many devils in woods, waters and wildernesses ready to hurt and prejudice people. In cases of melancholia, I conclude it is merely the work of the devil." His usually excellent critical ability deserted him if the subject was connected with the devil to whom he ascribed great power. His many complaints included giddiness, tinnitus, hallucinations (q.v.) of sight and hearing, depression, anxiety, and a multitude of psychosomatic disorders, all of which he attributed to demoniac possession or a tendency to epilepsy (q.v.).
Bibliography: Todd, J. M. 1964. *Martin Luther.*

LUYS, JULES BERNARD (1828-1897). A French neurologist. His reconstructions of cerebral structures were based on his own excellent drawings and photographs. He greatly contributed to the understanding of thalamic functions. Luys studied insanity, hysteria (q.v.), and hypnotism (q.v.) and was one of the founders of the Société d'Hypnologie et de Psychologie. He believed that patients could be treated by placing certain drugs near them. His main work was *The Brain and Its Functions,* which was translated into English in 1882.
Bibliography: Haymaker, W., and Schiller, F. 1970. *The founders of neurology,* 2d. ed.

LYCANTHROPY. A term derived from the Greek, literally meaning "wolfman," or Lycaon (q.v.). The individual affected behaves as if he were a wolf

or a wild animal. There are many examples in antiquity: Pliny the Elder (q.v.) referred to the case of Demaenetus, an Arcadian who was in this state for ten years. Nebuchadnezzar (q.v.) believed himself to be a beast for seven years. Virgil (q.v.) wrote about Moeris who was said to have become a wolf after ingesting some poisonous herbs. Herodotus (q.v.) believed that the Neuri became wolves for a short period every year. Marcellus, a third-century physician, and Aetius (q.v.), as well as the Arabs, described lycanthropy from clinical points of view. In the Middle Ages (q.v.) the belief in werewolves still persisted and even lingered on into the seventeenth century. It is to be found in the writings of physicians like Jean Fernel (q.v.) and Pierre Leloyer (q.v.).
See also ZOANTHROPY.
Bibliography: Pliny. *Natural History* 34, 22.
Zilboorg, G. 1941. *A history of medical psychology*.

LYCAON. In Greek mythology (q.v.), a king of Arcadia, who served Zeus a dish of human flesh and, in punishment, was changed into a wolf. The term lycanthropy (q.v.) has the same root as his name.
Bibliography: Eckels, R. P. 1937. *Greek wolf-lore*.

LYCOPODIUM. A variety of clubmoss. It was used in Russia in a form of aversion therapy (q.v.) for alcoholism (q.v.). A hot drink was made from it and given to the patient, who then had to drink a glass of vodka. Painful and violent vomiting resulted. This procedure was repeated two or three times in succession, causing great exhaustion and a permanent revulsion toward alcoholic drinks.
Bibliography: Kourennoff, P. M., and St. George, G. 1970. *Russian folk medicine*.

LYCURGUS. A king of the Edonians in ancient Thracia. Because he did not worship Dionysus (q.v.), the god punished him with madness. In a frenzy he killed his son with an axe, thinking that he was a vine.
Bibliography: Simon, B. 1978. *Mind and madness in ancient Greece*.

LYPEMANIA. A term coined by Jean Esquirol (q.v.) to indicate a form of insanity in which depression and mania (q.v.) are both present. He considered the condition usually to be hereditary and the lypemanic individual pale, lean and slender with black hair.
Bibliography: Esquirol, J.E.D. 1845. Reprint 1965. *Mental maladies: a treatise on insanity*.

LYSERGIC ACID DIETHYLAMIDE (LSD). A derivation of rye ergot. It was synthesized by Stoll and Albert Hofmann (q.v.) in 1938. Its hallucinogenic properties were accidentally discovered by Hofmann in

1943, when, during the course of laboratory work, he inhaled some of the substance and experienced "fantastic images of extraordinary plasticity." *See also* ERGOT POISONING.

Bibliography: West, L. J. 1968. Hallucinations. In *Modern perspectives in world psychiatry*, ed. J. G. Howells.

LYSSA. In Greek mythology (q.v.), the goddess of madness. She possessed (*see* POSSESSION) those who offended her and made them lose their minds.
Bibliography: Simon, B. 1978. *Mind and madness in ancient Greece.*